CARDIOVASCULAR IMAGING

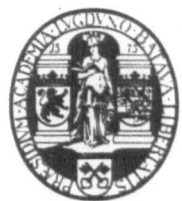 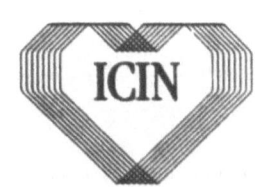 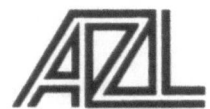

Developments in Cardiovascular Medicine

VOLUME 186

The titles published in this series are listed at the end of this volume.

Cardiovascular Imaging

Edited by

JOHAN H. C. REIBER
Laboratory for Clinical and Experimental Image Processing (LKEB),
Department of Diagnostic Radiology and Nuclear Medicine,
Department of Cardiology,
Leiden University Hospital,
The Netherlands
and
Interuniversity Cardiology Institute of the Netherlands (ICIN),
Utrecht, The Netherlands

and

ERNST E. VAN DER WALL
Department of Cardiology,
Leiden University Hospital,
The Netherlands
and
Interuniversity Cardiology Institute of the Netherlands (ICIN),
Utrecht, The Netherlands

This publication has been made possible with an educational grant from
Lorex Synthélabo, Maarssen, The Netherlands

LOREX SYNTHÉLABO

KLUWER ACADEMIC PUBLISHERS
DORDRECHT / BOSTON / LONDON

A C.I.P. Catalogue record for this book is available from the Library of Congress.

ISBN-13:978-94-010-6616-7   e-ISBN-13:978-94-009-0291-6
DOI:10.1007/978-94-009-0291-6

Published by Kluwer Academic Publishers,
P.O. Box 17, 3300 AA Dordrecht, The Netherlands.

Kluwer Academic Publishers incorporates
the publishing programmes of
D. Reidel, Martinus Nijhoff, Dr W. Junk and MTP Press.

Sold and distributed in the U.S.A. and Canada
by Kluwer Academic Publishers,
101 Philip Drive, Norwell, MA 02061, U.S.A.

In all other countries, sold and distributed
by Kluwer Academic Publishers Group,
P.O. Box 322, 3300 AH Dordrecht, The Netherlands.

Dedicated

to

Our Wives

Marjan and Barbara

and our Children

Beata   Hein

Sake and

Ernst Lucas

Table of Contents

Part Three: **Regression/progression of CAD and cardiovascular imaging**

Part Four: **DICOM and the filmless catheterization laboratory**

List of contributors

Richard G. Bach
J.G. Mudd Cardiac Catheterization Laboratory, Division of Cardiology, Department of Internal Medicine, St. Louis University Health Sciences Center, 3635 Vista Avenue at Grand, St. Louis, MO 63110, U.S.A.

Bruce H. Brundage
Division of Cardiology, Saint John's Cardiovascular Research Center, 1000 West Carson Street, Torrance, California 90509, U.S.A.

Paul B. Condit
Health Sciences Division, Cardiology Group, Eastman Kodak Company, 343 State Street, Rochester, New York, NY 14650-1133, U.S.A.
Co-authors: Gerry Pelanek and Terence Rourke

Stephanie Coulter
Cardiac Unit of the Massachusetts General Hospital and Harvard Medical School, Boston, MA 02114-2698, U.S.A.
Co-author: Michael H. Picard, Noninvasive Cardiac Laboratory

Jack T. Cusma
Division of Cardiology, Duke University Medical Center, P.O. Box 3012, Durham, NC 27710, U.S.A.
Co-author: Thomas M. Bashore

Eric de Groot
Interuniversity Cardiology Institute of The Netherlands (ICIN), P.O. Box 19258, 3501 DG Utrecht, The Netherlands
Co-authors: J. Wouter Jukema, Alexander D. Montauban van Swijndregt, Ad J. van Boven, Aeilko H. Zwinderman, Rob G.A. Ackerstaff, Anton F.W. van der Steen, Nicolaas Bom, Kong I. Lie and Albert V.G. Bruschke, on behalf of the REGRESS Study Group

Peter den Heijer
Department of Cardiology, University Hospital Groningen, Oostersingel 59, 9713 EZ Groningen, The Netherlands

Albert de Roos
Department of Diagnostic Radiology and Nuclear Medicine, Leiden University Hospital, Rijnsburgerweg 10, 2333 AA Leiden, The Netherlands
Co-authors: Ernst E. van der Wall, Rob van der Geest and Johan H.C. Reiber

Carlo Di Mario
EMO Centro Cuore Columbus S.r.l., via M. Buonarroti 48, 20145 Milano, Italy
Co-authors: Peter J. Fitzgerald and Antonio Colombo

André J. Duerinckx
Department of Cardiovascular MRI, West Los Angeles VA Medical Center (Wadsworth), 11301 Wilshire Blvd, Los Angeles CA 90073, U.S.A.

Eckart Fleck
Department of Cardiology and Angiology, German Heart Institute, Augustenburger Platz 1, D-13353 Berlin, Germany
Co-author: Helmut Oswald

Michel A. Galjee
Department of Cardiology, Medical Spectrum Twente, Ariënsplein 1, 7511 JX Enschede, The Netherlands

Bob Goedhart
Laboratory for Clinical and Experimental Image Processing (LKEB), Department of Diagnostic Radiology and Nuclear Medicine, Leiden University Hospital, P.O. Box 9600, 2300 RC Leiden, The Netherlands
Co-author: Johan H.C. Reiber

Günter Görge
Department of Cardiology, University Hospital Essen, Hufelandstrasse 5, D-45122 Essen, Germany
Co-authors: Jundo Gé, Michael Haude, Vijay Shah, Allen Jeremias, Helge Simon and Raimund Erbel

David M. Herrington
Section of Cardiology, The Bowman Gray School of Medicine, Medical Center Blvd., Winston-Salem, NC 21257-1045, U.S.A.

David R. Holmes Jr
Division of Cardiovascular Diseases and Internal Medicine, Mayo Clinic, 200 First Street SW, Rochester, MN 55905, U.S.A.
Co-authors: Merrill A. Wondrow, Kirk N. Garratt and Malcolm R. Bell

J. Wouter Jukema
Department of Cardiology, Leiden University Hospital, Rijnsburgerweg 10, 2333 AA Leiden, The Netherlands
Co-authors: Albert V.G. Bruschke and Johan H.C. Reiber

Thomas E. Kennedy
Camtronics Medical Systems, 900 Walnut Ridge Drive, Hartland, WI 53029, U.S.A.
Co-author: Eugene W. Bergholz

Charles Knight
Department of Invasive Cardiology, Royal Brompton Hospital, Sydney Street, Londen SW3 6NP, United Kingdom
Co-author: Ulrich Sigwart

Wenguang Li
Thoraxcenter, Erasmus University Rotterdam and the Interuniversity Cardiology Institute of the Netherlands, P.O. Box 1738, 3000 DR Rotterdam, The Netherlands
Co-authors: Nicolaas Bom, Clemens von Birgelen, Ton F.W. van der Steen, Chris L. de Korte, Elma J. Gussenhoven, Charles T. Lancée

Warren J. Manning
Cardiovascular Division, Beth Israel Hospital, 330 Brookline Avenue, Boston MA 02215, U.S.A.

Eric Maurincomme
GE Medical Systems Europe, 283 rue de la Minière, 78533 Buc Cedex, France
Co-author: Gérald Finet, Department of Hemodynamics, Cardio Vascular Hospital, 69394 Lyon Cedex, France

Michael V. McConnell
Cardiovascular Division, Department of Medicine, Brigham and Women's Hospital and Harvard Medical School, 75 Francis Street, Boston, MA 02115, U.S.A.
Co-authors: Peter Ganz, Richard T. Lee, Andrew P. Selwyn and Peter Libby

Gary S. Mintz
Washington Cardiology Center, 110 Irving Street N.W., Suite 4B1, Washington, DC 20010, U.S.A.
Co-authors: Augusto D. Pichard, Kenneth M. Kent, Jeffrey J. Popma, Lowell F. Satler, Carol L. Walsh, Paul R. Mackell and Martin B. Leon

Sharon L. Mulvagh
Cardiovascular Division, Mayo Clinic, 200 First Street S.W., Rochester, Minnesota 55905, U.S.A.

John F. Nealon
GE Medical Systems, P.O. Box 414, Milwaukee, WI 53210, U.S.A.

Jan A. Oomen
Department of Biomedical Technology, Thoraxcenter, Erasmus University Rotterdam, P.O. Box 1738, 3000 DR Rotterdam, The Netherlands
Co-authors: J.C. Hans Schuurbiers, Kenneth G. Lehmann*, Cees J. Slager and Patrick W. Serruys
* University of Washington, School of Medicine, Seattle, Washington, U.S.A.

Helmut Oswald
  Department of Cardiology and Angiology, German Heart Institute, Augustenburger
  Platz 1, D-13353 Berlin, Germany
Co-authors: Andreas Wahle, Ernst Wellnhofer and Eckart Fleck

Nico H.J. Pijls
  Department of Cardiology, Catharina Hospital, P.O. Box 1350, 5602 ZA Eindhoven,
  The Netherlands
Co-author: Bernard De Bruyne, Cardiovascular Center, Aalst, Belgium

Johan H.C. Reiber
  Laboratory for Clinical and Experimental Image Processing (LKEB), Department of
  Diagnostic Radiology and Nuclear Medicine, Department of Cardiology, Leiden
  University Hospital, P.O. Box 9600, 2300 RC Leiden, and Interuniversity Cardiology
  Institute of the Netherlands, Utrecht, The Netherlands
Co-authors Chapter 4: Lars R. Schiemanck, Pieter M.J. van der Zwet, Bob Goedhart,
Gerhard Koning, Martin Lammertsma, Martijn Danse, Jan J. Gerbrands*, Martin J. Schalij
and Albert V.G. Bruschke
* Information Theory Group, Delft University of Technology, Delft, The Netherlands

Martin J. Schalij
  Department of Cardiology, Leiden University Hospital, P.O. Box 9600, 2300 RC
  Leiden, The Netherlands
Co-authors: Pieter M.J. van der Zwet, Mariken J. Geldof and Johan H.C. Reiber

Axel Schmermund
  Department of Cardiology, University Hospital Essen, GHS, Hufeland Strasse 55, D-
  45122 Essen, Germany
Co-authors: Dietrich Baumgart, Günter Görge, Rainet Seibel, Dietrich Grönemeyer and
Raimund Erbel

Alexander M. Seifalian
  Division of Radiological Sciences, Guy's Hospital School of Medicine, London Bridge,
  London SE1 9RT, United Kingdom, and University Department of Surgery, Royal Free
  Hospital and School of Medicine, London, United Kingdom
Co-authors: David J. Hawkes, Christopher Bladin, Alan C. Colchester* and Kenneth E.
Hobbs
* Department of Neurology, Guy's Hospital School of Medicine

Simon H. Stertzer
  Division of Cardiovascular Medicine, Stanford University, 900 Welch Road, Suite 202,
  Palo Alto, CA 94304, U.S.A.
Co-authors Chapter 1: Eugene V. Pomerantsev, Jonas A. Metz, Peter J. Fitzgerald and
Paul G. Yock
Co-author Chapter 2: Eugene V. Pomerantsev

Ad van Boven
Department of Cardiology, Thoraxcenter, University Hospital Groningen, Oostersingel 59, 9713 EZ Groningen, The Netherlands
Co-author: Pascal Pfister, Sandoz Pharma Ltd., Basel, Switzerland

Ernst E. van der Wall
Department of Cardiology, Leiden University Hospital, Rijnsburgerweg 10, 2333 AA Leiden, The Netherlands
Co-author Chapter 32: Albert V.G. Bruschke

Albert C. van Rossum
Department of Cardiology, Free University Hospital Amsterdam, de Boelelaan 1117, 1081 HV Amsterdam, The Netherlands
Co-author: Johannes C. Post

Kitty Vreeswijk
Philips Medical Systems, P.O. Box 10.000, 5680 DA Best, The Netherlands

William Wijns
Cardiovascular Centre, OLV Hospital, 164 Moorselbaan, B9300 Aalst, Belgium, and Laboratory of Positron Emission Tomography, University of Louvain Medical School, Louvain-la-Neuve, Belgium
Co-authors: Anne Bol and Jacques A. Melin

Preface

In the past, coronary arteriography was the only modality available to provide high quality images of the coronary anatomy. Quantitative Coronary Arteriography (QCA) was developed, implemented, validated and extensively applied to obtain accurate and reproducible data about coronary morphology and the functional significance of coronary obstructions. In the previous volumes in this series of books we had limited our scope, therefore, to all the developments and applications which directly or indirectly had to do with (quantitative) x-ray coronary arteriography. However, over the last several years extensive basic technological research supported by clinical investigations has created ways to visualize the coronary morphology and the associated perfusion of the myocardial muscle by other competing modalities. As a result, time has come now to widen our scope and compare the feasibilities, strengths and limitations of these modalities in studying the presence, extent and consequences of coronary artery disease. Currently, the following modalities are available: x-ray coronary arteriography, intracoronary ultrasound, contrast- and stress-echocardiography, angioscopy, nuclear cardiology, magnetic resonance imaging, and cine and spiral CT imaging.

These marked technological developments have allowed the cardiologist to obtain complementary information about the coronary anatomy, ventricular function, and the myocardium relative to that obtainable with conventional imaging. For all these imaging modalities it is true that the application of dedicated quantitative analytical software packages enables the evaluation of the imaging studies in a more accurate, reliable, and reproducible manner. It goes without saying that these extensions and achievements have resulted in improved diagnostics and subsequently in improved patient care. Particularly in patients with ischemic heart disease, major progress has been made to detect coronary artery disease in an early phase of the disease process, to follow the atherosclerotic changes in the coronary arteries, to establish the functional and metabolic consequences of the luminal obstructions, and to accurately assess the results of interventional therapy. For instance, intravascular ultrasound permits the early detection of coronary artery disease and has been instrumental in the proper placement of interventional devices, contrast echocardiography has the potential for the assessment of the perfusion in the myocardial muscle, stress-echocardiography allows the detection of changes in regional wall motion at various stages of a pharmacological stress-test, coronary angioscopy is the only method that can provide "histopathological" data by the percutaneous route, magnetic resonance angiography can presently be used for screening of disease and potentially allows the measurement of all required data in a single imaging session ("one stop shop"), nuclear imaging techniques such as single-photon emission computed tomography and positron emission tomography, may well be applied for the evaluation of the functional and metabolic consequences of coronary artery lesions, cine and spiral CT may allow the noninvasive detection of calcium deposits, and quantitative coronary angiography allows the assessment of successful interventional therapy.

In line with our own interests and research activities at the Departments of Diagnostic Radiology and Nuclear Medicine, and of Cardiology, Leiden University Hospital, we wish to emphasize and cover both the engineering and image processing developments as well as the clinical applications in this book. Aside from all these high-tech developments in cardiac imaging techniques, the transition from the analog to the digital world has been going on now for some time. Through the efforts of the American College of Radiology (ACR), the National Electrical Manufacturers Association (NEMA), the American College of Cardiology (ACC), the European Society of Cardiology (ESC), and the representatives of the major imaging companies and university hospitals, it has been decided that the CD-R will be the exchange medium for cardiac images and DICOM-3 the standard file format. This has been a major achievement in the field of standardization activities. Since these developments have and will have a major impact on the way images will be stored, reviewed and exchanged in the near future, an important part of this book has been dedicated to DICOM and the filmless catheterization laboratory.

Cardiovascular imaging is a bibliographical "image" of a Symposium, held June 24-26, 1996, In Leiden. At this Symposium all the major advances in the areas mentioned above were addressed by the leading authorities in these fields. Based on the presentations of the invited Faculty, this book consists of a compilation of manuscripts related to each of these specific topics. As each chapter not only describes the state-of-the-art as of 1996, but also looks into the future, its content serves as a very valuable source of information for today and the years to come. We express our gratitude to all authors and co-authors for making great efforts in preparing their superb up-to-date chapters under a great time pressure so that this book would be available at the time of the Symposium. The authors are all excellent investigators in one or more fields of cardiac imaging and they have stimulated progress in cardiac imaging with the aim to improve patient care.

At the same time, this book may be considered as a mark of honor to prof.dr. A.E. van Voorthuisen, who retired June 1, 1996 after having been Head of the Department of Diagnostic Radiology and Nuclear Medicine of the Leiden University Hospital for over 25 years. In this capacity he has among others stimulated and supported the (cardiovascular) MRI developments from the early days, and recognized the additional benefits of quantitative analytical software developments by including the Laboratory of Clinical and Experimental Image Processing (LKEB) as a division to the Radiology Department.

We like to thank the significant contributions from mrs. N. Dekker (Kluwer Academic Publishers, Dordrecht, The Netherlands), mr. J. Schoones (Leiden University Medical Library), and mrs. A. van der Mey (Department of Cardiology, Leiden University Hospital), who all put a lot of effort in editing, preparing and completing Cardiovascular Imaging. Lastly, this book would not have been possible without a generous educational grant from Lorex Synthélabo (Maarssen, The Netherlands). We hope that this book will assist the cardiologist, the radiologist, the nuclear medicine physician, the image processing specialist, physicist, basic scientist, and the fellow who is in training for those specialties, in understanding the most recent achievements in cardiac imaging techniques and their impact on cardiovascular medicine.

The Editors,

Johan H.C. Reiber and Ernst E. van der Wall

1. The changing role of high speed rotational atherectomy in the present and future practice of coronary intervention

SIMON H. STERTZER, EUGENE V. POMERANTSEV, JONAS A. METZ, PETER J. FITZGERALD, PAUL G. YOCK

Summary

Eight hundred and fifty-two high speed rotational atherectomy (HSRA) procedures were performed in a single consecutive series of 769 patients. Stand alone HSRA was performed in 261 patients (29%). HSRA with adjunctive low pressure (≤ 2 ATM) balloon angioplasty (LP BA) was performed in 261 patients (34%), and HSRA with adjunctive high pressure (≥ 4 ATM) balloon angioplasty (HP BA) was performed in 216 patients (28%). Prognostically unfavorable Type B2 and C lesions dominated the study group (73.8%). Procedural success rate was 96%. Emergency coronary artery bypass surgery was performed in 1.3% of cases, Q-wave myocardial infarction occurred in 3.0% and death, related to procedure, was consequent in 0.4% of cases. Incidence of flow limiting dissections was 3.1%, distal spasm 5.2%, and "no reflow" phenomenon, 1.7%. The recent technique modifications included continuous advancer/guiding catheter infusion of the nitroglycerin - verapamil mixture, limitation of duration of lesion engagement by the burr, decrease of rotational speed, and strict control of rpm drop during lesion ablation. Evolution of the interventional technique involved trends towards decrease of the use of HP BA in conjunction with steady increase in the percentage of SA and LP BA procedures over time. During the last year a combination of HSRA and stents emerged. The "rotastenting" produces excellent results in longer and more frequently calcified lesions than the use of stents alone with higher degree of attainable stent expansion. These technique changes resulted in complete absence of "no reflow" in last two years, as well as a decrease in coronary vascular reactivity from all burr passes.

Introduction

High speed rotational atherectomy (HSRA) is a unique modality of atheroma debulking [1-11]. The clinical role of this technique has undergone significant evolutionary changes.

At the very first stage the concept of the creation of a "pilot hole" was dominant. One or two relatively small burrs were used just to provide for the subsequent passage of a PTCA balloon through a calcified lesion [2]. Subsequently, the advent of more aggressive lesion debulking led to the occurrence of the "no reflow" phenomenon, a complication which was observed in the absence of thrombus, dissection, intimal flap or embolus in affected arteries [9,12-15]. Despite the six years of worldwide application of this treatment modality, the

1

J.H.C. Reiber and E.E. van der Wall (eds.), Cardiovascular Imaging, 1-13.
© 1996 *Kluwer Academic Publishers.*

technique of HSRA is still subject to widely different individual operator variation, both in stand alone and in adjunctive balloon angioplasty procedures. The amount of atheroma debulking versus adjunctive barotrauma (high pressure balloon angioplasty, HP BA) varies amongst invasive cardiologists. The number of burrs utilized, the role of adjunctive balloon angioplasty, and the ultimate burr/artery ratios are, as yet, not standardized by interventionalists using HSRA.

The recent widespread acceptance of the intracoronary stents both as bailout and elective treatment have resulted in the HSRA/stent combination known as "rotastenting". This technique consists of variable degrees of debulking of a rigid lesion, with subsequent single or multiple stent deployment.

The subject of this communication is the effect of specific HSRA strategies on the immediate results. Herein represented is a technique analysis of a large series of consecutive procedures, performed by a single interventional group. The general strategy of rotational atherectomy represented in this series is to achieve as much ablation of atheroma as possible using a combination of techniques described below.

Procedure technique evolution

Three general HSRA treatment strategies have been used at Stanford University Hospital. The first is the stand alone procedure (SA), where the operator deploys sequential burrs, incrementally upsizing until an optimal effect is achieved. The second is HSRA followed by low pressure (<2 ATM) balloon inflation (LP BA), intended to improve border regularity or to relieve moderate spasm refractory to medications. Historically, the third strategy was HSRA followed by higher pressure (>4 ATM) balloon angioplasty (HP BA). This approach was employed when the "threatened no-reflow" phenomenon, forced cessation of further burr deployment, yet $\geq 50\%$ stenosis was still present. In the past year this strategy has changed significantly by the use of intracoronary stents. J&JIS stents are used for relatively straight and proximal coronary segments. When there is a significant tortuosity, diffuse or distal disease, the use of AVE Micro Stents becomes the treatment of choice.

Specific technical features of the procedure as currently practised are as follows:

1. An infusion line is piggybacked into the Rotablator advancer catheter. A mixture of 50 mg of dissolved nitroglycerin (Tridil®), and 5 mg of Verapamil in 500 cc of normal saline is infused by a constant infusion pump at 200 cc/hr [16]. During burr advances and withdrawals, high pressure saline infusion is carried out through the advancer in a standard fashion. Between passes, the infusion was switched back to the nitroglycerin - verapamil mixture at 200 cc/hr.

2. The duration of lesion engagement by the burr is limited to 10 - 15 seconds, depending on vessel size, lesion length and vascular reactivity. This represents a significant decrease in the time of burr engagement used prior to mid 1993, when 30-40 second runs were standard.

3. For burrs up to 2.00 mm in diameter, rotational speed is maintained at 175-180,000 rpm. For burrs of 2.00 mm in diameter and more, rotational speed is kept at 160-165,000 rpm.

4. Critical attention is paid to limiting the drop in speed of rotation during lesion

ablation to no greater than 5000 rpm.

Patients and procedural characteristics

Between October 1990 and January 1996, 769 patients with coronary artery disease underwent 852 coronary HSRA procedures. A detailed description of the procedure has been published previously [15]. Clinical indications for HSRA were stable or unstable angina, refractory to medical therapy, and/or inducible myocardial ischemia (EKG, Tl^{201}, stress Echo). Angiographically, the characteristic indications for the HSRA were significant calcification, bent segments, side branches, severe border irregularities and long, diffuse lesions. Initial burr sizes were chosen according to the most severe narrowing. Procedures were generally started with a 1.25 mm or 1.5 mm device, with incremental upsizing up to 2.38 mm or 2.5 mm, according to the size of the vessel and the vascular reactivity encountered during ablation runs. An average of 2.7 ± 0.9 burrs was used per procedure.

Two hundred twenty-three patients (29%) had stand alone HSRA, 261 patients (34%) underwent adjunctive low pressure balloon angioplasty, and in 215 patients (28%) HSRA was performed with adjunctive high pressure balloon angioplasty. Rotastenting was performed in 9% of the overall patient cohort (69 patients). However, stents were not available freely in the US until late 1994, so that in 1995, the average incidence of rotastent procedures rose to 28-40% of the quarterly HSRA procedures.

Qualitative angiographic lesion description

The qualitative description of lesion morphology included classification into eccentric, concentric or total occlusion subsets. Calcification at the lesion site and presence of irregularity of the borders were assessed. A lesion location was considered to be on a bend point if the diseased segment was angulated more than 90°. Characterization as discrete vs. diffuse disease and presence of significant side branches were recorded. Intraluminal filling defects or characteristic contrast staining before any intracoronary manipulation, were considered as signs of probable intracoronary thrombus.

Lesions were classified according to Ambrose [17] and ACC/AHA schemes. The Ambrose categories were: Class I lesions - concentric, smooth, local lesions; Class II lesions - uncomplicated eccentric focal stenoses with smooth borders. Class III lesions - complicated lesions: eccentric with irregular and/or overhanging borders. Class IV lesions - long (>2.5 cm) lesions, composed of several sequential narrowings in one complex lesion. The ACC/AHA classification of B lesions was subdivided into B1 (when only one B-criterion was present) and B2 (when more than one B-criterion was present).

Procedural definitions

Technical success: A reduction in percentage diameter stenosis after treatment to less than 50% and no in-hospital occurrence of major cardiac event.

Procedural success: Technical success in all treated lesions without occurrence of any major cardiac event during the hospital stay.

Major cardiac event: Occurrence during the hospital stay of death, a new Q-wave myocardial infarction, and/or need for emergency coronary bypass surgery.

No reflow phenomenon: Cessation of antegrade blood flow (TIMI 0-I) in major epicardial coronary artery without angiographic signs of significant intimal dissection, thrombus or emboli.

Intimal dissection: Any linear intimal defect observed post procedure, no matter how minor.

Spasm: Acute, diffuse and reversible decrease of the target vessel diameter post intervention.

Unstable angina [18]: Presence of at least one of the following three clinical features, accompanied by electrocardiographic changes:
1. Crescendo angina superimposed on a preexisting pattern of relatively stable, exertion-related angina pectoris;
2. Angina pectoris at rest as well as with minimal exertion;
3. Angina pectoris of new onset (within one month), which is induced by minimal exertion.

Baseline characteristics

The patients were predominantly male (Table 1). Seventy-eight percent were in Canadian Cardiovascular Society angina class III or IV, or had unstable angina. Fifty-seven and sixty-five percent presented with a history of hypertension or hypercholesterolemia, respectively. Forty-four percent had previous myocardial infarction. Three hundred eighty-four patients (50%) had previous PTCA. HSRA was used as the primary treatment method in 852 lesions.

Target lesion morphological characteristics

Four hundred and seventy-one lesions (55.3%) were de novo lesions (Table 2). Type B2 and type C lesions prevailed over simpler lesions of types B1 and A (28.9% and 44.9% vs. 14.3% and 11.6%, respectively). According to the Ambrose classification [17], local and eccentric lesions (Types II and III) were treated relatively infrequently, especially the so-called "unstable" lesions of type III. Local and concentric lesions of type I were treated more often, but diffuse multiple lesions of Class IV dominated in the study group (Table 2). Complete occlusions comprised 3.6% of lesions, whereas ostial and calcified lesions accounted for 10.3% and 16.7% of lesions, respectively. Quarterly analysis of treated lesion morphology failed to show any statistically significant changes in target lesion selection during the study period.

Procedure results

In this series of 852 lesions treated in 769 patients, technical success was achieved in 825 lesions (96.8%). The procedure was successful in 736 patients (96%).

Table 1. Clinical profile of 769 patients.

Index	n	%
Age (yr) Mean±SD, range	67.4±13	31-91
Gender, male	569	74
Diabetes	162	21
Hypertension	438	57
Hypercholesterolemia	499	65
Prior Smoking	361	47
Current Smoking	69	9
CCS Angina II	185	2
III	307	40
IV	78	10
Unstable	215	28
Prior Myocardial Infarction	338	44
Prior PTCA	384	50
Prior CABG	177	23

Table 2. Target lesion morphology according to Ambrose and AHA/ACC classifications.

	N	%
Ambrose I	272	32
Ambrose II	87	10.4
Ambrose III	51	6
Ambrose IV	408	48
Complete occlusions	31	3.6
Calcified	143	16.7
Ostial	88	10.3
AHA/ACC Type A	99	11.6
Type B1	122	14.3
Type B2	247	28.9
Type C	383	44.9
De Novo	471	55.5
Restenotic	335	39.3

Intimal dissection (Table 3) was the most frequent angiographic complication (10.9%). It should be noted that only in 3.1% of these lesions there was flow limitation. Adjunctive balloon angioplasty or stenting was highly effective in "retacking" dissections and improving luminal appearance. Significant distal spasm, refractory to intracoronary medications, and requiring additional balloon inflations, was noted in 5.2% of cases. Compromise of large side branches, observed in 12 cases (1.4%), was reversible in 10 cases without additional intervention (with complete restoration of the blood flow at the completion of procedure, or at 24 hr. restudy).

Coronary artery perforations (defined as any contrast extravasation) were observed in 5 cases (0.6%). None required surgical intervention or pericardiocentesis. In one case, extravasation was related to burr entrapment in a myocardial bridge.

Left main coronary artery injury, possibly related to guiding catheter manipulation, was observed in one case (0.1%). In another case, the procedure was complicated by fracture and discontinuity of the Rotablator C wire, requiring surgery to remove a remnant of the distal coil.

Acute closure of the target vessel was observed in 21 lesions (2.5%). "No reflow" phenomenon was observed in 13 of these lesions (1.7%). Acute thrombosis was observed in 4 of procedures (0.4%).

The overall rate of major cardiac events was 3.3%. Emergency CABG was performed in 1.3%. Death, related to the procedure, occurred in 3 patients (0.4%) of the series. It occurred in two cases after emergency bypass surgery, and in a third patient with an LVEF < 20%, after HSRA with elective cardiopulmonary support (CPS).

Table 3. Procedural complications.

	n	%
Major Cardiac Event	25	3.3
Emergency CABG	10	1.3
Death	3	0.4
Q-wave MI	23	3.0
Acute vessel closure	21	2.5
"No reflow" phenomenon	13	1.7
Filling defect, thrombus	4	0.4
Refractory spasm	44	5.2
Intimal dissection	93	10.9
Perforation	5	0.6
Side branch compromize	12	1.4
LMCA injury	1	0.1
Distal wire spring detachment	1	0.1

Stanford rotastent experience

In order to evaluate the impact of the combination of the HSRA and stent deployment (Rotastent group), we studied 33 patients prospectively with "rotastenting" of 40 coronary segments. All procedures were successful and uncomplicated. In order to evaluate the differences in baseline coronary lesion morphology and the acute results of procedure, we compared this group with 40 coronary segments of 34 patients treated with HSRA only (HSRA group). Forty diseased segments of 34 patients of a third comparison group were treated with Palmaz-Schatz J&JIS stent deployment (J&JIS Group). QCA assessment of the treated vessel was performed at baseline, after the use of the last burr, and post procedure using the QCAPlus software package developed and validated at Stanford [19]. Minimal luminal diameter (MLD), average intrastent diameter (AISD) , reference diameter (D ref.) and percent diameter stenosis (%D) were measured using the angiographic catheter for calibration. The patients of HSRA and J&JIS groups were selected retrospectively by matching angiographic D ref. In the Rotastent and J&JIS groups, ICUS was used to ascertain optimal stent expansion. ICUS was performed using the Insight system (CVIS, Sunnyvale, CA) with 2.9 F or 3.2 F catheters operating at 30 MHz. The recorded ultrasound imaging runs were analyzed off-line at the core laboratory at Stanford University. Quantitative parameters were derived from single frame analysis on the Tape Measure quantitation system (Indec Systems, Capitola, CA). The following lumen and vessel parameters were measured: minimum luminal diameter and area, reference luminal area, reference luminal diameter.

Measurements were taken from multiple locations in articulated Palmaz-Schatz stents. To assess stent expansion, the percent area expansion was calculated as a ratio between the minimal intrastent area and A ref. ICUS.

Qualitative angiographic description of lesion morphology revealed that the Rotastent group was characterized by extremely frequent calcification (Table 4). The frequency of angiographic calcification was significantly higher than in HSRA and J&JIS groups. Obviously, this reflects the lesion selection for the Rotastent. The occurrence of diffuse and tubular lesions was significantly highest in the HSRA group compared to the Rotastent and to the J&JIS group (80 vs. 67.5 vs. 45%, respectively, $p < 0.05$).

QCA assessment of baseline lesions (Table 5) revealed similar %D, MLD and D ref. Lesion length determined by QCA was significantly longer both in the HSRA and the Rotastent groups vs. the J&JIS group.

The size of the last used burr was similar in the HSRA and in the Rotastent groups (2.1 ± 0.3 vs 2.0 ± 0.3 mm). Nonetheless, the final MLD was higher in the Rotastent group (1.8 ± 0.4 vs. 1.4 ± 0.4 mm, $p < 0.05$). Doubtless, the HSRA procedure of more calcified lesions resulted in higher extent of debulking.

The final post procedure results (Table 5) demonstrated a highly significant increase in MLD, both in the J&JIS and the Rotastent groups, with less striking results in the HSRA cohort (MLD post was 3.0 ± 0.7 mm vs. 3.1 ± 0.5 mm vs 2.5 ± 0.7 mm, respectively $p < 0.01$). QCU assessment of the stent expansion demonstrated significantly better expansion in the Rotastent group compared to the J&JIS group ($91.9 \pm 4.4\%$ vs. $79.7 \pm 3.4\%$, $p < 0.03$).

These data demonstrate that rotastenting in longer and more frequently calcified

Table 4. Qualitative description of Rotastent groups.

	HSRA Group	%	Rotastent Group	%	p (HSRA-Rotastent)	J&JIS Group	%	p (Rotastent-J&JIS)	p (HSRA-J&JIS)
Calcifications	8	20	27	67.5	<0.01	5	12.5	<0.01	NS
Eccentric lesions	25	62.5	23	57.5	NS	25	62.5	NS	NS
Complete Occlusions	1	2.5	2	5	NS	1	2.5	NS	NS
Type A	1	2.5	2	5	NS	3	7.5	NS	NS
Type B1	5	12.5	6	15	NS	10	25	NS	NS
Type B2	13	32.5	12	30	NS	15	37.5	NS	NS
Type C	21	52.5	20	50	NS	12	30	NS	NS
Ulcerated	1	2.5	1	2.5	NS	4	10	NS	NS
Smooth	16	40	16	40	NS	18	45	NS	NS
Irregular	24	60	23	57.5	NS	19	47.5	NS	NS
Bend > 90 degrees	14	35	10	25	NS	7	17.5	NS	NS
Local <10 mm	9	22.5	13	32.5	NS	22	55	NS	<0.01
Diffuse >20 mm	17	42.5	14	35	NS	10	25	NS	NS
Tubular 10-20 mm	15	37.5	13	32.5	NS	8	20	NS	NS
Diffuse and Tubular	32	80	27	67.5	NS	18	45	NS	<0.01
Side Branch	10	25	14	35	NS	16	40	NS	NS
Thrombus	0	0	1	2.5	NS	2	5	NS	NS

Table 5. Quantitative coronary angiography and intravascular ultrasound data.

	HSRA Group		Rotastent Group		p (HSRA-Rotastent)	J&JIS Group		p (Rotastent-J&JIS)	p (HSRA-J&JIS)
	Mean	SD	Mean	SD		Mean	SD		
%D Baseline	63	14.3	61.7	12.4	NS	62.7	11.5	NS	NS
MLD Baseline, mm	1.2	0.5	1.2	0.4	NS	1.2	0.4	NS	NS
D ref., mm	3.0	0.7	3.1	0.7	NS	3.1	0.7	NS	NS
Length	20.9	9.4	21.1	12.3	NS	17.0	7.7	<0.05	<0.05
MLD HSRA, mm	1.4	0.4	1.8	0.4	<0.01				
MLD Final, mm	1.7	0.4	2.6	0.5	<0.01	2.6	0.7	NS	<0.01
%D Final	43.5	10.2	7.2	9.8	<0.05	8.3	10.7	NS	<0.01
Immediate Gain, %	18.6	17.7	46.5	17.5	<0.01	47.0	19.5	NS	<0.01
IVUS Area Expansion, %			91.9	19.4		79.7	18.7	<0.03	<0.01

lesions produces excellent results, compared to J&JIS placements alone in relatively simpler lesions. A very important finding is that better intravascular stent expansion is achieved after HSRA atheroma debulking.

The role of procedural technique modifications

An overall success rate of 96% in this series of 769 procedures on predominantly type C lesions is encouragingly high. The incidence of complications did not differ significantly from those published in our earlier series [15,16]. An analysis of the technique evolution, performed by our group in 1994 [16] reflected a trend toward a decline of high pressure adjunctive BA (Figure 2), while the percentage of stand alone procedures and low pressure adjunctive balloon angioplasty increased steadily (Figures 1,2). In the past year additional, significant changes have occurred. While the number of standalone and adjunctive high pressure balloon angioplasty have decreased, the number of rotastenting procedures increased significantly.

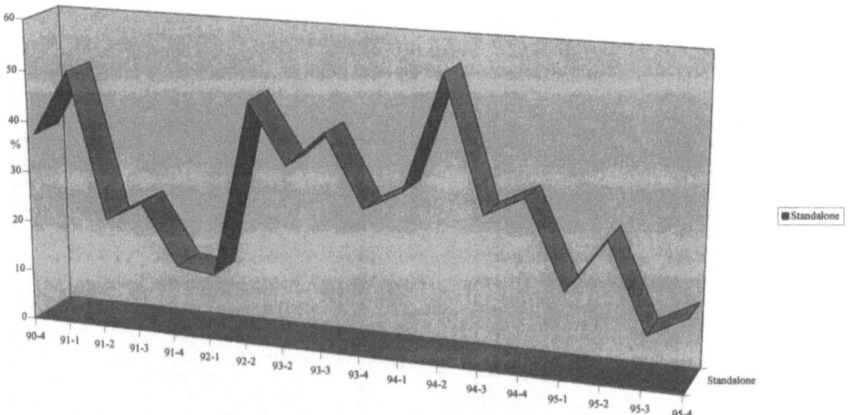

Figure 1. Quarterly dynamics of standalone HSRA procedures.

These trends reflect the operator's inclination to debulk more of each lesion by using the aforementioned technique modifications, by reducing the level of vascular reactivity from each burr pass. In case of significant dissection and/or large vessel size, the usage of adjunctive stenting has produced excellent results. Complications specific to HSRA include various degrees of vessel spasm and/or "no reflow" phenomena. Quarterly analysis of the incidence of spasm (Figure 3) showed a marked reduction in this phenomenon during study period. Lesion complexity by ACC/AHA gradation was the same during the study periods. Since the lesion selection was not a factor, the decrease in spastic complications may be considered to be a function of the operator technique, i.e., vasodilator infusion via the advancer, lower time of burr engagement, decreased rotation speed, and lower acceptable drop in rotation speed during ablative passes [16].

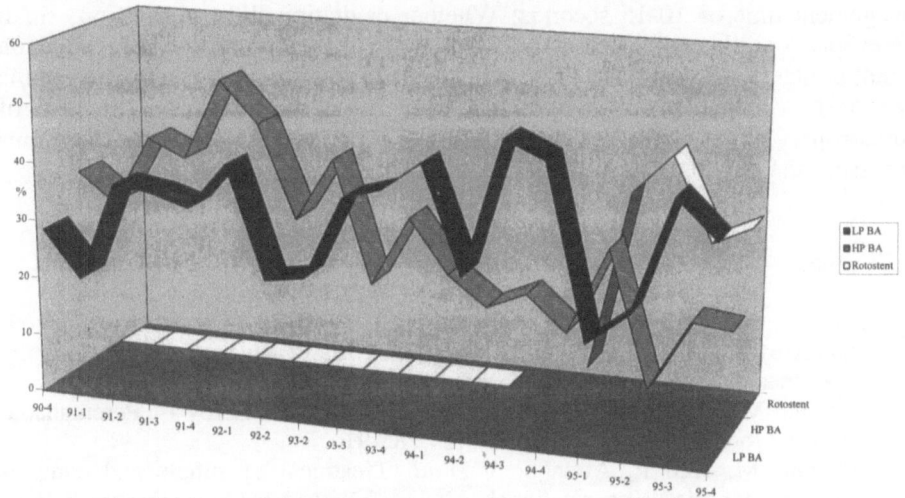

Figure 2. Quarterly dynamics of adjunctive PTCA and stenting.

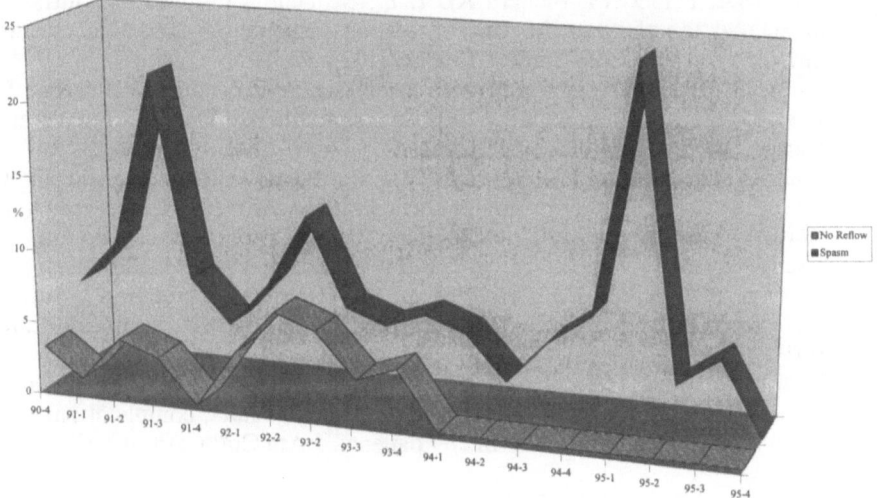

Figure 3. Quarterly dynamics of spasm and "No Reflow" incidence.

Figure 3 demonstrates the complete absence of the "no reflow" phenomenon in 1994 and 1995, when the last major changes in the technique were instituted. From our consecutive single center series we conclude that the two most important technique changes that have served to increase success rates in long, tight calcified lesions are the increased number of burrs used (2.7 ± 0.9 per lesion in 1993-1994 vs. 2.0 ± 1.0 in 1990-1992, $p < 0.01$), and the reduced burr engagement time of 10-15 seconds. Whether cavitation, heat generation, small vessel spasm or plaque burden is the major cause of the "no reflow" phenomenon cannot be stated with certainty. The adjustment of rotation speed, reduction in the time of burr engagement, incremental sequencing of burrs, and the use of intracoronary nitroglycerin-verapamil infusion mitigate spasm and slow flow, thus increasing the degree of debulking.

References

1. Ahn SS, Auth D, Marcus RD, Moore WS. Removal of focal atheromatous lesions by angioscopically guided high speed rotary atherectomy. Preliminary experimental investigations. J Vasc Surg 1988;7:292-300.
2. Bertrand ME, Lablanche JM, Fourrier JL, Bauters C, Leroy F. Percutaneous coronary rotary ablation. Herz 1990;15:285-91.
3. Borrione M, Hall P, Almagor Y *et al.* Treatment of simple and complex coronary stenosis using rotational ablation followed by low pressure balloon angioplasty. Cathet Cardiovasc Diagn 1993;30:131-7.
4. Gilmore PS, Bass TA, Conetta DA *et al.* Single site experience with high-speed coronary rotational atherectomy. Clin Cardiol 1993;16:311-6.
5. Kovach JA, Mintz GS, Pichard AD *et al.* Sequential intravascular ultrasound characterization of the mechanisms of rotational atherectomy and adjunct balloon angioplasty. J Am Coll Cardiol 1993;22:1024-32.
6. Mintz GS, Potkin BN, Keren G *et al.* Intravascular ultrasound evaluation of the effect of rotational atherectomy in obstructive atherosclerotic coronary artery disease. Circulation 1992;86:1383-93.
7. Smalling RW, Cassidy DB, Schmidt WA, Barrett R, Fulford S, Kirkeeide RL. Effects of rotational atherectomy in normal canine coronary and diseased human cadaveric arteries: potential for plaque removal from distal, tortuous, and diffusely diseased vessels. Cathet Cardiovasc Diagn 1991;24:300-7.
8. Teirstein PS, Warth DC, Haq N *et al.* High speed rotational coronary atherectomy for patients with diffuse coronary artery disease. J Am Coll Cardiol 1991;18:1694-701.
9. Warth DC, Leon MB, O'Neill W, Zacca N, Polissar NL, Buchbinder M. Rotational atherectomy multicenter registry: acute results, complications and 6-month angiographic follow-up in 709 patients. J Am Coll Cardiol 1994;24:641-8.
10. Zacca NM, Kleiman NS, Rodriguez AR *et al.* Rotational ablation of coronary artery lesions using single, large burrs. Cathet Cardiovasc Diagn 1992;26:92-7.
11. Stertzer SH, Pomerantsev EV, Fitzgerald PJ *et al.* Early changes of the coronary artery segment after high speed rotational ablation. Analysis of the procedure mechanics using 24 hr. restudies. Submitted for publication.
12. Ellis SG, Popma JJ, Buchbinder M *et al.* Relation of clinical presentation, stenosis morphology, and operator technique to the procedural results of rotational atherectomy and rotational atherectomy-facilitated angioplasty. Circulation 1994;89:882-92.
13. Henry M, Amor M, Ethevenot G, Henry I. Percutaneous peripheral rotational ablation using the Rotablator: immediate and mid term results. Single center experience concerning 146 lesions treated. Int Angiol 1993;12:231-44.

14. Safian RD, Niazi KA, Strzelecki M *et al* Detailed angiographic analysis of high-speed mechanical rotational atherectomy in human coronary arteries. Circulation 1993;88:961-8.

15. Stertzer SH, Rosenblum J, Shaw RE *et al*. Coronary rotational ablation: initial experience in 302 procedures. J Am Coll Cardiol 1993;21:287-95.

16. Stertzer SH, Pomerantsev EV, Fitzgerald PJ *et al*. Effects of technique modification on immediate results of high speed rotational atherectomy in 710 procedures on 656 patients. Cathet Cardiovasc Diagn 1995;36:304-10.

17. Ambrose JA, Winters SL, Arora RR *et al*. Angiographic evolution of coronary artery morphology in unstable angina. J Am Coll Cardiol 1986;7:472-8.

18. Rutherford JD, Braunwald E, Cohn PF. Chronic ischemic heart disease. In: Braunwald E, editor. Heart disease: a textbook of cardiovascular medicine. 3rd ed. Philadelphia: Saunders, 1988:1314-78.

19. Leung WH, Sanders W, Alderman EL. Coronary artery quantitation and data management system for paired cineangiograms. Cathet Cardiovasc Diagn 1991;24:121-34.

2. The AVE Micro Stents™

SIMON H. STERTZER & EUGENE V. POMERANTSEV

Summary

AVE Micro Stent is a stent model, recently introduced in clinical cardiology practice in Europe and undergoing currently multicenter clinical trials in USA. Both Micro Stent I and II are formed from a continuous segment of stainless steel wire in the zigzag design, and both display eight axial struts connected by eight radiused crowns. As the basic unitary element of the Micro Stent is either 3.0 or 4.0 mm in length (I&II, respectively), these devices are premounted on AVE delivery balloons as stents of : 6.0, 8.0, 9.0, 12.0, 15.0, 18.0, 21.0, 30.0 and 39.0 mm in length. Advantages of AVE Micro Stents include limited amount of metal, excellent x-ray opacity, highly customizable length and superior trackability. The degree of recoil is similar to the J&JIS stents. Stent profile allows passage through 6 and 7F guiding catheters. High flexibility of the AVE Micro Stent expands the range of accessible vessel segments. The analysis of the use of AVE Micro Stents in 1132 patients demonstrates the low complications rate as well as an overall restenosis rate of 20.9%.

Introduction

Clinical analysis of commercially available stent systems demonstrated some directions for improvement. The concept of using a minimal amount of implantable metallic material for intracoronary stenting emerged from the belief that stainless steel was dangerously thrombogenic. The idea was to create a scaffolding system using limited and adjustable amount of stainless steel. The way to do it was to create a subunit with enough mechanical stability to sustain a coaxial alignment in a hemodynamically active high pressure coronary vessel. Consequently, the modifiable zigzag four crown design seen in Figure 1 was first developed as a unitary device of 4.0 mm in length.

Another sensitive area is the radiopacity of the unit. First, it should be acceptably visible during the deployment procedure both in unexpanded and expanded state. Second, the x-ray opacity of the stent should not interfere with visual assessment of the resulting lumen.

The Micro Stent I

The basic design of the Micro Stent I is shown in Figure 1, and essentially consists of 4.0 mm length segments which expand to nominal diameters of 3.0, 3.5, and 4.0 millimeters. The Micro Stents are expandable to predetermined sizes by raising the delivery balloon pressures to variable levels explained below. Since the majority of the deployment balloons are compliant polyethylene, stents can

15

J.H.C. Reiber and E.E. van der Wall (eds.), Cardiovascular Imaging, 15-30.

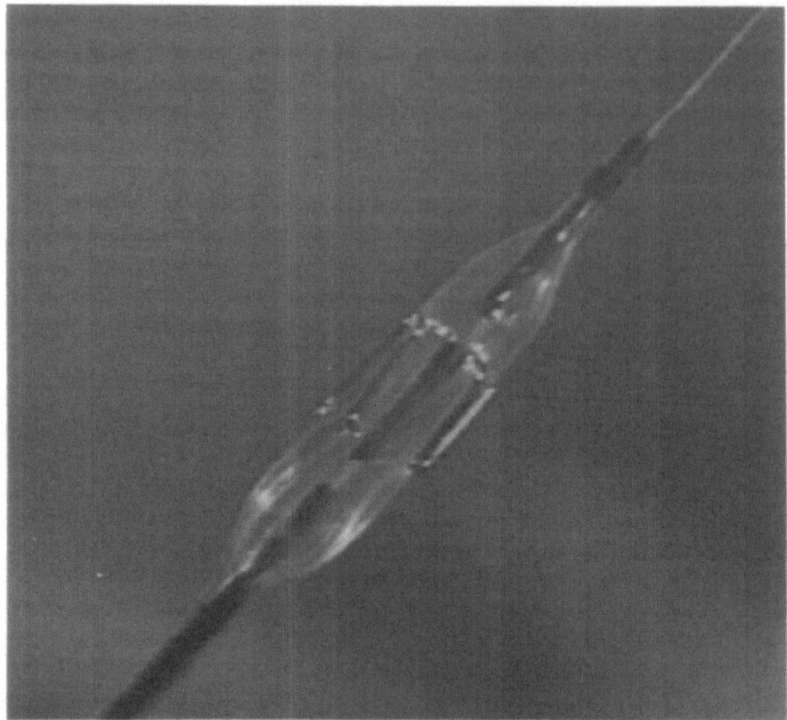

Figure 1. Single 4 mm length AVE Micro Stent I mounted on balloon.

be overexpanded beyond their nominal diameters by further increasing the balloon pressures as described in the deployment discussion.

The Micro Stent is fashioned into the zigzag crown configuration by processing an electropolished, 316L stainless steel wire of 0.008" (0.2 mm) in thickness. As a result of the mil thickness of the strut, the stent is moderately more radiopaque than most other similar clinical devices (Figures 2A, 2B). When deployed, the actual metallic surface area of the expanded state is approximately 9% (3.5 mm device). The strut design orients in a manner parallel to the blood flow, and shortens on expansion by about 2% (3.5 mm device). When the Micro Stent is mounted on the unexpanded balloon, it displays a maximal profile of 0.065"(1.65 mm), permitting its passage comfortably through a guiding catheter of 7 French size[1]. In addition to its low profile, the stent displays an extraordinary degree of longitudinal flexibility, such that it is expected to track wherever a PTCA balloon has passed first. This is especially true of the 4.0 and 8.0 mm unconnected segments (Figure 3). Clinical experience with this device today includes more than 28000 deployed stents worldwide.

---

[1] A 6 F compatible device is also available for brachial and radial approach.

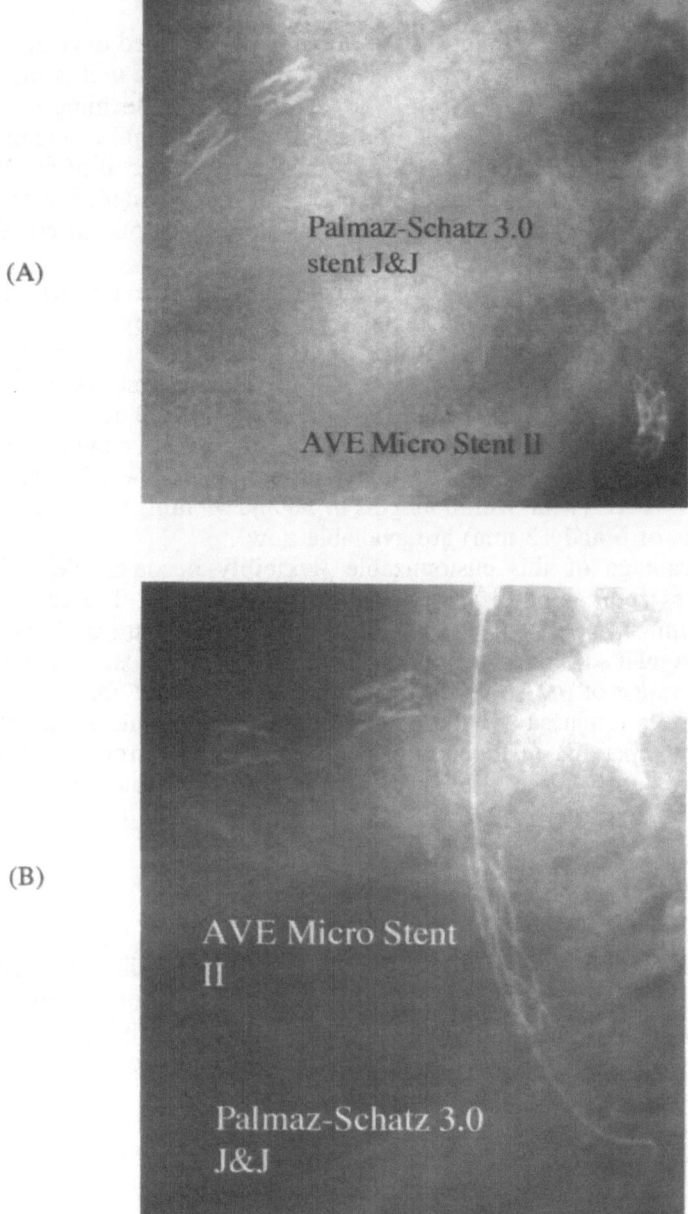

Figure 2. Comparative x-ray opacity study. (A) Two AVE Micro Stents I (3.5 mm
8 mm long) deployed into the animal left anterior descending coronary artery. One
3.5 - 15 mm J&JIS stent deployed into the mid circumflex. One 3.5 -15 mm AVE
Micro Stent II deployed into the distal circumflex. (B) Two AVE Micro Stents I (3.5
mm 8 mm long) deployed into the animal left anterior descending coronary artery.
One AVE Micro Stent II (3.5 mm 18 mm long) deployed into the mid circumflex.
One 3.5 - 15 mm J&J IS stent deployed into the distal circumflex.

The Micro Stent II

The Micro Stent II is a later iteration of the previously described device, in that although it is composed of precisely the same material, its basic unit is the three millimeter length segment (Figure 4). The effect of this seemingly minor modification on the stent is considerable in that the radial strength of the units is significantly increased. In this regard, whereas the degree of recoil of the Micro Stent I is 8.7%, the recoil propensity of the three millimeter length Micro Stent II is similar or less than Micro Stent I. As of now, more than 2500 Micro Stents II have been deployed worldwide.

Both Micro Stent I and II are formed from a continuous segment of wire in the zigzag design, and both display eight axial struts connected by eight radiused crowns. As the basic unitary element of the Micro Stent is either 3.0 or 4.0 mm in length (I&II, respectively) these devices are premounted on AVE delivery balloons as stents of: 6.0, 9.0, 12.0, 15.0, 18.0, and 21.0 mm in length. Moreover, these customizable lengths are available in various combinations of connected, i.e., welded (Figure 5), or unconnected units. Special application stents Micro Stent II XL (with overall lengths of 30 and 39 mm) as well as Micro Stent 2.5 (lengths of 6 and 12 mm) are available now.

The clinical advantage of this customizable flexibility becomes clear to the interventionalist as soon as he or she begins to use the device. The compliance curves for a 3.5mm Micro Stent I and II illustrate this in Figure 6. These data reveal the differential size changes in diameter of the stent and its delivery balloon over the range of pressures from subnominal to beyond nominal values. This translates into a remarkably wide range of lengths and diameters which can be elected by the operator in delivering stents to tortuous irregular, remote, dissected, and previously inaccessible areas of the coronary anatomy.

Delivery and deployment

The AVE Micro Stents I and II are premounted on a compliant balloon delivery system as is depicted in Figure 1. Radiopaque markers within the delivery balloon indicate the limits of the proximal and distal ends of the stent. An efficient, proprietary design firmly binds the stent to the underlying low profile balloon. This process is so reliable that the device neither injures the balloon on deployment nor loosens itself from the balloon on tracking. Consequently, the stent and its delivery system are sheathless. And this sheathlessness, in conjunction with the overall low profile contribute to the remarkable trackability that permits this stent to go wherever the balloon goes. Both the Micro Stent I and II are available in the over-the-wire and the monorail configurations.

Micro Stent deployment is generally carried out at nominal deployment pressure in the range of 9 to 11 atmospheres. If adequate debulking and balloon angioplasty have been done prior to stent deployment, post placement dilatation with a high pressure non-compliant balloon is usually unnecessary. Completely performed balloon PTCA accomplished before stent deployment is essential for optimal results with the Micro Stents, and represents a fundamental difference from the treatment strategies of some other stent devices. Indeed the policy of

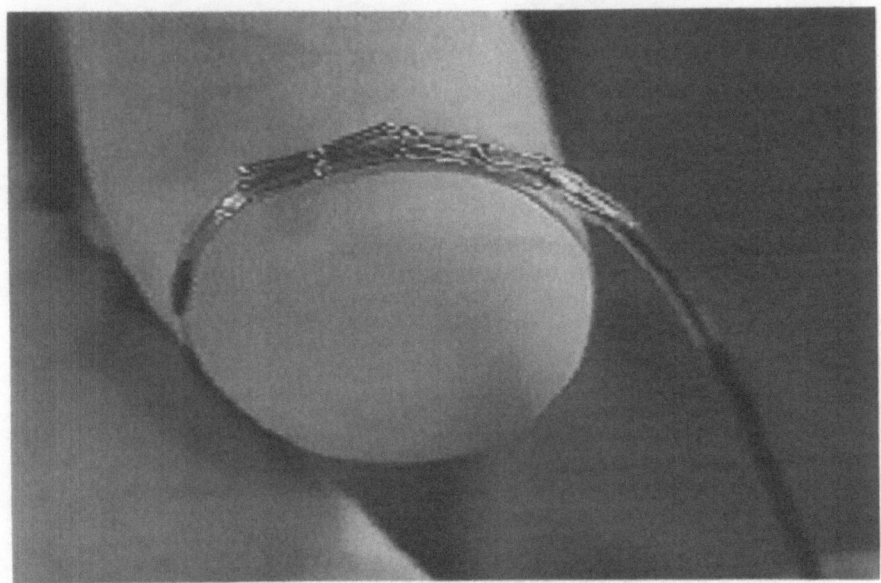

Figure 3. The demonstration of the AVE Microstent I flexibility in vitro.

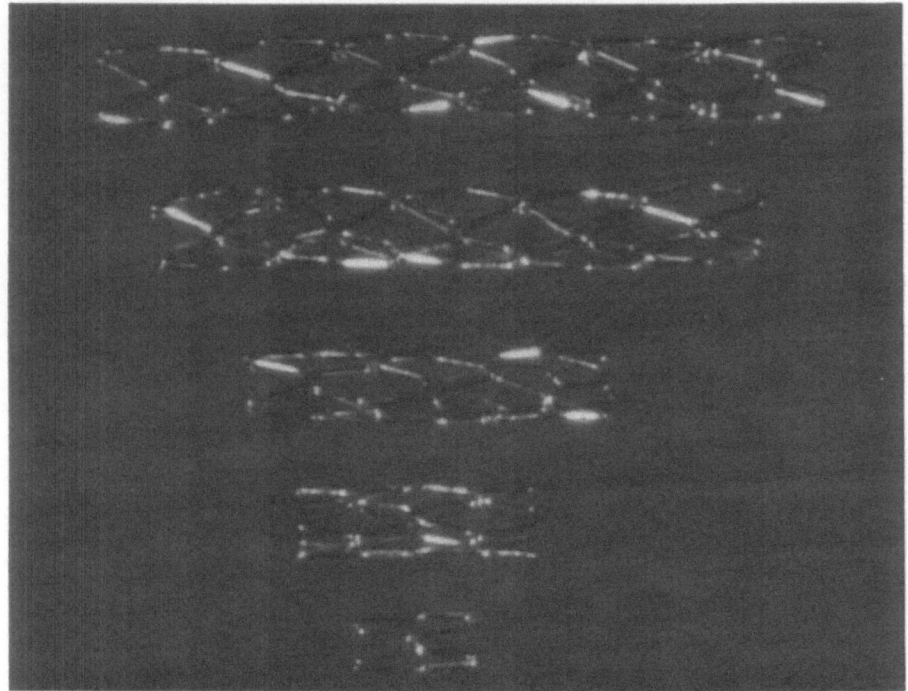

Figure 4. AVE Micro Stents II. Photograph represents 3.5 mm stents of 9, 12, 18, 30 and 36 mm long.

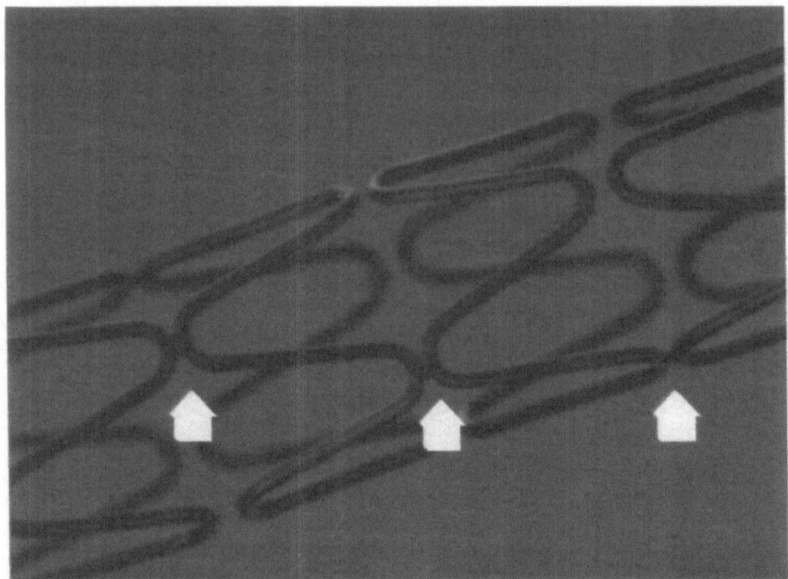

Figure 5. An example of the helical weld of the AVE Micro Stent II. White arrows indicate the welding sites.

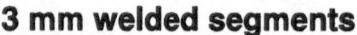

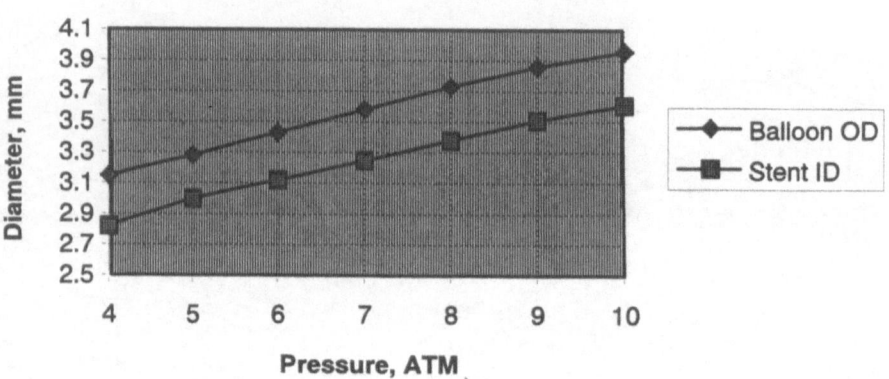

Figure 6A. Representation of delivery balloon/stent compliance relations of 3 mm welded segments.

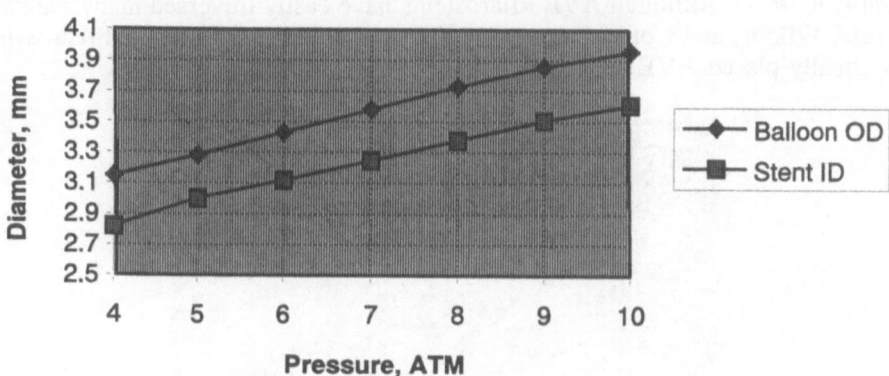

Figure 6B. Representation of delivery balloon/stent compliance relations of 4 mm welded segments.

underdilating lesions by a half size, i.e., 0.5 mm less than the desired stent size, and then fully expanding the stent with high pressure, completing the deployment at the same time, is clearly a contraindicated manner of installing an AVE device. Although post-deployment high pressure noncompliant balloon angioplasty is usually not required after placement of the Micro Stents, intracoronary ultrasound techniques have shown that in some lesions inadequately dilated, strut apposition is suboptimal, and further, higher pressure balloon expansion of the AVE stent is advisable. Nonetheless, as of March, 1995, in the vast majority of more than 29,000 Micro Stents that have been implanted outside the United States, IVUS was not employed. The authors however, prefer to verify the post-deployment result with IVUS where feasible, as we agree with Columbo et al. [2] that the requirement for anticoagulation with warfarin is doubtless superfluous if strut embedding is IVUS perfect. Intracoronary ultrasound study attempted after some instances of short (length) stent implantation, have been observed to partially displace the device. Although this may be operator error in some arteries, is almost always due to the rigid sheath of the IVUS, and not the imaging catheter itself. Hence if a stent placement was somewhat difficult, (e.g. small vessel, tortuous segment, large vessel with undersized stent) it is probably best to avoid IVUS, and simply deploy at higher pressure with the delivery balloon , or "sight unseen", to post-dilate with a high pressure noncompliant catheter.

Finally, in regard to delivery and deployment, one must emphasize a major clinical advantage of the Micro Stents I and II: i.e., they are nearly uniformly successful in traversing proximal stents already in place without being impeded by the previously placed device, and without dislodging an already implanted stent (Figure 7). Although AVE Microstents have easily traversed many Palmaz-Schatz, Wiktor, and Cordis stents, they are most reliable crossing and recrossing proximally placed AVE stents.

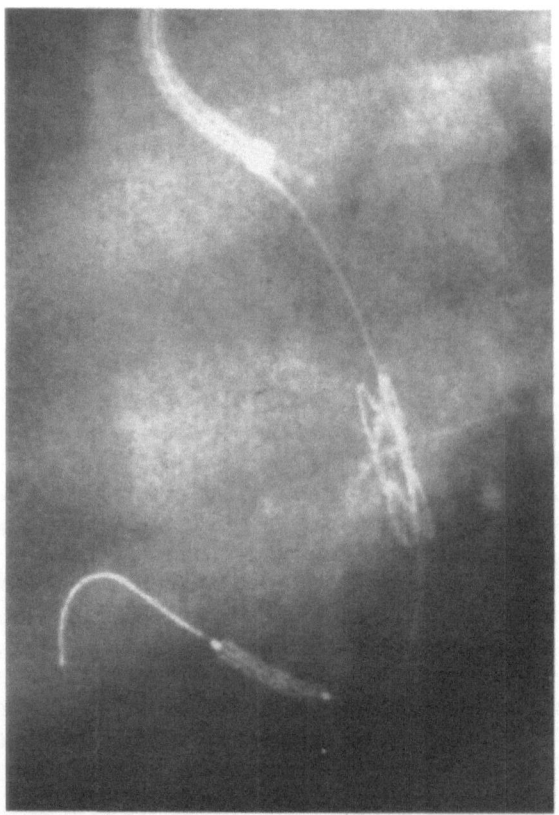

Figure 7. Animal experiment. AVE Micro Stent II (3.5 mm - 15 mm long) easily passed through previously deployed AVE Micro Stent II of the same size.

Comparative quantitative assessment

To assess comparative mechanical properties of AVE vs. Palmaz-Schatz stents, we performed matched QCA comparison. Our matching algorithm included lesion matching by reference diameter (D ref.), minimal luminal diameter (MLD) and lesion length (L). Matching process produced 40 matching coronary segments treated with primary deployment of AVE Micro Stents and 40 segments treated with the deployment of Palmaz-Schatz J&J coronary stents.

QCA was performed pre-procedure and post-stenting. QCA was used also to assess the real size of inflated balloon. Quantitative coronary angiography was performed using QCA Plus system, developed and validated at Stanford [7].

There was no difference in qualitative lesion description, including coronary artery, segmental location, lesion length, AHA/ACC class, presence of bends, side branches, lumen irregularities, etc.

Qualitative description of post-procedure lesion appearance also showed no differences in the frequency of acute closures, dissections, loss of side branches, spasm and recoil.

Basic QCA data presented in Table 1 demonstrate no difference in pre-procedure and post-procedure lesion dimensions. In both AVE and Palmaz-Schatz groups, stent deployment resulted in excellent lumen patency.

QCA derivatives, including the degree of stretch [8], recoil [8] and immediate gain demonstrate comparable amounts of recoil with high amount of immediate gain (Table 2).

Presented data demonstrate comparable mechanical properties of AVE Micro Stents and Palmaz-Schatz J&JIS stents in matched lesion subsets.

Table 1. QCA characteristics of 40 matched lesions treated by AVE Micro Stent deployment vs. 40 lesions treated by Palmaz-Schatz J&JIS stent deployment.

	MLD pre, mm (SD)	Length, mm (SD)	Dref. mm (SD)	%D pre (SD)	MLD post, mm (SD)	%D post (SD)
AVE Micro Stent	1.2 (0.4)	20.3 (13.9)	3.1 (0.7)	61.6 (9.6)	3.1 (0.7)	5.0 (11.0)
Palmaz-Schatz Stents	1.2 (0.4)	18.5 (10.6)	3.0 (0.7)	59.4 (10.1)	3.0 (0.8)	5.1 (12.9)
	NS	NS	NS	NS	NS	NS

Table 2. QCA Derivatives.

	Stretch %	SD	Recoil %	SD	Imm.Gain %	SD
AVE Micro Stent	51.5	43.5	11.1	47.9	62.6	22.9
Palmaz-Schatz Stents	46.7	34.6	13.9	47.3	60.6	38.9
	NS		NS		NS	

Clinical experience with the Micro Stent

By the first quarter of 1996, more than 30,000 Micro Stents have been implanted worldwide, most of the experience being accumulated in Europe, where the device was launched clinically in the fall of 1994. Serruys, in Rotterdam [3] and Columbo [2], in Milan, and Webb, in Vancouver have independently submitted

a total of over 300 cases for publication. Morice and Valeix in France, and
Reifart in Frankfurt , as well as Schalij in Holland [4-6] have also greatly
contributed to our understanding of this device.
Results of the clinical trials of the Micro Stents are shown in Tables 3-5. As is
demonstrated in this data the success rates are 96.3% for immediate implantation,
and the complication rates eminently acceptable, and similar to the experience
with other stents of identical composition. Although the cumulative long-term
results are still pending in most of the centers referred above, but the authors'
experience with the device from 1989 to the present time shows only 9 clinical
recurrences, i.e. 10.4%. These recurrence rates will probably rise as multicenter
trials increase the denominators to higher levels. However, Schalij et al. [6] now
report QCA analysis of 85 patients with 12.1 restenosis rate as of January 1996.
The analysis based on angiographic follow-up of 315 patients reported by 5
groups demonstrates overall restenosis rate of 20.9%.

Table 3. Multicenter clinical data on AVE Microstents.

Group	Date reported	Patients	Age, years	# of stents	Success	Restenosis reported
J.Webb, Vancouver	10/11/94	30	N/A	70	30	N/A
P.W.Serruys, Rotterdam	11/10/94	33	61	53	30	N/A
A.Colombo, Milan	10/14/94	36	64.4	51	29	N/A
Sweden	10/14/94	3	N/A	5	3	N/A
S.H.Stertzer, Stanford	4/4/95	87	67.3	219	86	9
M.Schalij, Leiden	9/15/95	155	61	155	151	10
N. Reifart, Frankfurt	9/11/95	150	N/A	186	147	N/A
B.Chevalier, G.Glatt, R.Royer, France	9/15/95	170	N/A	238	159	
D.Mathey, J. Schofer, Hamburg	9/22/95	397	N/A	666	384	38
J.J.Goy, Switzerland	10/23/95	101	N/A	123	101	7
Total		1132		17422	1090	
%					96.3	20.9%

Table 4. Summary data on complications, reported for 1008 patients.

Event	N	%
Q-wave MI	7	0.7
CABG	10	0.99
Thrombosis	11	1.1
Vascular Complications	9	0.9
Death	5	0.5
Total	42	4.1

Table 5. Multicenter summary data on clinical indications.

Indication	%
Restenosis	9.3%
SVG lesion	22.0%
Severe dissection	18.6%
Chronic occlusion	8.1%
Suboptimal PTCA	18.9%
Elective	21.9%

Table 3 summarizes the indications for stent implantation in the centers, reporting preliminary results in Table 1. Dissection and suboptimal PTCA are the major indication categories. Several prospective clinical and randomized evaluations of the AVE Micro Stents are presently being carried out in Europe.

Our experience shows that AVE Micro Stents are an extremely valuable tool for the treatment of tortuous vessels, especially when proximal tortuosity precludes the use of other scaffolding devices (Figures 8A, 8B). Adjunctive use of AVE Micro Stents is extremely important in diffusely diseased segments after the high speed rotational atherectomy (Figures 9A, 9B). It enables the operator to treat selectively remaining areas of residual recoil or dissection without creation of excessive areas of stented surface. Another valuable application of AVE Micro Stents is the adjunctive use after excimer laser recanalization of chronic occlusions (Figure 10). However in the interim, the ability of the device to complement high speed rotational atherectomy, and to track almost all balloon angioplasty sites, renders this device a welcome addition to the armamentarium of the interventionalist.

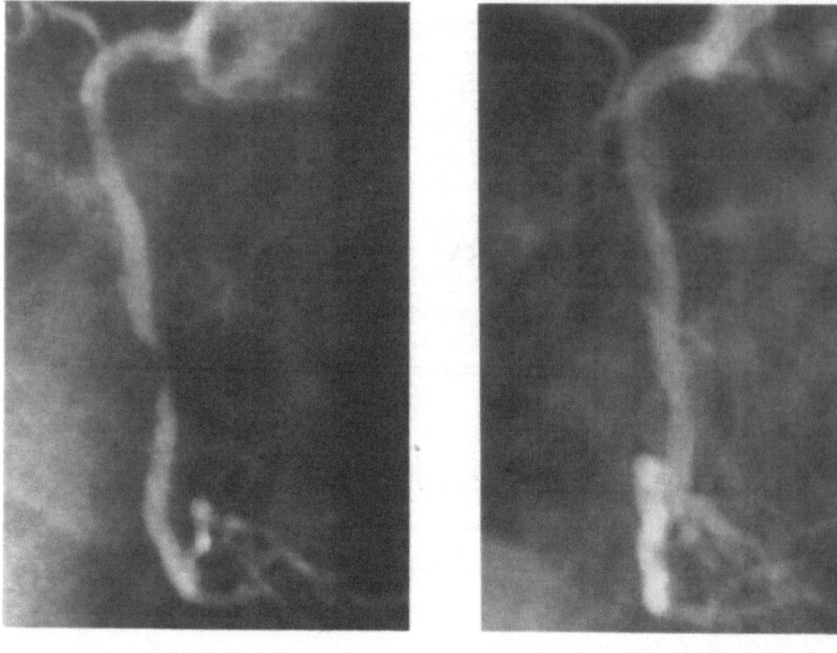

a   b

Figure 8. (A) Mid right coronary artery lesion before treatment. After predilatation, all attempts to deliver a J&JIS 3.0 mm 15 mm long stent were unsuccessful. The delivery of 3.0 mm 15 mm long AVE Microstent II was successful and uncomplicated. (B) Right coronary artery after adjunctive high pressure balloon inflation.

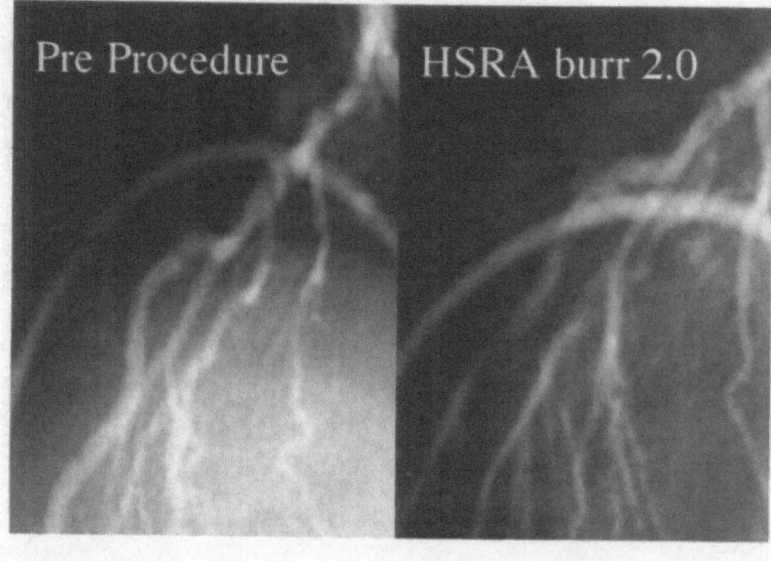

a

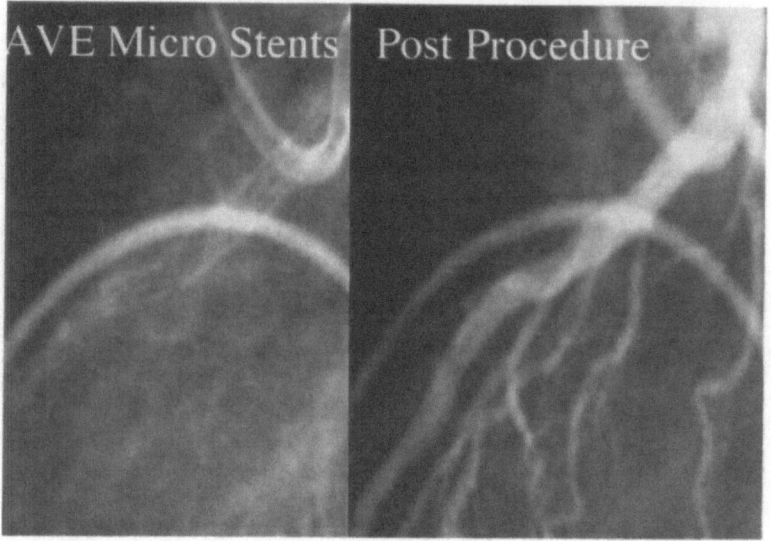

b

Figure 9. Top left: diffuse and calcified lesion of the mid left anterior coronary artery pre-procedure. Top right: after high speed rotational atherectomy with largest burr of 2.0 mm. There are a few sites of linear dissection and a "stop" lesion. Bottom left: a total of 4 AVE Micro Stents I deployed (overall stented length 44 mm). Bottom right: final angiographic appearance of the left anterior descending coronary artery.

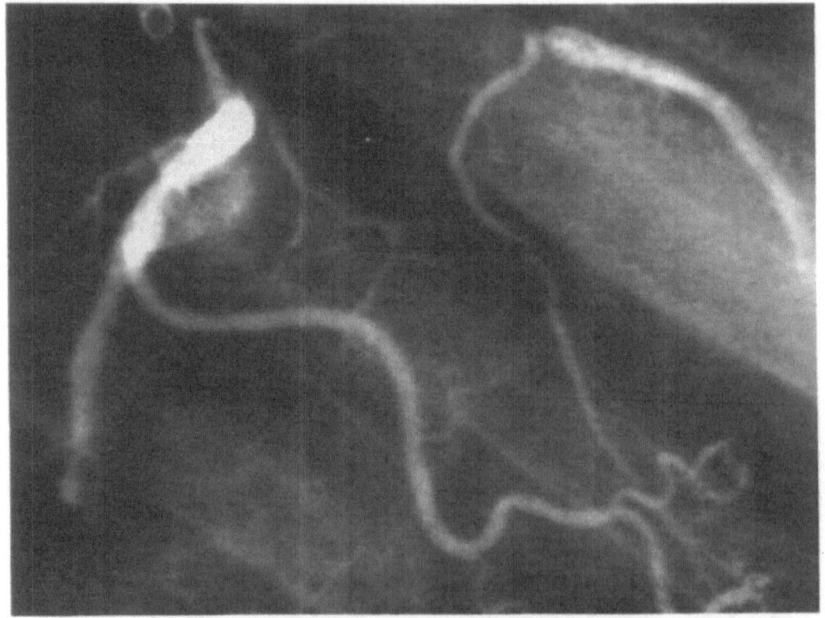

a

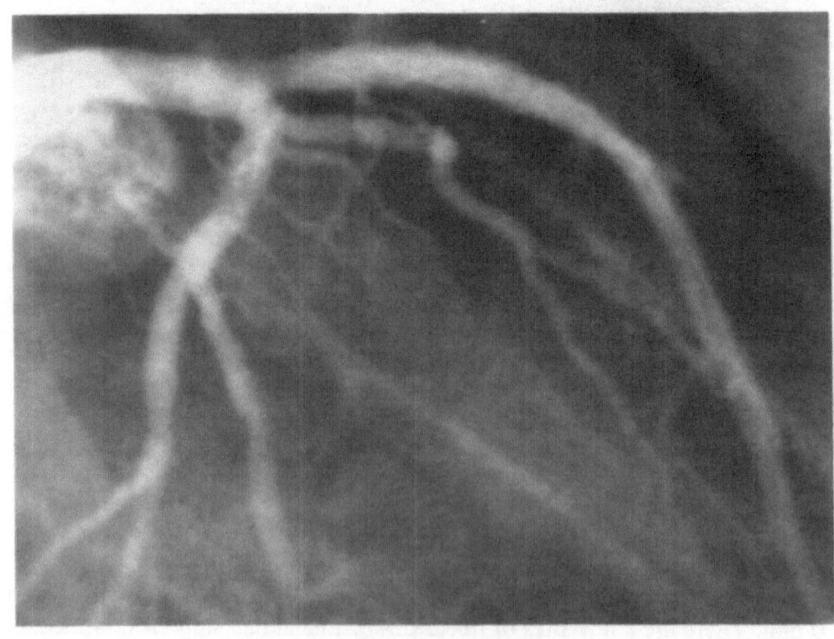

b

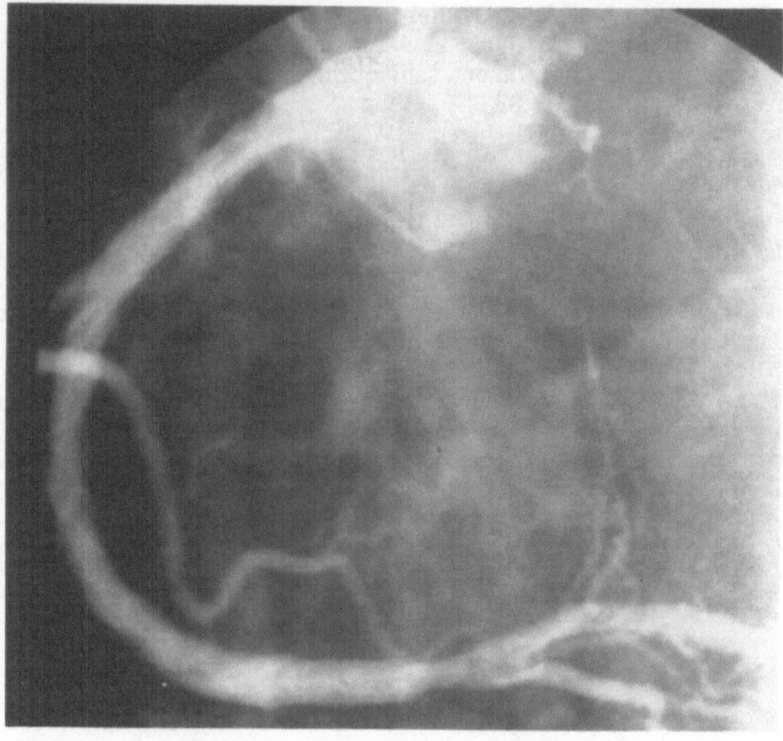

c

Figure 10. A combination of the excimer laser wire, balloon angioplasty and AVE Micro Stents II for the treatment of chronic coronary occlusions. (A) Baseline angiogram demonstrating chronic complete occlusions of the mid left anterior descending and distal right coronary arteries. (B) Final angiogram of the left coronary artery after the recanalization with 1.4 mm Spectranetics™ laser wire, predilation with 3.0 mm balloon and deployment of 3.0 mm 30 mm long AVE Micro Stent II followed by adjunctive high pressure balloon inflation. (C) Final angiogram of the right coronary artery after the recanalization with 1.4 mm Spectranetics™ laser wire, predilation with 3.5 - 40 mm balloon and deployment of 3.5 mm 15 mm long, 3.5 mm 39 mm long, and 3.5 mm 18 mm long AVE Micro Stents II followed by adjunctive high pressure balloon inflations.

References

1. Anwar A, Stertzer SH, Hidalgo BO *et al*. Coronary stenting with a new ultra-short balloon expandable device: early and late animal results. Cathet Cardiovasc Diagn 1994;31:85-9.
2. Colombo A, Maiello L, Nakamura S *et al*. Preliminary experience of coronary stenting with the Micro Stent™ [abstract]. J Am Coll Cardiol 1995;25(Special Issue):239A.
3. Ozaki Y, Keane D, Ruygrok P, de Feyter P, Stertzer S, Serruys PW. Acute clinical and angiographic results with the new AVE Micro coronary stent in

bailout management. Am J Cardiol 1995;76:112-6.

4. Savalle LH, Schalij MJ, Jukema JW, Reiber JHC. A prospective study of intracoronary stenting without subsequent anticoagulation, initial results. J Invasive Cardiol 1995;7:8A.

5. Tresukosol D, Schalij MJ, Jukema JW, Buis B, Reiber JHC. The micro stent: quantitative angiographic analysis and procedural results. J Invasive Cardiol 1995;7:8A.

6. Schalij MJ, Savalle LH, Tresukol D, Jukema JW, Reiber JHC, Bruschke AVG. The Micro Stent I, initial results and six months follow-up. Abstract for the presentation at ACC meetings, 1996

7. Leung WH, Sanders W, Alderman EL. Coronary artery quantitation and data management system for paired cineangiograms. Cathet Cardiovasc Diagn 1991;24:121-34.

8. Umans VA, Robert A, Foley D *et al*. Clinical, histologic and quantitative angiographic predictors of restenosis after directional coronary atherectomy: a multivariate analysis of the renarrowing process and late outcome. J Am Coll Cardiol 1994;23:49-58.

3. Non-surgical septum reduction in hypertrophic cardiomyopathy

CHARLES KNIGHT & ULRICH SIGWART

Summary

A novel treatment for relief of outflow tract obstruction in hypertrophic obstructive cardiomyopathy is described. Reduction in septal mass is achieved via transluminal induction of focal septal infarction by intracoronary alcohol injection, rather than by surgical myomectomy. The results of the first three patients treated in this fashion have been reported recently; in this preliminary series the procedure produced a dramatic reduction in the extent of left ventricular outflow tract obstruction. The procedure is well tolerated and, in the limited number of patients treated so far, has minimal morbidity. Gradient reduction appears to be maintained over follow-up. Further studies are underway to fully evaluate the role of the technique in treating symptomatic patients with hypertrophic cardiomyopathy.

Current therapies for symptoms in hypertrophic cardiomyopathy

A significant minority of patients with hypertrophic cardiomyopathy, around 25%, have evidence of a left ventricular outflow gradient [1]. Such patients may suffer symptoms of angina, dyspnoea and syncope as a consequence of dynamic left ventricular obstruction consequent upon asymmetrical septal hypertrophy and systolic anterior motion of the mitral valve [2].

Negative inotropic drugs, dual chamber pacing and surgical resection make up the current therapeutic options for relief of such symptoms in hypertrophic obstructive cardiomyopathy.

Beta-blockers reduce overall myocardial contractility and thus reduce systolic thickening of the septal bulge. This can reduce left ventricular outflow tract obstruction [2,3]. The effect of betablockade is most pronounced on exercise, as the degree of obstruction depends to a large extent on the levels of circulating catecholamines. Other negatively inotropic drugs, such as verapamil [4] and disopyramide [5] have also been shown to reduce left ventricular outflow obstruction. However, despite drug therapy with these agents, many patients remain symptomatic.

Dual chamber pacing can also reduce left ventricular outflow tract obstruction in hypertrophic cardiomyopathy [6,7]. Pacing has two mechanisms of action; in addition to altering the pattern of left ventricular excitation, the timing of atrial contraction can also be optimized [8]. Pacing would commonly be recommended to patients with symptoms persisting despite medical therapy, before consideration of surgery. The relative benefits of dual chamber pacing and surgical resection are currently being assessed by the European Pacing in Cardiomyopathy (PIC) study.

J.H.C. Reiber and E.E. van der Wall (eds.), Cardiovascular Imaging, 31-37.

A degree of controversy has always surrounded surgical treatments for hypertrophic cardiomyopathy as not all patients with significant gradients are symptomatic, and patients without gradients may suffer similar symptoms as a result of diastolic dysfunction and abnormalities of the small coronary arteries [9]. Some authors have therefore argued that the degree of outflow tract obstruction is irrelevant to the production of symptoms [10]. However, in those patients with large gradients that are symptomatic despite medical treatment, surgical relief of obstruction has been shown to improve quality of life [11,12], even if, in the absence of prospective randomized control trials, its prognostic effects remain uncertain. There are several techniques for the surgical removal of the offending portion of the interventricular septum [13-15]. The majority of patients derive long-term symptomatic benefit without significant impairment of left ventricular function [16]. However, surgery requires extracorporeal circulation and is associated with a moderate surgical risk of at least 5% [13,17].

An alternative approach to septal reduction

The concept of septal reduction by focal infarction using catheter techniques was first conceived following observations on the effect of balloon occlusion on the function of focal areas of the myocardium [18,19].

The first septal branch of the anterior descending coronary artery supplies the myocardium of the proximal interventricular septum; the area of myocardium whose abnormal structure and function is responsible for the production of the left ventricular outflow tract obstruction in hypertrophic obstructive cardiomyopathy. In patients with hypertrophic obstructive cardiomyopathy, temporary occlusion of the first septal artery was shown to produce favourable hemodynamic effects, with marked reduction in intracavity gradients upon occlusion of the first major septal artery [19]. These findings have been confirmed by others [20].

Following these preliminary observations we have recently reported [21] the development of a non-surgical technique to achieve a reduction in septal mass, by producing septal infarction using catheter techniques. Intracoronary alcohol injection was shown to be effective in permanently reducing gradients in three patients with severe hypertrophic obstructive cardiomyopathy.

Preliminary observations

Occlusion of a coronary artery with an angioplasty balloon during coronary angioplasty results in selective suppression of the systolic and diastolic function of the supplied area of the myocardium [18,19]. The area of myocardium responsible for the production of the left ventricular outflow tract obstruction in hypertrophic obstructive cardiomyopathy is the proximal interventricular septum. This area is supplied by the first septal branch of the anterior descending coronary artery. The first phase of our investigation was therefore to observe the effect of temporary occlusion of the first septal artery on the degree of outflow tract obstruction in patients with hypertrophic cardiomyopathy.

Patients were studied using retrograde and transeptal cardiac catheterization to ensure reliable measurements of the intracavity gradient. Pressures were measured by fluid filled catheters in the ascending aorta and simultaneously in different locations within the left ventricle, via a transeptally introduced Brockenborough catheter placed in the left ventricular inflow tract. The left ventricular outflow tract pressure gradients were measured at rest, during dynamic bicycle exercise, during the Valsava manoeuvre, following induction of premature ventricular contraction, after administration of amyl nitrate and during isoproterenol infusion. Once these baseline measurements had been obtained, the left coronary ostium was intubated using an 8 French coronary angioplasty guiding catheter and, after heparinization, the first major septal artery was intubated with a 0.014 " guide wire and a small diameter over-the-wire angioplasty balloon was advanced to the artery's origin. Contrast was injected through the lumen of the balloon catheter to delineate the area of the interventricular septum supplied. The artery was then occluded by inflation of the balloon to pressures of between 3 and 5 bar for up to five minutes. During the period of occlusion, the left ventricular outflow gradient was remeasured at rest and during the provocations described above. Three patients were studied. At baseline, the intraventricular gradients increased markedly with preload reduction as well as during the Valsalva manoeuvre and isoproterenol infusion. Post-extrasystolic beats showed very large gradients. There was a decrease in the gradient just prior to exercise, probably as a result of increased preload from leg raising [22].

In all three patients the effect of balloon occlusion of the first major septal artery was to markedly reduce the left ventricular outflow gradient from 67 ± 37 mmHg to 12 ± 6 mmHg. The gradient remained low even during provocation: 26 ± 14 mmHg in the post-extrasystolic beat, 18 ± 11 mmHg during the Valsalva and 21 ± 13 mmHg during isoproterenol infusion. Upon balloon deflation, these beneficial effects were immediately reversed, the gradients returning to baseline levels.

In two patients, 0.5 mg of verapamil was injected through the central balloon lumen into the artery. This prolonged the effects of occlusion - the gradients remaining low for around thirty minutes following balloon deflation.

Myocardial ablation

The preliminary studies detailed above demonstrated that occlusion of the first septal artery temporarily reduced the intraventricular gradient in patients with hypertrophic obstructive cardiomyopathy. However, the effects of balloon occlusion were temporary and in order to produce any lasting gradient reduction it was clear that it was necessary to induce an area of permanent septal necrosis rather than transient septal ischaemia.

Ethical approval for treatment of a limited series of patients with hypertrophic cardiomyopathy in this way was obtained from the Ethics Committee of the Royal Brompton Hospital. The results of the first three permanent non-surgical septal ablations have recently been reported [21]. We have subsequently performed the procedure in further patients with similar results.

Indications and patient selection

As with any novel therapy, prognostic effects are as yet unknown. ·At our institution, therefore, non-surgical septal reduction has only been performed in patients with hypertrophic obstructive cardiomyopathy with disabling symptoms of angina and dyspnoea despite medical treatment and/or pacemaker therapy. In all cases, evidence of significant outflow tract obstruction on baseline echocardiography had to be present before the procedure was considered. Consent for the new procedure was obtained only after careful explanation of the proposed technique of ablation and discussion of the surgical alternatives.

Description of the technique

Retrograde and transeptal cardiac catheterization is performed as previously described. Resting measurements of the left ventricular gradient are recorded and then the patients undergo provocation with Valsalva manoeuvre and dobutamine/isoproterenol infusion when measurement of the gradient is repeated. Gradients are also recorded after extrasystoles. In addition a temporary pacing wire is inserted into the right atrium and the patients paced atrially at rates of 100 and 120 bpm. The effect of increased heart rate on the gradient is recorded.

The first major septal branch of the anterior descending coronary artery is then identified and catheterized with a 2mm angioplasty balloon after the administration of 10,000 units heparin. The balloon is inflated and the gradients remeasured at rest and on provocation. In most cases, this results in a marked reduction in the degree of left ventricular outflow tract obstruction, disappearing immediately upon balloon deflation. In some patients intubation of several septal branches may be necessary before finding an artery which, when occluded, produces the desired reduction in gradient. Occasional patients have less favourable coronary anatomy, the proximal interventricular septum being supplied by a number of small branches rather than by a single large septal artery. In such cases, temporary occlusion of a small branch may have no effect on the gradient.

Following observation of the effects of temporary occlusion, the balloon is re-inflated and the guide wire withdrawn. The temporary pacing wire should be repositioned into the right ventricle. After the administration of 5 mg diamorphine, 5 ml of absolute alcohol is slowly injected into the septal artery through the central lumen of the angioplasty catheter, and left in situ for 2-5 minutes, with the balloon remaining inflated at the origin of the septal artery.

After ablation, a repeat angiogram is performed to demonstrate occlusion of the target artery. The gradient is remeasured at rest and on provocation.

In patients with a number of small branches, injection of alcohol into more than one branch may be necessary to produce the desired reduction in gradient.

Results

There is an immediate reduction in left ventricular outflow gradient in the vast majority of patients. The gradient does not reappear after balloon deflation. The gradient on provocation is also substantially reduced.

Over the longer term it is clear that the reduction in gradient is maintained. In the first three patients treated, three month echocardiography showed mean resting gradients at rest of 11 mmHg and 58 mmHg on maximal provocation, compared with 56 mmHg (rest) and 154 mmHg (provocation) before the procedure [23]. Symptomatically, all patients report substantial benefit, with reductions in symptoms of angina and dyspnoea.

Complications

Patients report chest pain of a moderate degree immediately after the alcohol injection, but this is short-lived. Transient complete heart block is relatively common and underscores the importance of performing the procedure under cover of a temporary pacing wire. We have not observed heart block to persist for longer than a few minutes. One patient developed ventricular fibrillation secondary to bradycardia on sheath removal, a few hours after the procedure, but this responded to a single DC shock, and there were no adverse sequelae.

After the procedure all patients have had uneventful post-operative courses. Creatinine phosphokinase levels are typically raised to around 2500 IU. Patients can be discharged on the second post-operative day.

Future directions

Non-surgical septal reduction has a number of attractive features which are not shared by alternative modes of therapy: it is simple, predictable - the hemodynamic outcome of the definitive ablation can be determined in advance by temporary occlusion of the target vessel - and appears to have minimal morbidity. The induction of permanent septal damage in patients with hypertrophic cardiomyopathy appears to be surprisingly well tolerated, and no serious complications have been observed in the limited number of patients treated so far. Although heart block has occurred, it has only been a temporary phenomenon, and we have not observed any late brady- or tachy-arrhythmias.

It has become clear that a component of the spectacular immediate reduction in gradient may be the result of a degree of global myocardial stunning, as gradients are invariably higher on the first post-operative day (echocardiography) compared with immediately at catheterization. However, there is also scope for late reduction in outflow tract obstruction as a consequence of fibrosis and thinning of the septum as the infarct heals. The late hemodynamic results obtained will be a balance between these two competing processes.

Non-surgical septal reduction is still in its infancy and the long term benefits and complications are unknown. The function of the septum may recur over time, and scarring produced by the infarction may set up a late arrhythmogenic focus. Careful patient selection and postoperative monitoring are essential if the true effectiveness of the technique is to become clear. As the procedure is now being performed in a small number of other centers, an international registry of patients treated in this fashion is being set up to optimize data collection. We hope that prospective randomized trials can be instituted to allow a proper comparison between non-surgical reduction and existing forms of therapy such as pacing and surgery.

References

1. Ciro E, Nichols PF 3rd, Maron BJ. Heterogeneous morphologic expression of genetically transmitted hypertrophic cardiomyopathy. Two-dimensional echocardiographic analysis. Circulation 1983;67:1227-33.
2. Maron BJ, Bonow RO, Cannon RO 3rd, Leon MB, Epstein SE. Hypertrophic cardiomyopathy. Interrelations of clinical manifestations, pathophysiology and therapy (2). N Engl J Med 1987;316:844-52.
3. Flamm MD, Harrison DC, Hancock EW. Muscular subaortic stenosis. Prevention of outflow obstruction with propranolol. Circulation 1968;38:846-58.
4. Chatterjee K. Calcium antagonist agents in hypertrophic cardiomyopathy. Am J Cardiol 1987;59:146B-152B.
5. Sherrid M, Delia E, Dwyer E. Oral disopyramide therapy for obstructive hypertrophic cardiomyopathy. Am J Cardiol 1988;62:1085-8.
6. Grbic M, Sigwart U, Kappenberger L, Goy JJ. Reduction du gradient intraventriculaire en presence de la cardiomyopathie obstructive par le pacing atrio-ventriculaire avec P-R raccourci [abstract]. Schweiz Med Wochenschr 1987;117(Suppl.21):29.
7. McDonald K, McWilliams E, O'Keefe B, Maurer B. Functional assessment of patients treated with permanent dual chamber pacing as a primary treatment of hypertrophic cardiomyopathy. Eur Heart J 1988;9:893-8.
8. Jeanrenaud X, Goy JJ, Kappenberger L. Effects of dual-chamber pacing in hypertrophic obstructive cardiomyopathy. Lancet 1992;339:1318-23.
9. Frank S, Braunwald E. Idiopathic hypertrophic subaortic stenosis. Clinical analysis of 126 patients with emphasis on the natural history. Circulation 1968;37:759-88.
10. Oakley CM. Non-surgical ablation of the ventricular septum for the treatment of hypertrophic cardiomyopathy. Br Heart J 1995;74:479-80.
11. Maron BJ, Merrill WH, Freier PA, Kent KM, Epstein SE, Morrow AG. Long-term clinical course and symptomatic status of patients after operation for hypertrophic subaortic stenosis. Circulation 1978;57:1205-13.
12. Bonow RO, Maron BJ, Leon MB. Medical and surgical therapy of hypertrophic cardiomyopathy. Cardiovasc Clin 1988;19:221-39.
13. McIntosh CL, Maron BJ. Current operative treatment of obstructive hypertrophic cardiomyopathy. Circulation 1988;78:487-95.
14. Seiler C, Hess OM, Schoenbeck M et al. Long term follow-up of medical versus surgical therapy for hypertrophic cardiomyopathy: a retrospective study. J Am Coll Cardiol 1991;17:634-42.
15. Chahine RA. Surgical versus medical treatment of hypertrophic cardiomyopathy: is the perspective changing? J Am Coll Cardiol 1991;17:643-5.
16. Borer JS, Bacharach SL, Green MV et al. Effect of septal myotomy and myectomy on left ventricular systolic function at rest and during exercise in patients with IHSS. Circulation 1979;60(2 pt 2):82-7.
17. Mohr R, Schaff HV, Danielson GK, Puga FJ, Pluth JR, Tajik AJ. The outcome of surgical treatment of hypertrophic obstructive cardiomyopathy. Experience

over 15 years. J Thorac Cardiovasc Surg 1989;97:666-74.

18. Sigwart U, Grbic M, Essinger A, Rivier JL. L'effet aigu d'une occlusion coronarienne de la dilatation trans luminale [abstract]. Schweiz Med Wochenschr 1982;112:lors 1631.

19. Sigwart U, Grbic M, Payot M *et al*. Wall motion during balloon occlusion. In: Sigwart U, Heintzen PH, editors. Ventricular wall motion, New York:, Georg Thieme, 1983:206-10.

20. Gietzen F, Leuner C, Gerenkamp T, Huhn K. Relief of obstruction in hypertrophic cardiomyopathy by transient occlusion of the first septal branch of the left coronary artery [abstract]. Eur heart J 1994;15 Abstract Suppl:125.

21. Sigwart U. Non-surgical myocardial reduction for hypertrophic obstructive cardiomyopathy. Lancet 1995;346:211-4.

22. Grbic M, Sigwart U. Relationship between preload and afterload and gradient in hypertrophic obstructive cardiomyopathy [abstract]. Circulation 1982;66(Suppl.II):II-268.

23. Knight CJ, Gunning M, Henein M *et al*. Follow-up after non-surgical septum reduction in hypertrophic obstructive cardiomyopathy [abstract]. Circulation 1995;92(Suppl.I):I-781.

4. State of the Art in Quantitative Coronary Arteriography as of 1996

JOHAN H.C. REIBER, LARS R. SCHIEMANCK, PIETER M.J. VAN DER ZWET, BOB GOEDHART, GERHARD KONING, MARTIN LAMMERTSMA, MARTIJN DANSE, JAN J. GERBRANDS, MARTIN J. SCHALIJ & ALBERT V.G. BRUSCHKE

Summary

In this chapter the important developments which have led to the third generation in quantitative coronary arteriographic (QCA) analytical software are presented, as well as current developments in the fields of image compression and storage. The conventional QCA approaches with automated contour detection techniques based on Minimum Cost contour detection Algorithms (MCA) have been well established and validated. However, further improvements in the calculations of the diameter and reference diameter functions were needed, especially for complex morphology and for stent applications. The development of the Gradient Field Transform (GFT^R) approach for the quantitation of complex lesions represents a major step forward in QCA. With the advent of the cineless catheterization laboratory, the issue of image compression has become of major relevance. Phantom studies with lossy JPEG image compression at 512^2 matrix size demonstrate that the compression factor (CF) should not exceed the level of 10. On the other hand, if JPEG and LOT lossy compression schemes (CF's of 5,8 and 12) are applied to routinely acquired coronary angiographic image results, QCA measurements demonstrate that all three compression factors lead to significantly increased random differences in the measurements. These results suggest that even the JPEG and LOT compression ratio of 5 is not acceptable for QCA. Finally, an extensive QCA study has demonstrated that S-VHS video tape is unacceptable for QCA and should be excluded from quantitative angiographic clinical trials.

Introduction

Since the first papers on quantitative coronary arteriography (QCA) were published in 1977 and 1978, this field has grown substantially [1,2]. Two major clinical developments which started in the early eighties have stimulated this growth: 1) the enormous innovation and applications in coronary recanalization techniques (PTCA, atherectomy, thrombolysis, stent, laser, etc.); and 2) the increasing interest to study the effects of new drugs directed at the regression or no-growth of existing coronary artery disease, or the delay in the formation of new lesions [3]. This means that until recently these analytical approaches were used predominantly in clinical research trials [4,5].

Over the last few years an increasing interest has been noted in applying QCA before and during coronary interventions. This enables the operator to size the

39

J.H.C. Reiber and E.E. van der Wall (eds.), Cardiovascular Imaging, 39-56.
© 1996 *Kluwer Academic Publishers.*

optimal balloon or stent diameter and length for a particular procedure and to assess the success of the procedure in an objective manner. It has also been demonstrated that rest stenoses < 20% measured objectively after the procedure, lead to less events after 6 months [6]. Such applications are certainly facilitated by the ongoing improvements in computer hardware (roughly a 100% increase in performance every 2 years) and software, by the improvement and invention of better suited algorithms for the analysis of coronary lesions, and the optimization of the user interfaces, so that results become available within seconds, thereby minimally delaying the angiographic procedure. On the other hand, the on-line applications also significantly increase the demands on the QCA analytical software packages, in terms of robustness, accuracy and precision, and the capability to follow the irregular morphology that is often seen during the interventional procedures. If these demands are not or will not be met in the near future, these packages will not be used. Taking into account the high costs of the interventional devices, these on-line applications are likely to expand as health insurance companies and government agencies will follow with increasing interest the cost-benefit aspects of intervention procedures. In the first part of this chapter the new developments which have led to the third generation QCA system will be presented.

Until the late eighties, 35 mm cinefilm was the only practically useful medium for the storage of the coronary arteriograms. In the second half of the eighties digital x-ray systems were introduced for cardiac applications. It became possible to store the images in digital format in real-time on the large Winchester disks of these systems and to retrieve and display selected images and cineruns on the video monitors in the catheterization laboratory. These digital systems have played a major role in the clinical development of intervention cardiology. If such digital facilities are not available, the complex intervention procedures cannot be performed without adding significant additional risks to the patient. Now that we are entering the era of the cineless catheterization laboratories, the review, storage and exchange of the enormous amounts of digital data are subjects of new developments and discussions. Now that the CD-R as the exchange medium and the DICOM-3 as the exchange format have been accepted, the new question is which level of lossy image compression is still acceptable without affecting the diagnostic interpretation and the QCA results. The preliminary results of QCA pilot studies on different image compression schemes and ratios carried out in our laboratory and the use of S-VHS video tape as an archive medium will be presented in the second half of this chapter.

State-of-the-art in quantitative coronary arteriography

Basic principles of QCA

Over the past five to seven years, we have developed and validated two analytical QCA software packages [7]:
1)   the Automated Coronary Analysis (ACA) software package for the digital

Philips[1] DCI and Integris 3000H systems, referred to as ACA-DCI;

2) the QCA-packages on the cinefilm and digital based Cardiovascular Measurement System (CMS) of MEDIS[2]; the cinefilm-based application is referred to as the off-line QCA-CMS system, the on-line application whereby the CMS system is connected to the output of the digital x-ray system, the on-line QCA-CMS system.

In November of 1995 the 3rd-generation QCA-CMS package was released with state-of-the-art features. Before describing the new features, a short description of the basic principles of the QCA-technique will be given. The selection of the coronary segment to be analyzed requires the user to simply indicate the beginning and end point of that segment. Next, an arterial pathline through the segment of interest is computed automatically [8]. In the rare cases that an appropriate path is not found, two alternative solutions exist. The first one is that the user defines an intermediate point in the vessel which must belong to the pathline; the algorithm now searches for a new path from the starting point through this edited point to the end point. A second alternative is that the user indicates a number of points in the arterial segment, which are subsequently connected by straight lines followed by a smoothing procedure. In all instances, a pathline through the vessel segment is obtained. Next, the contour detection procedure is carried out in two iterations relative to a model. In the first iteration the detected pathline is the model. The individual left and right vessel contours detected in the first iteration function as models in the second iteration. The contour detection technique that we use is the Minimum Cost Algorithm (MCA), which searches for an optimal contour path along the entire segment through an edge strength data matrix based on the weighted sum of first and second derivative values. To correct for the limited resolution of the entire x-ray system, the edge strength data is modified in the second iteration based on an analysis of the point spread function of the imaging chain, which is of particular importance for the accurate measurement of small diameters as in obstructions. If such correction is not applied, significant overestimation of vessel sizes below approximately 1.2 mm would occur. It must be stressed that the MCA algorithm must be optimized for the image modality used, i.e. either for the 35 mm cinefilm images, or the digital images. Aside from the fact that on 35 mm cinefilm the vessels are visible as bright structures against a dark background, and the digital images the other way around, additional differences include spatial resolution, pixel sizes, noise patterns and the nonlinear relation between the observed grey level and contrast density.

Calibration of the image data is usually performed on a nontapering part of the contrast catheter following a similar edge detection procedure as for the arterial segment. However, in this case, the additional information that the projection of a circle-cylindrical structure is characterized by parallel boundaries is used in the definition of the catheter contours. During film analysis, regions of interest (ROI's) are magnified optically ($\pm$ 2.3 fold) resulting in calibration factors in the

---

[1] Philips Medical Systems, Best, The Netherlands

[2] MEDIS Medical Imaging Systems, Nuenen, The Netherlands

range of 0.08-0.10 mm/pixel, which is optimal for the edge detection algorithm used for the cinefilm application. During digital analysis, the ROI's are obtained by a bicubic two-fold interpolation approach resulting in calibration factors typically in the same range as for cinefilm for images acquired with a 7" image intensifier.

From the left- and right-hand contours of the arterial segment a diameter function is determined, on the basis of which the following parameters are automatically calculated: the site of maximal percent diameter stenosis, the obstruction diameter, the corresponding automatically determined reference diameter and the extent of the obstruction. Additionally derived parameters include obstruction symmetry, inflow and outflow angles, area of the atherosclerotic plaque and functional information in terms of the radiographic Stenotic Flow Reserve (SFR-) value and transstenotic pressure gradients. The QCA-CMS provides in addition (sub)segment related data, such as the mean and standard deviation of diameter measurements, and projected vessel areas in the proximal, obstructed and distal subsegments.

New Features 3rd generation QCA-CMS

1. New Diameter Function
Calculation of the width of a vessel segment along its trajectory from proximal to distal resulting in a diameter function is not a trivial task [9]. In the following, the line defining the width or diameter of the vessel at a certain location, will be denoted a measurement chord. Inappropriate designs of diameter functions can lead to overestimation of vessel dimensions, increased variabilities due to instable measurement chord directions (staggering) between the left and right contours, etc. In an attempt to further improve the accuracy and precision of the vessel diameter measurement, it was felt necessary to design a new Diameter Function based on the following requirements: 1) a more stable and smoothly changing course of the measurement chords along the vessel's trajectory; 2) chords should be parallel to the wavefront of the flowing blood to provide the most realistic results and to prevent overestimations at certain positions along a vessel segment; 3) suitability for complex vessel morphology; and 4) a high sampling rate, i.e. distance between neighboring chords at roughly the pixel size [9].

From the Diameter Function the socalled Reference Diameter Function is derived which has two functions: 1) to allow for the automated assessment of the reference diameter value (often denoted Interpolated Reference Diameter) at the site of the obstruction (Figure 1); and 2) to allow for the reconstruction of the original dimensions of the vessel segment to mimick the situation before the focal disease occurred. The Automated Reference Diameter approach has been found to be a very robust and reproducible technique. The reconstruction of the original vessel boundaries can lead to very erroneous results, particularly in curved vessels, if the proper algorithm is not used. In our design, an iterative approach is followed. From the arterial contours, an initial arterial diameter function is assessed. By using a modified linear regression analysis, the reference diameter function can be calculated, and the reference contours reconstructed. Based on these initial reference contours in combination with the arterial contours, a new arterial diameter function can be derived, which is characterized by much more

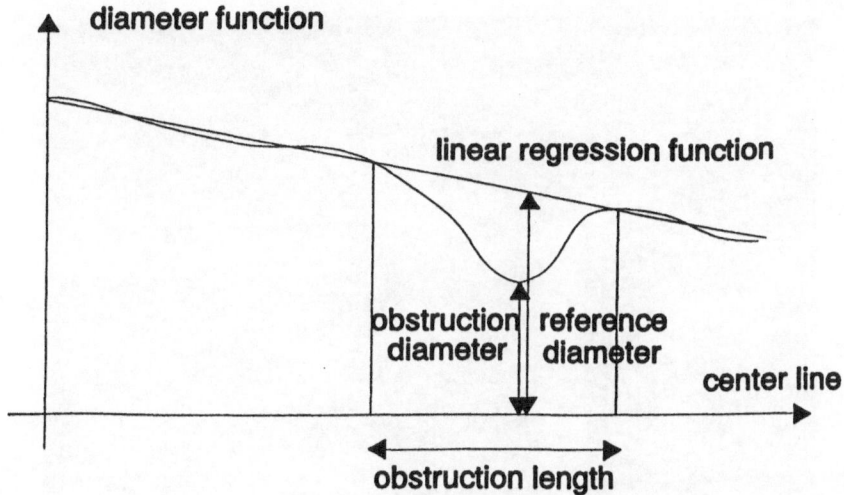

Figure 1. Schematic drawing of Diameter Function and the Reference Diameter Function. The Reference Diameter equals the value of the Reference Diameter Function at the site of the obstruction.

stable measurement chords; this is due to the fact that these chords were derived from the much smoother reference contours. From this new arterial diameter function the process of calculation of reference diameter function and reference contours is repeated, until a stable situation has been reached. In general, one or two iterations suffice. The correctness of this approach has been verified based on the visual interpretation of the results from many analyses of vessels with very different patterns. Of course, there is no gold standard to compare the results with. Figure 2A is an example of a curved vessel with a nicely reconstructed vessel contour. On the other hand, an incorrect result in the proximal portion of the vessel (arrow) is demonstrated in Figure 2B. The differences between the true luminal boundaries and the reconstructed vessel dimensions represent the area of the atherosclerotic plaque in this view.

With the advent of the overdilated stents as proposed by Colombo et al. [10] and the straightforward application of the Reference Diameter Function approach, incorrect results could be obtained. This is illustrated in Figure 3A. It is clear that the overdilated stent causes the reference diameter function to taper significantly, such that neither the normal vessel size nor the overdilated stent size is measured correctly over the stented portion of the vessel. In this case a stenosis of -0.7% would be measured (obstruction diameter 4.45 mm, reference diameter 4.42 mm). This is a very undesirable situation. We have developed the following practical solution for this. In such cases of overdilated vessel segments, but also in cases of areas of ectasia, overlap of vessel segments, etc., the user can 'flag' the portion of the vessel segment, and the corresponding diameter values are excluded in the subsequent calculation of the Reference Diameter Function. The correctly calculated Reference Diameter Function and reconstructed reference contours are presented in Figure 3B, which is more in line with what one would

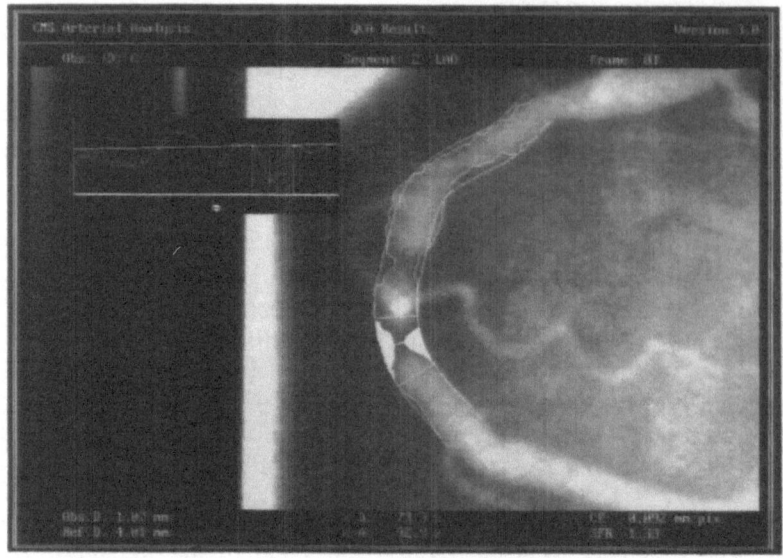

a

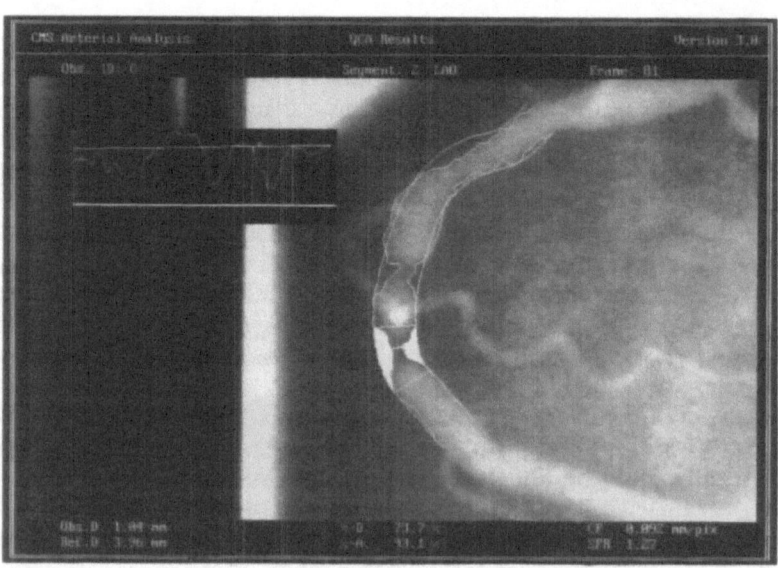

b

Figure 2. From the luminal contours the vessel's original boundaries are reconstructed. Figure 2A shows an example of a curved vessel with a perfectly reconstructed vessel contour. An inappropriate reconstruction in the proximal portion of the vessel is given as an example in Figure 2B.

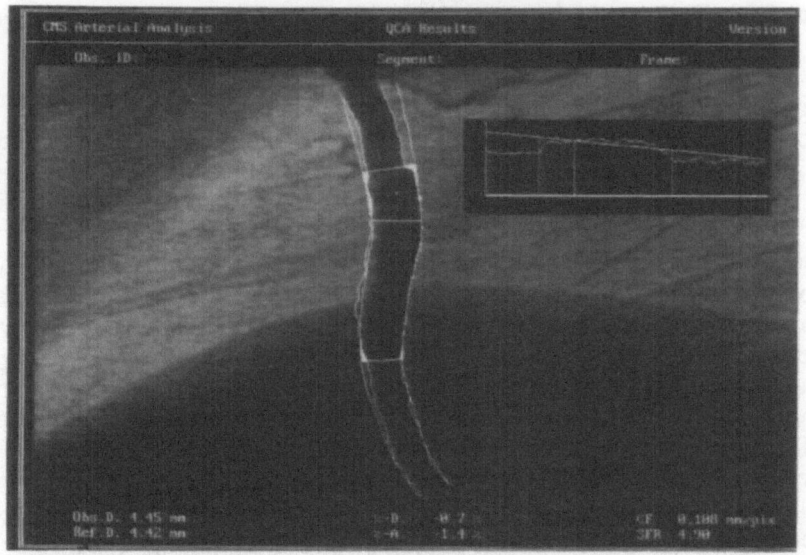

a

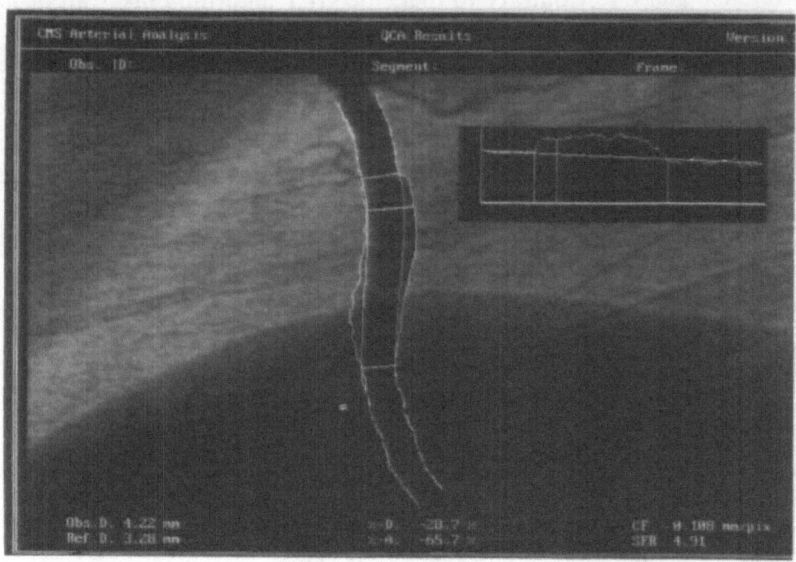

b

Figure 3. Example of a vessel with an overdilated stent. Straight forward application of the Reference Diameter Function would lead to arbitrary, erroneous results, in this case a significant tapering of the Reference Diameter Function (Figure 3A). By 'flagging' the stented area, a nontapering Reference Diameter Function results and appropriately reconstructed reference contours (Figure 3B). Images made available by Jacques Lespérance, M.D., Montreal Heart Institute, Canada.

expect [11]. This results in a narrowing of -28.7% (obstruction diameter 4.22 mm, reference diameter 3.28 mm).

2. Complex Vessel Morphology

The conventional contour detection method as implemented on the DCI and CMS systems is based on the so-called Minimum Cost Algorithm (MCA), which has been demonstrated to be very fast and robust for images which can significantly vary in image quality. This approach has been demonstrated to work very well in QCA as long as the contours are relatively smooth in shape. However, complex vessel morphology may occur post-coronary intervention, for example, when a dissection occurs. Also before intervention, obstructions with very sharp corners are found. The MCA technique by its design is hampered in tracing very irregular boundaries. To be able to adequately analyze such very irregular stenoses, we have developed a novel algorithm, the Gradient Field Transform (GFT^R), which does not have the disadvantages of the MCA algorithm [12].

The essential differences between the MCA and GFT algorithms can be explained briefly with the graphical example illustrated in Figure 4. The closed circles represent pixels along the scanlines (straight lines) defined perpendicular to the arterial's pathline. Pixel A is a contour point under consideration. In search for the next point of the arterial boundary, the MCA algorithm would only consider points C7, C8 and C1. Contrary to that, the GFT algorithm takes all of its eight neighbour points (C1 - C8) into account. This approach enables the GFT algorithm to follow more irregular arterial boundaries and even allow reversal of the contour direction, e.g. to follow flaps.

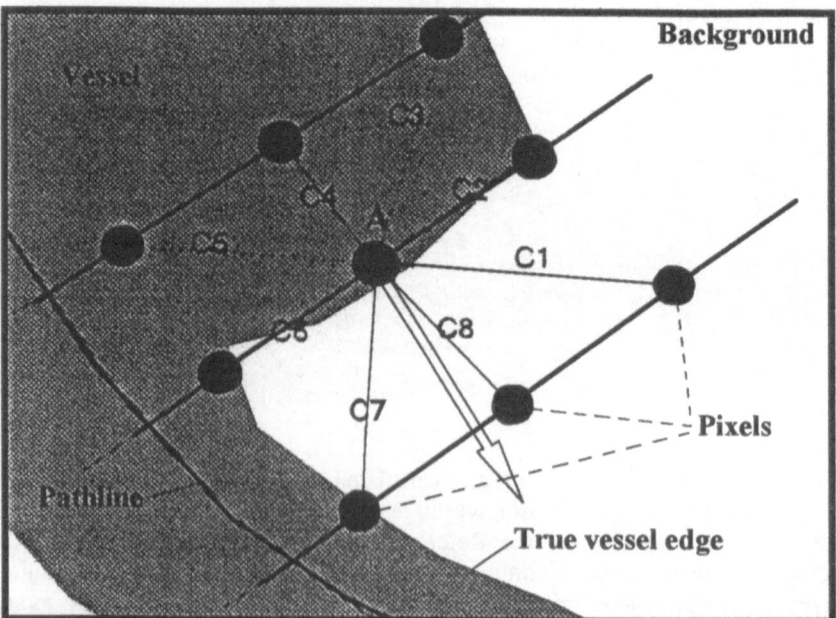

Figure 4. Schematic representation of a vessel with its pathline, the scanlines and the search directions for the GFT^R algorithm.

This GFT has been validated extensively on phantom images and on digital coronary arteriograms [12]. These and later evaluation studies have demonstrated that obstruction diameters as assessed by the GFT are on the average 0.25 mm smaller than those detected by the MCA algorithm. The detected contours are a little bit more irregular due to the fact that the algorithm is more sensitive to noise in all possible directions. However, we believe that these data represent a correct reflection of the vessel's morphology. These irregularities may also provide prognostic information as suggested earlier by Kalbfleisch et al. [13]. This needs to be investigated in future studies.

The GFT has been incorporated into the QCA-CMS software package (Version 3.0) in the following manner. The first step in a typical QCA analysis is always carried out following the conventional MCA-approach. Based on the detected contours, the user or the program itself may decide whether certain parts of the coronary segment are so irregular or complex, that an additional GFT-search is warranted. If so, the user indicates the beginning and the end of the part to be reanalyzed. Next, the GFT contour detection is carried out in between these boundaries; the GFT contours subsequently replace the local MCA contours. In the usual manner, the user can make further manual corrections. Such a combined effort exploits the advantages of both algorithms. Despite the much higher mathematical and computational complexity of the GFT algorithm, a typical GFT analysis does not take longer than a few seconds. The higher sensitivity of the GFT for irregularities is precisely the reason why we have implemented the current version as an additional iteration on part or the entire MCA-contour. Since complex lesions represent, in general, only a minor percentage of the cases to be quantified, this approach will speed up the analysis of the more regular stenoses.

Our experiences with the GFT indicate that this approach may be very useful for the analysis of ostial lesions, and for the analysis of radiopacque stents. With the appropriate optical zooming (in an off-line configuration), the GFT is able to follow the outer boundaries of the stent struts and the contrast lumen in between the stent struts. An example of an analysis of the Wiktor stent by the MCA and GFT techniques is given in Figures 5A (MCA) and 5B (GFT). It is clear that the GFT indeed results in a smaller obstruction diameter (2.42 by GFT versus 2.53 by MCA), a larger reference diameter (3.13 mm versus 3.01 mm), and therefore a more severe percent diameter obstruction (22.7% versus 15.9%). The mean diameters over the entire segment are approximately the same (2.92 mm versus 2.90 mm).

Validation of QCA

Desmet et al. [14] have compared 3 different QCA systems (Polytron 1000, the AWOS Workstation and the CMS(V2.0)) and found significant differences in outcomes when applied to a PTCA study. Due to the correction for the limited resolution of the x-ray system, they indeed found that the CMS exhibited a tendency to yield lower values for very small diameters and higher values for larger vessels. The long-term gain as assessed by CMS was almost twice the value obtained with AWOS; significant differences were also found in the acute gains. They concluded that their findings underscore the continuing need for a

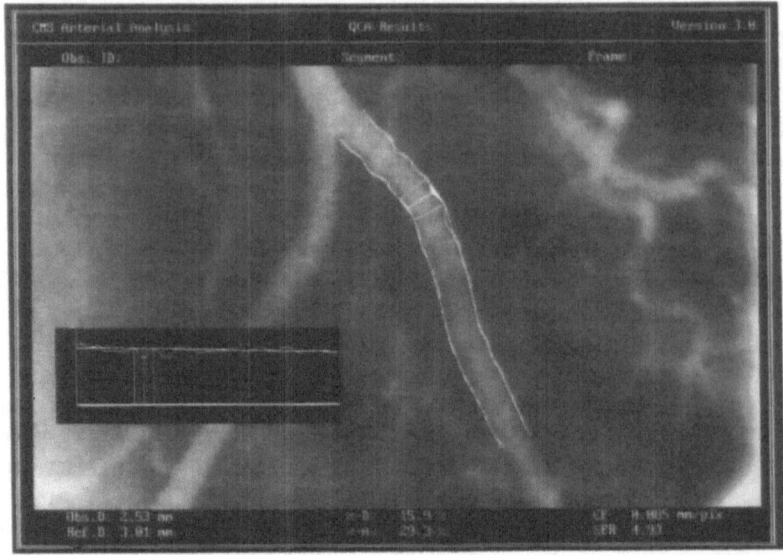

a

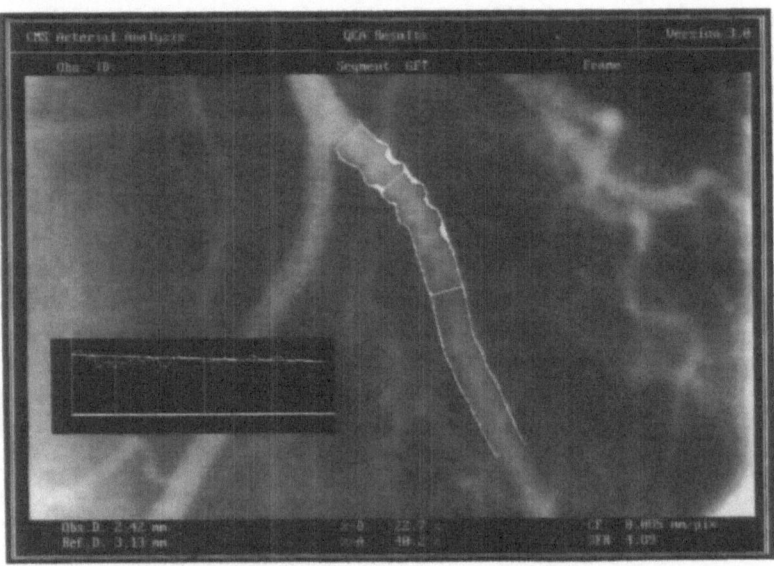

b

Figure 5. Example of an analysis of the Wiktor stent by the conventional Minimum Cost Algorithm (MCA) in Figure 5A and the new Gradient Field Transform (GFT^R) in Figure 5B.

central core laboratory in multicenter trials in order to optimize consistency. One major limitation of the study by Desmet et al. [15] is that no objective comparative data on the three systems is available.

Recently Hausleiter et al. [16] have compared the QCA-CMS (Version 1.11) with the CAAS and ARTREK analytical software packages. The study material included phantoms comprised of 19 stenotic and nonstenotic glass tubes with a diameter range from 0.54 to 4.9 mm, and a clinical study including 322 coronary segments. In the cinefilm-based phantom study the overall accuracy of the QCA-CMS was found to be -6 μm (ARTREK: 39 μm; CAAS: 35μm) with an overestimation of small vessels (<1.5 mm) of only -11μm (ARTREK: 38 μm; CAAS: 51 μm); for an additional digital-based ARTREK-study the overall accuracy was 85 μm and the small vessel accuracy 97 μm. The clinical study also confirmed that the QCA-CMS corrected the usually occurring overestimation of small vessel sizes.

Pincushion distortion

Often the question comes up whether the images should be corrected for the pincushion distortion introduced by the image intensifier. However, it has been shown by various investigators that the amount of pincushion distortion depends on the rotation and angulation of the x-ray gantry [17]. Since the distortion vectors are usually derived from centimeter-grid measurements in the antero-posterior projection, artefacts may be created when the same correction vectors are applied to contour data derived from other angiographic views. With so many disturbing issues left open, we decided to further investigate this problem [18]. Therefore, a cm-grid was fixed onto the input screen of the image intensifier, and the gantry was rotated to span all possible geometric positions of the system (rotation: RAO90-LAO90, angulation: Cranial 40-Caudal 40). The corresponding x-ray images (either from cinefilm or digital) were analyzed with a specially developed analytical package, which automatically located all intersection points of the copper wires of the cm-grid. For each pixel position in a frame a distortion vector and a gradient vector could be derived, with the gradient vector denoting the local inhomogeneities in the distortion field. It can be demonstrated that a distorted, although homogeneous region of interest has no effect on the calibration factor. The results from this evaluation study showed that the distortion (in absolute terms as well as the gradients) is highly dependent upon the rotation and angulation of the x-ray system. Both the earth magnetic field as well as other electromagnetic sources may influence the distortion. Therefore, it was concluded, that in QCA correction for pincushion distortion is not to be advised, as the errors caused by the corrections may be larger than the errors associated with the original uncorrected data. It should also be realized that modern image intensifiers used in the 7" mode have relatively little distortion.

The cineless catheterization laboratory

With the ACC '95 and '96 and the ESC '95 demonstrations of the exchange of cardiovascular images on CD-R according to the DICOM-3 standard as proposed by the ACC/ACR/NEMA/ESC Committee, a major step forward has been made towards the realization of the cineless catheterization laboratory [19,20]. The amount of digital data involved in coronary arteriography is enormous. At an acquisition speed of 30 frames/s and a matrix size of 512x512x8 bits, 7.5 Mbytes of data is generated per second. A study with a maximal number of 4800 frames, requires 1200 Mbytes of digital data to be stored. Although the expenses of the storage media, communication systems, etc. are likely to decrease significantly in the future, compression techniques have been suggested to ease the storage and transfer demands.

One of the major questions still to be resolved is how much image compression is allowed. Currently, the DICOM standard allows the storage of compressed data at a maximum compression ratio of 5 using the widely available JPEG compression scheme, which has been accepted as a standard. The highest acceptable lossy compression ratio will be determined by noticeable effects on the diagnostic interpretation of these images, and whether QCA will be affected. The ACC/ACR/NEMA/ESC Committee has agreed to carry out a large combined study including a minimum of 100 angiographic runs to answer the following pertinent questions:

1. Is the detection of specific coronary features hampered by the lossy image compression?
2. What are the effects on QCA?
3. At which level are differences noticeable on a side-by-side comparison?

In two pilot studies we have attempted to find out in which directions the answers will be found. The designs and the results of these studies will be discussed below.

Phantom compression study

The goal of this pilot study was to investigate the effect of JPEG lossy compression with compression factors (CFs) of 6, 10 and 14 on digital images of stereolytographically produced resin phantoms (from Dr. Revel, Lyon, France) containing asymmetric obstructions, which were positioned such that symmetric projections were obtained. The phantom consisted of 6 tubes with obstruction diameters in the range of 1-9 mm and with a reference diameter of 9 mm. The images were acquired at the 5" and 7" modes of the image intensifer, at 512x512 and 1024x1024 matrix sizes, compressed and decompressed with the 3 compression factors and analyzed with the conventional Minimum Cost Algorithm (MCA) as well as with the Gradient Field Transform (GFT) on the CMS system (Version 3.0). To be able to compare the quantitative measurements of the analyzed segments in corresponding compressed/decompressed images, which only differ in compression factor, a standardized approach was used in the sense that the same start and end points of the pathlines were used in the corresponding compressed/decompressed images; no corrections to the contours were allowed. By this approach any differences observed would only be due to the actual differences in the arterial dimensions as influenced by the different compression factors. All images were analyzed twice by the same observer with an interval of one week to assess the intra-observer variabilities; of course, in the repeated analyses the observer set new beginning and end points for the pathlines. The calibration procedure was performed of the basis of a cm-grid, acquired at the same geometric level as the centers of the phantom tubes.

The mean signed differences between the average values of the first and second measurements in the images with data compression, and the first and second measurements in the original non-compressed images, and the standard deviation of these differences were calculated to express the inter-compression systematic and random errors for each compression factor (Figure 6). The results are given in Tables 1A and 1B.

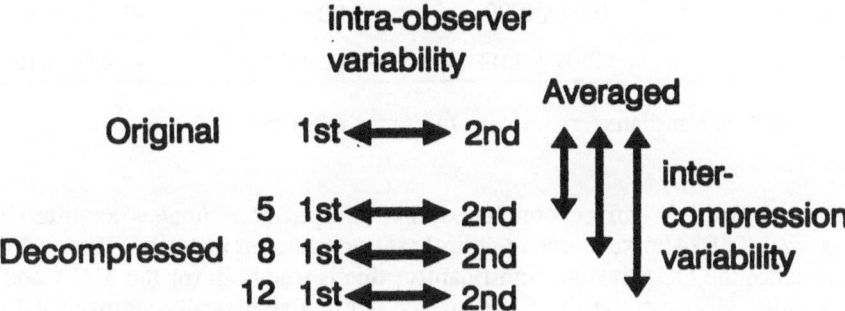

Figure 6. Schematic diagram illustrating the type of comparisons carried out in the QCA-compression studies.

Table 1A. The inter-compression variabilities expressed in terms of systematic $\pm$ random errors in the QCA of phantom images acquired at 512^2 and 1024^2 matrices and carried out with the MCA-algorithm.

MCA-algorithm N = 39 512^2 images	CF 6 - original	CF 10 - original	CF 14 - original
Dobs (mm)	0.02±0.08	0.01±0.09	0.03*±0.12
Dref (mm)	0.01±0.06	0.01±0.03	0.00±0.04
1024^2 images			
Dobs (mm)	0.00±0.06	-0.02±0.07	-0.02±0.06
Dref (mm)	-0.01±0.05	-0.01±0.05	-0.01±0.03

*p<0.05
Dobs = obstruction diameter; Dref = reference diameter

Table 1B. The inter-compression variabilities expressed in terms of systematic $\pm$ random errors in the QCA of phantom images acquired at 512^2 and 1024^2 matrices and carried out with the GFT-algorithm.

GFT-algorithm N = 40 512^2 images	CF 6 - original	CF 10 - original	CF 14 - original
Dobs (mm)	0.02 ± 0.10	-0.02 ± 0.09	0.03 ± 0.11
Dref (mm)	0.01 ± 0.05	0.01 ± 0.03	0.00 ± 0.04
1024^2 images			
Dobs (mm)	0.01 ± 0.09	-0.00 ± 0.10	-0.04 ± 0.13
Dref (mm)	-0.01 ± 0.03	-0.02 ± 0.10	-0.03 ± 0.12

Dobs = obstruction diameter; Dref = reference diameter

From these data, it can be concluded that for phantom images acquired at a matrix size of 1024^2 pixels, even the highest compression factor of CF = 14 does not influence the QCA results significantly; this is true both for the MCA and the GFT results. However, at the 512^2 matrix sizes, a statistically significant (p < 0.05) systematic difference is found at CF = 14 using the MCA algorithm; these differences were not found using the GFT algorithm. In other words, at the 512^2 matrix size, the compression factor should not exceed 10.

Angiographic compression study

Under ideal circumstances with homogeneous backgrounds high compression ratios apparently are still acceptable. The question, of course, is whether the same will be true under clinical conditions. To obtain the appropriate answers, we compared the influence of two compression schemes (LOT and JPEG) at CFs of 5, 8 and 12 on coronary measurements assessed with the ACA-DCI package. The Lapped Orthogonal Transform (LOT) scheme was developed by Philips Medical Systems [21,22]. The main difference with the JPEG algorithm is that the 8x8 blocks used in the LOT algorithm overlap each other, while that is not the case with JPEG.

A set of 30 routinely acquired coronary arteriographic runs was used, showing a total of 37 obstructions. This data set was taken from a large data set acquired on a Philips DCI-S at l'Hopital Cardiologique de Lille, which has been used for a quantitative study on the effects of image compression on the visual interpretation of coronary angiograms.

During the acquisition procedures, the images were stored on streamer tape without any compression. At the Philips Research Laboratory in Eindhoven, the images were read into a computer system, frame by frame, compressed and again thereafter decompressed using the JPEG and LOT schemes at ratios of 5, 8 and 12. After decompression the new image series were stored on tape for later analysis.

The analysis of the set of clinical images was performed in the same manner as the set of phantom images, i.e. 1) the same start and end points of the pathlines were used in the corresponding compressed/decompressed images; 2) no corrections to the detected contours were allowed; and 3) all images were analyzed twice by the same observer with an interval of one week to assess the intra-observer variabilities. The calibration procedure was performed on the basis of the catheter, prior to every measurement. In the corresponding catheter images, which only differ in compression scheme and ratio, the same coordinates of the start and end points were used.

The mean signed differences (accuracy or systematic error) between the first and second measurements in images with the same compression factor and scheme, and the standard deviation of these differences (precision or random error) were calculated to express the intra-observer variability for the original image series and for each of the compressed/decompressed series. The F-test was used to determine the significance of the differences in the intra-observer random errors for the compressed image series versus those of the original image series. The intra-observer variabilities for the obstruction and reference diameter measurements assessed from the original and compressed/ decompressed image series are given in Table 2 for both the LOT and JPEG compression schemes. From this table it can be observed that the random errors in the absolute diameter measurements increase significantly for the JPEG scheme at a compression factor of 5 for the obstruction diameter, and for LOT for the reference diameter at a compression factor of 12.

Table 2. Intra-observer variabilities expressed in terms of systematic $\pm$ random errors for the original images and the JPEG and LOT compressed/decompressed images with compression factors of 5, 8 and 12.

LOT N = 37	Original	CF = 5	CF = 8	CF = 12
Dobs (mm)	0.01 ± 0.11	-0.01 ± 0.12	0.03 ± 0.14	0.02 ± 0.16
Dref (mm)	-0.02 ± 0.13	0.03 ± 0.15	0.04 ± 0.18	0.02 ± 0.21*
JPEG N = 37	Original	CF = 5	CF = 8	CF = 12
Dobs (mm)	0.01 ± 0.11	0.02 ± 0.19*	-0.07 ± 0.15	-0.02 ± 0.14
Dref (mm)	-0.02 ± 0.13	0.00 ± 0.14	-0.03 ± 0.15	0.01 ± 0.18

*$p<0.005$

The inter-compression variability data are presented in Table 3 in the same format as was used in Table 1.

Table 3. The inter-compression variabilities expressed in terms of systematic ±
random errors for corresponding measurements performed on 37 coronary
obstructions with and without the JPEG or LOT data compression at different
compression factors.

JPEG compression N = 37	CF 5 - original	CF 8 - original	CF 12 - original
Dobs (mm)	0.02 ± 0.24	-0.05 ± 0.23	0.01 ± 0.26
Dref (mm)	-0.03 ± 0.23	-0.03 ± 0.31	-0.07 ± 0.29
LOT compression N = 37	CF 5 - original	CF 8 - original	CF 12 - original
Dobs (mm)	-0.03 ± 0.23	0.03 ± 0.23	0.00 ± 0.26
Dref (mm)	-0.05 ± 0.26	0.04 ± 0.25	0.00 ± 0.28

The results in Table 3 clearly demonstrate that these lossy compression techniques
do not lead to statistically significant over- or underestimations in absolute
dimensions in coronary angiograms, but rather to significantly increased random
differences (in comparison with data presented in Table 2). These results suggest
that even the JPEG and LOT compression factor of 5 is not acceptable for QCA.

S-VHS archive medium

In the transition period between cinefilm and digital, many hospitals have decided
to use S-VHS video tape as the long-term storage medium. Economics apparently
play the major or only role in these decisions, thereby completely ignoring the
poor specifications of S-VHS devices. In practice, copies of these tapes are also
made for exchange with other departments/hospitals. This situation should be
avoided at all times, due to the deteriorated image quality of copies of the tapes.
The ESC Task Force on Digital Imaging in Cardiology has also strongly
recommended against the use of S-VHS and U-Matic video-tapes and other
devices comparable in quality for these purposes [23]. Taking into account the
current practice in hospitals and possibly in QCA Core Laboratories, we were
interested in finding an objective manner to study the influence on the QCA
results when using this storage medium. For that purpose, we carried out an
evaluation study using a plexiglass phantom of known dimensions, which was
positioned horizontally as well as vertically in the field of view [24]. The digital
images were stored on S-VHS tape and the stored images were redigitized and
analyzed. The following objective observations were made: 1) large
overestimations (up to 0.87 mm) occur for tube sizes below 1 mm for vertically
positioned tubes; 2) random errors in measurements are much larger for vertically
positioned tubes (0.36 mm, at 7" image intensifier (II)) than for horizontally
positioned tubes (0.17 mm, 7" II); and 3) little differences in results between
enhanced and nonenhanced images were found. All these deviations can be
explained by the poor signal-to-noise ratio and the limited bandwidth of the S-

VHS video tape. Therefore, it can be concluded, that S-VHS video tape is unacceptable for QCA and should be excluded from quantitative angiographic clinical trials.

References

1. Brown BG, Bolson E, Frimer M, Dodge HT. Quantitative coronary arteriography: estimation of dimensions, hemodynamic resistance, and atheroma mass of coronary artery lesions using the arteriogram and digital computation. Circulation 1977;55:329-37.
2. Reiber JHC, Booman F, Tan HS *et al*. A cardiac image analysis system. Objective quantitative processing of angiocardiograms. Comput Cardiol 1978;239-42.
3. Reiber JHC, Serruys PW, editors. Advances in quantitative coronary arteriography. Dordrecht: Kluwer Academic Publishers, 1993.
4. Jukema JW, Bruschke AVG, van Boven AJ *et al*. Effects of lipid lowering by pravastatin on progression and regression of coronary artery disease in symptomatic men with normal to moderately elevated serum cholesterol levels. The Regression Growth Evaluation Statin Study (REGRESS). Circulation 1995;91:2528-40.
5. Bruschke AVG, Jukema JW, van Boven AJ, Bal ET, Reiber JHC, Zwinderman AH. Angiographic endpoints in progression trials. Submitted.
6. Waksman R, Weintraub WS, Ghazzal ZMB *et al*. Directional Coronary Atherectomy (DCA): is much bigger much better? [abstract] Circulation 1995;92(Suppl.I):I-329.
7. Reiber JHC, von Land CD, Koning G *et al*. Comparison of accuracy and precision of quantitative coronary arterial analysis between cinefilm and digital systems. In: Reiber JHC, Serruys PW, editors. Progress in quantitative coronary arteriography. Dordrecht: Kluwer Academic Publishers, 1994:67-85.
8. Van der Zwet PMJ, von Land CD, Loois G, Gerbrands JJ, Reiber JHC. An on-line system for the quantitative analysis of coronary arterial segments. Comput Cardiol 1990:157-60.
9. Reiber JHC, Koning G, von Land CD, van der Zwet PMJ. Why and how should QCA systems be validated? In: Reiber JHC, Serruys PW, editors. Progress in quantitative coronary arteriography. Dordrecht: Kluwer Academic Publishers, 1994:33-48.
10. Colombo A, Hall P, Nakamura S *et al*. Intracoronary stenting without anticoagulation accomplished with intravascular ultrasound guidance. Circulation 1995;91:1676-88.
11. Reimers B, Di Francesco L, Di Mario C *et al*. A new approach to the assessment of residual stenosis after stent implantation with quantitative angiography [abstract]. Submitted to ESC 1996.
12. Van der Zwet PMJ, Reiber JHC. A new approach for the quantification of complex lesion morphology: the gradient field transform; basic principles and validation results. J Am Coll Cardiol 1994;24:216-24.
13. Kalbfleisch SJ, McGillem MJ, Simon SB, DeBoe SF, Pinto IMF, Mancini GBJ. Automated quantitation of indexes of coronary lesion complexity. Comparison between patients with stable and unstable angina. Circulation 1990;82:439-47.
14. Desmet W, De Scheerder I, Beatt K, Huehns T, Piessens J. In vivo comparison

of different quantitative edge detection systems used for measuring coronary arterial diameters. Cathet Cardiovasc Diagn 1995;34:72-80.

15. Reiber JHC Editorial Comment. Cathet Cardiovasc Diagn 1995;34:81.
16. Hausleiter J, Nolte CWT, Jost W, Wiese B, Sturm M, Lichtlen PR. Comparison of different quantitative coronary analysis systems: ARTREK, CAAS, and CMS. Cathet Cardiovasc Diagn 1996;37:14-22.
17. Solzbach U, Wollschläger H, Zeiher A, Just H. Optical distortion due to geomagnetism in quantitative angiography. Comput Cardiol 1988:355-7.
18. Van der Zwet PMJ, Meyer DJH, Reiber JHC. Automated and accurate assessment of the distribution, magnitude and direction of pincushion distortion in angiographic images. Invest Radiol 1995;30:204-13.
19. Cardiac angiography without cinefilm: erecting a "Tower of Babel" in the cardiac catheterization laboratory. American College of Cardiology Cardiac Catheterization Committee. J Am Coll Cardiol 1994;24:834-7.
20. American College of Cardiology, American College of Radiology and industry develop standard for digital transfer of angiographic images. ACC/ACR/NEMA Ad Hoc Group. J Am Coll Cardiol 1995;25:800-2.
21. Koning G, Baretta P, Zwart P, Reiber JHC. Effect of lossy image compression on QCA results [abstract]. Circulation 1995;82(Suppl.I):I-22.
22. Breeuwer M, Heusdens R, Klein Gunnewiek R, Zwart P, Haas HPA. Data compression of x-ray cardio-angiographic image series. Int J Card Imaging 1995;11(Suppl.3):179-86.
23. Simon R, Brennecke R, Heiss O, Meier B, Reiber H, Zeelenberg C. Report of the ESC Task Force on Digital Imaging in Cardiology. Recommendations for digital imaging in angiocardiography. Eur Heart J 1994;15:1332-4.
24. Reiber JHC, Koning G, van der Zwet PMJ, Schiemanck L. Inaccuracy of quantitative coronary arteriography when analyzed from S-VHS videotape. Cathet Cardiovasc Diagn 1996;37:32-8.

5. 3-D Coronary angiography for quantitative analysis of coronary morphology

HELMUT OSWALD, ANDREAS WAHLE, ERNST WELLNHOFER & ECKART FLECK

Introduction

Quantitative evaluations of coronary vessel systems are of increasing importance in cardiovascular diagnosis, therapy planning and quality control. Whereas local evaluations, such as stenosis analysis, are already available with sufficient accuracy, global evaluations of vessel segments or vessel subsystems are uncommon today. Especially for the diagnosis of diffuse coronary artery diseases, we combined a 3-D reconstruction system operating on biplane angiograms with a length/volume calculation. The 3-D reconstruction results in a 3-D model of the coronary vessel system, consisting of the vessel skeleton and a discrete number of contours. To obtain an utmost accurate model, we focussed on exact geometry determination. Several algorithms for calculating missing geometric parameters and correcting remaining geometry errors were implemented and verified. The length/volume evaluation can be performed either on single vessel segments, on a set of segments, or on subtrees. A volume model based on generalized elliptical conic sections is created for the selected segments. Volumes and lengths (measured along the vessel course) of those elements are summed up. In this way, the morphological parameters of a vessel subsystem can be set in relation to the parameters of the proximal segment supplying it. These relations allow objective assessments of diffuse coronary artery diseases.

Problem domain

Atherosclerotic coronary artery disease is a major epidemiological problem associated with functional impairment, expensive treatment and fatal outcome in many patients. Whereas the diagnosis of local stenosis is well established and often amenable to invasive therapy, diffuse disease is a domain of conservative therapy. A quantitative assessment of progression of the latter is desirable in order to judge the effects of different modalities of medical treatment and epidemiologic interventions decreasing risk factors. This remains true, even if stress tests and other clinical information supply additional data for evaluating disease and help in decision making.

Angiographic images of the coronary tree convey the impression that diffuse disease might be associated with remodelling of the coronary vascular branches. Absolute measurements of diameters, lengths or volumes of the segments of the artery requires 3-D reconstruction of the tree. Since these absolute dimensional values are of limited use due to large physiological variation in the size of coronary arteries, we aimed to construct a set of nondimensional measures. This set needs to be independent of size and functional state of the coronary vessel

J.H.C. Reiber and E.E. van der Wall (eds.), Cardiovascular Imaging, 57-78.

allowing for quantification of morphological changes in the 3-D tree. The spatially reconstructed vessel trees were decomposed hierarchically, analyzing stems and crowns of the derived subtrees.

Modelling and Evaluation

Within the last decade, much work has been performed in the field of vessel detection and three-dimensional reconstruction of the coronary system of the heart. Thus, in this section we primarily figure out differences and enhancements in relation to earlier works of other authors. A rather theoretical presentation of the model generation and evaluation process is followed by a validation in several phantom studies and the verification of the entire system.

3-D Reconstruction

The Reconstruction Pipeline

The reconstruction process (Figure 1) starts with the image acquisition, where biplane images are mandatory. The problem of handling distortions such as pincushion and sigmoidal effects has already been solved. In this section, we assume that the biplane angiograms are rectified, centered (i.e., the central beam is located in the center of each image) and free of axial rotations. The sizes of the image intensifier entrance fields are assumed to be known.

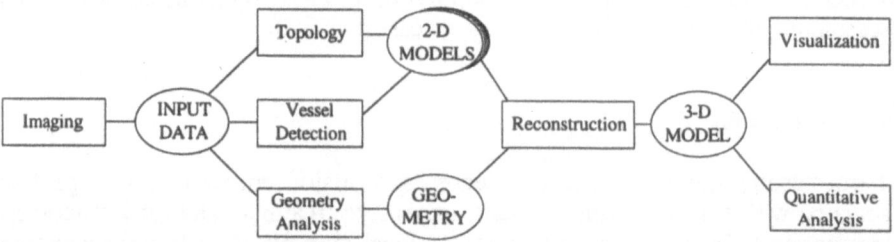

Figure 1. The reconstruction pipeline

By a combination of interactive topology marking and automatic vessel detection, for each projection a 2-D model is generated. A complex imaging geometry analysis and approximation system was developed to reconstruct a 3-D model as accurately as possible. This model can then either be visualized to obtain a realistic impression of the vessel morphology, or quantitative analyses can be performed with high accuracy. Especially in those evaluations that cannot be performed by simple manual measurements on angiograms, 3-D evaluations are indispensable to obtain important morphological parameters. Thus, we focussed on imaging geometry analysis and on finding an optimum model for volume representation. An additional application area can be found in the calculation of the optimal views for interventional procedures.

Imaging geometry

Standard biplane angiographic equipment consists of two x-ray systems having a common coordinate system. The geometries of biplane imaging devices were analyzed by Wollschläger et al. [1]. They assumed a fixed rotational origin of both systems, the isocenter: the projection axes intersect at this isocenter. The geometry is derived from the known angulation parameters and the distances of the x-ray sources and image intensifiers to the origin. Several evaluation systems are based upon these and other idealized assumptions, e.g., performing an isocentric calibration for diameter analyses on local stenoses [2-4].

For our purpose of accurate 3-D reconstruction, we need a very high reconstruction accuracy, because linear reconstruction errors raise up to the third power in the following analysis steps. The classic isocentric model could not satisfy this requirement due to various mechanical influences:

first, a significant amount of gantry sag during rotation causes the projection axes not to intersect, thus the isocenter becomes blurred;

second, there is no adequate way to measure the required distances manually in medical routine; distances assumed to be fixed also vary due to gantry sagging [5]. In phantom studies instabilities of the isocenter were demonstrated.

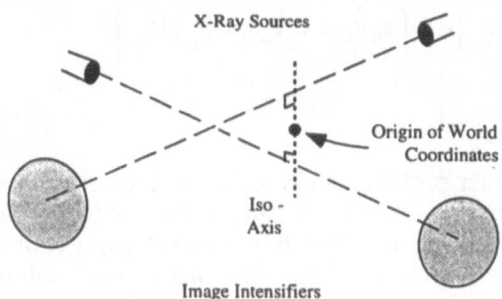

Figure 2. Iso-axis imaging geometry model

In our imaging geometry model, we use a variable iso-axis instead of a fixed isocenter to consider the real mechanical properties. The distance of the projection axes creates a unique iso-axis orthogonal to both of them (Figure 2). The locations of x-ray sources and image intensifiers are determined in terms of distances to this iso-axis. The origin of the world coordinate system is defined as the weighted middle of the intersections of both projection axes with the iso-axis. The angulation is obtained conventionally as a sequence of rotations, considering the shift. Since the orientation of the iso-axis depends on the angulation, the iso-axis may vary between different acquisitions. Since the distance of the projection axes is not constant - even in acquisitions with the same angulations - the location of the origin may slightly vary between acquisitions as well. This fact has relevant influence for our purposes.

The transformation of a point from metric world (WC) via x-ray system (XC) to the image (IC) coordinates of projection p is:

$$[x_{xc}, y_{xc}, z_{xc}] = \left([x_{wc}, y_{wc}, z_{wc}] + \vec{I}_p \right) \cdot \mathbf{R}_p \qquad (1a)$$

$$[u_{ic}, v_{ic}] = [x_{xc}, y_{xc}] \cdot \frac{D_{S_p} + D_{I_p}}{s_p \cdot \left(D_{S_p} + z_{xc} \right)} \qquad ,\text{where} \qquad (1b)$$

I   is a 3-D translation vector (iso-axis portion);
R   is a 3x3 rotation matrix (angulation);
D_S is the distance between x-ray source and iso-axis;
D_I distance image intensifier input surface to iso-axis;
s   is the scaling factor of the image intensifier.

Point reconstruction

While the imaging process results in unique projections of a point, the inverse is ambiguous. Due to the loss of one dimension, only one ray per projection can be reconstructed that pierced the object point during imaging. The ray q(t) with $0 \leq t \leq 1$ of a projected point [u,v] is then:

$$q_{xc}(t) = \left[0, 0, -D_{S_p} \right] + t \cdot \left[s_p u_{ic}, s_p v_{ic}, D_{S_p} + D_{I_p} \right] \qquad (2a)$$

$$q_{wc}(t) = q_{xc}(t) \cdot \mathbf{R}_p^{-1} - \vec{I}_p \qquad (2b)$$

Similar to the isocenter problem, there exist no intersection point. The two rays do not intersect due to several possible error sources. The definition of a generalized intersection point solves this problem [6,7]. For both projections a point Q_p on ray q_p is searched, where their distance is minimum. The weighted middle of these points is the desired object point P (Figure 3).

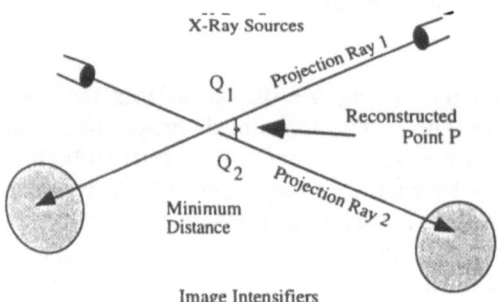

Figure 3. Point reconstruction

In the next section we show how to use this reconstruction error for a global error detection and correction; nevertheless the generalized intersection point has to be used for local error considerations, because a global correction can only minimize the mean errors.

Analysis and approximation of the imaging geometry

Fencil and Metz [8] have developed algorithms to determine the imaging geometry from 8 points, including angulation, distances and isocentric shifts (i.e., the deviation of the projection axes from the rotational origin). Again, this method is not applicable in clinical routine, thus we have to make some obvious assumptions and restrict ourselves to points or objects visible in the angiograms without additional artificial markers.

Some parameters are mainly a matter of adjustment. Once fixed, they are either constant (e.g., image intensifier size), or they can be easily determined by rulers, etc. (angulation). The spatial locations of x-ray sources and image intensifiers must be calculated as accurately as possible, but they cannot be determined by rulers or manual measurements. Unavoidable inaccuracies of the given parameters must be detected and corrected. Our method uses both known imaging parameters and at least two to five interactively marked reference points of known correspondence in the angiograms. From the known geometric parameters an initial imaging geometry is calculated. In an iterative process this initial geometry is improved by a mean-value based statistical approach, analyzing the errors from reconstructing the reference points [5].

The total error in $y_i = f(x_i, t_i)$ projection p of the i-th reference point is a function of the distance x_i of the reconstructed point to the projection axis in the direction of the iso-axis, and the relative location t_i of the point in direction of the projection axis (Figure 4). The total error is:

$$y_{i_p} = \sum_{j=0}^{m-1} y_{ij_p} = \sum_{j=0}^{m-1} f_j\left(x_{i_p}, t_{i_p}\right) \tag{3}$$

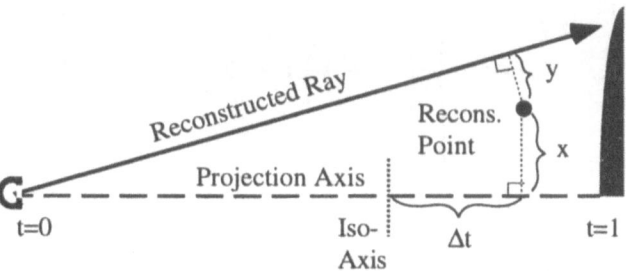

Figure 4. Diagram explaining the calculation of the projection errors.

The extraction of a component delivers one correction coefficient to apply to the actual geometry. Afterwards, this component Δy_j is subtracted from the original error. The next error component is extracted, and so on. The dimension-less correction coefficients k_0 for the iso-axis portion, k_1 for the magnification and k_2 for the perspective distortion are determined as follows:

$$k_{0_p} = \frac{\sum\limits_{i=1}^{n} y_{i_p}^{\langle 0 \rangle}}{\sum\limits_{i=1}^{n} 1[m]} \quad ; \quad k_{1_p} = \frac{\sum\limits_{i=1}^{n} \left(y_{i_p}^{\langle 1 \rangle} \cdot \mu_{x_p}(x_{i_p}) \right)}{\sum\limits_{i=1}^{n} \left(t_{i_p} \cdot x_{i_p} \cdot \mu_{x_p}(x_{i_p}) \right)}$$

$$k_{2_p} = \frac{\sum\limits_{i=1}^{n} \left(y_{i_p}^{\langle 2 \rangle} \cdot \mu_{\Delta t_p}(\Delta t_{i_p}) \cdot \mu_{x_p}(x_{i_p}) \right)}{\sum\limits_{i=1}^{n} \left(\Delta t_{i_p} \cdot x_{i_p} \cdot \mu_{\Delta t_p}(\Delta t_{i_p}) \cdot \mu_{x_p}(x_{i_p}) \right)}$$

(4a-c)

where

$$y_{i_p}^{(j)} = y_{i_p} - \sum\limits_{j^*=0}^{j-1} \Delta y_{j^*_p} \quad ; \quad \Delta t_p = t_p - t_{I_p} \quad ; \quad t_{I_p} = \frac{D_{S_p}}{D_{S_p} + D_{I_p}}$$

$\mu(\ )$: weighting functions; [m]: length dimension.

The functions $\mu(\ )$ are required to ensure that points near the projection axes (x) and the iso-axis (Δt) are weighted less than those of higher informational value. Without this weighting, the algorithm may not properly approximate if many of the reference points are of less significance. The applied functions preserve the sign and are continuous:

$$\mu(v, r_1, r_2 r_3) =$$

$$\begin{cases} \left\{ \begin{array}{ll} 1 - \dfrac{1}{2\left(1 + \frac{v - r_1}{r_2}\right)} & \text{if } v > r_1 \\[2mm] \dfrac{1}{2} & \text{if } v = r_1 \\[2mm] \dfrac{1}{2\left(1 - \frac{v - r_1}{r_2}\right)} & \text{if } v < r_1 \end{array} \right\} \cdot \left(1 - \dfrac{1}{1 + \frac{v}{r_3}}\right) & \text{if } v > 0 \\[14mm] \quad 0 & \text{if } v = 0 \\[8mm] \left\{ \begin{array}{ll} -1 + \dfrac{1}{2\left(1 - \frac{v + r_1}{r_2}\right)} & \text{if } v < -r_1 \\[2mm] -\dfrac{1}{2} & \text{if } v = -r_1 \\[2mm] -\dfrac{1}{2\left(1 + \frac{v + r_1}{r_2}\right)} & \text{if } v > -r_1 \end{array} \right\} \cdot \left(1 - \dfrac{1}{1 - \frac{v}{r_3}}\right) & \text{if } v < 0 \end{cases}$$

(4d)

v   is the input value to weight;

r_1 is a fixed parameter for $\mu(v) = \pm\ 0.5$ threshold;

r_2 is a fixed parameter for the steepness at $\mu(v) = \pm\ 0.5$;

r_3 is a fixed parameter for overall curve steepness.

After extracting all components, the actual geometry is corrected by application of the coefficients, and the reference points are reconstructed again. If the mean reconstruction error is less than a self-adjusting threshold, the iteration stops and the actual geometry is used as the final approximation.

While the approximation algorithm is able to correct errors relatively between projections, there is no absolute measure for magnification. Thus, at least one object of given size within the images has to be known. Conventional methods use the projected radius of a catheter in one projection for calibration, which leads to errors in later quantitative evaluations.

To get a reliable reference size, we either use markers on a catheter with known distances (cardio-markers) or the outer diameter of the pigtail catheter loop. During the geometry approximation process, the object is reconstructed with the actual geometry. The relation between the calculated and the real spatial sizes of the calibration object results in an additional correction coefficient for the geometry approximation [5].

2-D hierarchical model generation

To obtain a 3-D model, for each projection a 2-D model has to be generated. This is done by interactive marking of the vessel topology. The operator selects corresponding points in both projections, called nodes: the vessel ostii, branches, leaves (where to stop reconstruction) or other striking points (Figure 5). The biplane correspondence is defined during this step, assigning for each vessel in one projection the corresponding vessel in the other projection.

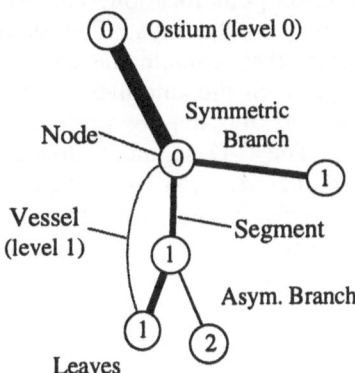

Figure 5. Vessel hierarchy.

A structural attribute of a node is its level, indicating the membership to a vessel segment and the tree hierarchy. A vessel segment is defined as a set of connected nodes of the same level. From each node other vessels segments of a lower level may branch. The nodes split the vessels up into different segments. While the nodes are set interactively, the vessel course and edges are determined automatically by using the nodes as guide points for a vessel detection algorithm [9]. As a result, each segment consists of a discrete number of elements, containing the 2-D image coordinates of centerline and both edge points.

Tagged compound model

After generating the 3-D model of the coronary vessel system, this model has to be available for further analysis processes and archiving. Therefore a flexible, hardware-independent representation of the geometry and both 2-D / 3-D models was developed [10]. The vessel tree is linearized by a recursive depth-first-search method, which preserves the vessel hierarchy. Each portion of information is packed into a multi-level tag stream. The stream starts with an identification tag, indicating the type of description (e.g. device parameters, imaging geometry, or vessel tree). Depending on this type the tag hierarchy may change. For instance, a device description needs a tag referring to the order of rotations, which may be skipped when the imaging geometry has been established for an individual image series. It is a main characteristic of our interface, that only those tags of importance to the specific application are extracted. Thus, for example, a stenosis analysis system does not need to take care of the vessel hierarchy, but can add further tags for its analysis results.

Tag hierarchy for a completely reconstructed vessel tree contains the imaging geometry in terms of locations of x-ray sources and image intensifiers rather than plain rotation angles and distances. For each node, entries of their 2-D and 3-D attributes are included. Each set of attributes is subdivided into node and segment portions. Whilst the node attributes contain single values or vectors, segment attributes are lists of items.

For each node, the interactively marked points are stored as well as the reconstructed rays and the object point location. The 3-D set additionally contains the points of nearest distance on the rays. The segment attributes are more complex. In the 2-D models, they contain the centerline and both edge point coordinates. Manual corrections of the automatic vessel detection are notified in optional tags. Due to lesions, vessels may be partially invisible. For these cases special tags were included. The 3-D segment attributes contain the centerline coordinates as well as the radius vectors. The radius tags may be replaced, e.g. by the results of contour detection on intravascular ultrasound images. A special tag indicates the relation between the 2-D models and the 3-D model. Thus, if a specific element in one projection was selected, its corresponding element in the second projection and the 3-D element can easily be found. The optional tag can be used to emphasize regions of interest.

Models can be mixed, e.g. separate vessel systems from left and right coronary arteries . Thus the morphological information of multiple image series can be combined in a single model (Figure 6).

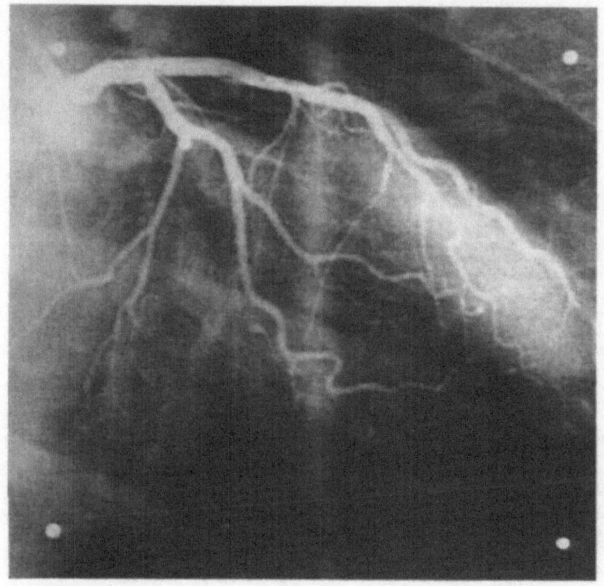

a

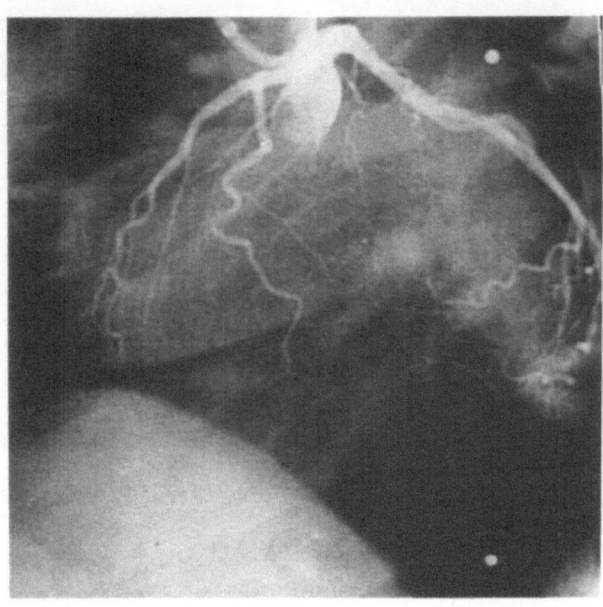

b

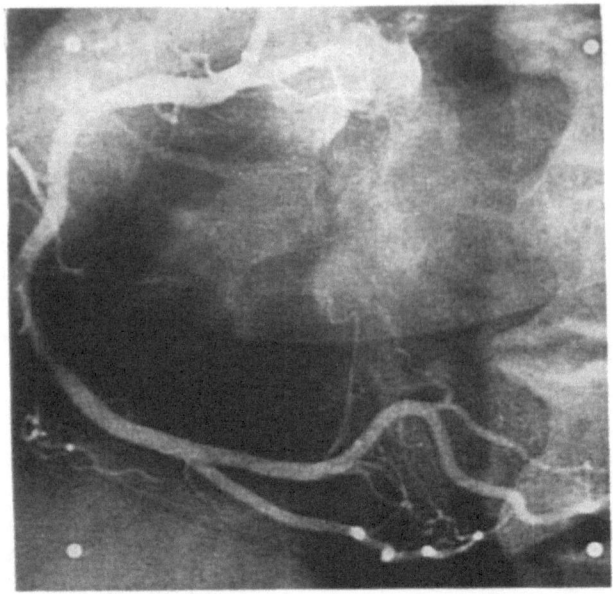

c

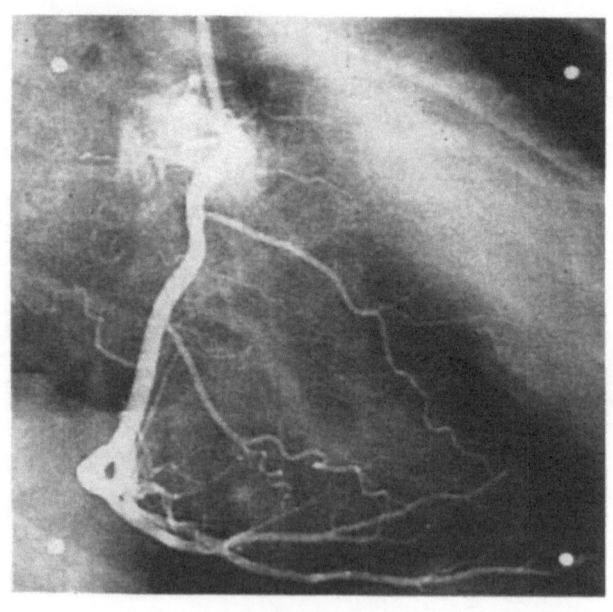

d

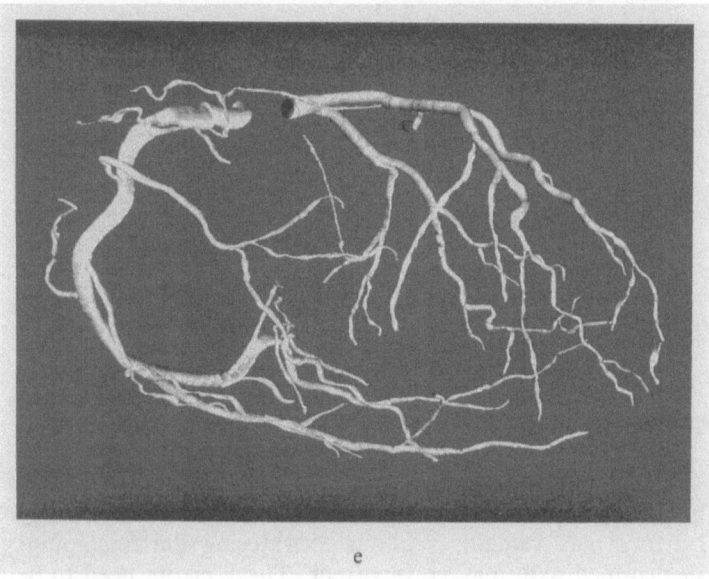

e

Figure 6A t/m E. 1A, 1B, 1C, 1D: Biplane angiograms of right and left coronary vessel System 1e: Shaded display of reconstructed and fit together of the right and left Coronary System based on 1A, 1B, 1C, 1D angiograms

Segment reconstruction

After geometry and vessel topology have been determined and the nodes of the vessel system have been reconstructed, the vessel segments found during the vessel detection algorithm have to be reconstructed. Segments are always enclosed by two nodes. While node points create only one ray per projection, segments create ray bundles, where the corresponding ray pairs have to be found. A cost matrix is generated, which contains the distances of the rays for each pair of segment elements (Figure 7).

This is done by calculating the points of the minimum distance. The correspondence is defined by the path of lowest distances from matrix elements (0,0) to (n-1,m-1).

Parker et al. developed a method where the elements are discretely assigned and reconstructed [11]. We created a new algorithm with additional interpolation of missing elements to any desired segment length. The resulting 3-D segment contains at least the number of elements of the longer 2-D segment. The diagonal represents the simplest case of linear assignment. Bilinearly interpolated profiles of the cost matrix are obtained orthogonally to the diagonal, then descent and minima on the profile are evaluated, resulting in an element of the optimum path. Difficult shapes of the vessel segment (e.g., S-curvatures) may cause local ambiguities in the matrix. In extreme cases a plateau of same values is created, when several projection rays are in the same level. As a fallback solution, linear assignment with additional smoothing is performed then. Thus, the cost minima are not necessarily zero for all matches.

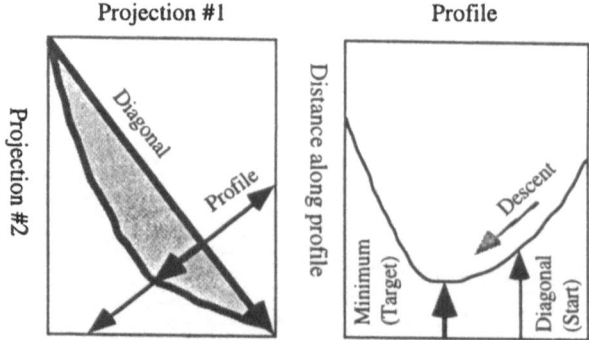

Figure 7. Optimum correspondence path

The global geometry approximation algorithm can minimize only the global mean error, local errors may remain. Without considering the remaining geometric errors, the determined path may be incorrect. These errors need to be corrected before performing the element matching. The geometric error vectors derived from the nodes enclosing the segment are interpolated along the error direction. The error direction in a node P is orthogonal to both projection rays. It consists of a constant portion orthogonal to the projection axes, and a variable portion dependent on the distortion due to perspective. Thus, error directions of nodes that are close to each other are nearly collinear. The mean error direction of two or more neighbouring nodes is defined as the intermediate of their local error directions:

$$\overline{e_{MEAN}} = \begin{cases} \overline{e_A} + \overline{e_B} & \text{if } \overline{e_A} \cdot \overline{e_B} \geq 0 \\ \overline{e_A} - \overline{e_B} & \text{else} \end{cases} \tag{5}$$

$$\overline{e_A} = \overline{P_A Q_{A_p}} \quad \text{and} \quad \overline{e_B} = \overline{P_B Q_{B_p}}$$

For each projection p the error vectors $\overline{e}$ from the reconstructed node P to the nearest points Q_p on their rays are extracted for both surrounding nodes A and B of a segment. Along the mean error direction $\overline{e_{MEAN}}$, for each element an individual error vector $\overline{e_{ELEM}}$ is interpolated (Figure 8). This is performed by obtaining the scalar products of the reconstructed world coordinates of both nodes and the desired element with the mean error direction vector.

Weighted by the element's distances to A and B, their local error vectors are interpolated:

$$\overline{e_{ELEM}} = (1-t) \cdot \overline{e_A} + t \cdot \overline{e_B} \; ; \; t = \frac{\overline{e_{MEAN}} \cdot \left(\overline{q_A} - \overline{q_{ELEM}} \right)}{\overline{e_{MEAN}} \cdot \left(\overline{q_A} - \overline{q_B} \right)} \tag{6}$$

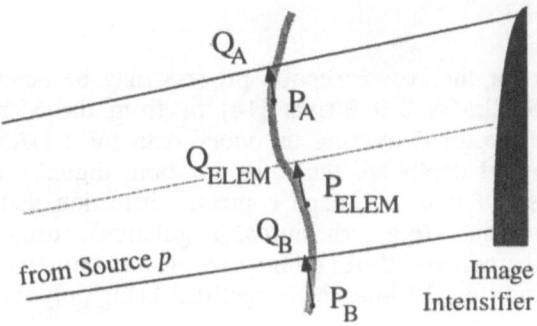

Figure 8. Local error correction

The points Qp of an element are then shifted in the opposite direction of the error vectors. The minimum distance between the two ray candidates has now the best fit to the surrounding nodes [7].

Modelling of vessel cross sections

The vessel detection algorithm delivers both centerline and edges in 2-D images. They can be reconstructed to a radius vector for each projection, i.e., for biplane views there are two vectors available. Thus, there is no need to restrict ourselves to circular contours (e.g., as done in [4]). However, it is necessary to consider some ambiguities when calculating elliptical cross sections.

For each element of a vessel the 3-D centerline points are calculated. For each projected centerline point P two edge point pairs E exist with symmetrical distance from P. Their image points can be used to reconstruct the radius vectors: The distance B_{Edge}-B_{Point} in world coordinates multiplied by the factor t for object point P yields the radius r. Due to an oblique entering of the ray by angle α, this radius is radially lengthened by $1/\cos\alpha$. More significant are errors due to point-spreading for small vessels. These can be corrected empirically by phantom measurements [9].

As already described the 2-D coordinates of the segment elements are interpolated. This requires the additional interpolation of the edge information. Although we can achieve a high correspondence of the selected radius vectors, small errors in the correspondence remain due to tolerances in setting of the nodes, etc.

After establishing both radius vectors, they can be used to form the elliptic contour. Only in the case of triple orthogonality [12,13] can the radius vectors be used directly as the axes, otherwise the form of the ellipse is ambiguous due to a systematic loss of spatial information. To compensate for this effect, we continuously change the shape of the contour from elliptic to circular depending on the amount of spatial information for each element (Figure 9).

Data acquisition

The image data for the reconstruction process may be acquired in two ways: directly in ACR-NEMA 2.0 format [14] or from the 35mm films using an ARRIPRO 35 projector delivering the video data for a DASM frame grabber. Pixel resolution and depth are the same for both digitally and conventionally acquired images. Of course, image contrast, distortion and noise differ. The required imaging data (e.g., distances, angulations, used catheters) can be retrieved from the patient information system (interventional data protocol).

In a preprocessing step the images are rectified using polynomial equations [9].

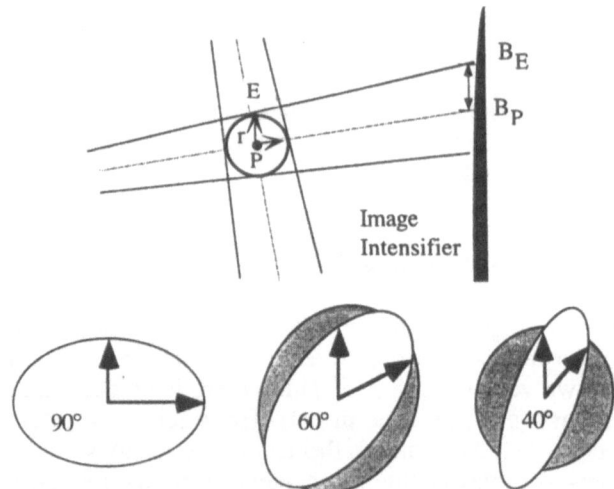

Figure 9. Radius reconstruction and ellipse deformation

Errors are eliminated that were caused by the convex shape of the image intensifier entrance fields and the geomagnetic field, or by other effects during the acquisition and digitization process. Four lead markers mounted on the image intensifier entrance fields in known distances and orientations are used for further dewarping to obtain the correct image centers and orientations [15]. Also, the real image intensifier sizes can be determined by these markers.

For each chain of image acquisition (used device, media, and correction processes) a unique set of device parameters is generated. Using these base parameters, for individual image series the imaging geometry is derived.

Validation

Quantitative verifications were performed in several phantom studies. The imaging geometry approximation system was tested with both synthetically generated and real images. A virtual cube phantom with 40 mm edge length was used with a significantly distorted set of imaging parameters; the original parameters could be restored with a maximum remaining error of 0.012 mm in iso-axis distances [5].

In a further study we used a hexagonal phantom to determine the gantry sags. In standard frontal and lateral orientation, we measured an isocentric shift (i.e., distance of a projection axis to the rotational origin) of 10.4 mm for both systems. After establishing an exact isocenter in frontal/lateral orientation, and moving the systems to 30°RAO/30°caud and 60°LAO/30°cran, a shift of 2.7 mm was found. Even when using the frontal system for both angulations, there was still a sag of 1.7 mm. Significant distortions could be measured in longitudinal direction related to the projection axes: in theory, as far as our equipment is concerned, the distance of each focal spot to the isocenter is assumed to be constant ($D_S \approx 700$ mm) and not dependent on either rotation or total distance to the image intensifier. We found that the focal spot of the lateral system shifted by ± 9.5 mm during rotation, while the frontal focal spot had a tolerance of ± 20.1 mm in D_S. In general, these distortions are not reproducible.

A comparison between the different single- and biplane calibration methods was performed using a cylindric solid phantom (40 mm in length by 6 mm in diameter) imaged in triple orthogonality. For calibration, a 7F pigtail catheter was available with 3 markers of each 20 mm distance, and a loop of 14.5 mm in diameter. This pigtail catheter was inserted: 1) in triple orthogonality; 2) oblique by approx. 30° and slightly curved; and 3) in a strong S-shaped curve with oblique orientations up to 60°. Additionally, angulated images with down to 70° inclination angle between the systems and $\pm 15°$ of skew were taken. After performing each calibration method, we reconstructed the cylinder and determined the errors in diameter and volume.

Using the conventional single-plane catheter diameter calibration method, volume measurement errors were in the range of 21-29 %. The single-plane cardio-marker method yields good results only if the catheter is in triple orthogonality and adjusted in isocenter level; gross errors were caused by oblique catheters, thus the volume errors were in the range of 15-66 %. The biplane methods should raise better results. As proposed by Büchi and Kirkeeide [3], the isocenter method yielded a mean volume error of 3.1 %, whereas a maximum error of 9.7 % was measured due to gantry sagging. Our biplane cardio-marker calibration (with edge detection applied to follow the catheter curvature) resulted in a comparable mean error of 3.5 %, but within a more stable range of 3.0-4.6 %. Finally, the biplane calibration using the pigtail loop minimized the volume errors to 0.8-4.4 % (mean 2.6 %).

While parallaxes do not cause significant further errors (volume errors using a spiral phantom of 76 mm in length and 5 mm in diameter: triple orthogonality 1.6 %, 60° oblique to iso-axis 1.9 %), inclination angles less than 30° between the x-ray systems raised the measured errors dramatically due to a high loss of spatial information. Within the inclination range of 60-120° used in medical practice, the additional volume errors kept below 1.5 % (70°). In absence of overlapping, differences due to changes of the object position and orientation resulted in errors below 1 %. Overlapping vessels, or if the vessels are strongly shortened in one or both projections, significant errors occur due to ambiguities and incorrect edge recognition (up to 8 % in local diameters, and up to 3 % in vessel volumes). The real phantom dimensions were obtained by manual measurements and/or water displacement.

Medical application

There are many patients suffering from coronary artery disease without significant local stenosis, and even more, who have qualitatively obvious diffuse disease in addition to local stenoses. Qualitative alterations in the angiographic appearance of the coronary tree are of unknown significance. The assessment of their clinical impact implies the development of tools defining and quantifying these alterations. Even in patients with obvious diffuse disease, as in patients with dilating atherosclerotic arteries or with diffuse vessel narrowing (e.g., in diabetic patients) there is only a qualitative description possible, presented as an obstacle to assessment of severity of disease and the impact of therapeutic intervention on the progression.

Whereas the diagnosis and treatment of local stenosis are well established, assessment of diffuse disease remains difficult and time consuming. There have been several approaches each suffering from various limitations. Conventional approach is usually serial measurement of absolute luminal diameters or cross-sections [16].

Recently it was proposed to compare cross-sectional luminal area with the total distal length of the vascular tree, since there is a strong correlation between the size of the coronary tree and regional mass perfused [17].

Chronic reduction in perfusion or progression in atherosclerosis should be associated with re-modelling of trees and subtrees. The vascular tree in patients without atherosclerotic disease seems to follow certain scaling laws [17-19] complying with the principles of minimum viscous energy loss and limited adaptive vascular shear-stress [17]. The extent of deviation from this normal pattern should reflect the severity of disease. The observation that even diffuse disease is often not homogeneously distributed, suggests that correlation analysis of dimensions in sets of coronary subtrees might be a suitable approach to measure progression in diffuse disease.

The purpose of this study is to quantify diffuse disease overall on total trees, which is to be well discerned from evaluating stenosis or reconstructing plaque locally. Thus, for testing this approach, LCA and RCA trees were analyzed retrospectively from three groups of patients selected according to clinical diagnosis:

o Patients having no visible disease (controls);

o Patients with CAD of the localized type post-PTCA (CAD);

o Patients with severe diffuse and dilating coronary artery disease (DCAD).

The patients, routinely imaged in the years 1992 and 1993 due to various diseases, were selected by their findings using the local patient information system. They had been imaged in standard projections (0-45°RAO, 45-90°LAO, with up to ±20° skew) using either 6", 7" or 9" (general views) image intensifier diameters. Patients had been catheterized by Judkins technique in local anaesthesia without special additional preparation. Manually injected Ultravist™ had been used as contrast agent. Analysis was done on end-diastolic frames, except a special study with 11 selected biplane angiographic pairs of different heart cycle phases of the same patient.

After performing the reconstruction process, the visible parts of the arteries are available as a 3-dimensional tree (Figure 10). This tree can be decomposed into

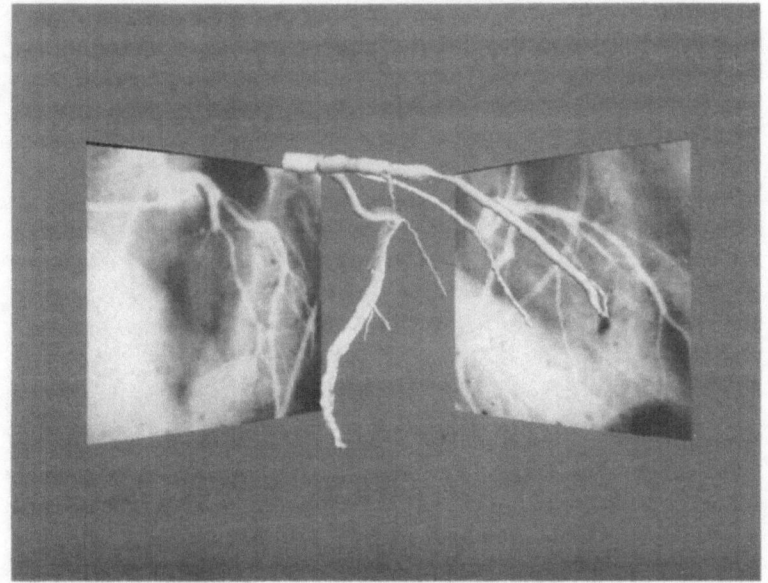

a

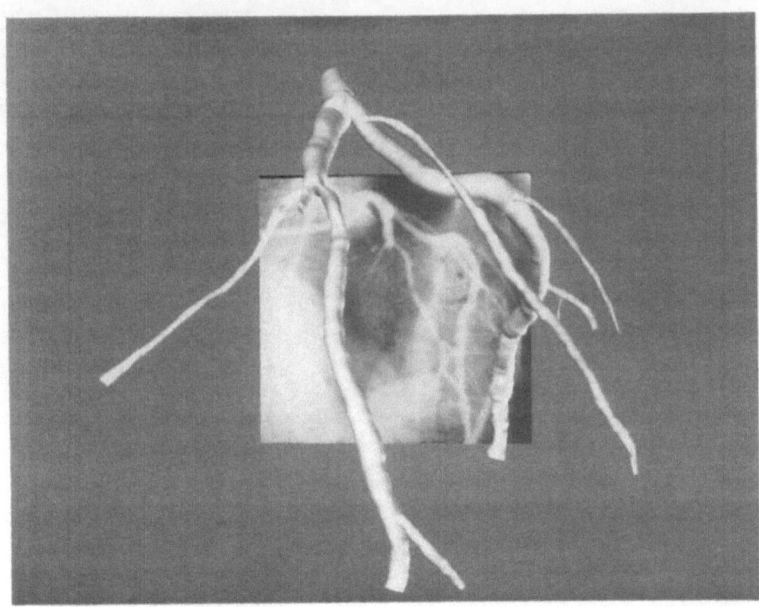

b

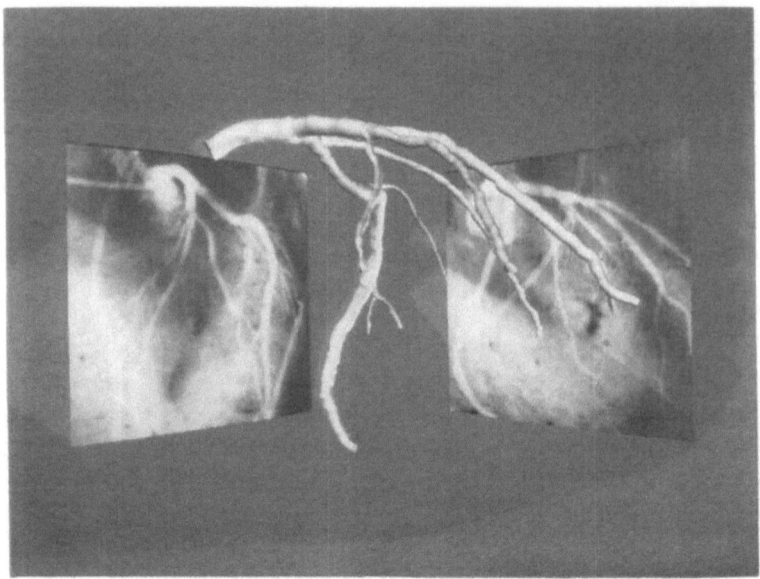

c

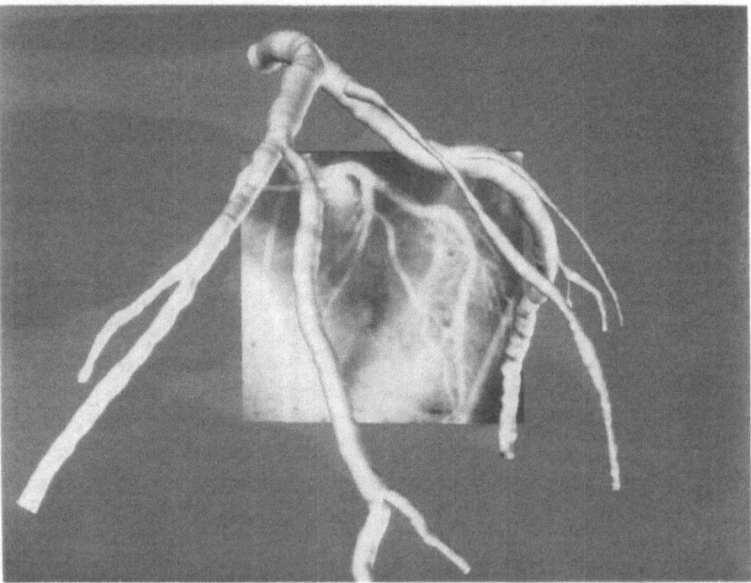

d

Figure 10. 10A and 10B: Shaded display of reconstructed left coronary system with occluded LAD. 10C and 10D: Shaded display of reconstructed left coronary system after reopening of LAD by laser-angioplasty.

a "stem" containing the segments from the root to the first bifurcation, and a corresponding "crown" consisting of the branches below the bifurcation. For example, the LCA is decomposed into the left main as the stem, and the combination of LAD and Cx as the crown. The principal branches of a crown containing at least one additional bifurcation may be regarded as subtrees and are decomposed into stems and crowns in the same way as described above. A crown without any bifurcating branch cannot be decomposed. By the recursive application of this decomposing algorithm, every tree gives rise to a family of subtrees consisting each of a stem and a corresponding crown.

Assessment of tree destruction

Supposing a fractal vessel geometry in controls, the dimensions of the subtrees in terms of lengths, diameters and volumes are scaled in a similar way [17-19]. Atherosclerotic disease due to inhomogeneous distribution is expected to be associated with increased variance in the scaling of individual subtrees. Angiographically visible destruction of the arterial tree seen in dilating coronary artery disease implies virtual abolishment of the normal fractal geometry. Thus, an effective measure for assessment of progressive destruction of fractal order in a coronary tree should assume well-separated values in the tree groups of patients, and has to quantify the amount of similarity of scaling relations within a subtree. Correlations of the dimensions of the subtrees are suitable measures [20].

Results

For every subtree, there are six corresponding values (length, diameter and volume, both for stem and for crown) which should be correlated. Graphical and numerical analyses showed that the relations are non-linear. Logarithmic transformation turned out to be an appropriate preprocessing step linearizing data. Analysis using Bravais Pearsons correlation coefficient [20] was done in 67 RCA and 62 LCA subtrees in controls, 35 RCA and 83 LCA subtrees in the CAD group, and in 30 RCA and 42 LCA subtrees in the DCAD group.

There are 15 different combinations available to select a pair out of the six parameters mentioned above for a correlation analysis. The sum of these correlations gives a rough assessment of the degree of order inherent in the set of analyzed subtrees. Since some of these correlations are partially trivial (e.g., diameter of stem in relation to the volume of stem), retaining them is to be considered as giving additional weight to good correlations. We applied a weighting factor of zero to those correlations smaller than 0.5 in this sum to suppress bad correlations. The weighted sum of these 15 correlations (SUM) proved to be an effective measure of progressive destruction of order in the coronary tree with severity of atherosclerotic disease, as can be seen from Table 1. Since weighted adding of measures yields again measures according to mathematical theory, the empirically defined parameter SUM remains a measure [21]. It is decreased, if variance in the dimensions of the subtrees increases. Intervention with ergonovine (a test agent producing vascular spasm) decreases

SUM by approx. 13%, whereas intervention with nitroglycerin (a vasodilating agent) increases SUM by approx. 12%.

Table 1. Correlation analysis.

Group	n	Length	Volume	Diam.	SUM
RCA					
Control	67	0.45	0.48	0.82	3.67
CAD	35	0.30	0.35	0.81	2.80
DCAD	30	0.25	0.28	0.40	1.50
LCA					
Control	62	0.57	0.61	0.82	4.73
CAD	83	0.42	0.45	0.79	3.51
DCAD	42	0.23	0.23	0.50	1.65

Apart from the weighted sum of correlations, the correlations of the diameter of the stem with the diameter (D), length (L) and volume (V) of the corresponding crown are statistically significant (Table 1). The correlations were generally better in the left coronary artery than in the right coronary artery.

Discussion

Since ordinarily decomposition of the coronary tree yields more than ten subtrees, calculating SUM on an individual basis seems feasible. Nevertheless it would be desirable to have a local measure requiring only the evaluation of a part of the coronary tree.

The amount of time spent by the operator in evaluating a total tree varies widely according to the experience of the operator, complexity of the coronary anatomy, and technical factors, e.g., quality of the angiograms and the precision of the technical equipment and the interventional data protocol. A realistic estimation per total evaluation is 1 to 2 hours.

Seiler et al. [17] found a correlation between area measured at any location in LCA and the total summed length of distal branches of $r = 0.93$ in controls and $r = 0.88$ in all patients. This parameter roughly corresponds to L. In a smaller series of 53 subtrees previously reported [22], we found correlations of $r = 0.802$ for L, whereas now in controls this value was only 0.57 in LCA subtrees. The difference is attributed to several reasons. Apart from variance of r within a confidence interval due to sampling, Seiler's area calculation was based on diameters from selected segments of the coronary angiogram suitable for QCA, whereas our data include all segments (even those with ambiguous nodes, overlapping regions, areas of overexposure and those containing stenoses). Correlation was worse in subtrees approaching the limits of angiographic resolution. Thus, suppressing the highest order of subtrees improves correlations. Based on our experience, ignoring subtrees with an order of higher than 6, or - in other terms - with mean stem and crown diameters less than 0.5 mm, is recommended.

Comparing different phases of the cardiac cycle, there was a slight reduction of diameter and volume (2.31 mm, 0.865 ml) in early diastole as compared to systole (2.58 mm, 1.059 ml). The length of the tree varied about 3.4%. This variance was not systematic as in diameters and volumes, and is within the limits of reproducibility.

More extensive clinical testing in different groups of patients is necessary to address these problems and to evaluate this approach further.

References

1. Wollschläger H, Lee P, Zeiher A, Solzbach U, Bonzel T, Just H. Mathematical tools for spatial computations with biplane isocentric x-ray equipment. Biomedizinische Technik 1986;31:101-6.
2. Wollschläger H, Lee P, Zeiher A, Solzbach U, Bonzel T, Just H. Improvement of quantitative coronary angiography by calculation of exact magnification factors. Comput Cardiol 1985/86:483-6.
3. Büchi M, Hess OM, Kirkeeide RL *et al.* Validation of a new automatic system for biplane quantitative coronary arteriography. Int J Card Imaging 1990;5:93-103.
4. Peifer JW, Ezquerra NF, Cooke CD *et al.* Visualization of multimodality cardiac imagery. IEEE Transactions on Biomedical Engineering. IEEE press 1990;37:744-56.
5. Wahle A, Wellnhofer E, Oswald H, Fleck E. Biplane coronary angiography: accurate quantitative 3-D reconstruction without isocenter. Comput Cardiol 1993/94:97-100.
6. Parker DL, Pope DL, White KS, Tarbox LR, Marshall HW. Three dimensional reconstruction of vascular beds. Information processing in medical imaging. Nihoff Boston 1986:414-30.
7. Wahle A, Oswald H, Schulze GA, Beier J, Fleck E. 3-D reconstruction, modelling and viewing of coronary vessels. Comput Assis Radiol CAR'91, Springer Verlag Berlin 1991:669-76.
8. Fencil LE, Metz CE. Propagation and reduction of error in 3-D sStructure dDetermined from biplane views of unknown orientation. Med Physics 1990;17:951-61.
9. Beier J, Oswald H, Fleck E. Edge detection for coronary angiograms: error correction and impact of derivatives. Comput Cardiol 1991, Venice IT, IEEE press 1991:513-6.
10. Wahle A, Oswald H, Fleck E. A new 3-D attributed data model for archiving and interchanging of coronary vessel systems. Comput Card 1993, London UK, IEEE press 1993/94:603-6.
11. Parker DL, Pope DL, van Bree R, Marshall HW. Three dimensional

reconstruction of moving arterial beds from digital subtraction angiography. Comput Biomed Res 1987;20:166-85.

12. Wollschläger H, Zeiher A, Lee P, Solzbach U, Bonzel T, Just H. Computed triple orthogonal projections for optimal radiological imaging with biplane isocentric multidirectional x-ray systems. Comput Cardiol 1986, Boston MA, IEEE press 1986/87:185-8.

13. Dumay ACM, Reiber JHC, Gerbrands JJ. Determination of optimal angiographic viewing angles: basic principles and evaluation study. IEEE Transactions on Medical Imaging, IEEE press 1994;13:13-24.

14. ACR-NEMA 300-1988. Digital imaging and communications. Nat Electr Manufacturers Association 1989, Washington DC, pp. 11-20/59-84.

15. Onnasch DGW, Prause GPM. Geometric image correction and isocenter calibration at oblique biplane angiographic views. Comput Cardiol 1992, Durham NC, IEEE press 1992/93:647-50.

16. De Feyter PJ, Serruys PW, Davies MJ, Richardson P, Lubsen J, Oliver MF. Quantitative coronary angiography to measure progression and regression of coronary atherosclerosis. Circulation 1991;84:412-23.

17. Seiler CH, Kirkeeide RL, Gould KL. Basic structure function relations of the epicardial coronary vascular tree: basis of quantitative coronary arteriography for diffuse coronary artery disease. Circulation 1992;85:1987-2003.

18. Zhou SH, Mateeva E, Collins R. The anatomy of human coronary vessels. 2nd Int Symp Biofluid Mechanics and Biorheology, Liepsch D ed. Springer 1990:463-70.

19. Van Beek JHGM, Roger SA, Bassingthwaighte JB. Regional myocardial flow heterogeneity explained with fractal networks. Am J Physiol 1989;257:H1670-80.

20. Armitage P, Berry G. Statistical methods in medical research. Blackwell Scientific Publications, London UK, 2nd ed. 1987:150.

21. Bauer H. Wahrscheinlichkeitstheorie und Grundzüge der Maßtheorie. Walter de Gruyter Verlag, Berlin/New York, 2nd ed. 1974:22-3.

22. Wahle A, Wellnhofer E, Mugaragu I, Sauer HU, Oswald H, Fleck E. Quantitative volume analysis of coronary vessel systems by 3-D reconstruction from biplane angiograms. IEEE Medical Imaging Conference 1993, San Francisco CA, IEEE press 1993/94;2:1217-21.

6. State of the art in ICUS quantitation

WENGUANG LI, NICOLAAS BOM, CLEMENS VON BIRGELEN, TON F.W. VAN DER STEEN, CHRIS L. DE KORTE, ELMA J. GUSSENHOVEN & CHARLES T. LANCÉE

Summary

IntraCoronary UltraSound (ICUS) data are the basis of two-dimensional (2D) quantitative information and three-dimensional (3D) reconstruction. A method for semi-automatic 3D image quantification for volumetric study of series of echo slices has been developed. The semi-automatic contour detection method was tested in-vitro in tubular phantoms of known dimensions. Intra- and interobserver variability was evaluated in-vivo for area and volume measurements of diseased human coronary arteries.

High blood backscatter level at ICUS imaging frequencies appears to be a major limiting factor for automatic contour procedures and 3D reconstruction. Video-frame averaging methods have shown to be helpful for reducing intra- and interobserver variability of the manual lumen definition, but not sufficient to enhance the image for automatic contour detection.

New technologies to use the RadioFrequency (RF) ultrasonic signal for image improvement, although still in their early development stage, are looking promising. A RF processing technique based on correlation of a time sequence of RF echo traces can yield a high value at the wall region against a low value in the lumen region. With the RF correlation technique, the image can be improved drastically, thus facilitating application of fully automated image segmentation techniques. Furthermore, the RF processing methods may provide other quantitative parameters about functions of the vessel. These methods include:

1. Flow estimation. The de-correlation procedure of blood scattering signals is related to the velocity of blood particles traveling across the ultrasound beam. Quantifying this procedure may provide an estimation of 2D velocities distribution for the blood flow;
2. Intravascular elastography. Tissue with different elastic properties will reveal different strains to an applied stress. This is currently used for functional imaging.

Introduction

High frequency intracoronary ultrasound (ICUS) permits visualization and quantitation of coronary atherosclerotic diseases [1-3] and assessment of catheter-based intervention [4-7]. In comparison to angiography, this technique provides a more accurate measure of the cross-sectional lumen and plaque areas. Furthermore, the tomographic nature of the ICUS imaging technique allows three-dimensional (3D) reconstruction and quantification of the vessel over the

J.H.C. Reiber and E.E. van der Wall (eds.), Cardiovascular Imaging, 79-92.
© 1996 *Kluwer Academic Publishers.*

entire narrowed segment [8-12]. Fully automated image segmentation methods have been developed in order to reduce the time and the subjectivity of manual tracing on a 3D ICUS data set. A simple approach is the image threshold method which separates the lumen and tissue based on grey intensities [10]. A more elaborate solution is to identify the time or spatial characteristics of blood speckles. Based on random features in the spatial distribution of blood speckles, a so-called "blood speckle identification algorithm" was developed with statistical pattern recognition [8]. The other approach is a combination of an image subtraction method to extract the time-varying features of blood with a 3D region growing algorithm [13]. All these methods, however, are limited to the detection of the arterial lumen. An alternative approach is the sequential contour detection based on dynamic programming techniques [14,15]. This technique uses a global optimization rule to find the boundary and can be used to detect the lumen and media contours. Since the optimization technique is robust to image noise, it has been widely used in several fields of medical image processing, particularly in contour detection on ultrasound images [16-18]. The success rate of applying these fully automated techniques, however, is not infrequently restricted by factors such as lack of sharpness of the lumen-wall interface, the similar acoustic properties of the plaque and adventitia and interference from blood scattering. To provide an efficient method which is able to deal with images of various quality, a semi-automatic approach has been developed and tested through in-vitro and in-vivo studies.

3D quantitative ICUS system

Computer System

The analysis program utilizes the Microsoft Windows operating system on a Pentium personal computer with 16 Mbytes of internal RAM. A framegrabber is installed (DT-3852; resolution: 800 x 600 x 8 bits) to digitize a user-defined region of interest from the video images. A maximum of 200 ICUS images can be digitized at a user-defined digitization frame rate (maximum: 20/s). The reconstructed segment length is thus defined by the speed of the motorized pull-back during the basic image acquisition and by the digitization frame rate. In the present study a pull-back speed of 1.0 mm/s and a digitization frame rate of 8 images/s (in-vitro) and 10 images/s (in-vivo) were used, resulting in a reconstructed segment length of 25 and 20 mm, respectively. The pixel size, which depends on the magnification applied by the basic ICUS imaging system, ranged from 26 μm to 36 μm.

Semi-automatic Contour Detection

The purpose of the image segmentation procedure is to define the regions of the vessel lumen and lesion on each ultrasound cross-section. The luminal area is defined by the leading edge of the arterial wall. To estimate the size of the total cross-sectional area of the artery, the interface between intima-media complex and adventitia is identified.

The semi-automatic contour detection is based on a minimum cost algorithm, previously applied and described in cross-sectional ICUS images [17,19,20]. By this approach the digitized ICUS images are resampled according to a radial image reconstruction (64 radii in the cross-sectional images; 200 rows in the longitudinal sections). A cost matrix which represents the edge strength is calculated from the image data. For the detection of the boundary between lumen and plaque the cost value is defined by the spatial first-derivative. In order to detect the external boundary of the total vessel, a pattern matching process by cross-correlation is adopted for the cost calculations. Through the cost matrices a path with the smallest accumulated value is determined by dynamic programming techniques.

The semi-automatic contour detection approach consists of three steps. First, two perpendicularly cut planes which are parallel to the longitudinal axis are interactively selected. Data located at the interception of the cut planes and the voxel volume are derived to reconstruct two longitudinal images. The angle and location of the cut planes can be interactively changed by the user to obtain an optimal quality of the longitudinal images.

The second step is an interactive tracing procedure which defines the contours of the lumen and plaque in the longitudinal images. The program starts with an automatically detected contour by the minimum cost algorithm. To modify the detected contour, points can be added manually to force the contour passing through the desired positions. Since the cost matrix has been pre-calculated and stored in the memory, the longitudinal contour can be interactively retraced and updated on both the longitudinal and transverse displays. For each longitudinal image, two lumen contours and two media contours are traced (Figure 1).

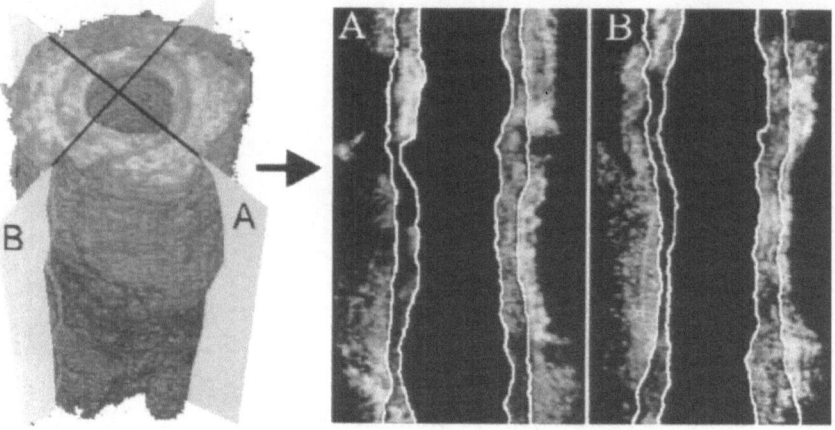

Figure 1. 3D ICUS image volume (left) is intercepted by two perpendicular planes A and B to generate two longitudinal views (right). The detected contours of the lumen and the total vessel are superimposed on the longitudinal images.

The third step is the contour detection on each cross-sectional image with information from the longitudinal contours. By transforming the contours from the two longitudinal planes to the transverse plane, four pre-defined points become available for each cross-section. These points indicate the edge positions where the contour should pass through. A cost matrix having a very low value at the four pre-defined positions is yielded from the resampled image data. An optimal path passing through the four edge points is then determined by applying the minimum cost algorithm. Finally, the optimal path is interpolated and converted back to the original coordinates to form a continuous contour in the cross-sectional plane (Figure 2, left).

Volumetric Quantification

Volumetric measurements of ICUS images can be derived from the detected contours of the lumen and the total vessel area. The cross-sectional area of the lumen and the total vessel are calculated on each echographic slice. The plaque area is calculated by subtracting the free lumen area from the total area of the vessel. The volumes of the lumen and plaque are then calculated from the following formula:

$$V = \sum_{i=0}^{N} Ai * Hi$$

where Ai is the cross-sectional area, Hi is the thickness of the slice and N is the number of slices. Resulting quantitative data such as the lumen area, plaque area and % area stenosis can be plotted as a function of vessel position to provide immediate assessment of the lesion distribution along the length of the vessel (Figure 2, right).

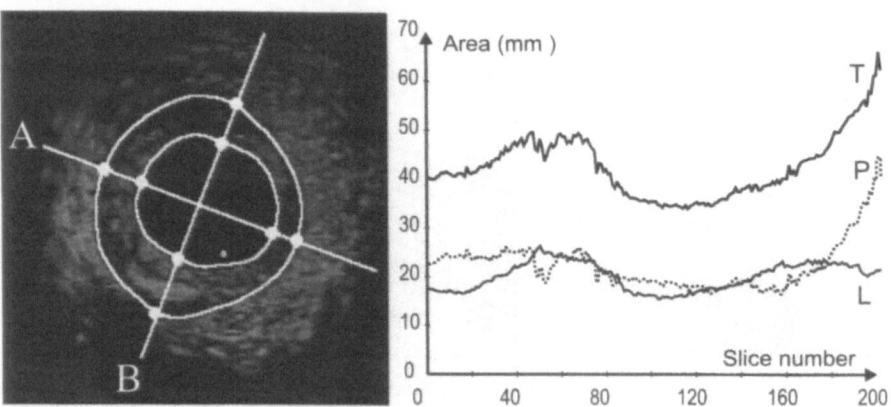

Figure 2. Left: Contour detection of a cross-sectional image on the 3D ICUS data set with 200 slices. Lines A and B indicate the intercepting positions of the two longitudinal views. The corresponding positions of the longitudinal contours are marked by the circles. The contours of the lumen and the total vessel are derived by finding an optimal contour passing through the longitudinal markers.
Right: Cross-sectional area measurements of the lumen (L), total vessel (T) and plaque (P) plotted as a function of the vessel position. The volumes of the lumen and plaque measured over a vessel length of 4 cm are 815.9 mm³ and 1715.5 mm³, respectively.

Three-Dimensional Display

Once the image segmentation has been performed, the 3D arterial objects can be reconstructed using the voxel modeling method. In this modeling approach, a pixel on the 2D echo image is extended to a 3D volume element or so-called "voxel". Each voxel is classified as a member of either the lumen or the wall structures by the detected contours. The reconstructed data sets are rendered by the depth-gradient shading method. The brightness of the voxel is computed from both the depth of the voxel to provide distance perception, and the gradient vector of the voxel to enhance the orientation of the voxel surface.

To visualize the interior structure of the vessel segment, the reconstructed arterial wall can be cut and opened longitudinally. Figure 3 shows a "clam-shell" view of a coronary artery reconstructed from 200 ultrasound images. The 3D display provides the details of the lumen surface and the longitudinal structure of the plaque.

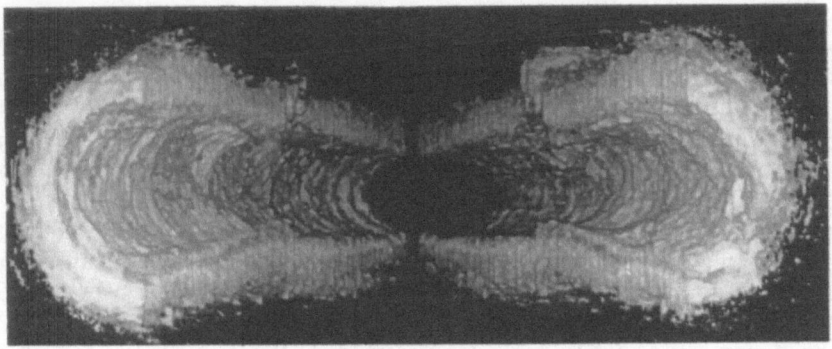

Figure 3. 3D display by opening up the ICUS volume along the sagittal plane.

Validation of the 3D system

ICUS imaging system

A mechanical rotating ICUS catheter (Microview CVIS, Sunnyvale, CA) with a distal external diameter of 2.9F was used. This ICUS imaging system is equipped with a transparent distal sleeve, covering the rotating imaging core. Using a motorized pull-back system the imaging core is withdrawn inside this sleeve. The design of the catheter and pull-back system minimizes the risk of catheter rotation and facilitates several pull-backs of the echo-transducer without increasing the risk of vessel damage, as the echo-transparent distal sleeve prevents the ICUS-transducer from coming into direct contact with the vessel wall.

In-vitro phantom study

A tubular paraffin-phantom was constructed and fixed inside a tube of acrylate. The phantom has a circular lumen with a stepwise increase in diameter (2, 3, 4, and 5 mm) each of 5 mm length. A paraffin phantom was used as its properties with regards to reflection and absorption of ultrasound are similar to those of vessel tissue. Five motorized uniform pull-backs (1 mm/s) of the ultrasound imaging transducer through the paraffin phantom were performed in water.

The mean differences in area measurements (n = 600) for all phantom segments ranged from -0.6 to 1.2%. The measured volumes (n = 20) showed a good agreement with the true phantom volume (true: 212.1 mm³, measured: 214.6 + 2.5 mm³).

In-vivo study

Intraobserver and interobserver variability of the quantification method were studied in 20 ICUS examinations of diseased, non-wedged human coronary segments in-vivo [21]. Segments with short calcifications or single major side-branches were included in the study, while an ICUS study with excessive systolic-diastolic movement was not considered for analysis. Since the imaging core is straightened during the first seconds of withdrawal, care was taken to start the pull-back 1 cm distal to the segment analyzed. The ICUS examinations were recorded on video-tape and analysis was performed off-line by the new quantitative ultrasound analysis system, using a digitization frame rate of 10 images/s. Thus, 20 mm long coronary artery segments were reconstructed and measured, utilizing the maximum memory capacity of the system which is currently 200 images.

The results of the intra- and interobserver reproducibility study are shown in Figure 4. A high correlation value (0.99) was found for coronary lumen, total vessel and plaque area measurements in both intra- and interobserver tests. The mean intraobserver differences of the volume measurements were -0.8% $\pm$ 2.1% for the lumen, -0.4$\pm$0.6% for total vessel and -0.1% $\pm$ 1.7% for plaque, respectively (M $\pm$ SD, all p = NS). Similar results were found between the two independent observers (M $\pm$ SD: lumen: -0.7% $\pm$ 2.7%, total vessel: 0.2% $\pm$ 0.7%, plaque: 1.0% $\pm$ 2.8%, all p = NS).

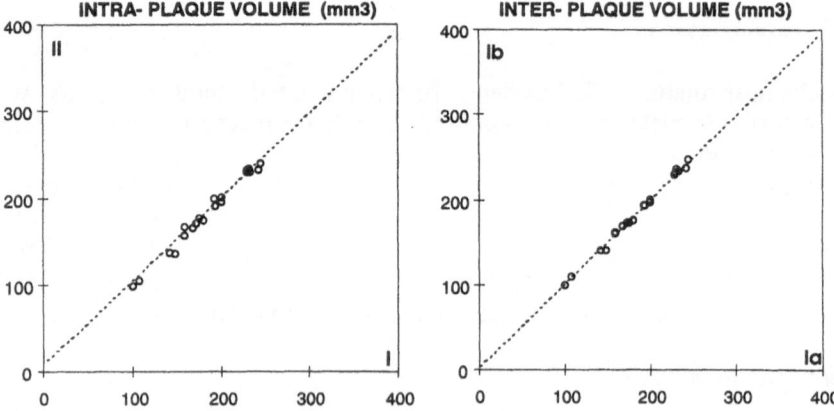

Figure 4. Plots of plaque volume measurements from 20 patient studies showing a good agreement for both intra- and interobservation.

Given the importance of direct imaging as well as quantitative analysis as described above, a number of limitations exist. Interference from strong blood scattering signals, for instance, has presented a major difficulty for automated contour detection. One of the approaches which allow to improve the image quality is to make use of the specific characteristics of blood scattering signals.

ICUS Image Enhancement

Video averaging method

From real-time ICUS imaging, it can be seen that the backscatter pattern of flowing blood varies randomly during the cardiac cycle whereas echoes of arterial tissues present a relative static pattern; this phenomenon facilitates a temporal averaging method to enhance the luminal boundary for off-line analysis [22]. Averaging a number of consecutive images over time may smoothen the changing blood scatters while preserving the relatively stable structure of the arterial wall, and thus enhance the contrast at the luminal interface on a still-frame image. The effect of averaging 8 video frames is demonstrated in Figure 5.

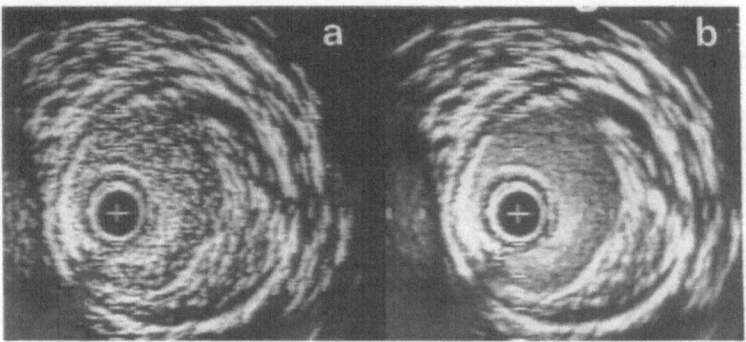

Figure 5. Image enhancement by the video averaging method. a) original single-frame image containing blood scatters; b) image obtained by averaging 8 video frames. The visibility of the arterial lumen is significantly improved on the averaged image, particularly the edge of the ruptured lesion which is difficult to recognize on the single-frame image.

The accuracy of this method was tested by comparing the lumen area measurements on the temporal-averaged image with the data of the same cross-section obtained from the single-frame images. The mean lumen area measured on the temporal-averaged images was similar to that measured on the single-frame images (mean difference: $-0.02 + 1.16$ mm^2, p = NS). Intra-observer variation in the averaging method were 2.4 times smaller than the measurements of the single-frame images (variation coefficient: single-frame: 8.8% vs averaged image: 3.6%). As main result, the temporal averaging method has shown to be helpful for off-line quantification of the luminal dimensions from images with blood scattering echoes.

One of the major concerns for the video processing method is the possible blurring effect caused by the motion of the wall or the catheter tip. Rapid motion of wall or flaps tend to disappear when applying the averaging technique in real-time. Studies on better image processing methods are therefore directed towards the more powerful possibilities using the radio-frequency (RF) echo data where faster processing can be applied, thus avoiding the time lag between the video frames.

RF Processing Method

Because blood particles usually move at a higher speed than vessel wall, the temporal characteristics of blood scattering signals will be different from those generated by the wall tissue [23]. Five in-vivo animal experiments were carried out to study temporal correlation properties of the RF data obtained from blood and tissue. After positioning the echo catheter inside the iliac artery, M-mode data were acquired at the same transmission angle with a high pulse repetition rate (Figure 6, left) and a sequence of 30 RF traces (T1, T2, ... T30) was obtained (Figure 6, middle). The correlation coefficient between the first and the subsequent RF traces was measured in the selected regions of blood and the arterial wall. The results show the blood regions have a shorter correlation time than that measured from the wall regions (Figure 6, right).

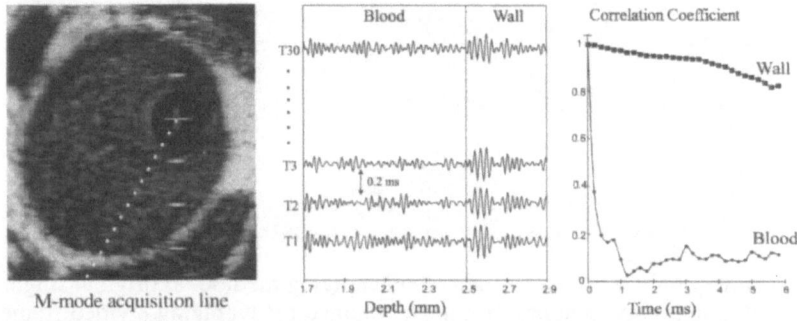

Figure 6. Illustration of RF data acquisition and correlation measurement. Left: intravascular cross-sectional image of an iliac artery. Middle: RF traces collected from the beam position indicated by the dotted line. The regions of blood and wall are defined. Right: Correlation coefficient calculated from the two regions. The curve of the blood region drops rapidly in a short delay time while the output of the wall region maintains a high value throughout the data acquisition period.

Based on the observation that blood scattering signals vary faster over time than echoes from tissue, we have developed an RF correlation weighting method for suppression of the blood echo intensity. The principle is to generate a weighting function which has a low value for blood signals against a high value elsewhere. When the correlation is calculated with a small moving window in a set of RF traces, the output of tissue regions will be highly correlated while that of blood regions will have a low value. Using this information as a weighting factor to modify the amplitudes of the RF signals, the blood echo intensity can be significantly reduced. Figure 7 illustrates an example of image enhancement by means of the correlation weighting method.

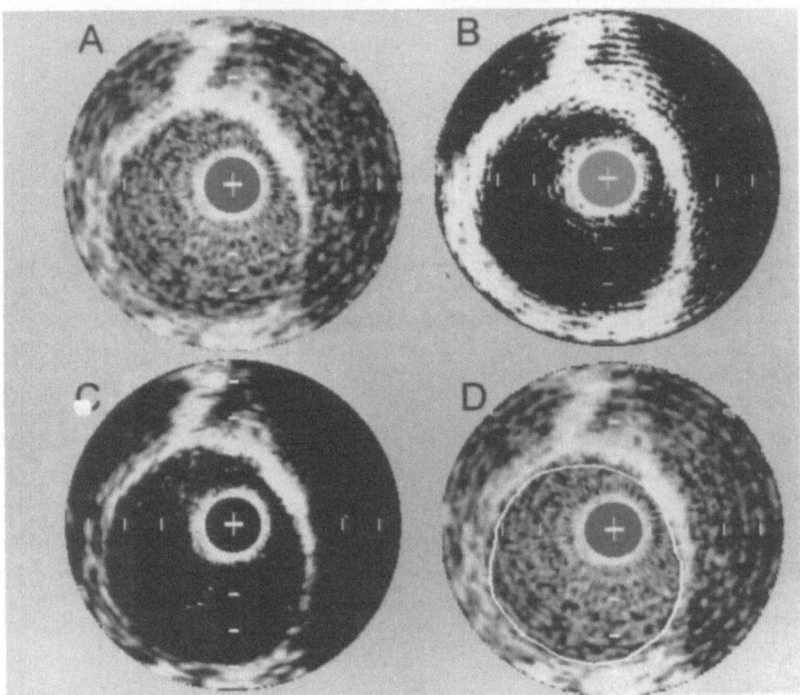

Figure 7. Image enhancement by RF correlation processing. A: image constructed with the first RF trace of each scan angle showing strong blood scattering inside the lumen. B: image constructed from the correlation weighting function obtained from 8 RF traces per angle. C: enhanced image by the RF correlation method. The blood scattering echoes are completely removed while the details of the arterial wall are preserved D: automated contour superimposed on image A. The binary structure of the weighting function allows automated image segmentation with a simple threshold method.

Quantitation of functional parameters

Flow estimation

For ICUS imaging in which the ultrasound beam is always perpendicular to the direction of blood flow, the de-correlation of blood signals is due mainly to transverse flow which causes blood particles to wash in and out of the ultrasound beam. The correlation time is thus related to the velocity of blood flow and the beam width; the faster blood particles move, the shorter the correlation time will be. This relationship could be used to estimate the flow velocity by measuring the de-correlation speed of the RF sequence. This hypothesis has been tested in an in-vitro experiment where the velocity of the blood phantom was changed by controlling the flow rate. Results show that the correlation output indeed decreases with an increase of the flow (Figure 8). An exact relationship between de-correlation and velocity needs yet to be determined.

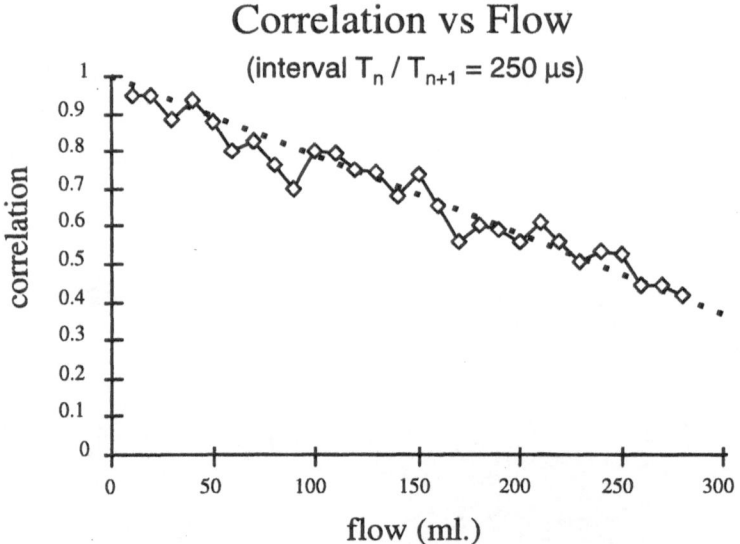

Figure 8. Relation between correlation outputs and flow rates measured in-vitro from a parabolic flow phantom.

When the de-correlation time would be measured with a moving window along the depth for all angular positions, a 2D velocity profile map could be derived from the relationship between correlation and velocity and displayed as a cross-sectional image. Since the cross-sectional area can be determined accurately with ICUS, it might become possible to estimate volumetric flow without making assumption of vessel geometry and velocity distribution. Figure 9 illustrates velocity profiles estimated from the in-vivo cross-sectional RF data set with the correlation method. The estimated profiles seem to be corresponding to an expected parabolic flow.

Intravascular elastography

It is known that the mechanical properties of tissue such as elasticity and the mechanical impedance differ for different kinds of tissue and change depending on the condition of the tissue. Two approaches to the ultrasonic measurement of these properties of intravascular tissue are being investigated.

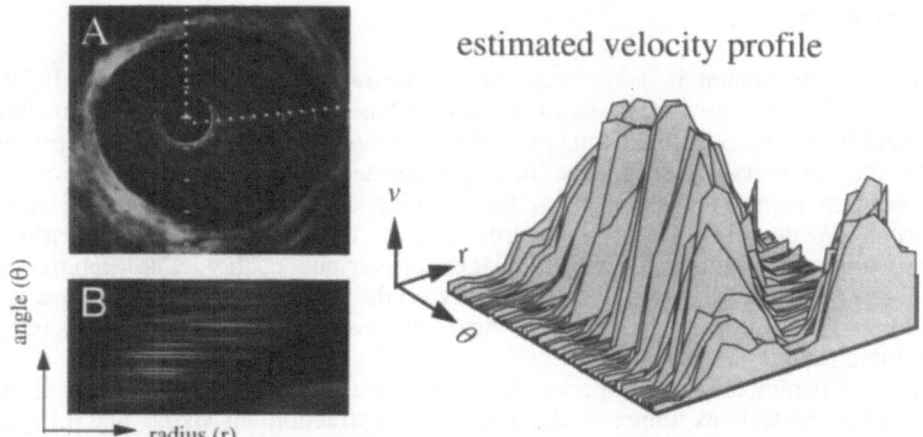

Figure 9. Example of flow estimation from the cross-sectional RF data. Left A: the original grey-scale image. Two dotted lines indicate the sector where velocity profiles were estimated. Left B: two-dimensional de-correlation map displayed in polar co-ordinates. A high image intensity presents a fast de-correlation speed. Right: Plot of the estimated velocity profiles showing a parabolic-like structure (with permission from W. Li et al. proceedings IEEE Ultrasonics Symposium 1995).

In the first approach the local radial strain is estimated as a measure of local tissue hardness. Based on the principle [24] that softer tissue will deform relatively more than harder tissue when a pressure is applied to the tissue, RF signals are acquired using two levels of endoluminal pressure. The resulting local tissue displacements are estimated by calculating the timeshift between the gated RF signals using cross correlation. The local strain is determined by calculating the finite difference of the timeshift and displayed as grey level images. Preliminary data obtained from phantoms showed the feasibility of intravascular ultrasonic hardness imaging. Hard and soft plaques can be identified from the strain images independently of the echogenicity contrast between the plaque and vessel wall, showing the potential of hardness imaging to depict information that is not available from intravascular echograms alone [25,26].

Another possible approach is a dynamic one. When an outside sound source is used, local vibration properties will differ depending on tissue properties. Studies are ongoing to calculate the possible feasibility of such an approach. The tissue will be forced to vibrate as a result of a sound wave of, for instance, 20 kHz. The amplitude of a local movement is directly related to the local mechanic properties, which can be detected using an RF signal leading to small time differences. Experiments showed that it is possible to track the local tissue displacement as a function of the 20 kHz sound field [27].

Elastography in intravascular imaging should lead to detection of local "elasticity" of the vessel wall and the atherosclerotic lesions to generate a complementary image in addition to the normal intravascular ultrasound image. This allows differentiation of plaques in a more quantitative way than just in "hard" or "soft" plaques.

Conclusion

Image segmentation is a key step for an accurate 3D quantification of ICUS images. The proposed semi-automatic method has two advantages. First, it makes use of information from the longitudinal reconstruction to guide contour detection on the transverse images. The four pre-defined longitudinal points provide important prior knowledge about the position and shape of the boundaries. Secondly, user interaction is incorporated in the minimum cost algorithm, providing possibilities to handle images of various quality. The amount of required manual definition depends mainly on the image quality; for high quality images, such as those obtained in-vitro, the contour detection can run fully automatically.

It is of paramount importance to improve the image quality in intracoronary imaging as well as improve the parameter extraction on tissue and plaque morphology. This will further simplify techniques for quantitative analysis of ICUS images. New RF signal processing methods will extend quantitative ICUS from basic morphologic parameters towards quantitation of functional parameters, such as blood flow and vessel elasticity of the coronary system.

References

1. Hodgson JMcB, Reddy KG, Suneja R, Nair RN, Lesnefsky EJ, Sheehan HM. Intracoronary ultrasound imaging: correlation of plaque morphology with angiography, clinical syndrome and procedural results in patients undergoing coronary angioplasty. J Am Coll Cardiol 1993;21:35-44.
2. Losordo DW, Rosenfield K, Kaufman J, Pieczek A, Isner JM. Focal compensatory enlargement of human arteries in response to progressive atherosclerosis. In vivo documentation using intravascular ultrasound. Circulation 1994;89:2570-7.
3. St-Goaur FG, Pinto FJ, Alderman EL *et al*. Intracoronary ultrasound in cardiac transplant recipients: in vivo evidence of "angiographically silent" intimal thickening. Circulation 1992;85:979-87.
4. Mintz GS, Potkin BN, Keren G *et al*. Intravascular ultrasound evaluation of the effect of rotational atherectomy in obstructive atherosclerotic coronary artery disease. Circulation 1992;86:1383-93.
5. Nakamura S, Colombo A, Gaglione A *et al*. Intracoronary ultrasound observations during stent implantation. Circulation 1994;89:2026-34.
6. Tenaglia AN, Buller CE, Kisslo KB, Stack RS, Davidson CJ. Mechanisms of balloon angioplasty and directional coronary atherectomy as assessed by intracoronary ultrasound. J Am Coll Cardiol 1992;20:685-91.
7. Tobis JM, Mallery JA, Gessert J *et al*. Intravascular ultrasound cross-sectional arterial imaging before and after balloon angioplasty in vitro. Circulation 1989;80:873-82.
8. Hausmann D, Friedrich G, Sudhir K *et al*. 3D intravascular ultrasound imaging with automated border detection using 2.9 F Catheters [abstract]. J Am Coll Cardiol 1994;23(Special Issue):174A.
9. Li W, Bom N, van Egmond FC. Three-dimensional quantification of intravascular ultrasound images. J Vasc Invest 1995;1:57-61.

10. Matar FA, Mintz GS, Douek P *et al*. Coronary artery lumen volume measurement using three-dimensional intravascular ultrasound: validation of a new technique. Cathet Cardiovasc Diagn 1994;32:214-20.
11. Roelandt JRTC, Di Mario C, Pandian NG *et al*. Three-dimensional reconstruction of intracoronary ultrasound images. Rationale, approaches, problems, and directions. Circulation 1994:90:1044-55.
12. Rosenfield K, Losordo DW, Ramaswamy K *et al*. Three-dimensional reconstruction of human coronary and peripheral arteries from images recorded during two-dimensional intravascular ultrasound examination. Circulation 1991;84:1938-56.
13. Li W, Bouma CJ, Gussenhoven EJ *et al*. Computer-aided intravascular ultrasound diagnostics. In: Roelandt J, Gussenhoven EJ, Bom N, editors. Intravascular Ultrasound. Dordrecht: Kluwer Academic Publishers, 1993:79-90.
14. Gerbrands JJ, Hoek C, Reiber JHC, Lie SP, Simoons ML. Minimum cost contour detection in technetium-99m gated cardiac blood pool scintigrams. Comput Cardiol 1982:253-6.
15. Reiber JHC, Serruys PW, Kooijman CJ *et al*. Assessment of short-, medium-, and long-term variations in arterial dimensions from computer-assisted quantitation of coronary cineangiograms. Circulation 1985;71:280-8.
16. Bosch JG, Reiber JHC, van Burken G *et al*. Automated endocardial contour detection in short-axis 2-D echocardiograms: 'methodology and assessment of variability. Comput Cardiol 1988:137-40.
17. Li W, Bosch JG, Zhong Y *et al*. Semiautomatic frame-to-frame tracking of the luminal border from intravascular ultrasound. Comput Cardiol 1991:353-6.
18. Sonka M, Zhang X. Siebes M *et al*. Automated segmentation of coronary wall and plaque from intravascular ultrasound image sequences. Comput Cardiol 1994:281-4.
19. Di Mario C, The SHK, Madretsma S *et al*. Detection and characterization of vascular lesions by intravascular ultrasound: an in vitro study correlated with histology. J Am Soc Echocardiogr 1992;5:135-46.
20. Li W, von Birgelen C, Di Mario C *et al*. Semi-automatic contour detection for volumetric quantification of intracoronary ultrasound. Comput Cardiol 1994:277-80.
21 Von Birgelen C, Di Mario C, Li W *et al*. Volumetric quantification in intracoronary ultrasound: validation of a new automatic contour detection method with integrated user interaction [abstract]. Circulation 1994;90(4 pt 2):I-550.
22. Li W, Gussenhoven EJ, Zhong Y *et al*. Temporal averaging for quantification of lumen dimensions in intravascular ultrasound images. Ultrasound Med Biol 1994;20:117-22.
23. Li W, van der Steen AFW, LancJe CT, Honkoop J, Gussenhoven EJ, Bom N. Temporal correlation of blood scattering signals in vivo on radio frequency intravascular ultrasound. Ultra-sound Med Biol. In press.
24. Ophir J, Cespedes I, Ponnekanti H, Yardi Y, Li X. Elastography: a quantitative method for imaging the elasticity of biological tissues. Ultrason Imaging 1991;13:111-34.
25. Cespedes I, de Korte CL, van der Steen A.F.W., Lancée CT. Intravascular ultrasound system for characterization and imaging of atherosclerotic plaque hardness [abstract]. In: Fourteenth annual Houston conference on biomedical engineering research, Houston: S.N, 1996;147.

26. Cespedes I, de Korte CL, van der Steen AFW, Lancée CT. Imaging atherosclerotic plaque hardness using intravescular ultrasound [abstract]. Ultrason Imaging. In press.
27. De Korte CL, Cespedes I, van der Steen AFW, Lancée CT. Local compressibility assessment using 20 kHz sound excitation [abstract]. Ultrason Imaging. In press.

7. Imaging atherosclerosis: lesion vs. lumen

MICHAEL V. MCCONNELL, PETER GANZ, RICHARD T. LEE,
ANDREW P. SELWYN & PETER LIBBY

Summary

Conventional coronary imaging, in the form of coronary angiography, does not
directly image the atherosclerotic lesion. Despite a marked reduction in acute
coronary events with lipid-lowering ("regression") therapy, angiography has
failed to detect significant improvement in the coronary lumen. Recent clinical
and pathobiologic data point to features within the atherosclerotic plaque, such
as the fibrous cap, lipid pool, inflammatory cell infiltrate, and extracellular
matrix, that are critical to plaque disruption and acute coronary events. Lipid-
lowering therapy may ameliorate these structural and biologic features of the
vulnerable atherosclerotic plaque. Advanced imaging techniques capable of
identifying features of the vulnerable atherosclerotic lesion are needed to elucidate
further the mechanisms of atherosclerosis progression, to identify patients at risk
for acute coronary events, and to provide a means to study novel plaque
stabilizing therapies. Ultrasound, nuclear scintigraphy, x-ray, magnetic
resonance, and light-based imaging techniques all have the potential to image
plaque components and provide more direct information about atherosclerotic
lesion vulnerability.

Background

Angiography has until recently remained unchallenged as the reference or "gold
standard" in the definition of coronary artery disease [1]. Over one million
diagnostic coronary angiograms are currently performed each year [2] and the
degree of angiographic stenosis has served as the measure of disease severity for
generations of cardiologists. The angiographic technique provides silhouette
images of the coronary lumen formed by x-ray absorption of contrast medium
dissolved in blood and works well for visualizing highly stenotic lesions.
Visualization of such high-grade stenoses has provided the criteria for
determining coronary interventions, including percutaneous transluminal coronary
angioplasty (PTCA) and coronary artery bypass grafting (CABG). Much of
contemporary cardiology and cardiac surgery rests on the axiom: the greater the
stenosis, the greater the risk of an acute clinical event such as myocardial
infarction or unstable angina.

The last decade has witnessed a profound evolution in our understanding of the
pathophysiology of coronary artery disease and acute coronary syndromes,
forcing a reassessment of our reliance on angiography. We have come to
appreciate that highly stenotic coronary atheroma, commonly associated with
stable exertional angina, are actually less frequently the cause of acute myocardial
infarction or unstable angina than mild-to-moderate coronary stenoses [3-5].

J.H.C. Reiber and E.E. van der Wall (eds.), Cardiovascular Imaging, 93-107.
© 1996 *Kluwer Academic Publishers.*

Indeed, while revascularization of high-grade stenoses effectively relieves angina, it does not necessarily prevent myocardial infarction [6]. In addition, despite substantial reductions in acute coronary events with lipid-lowering therapy, angiographic data have shown minimal change in the coronary lumen [7,8]. Finally, pathologic and biologic data have identified features of atherosclerotic plaques, such as thin fibrous caps, large lipid pools, and localized "inflammation," that are associated with plaque disruption and acute coronary syndromes [9-11]. These characteristic features of the "vulnerable" atherosclerotic plaque are invisible to angiography as this modality does not image the arterial wall and thus cannot provide direct information about plaque structure, composition, function, or biology. Better understanding of the pathobiology of atherosclerotic plaque progression and regression, and the corresponding improvement in our treatment of patients, will require imaging modalities that directly visualize the arterial wall and its salient features.

Mechanisms in the progression of coronary atherosclerosis

Endothelial dysfunction

One of the earliest features of coronary atherosclerosis is the impairment of endothelium-dependent vasodilation in both conduit and resistance coronary vessels. Even apparently healthy, asymptomatic subjects with risk factors for atherosclerosis exhibit impaired coronary vasomotion in response to endothelial-dependent stimuli [12,13]. This endothelial dysfunction is more pronounced at coronary branchpoints and stenoses and predicts more rapid development of coronary atherosclerosis in cardiac transplant patients [14,15]. Coronary endothelial dysfunction may thus provide an early indicator of patients who are prone to progress to clinical disease and may also be a marker of "active" disease - identifying patients at higher risk for acute ischemic events [16].
Impaired endothelial-dependent vasodilation is thought to result from the reduced bioavailability of nitric oxide (NO), which has both anti-atherogenic and anti-thrombotic effects in addition to being a potent vasodilator. Atherosclerosis is associated with the local generation of oxygen free radicals, which can neutralize NO activity. Thus, endothelial dysfunction may be an indicator of the oxidative "stress" to the endothelium [16]. Indeed, lipid-lowering therapy with or without antioxidant therapy improved endothelial-dependent vasomotor responses in individuals with coronary endothelial dysfunction [17,18].

Compensatory enlargement

Careful pathologic studies have shed considerable light on the mechanisms of atherosclerosis progression. Much of the growth of an atherosclerotic plaque occurs by outward, abluminal expansion. This compensatory enlargement, so-called "remodeling," of coronary arteries associated with plaque formation was first observed in monkeys fed an atherogenic diet [19,20]. This phenomenon was first reported in humans by Glagov and colleagues [21], who studied histologic sections of the left main coronary artery obtained at autopsy. It was noted that the area circumscribed by the internal elastic lamina increased as the area of the plaque contained within the lumen increased, thus preserving luminal area up to a critical point (40% area stenosis). At this point the artery appeared unable to continue to enlarge to a degree sufficient to prevent significant luminal narrowing. Similar findings were noted by other investigators in the left anterior descending, right and circumflex coronary arteries [22-24]. Angiography, by visualizing only changes in the lumen, cannot evaluate this important component of atherosclerosis progression.

Plaque rupture

Over the past 15 years, pathologic studies have confirmed that atherosclerotic plaque rupture commonly initiates unstable coronary syndromes [9,25]. Atherosclerotic plaques typically consist of a lipid-rich core in the central portion of an eccentrically thickened intima (Figure 1). The lipid core is separated from the coronary lumen by a fibrous cap, the edges of which are referred to as the "shoulder" region. The lipid-rich core typically contains many lipid-laden

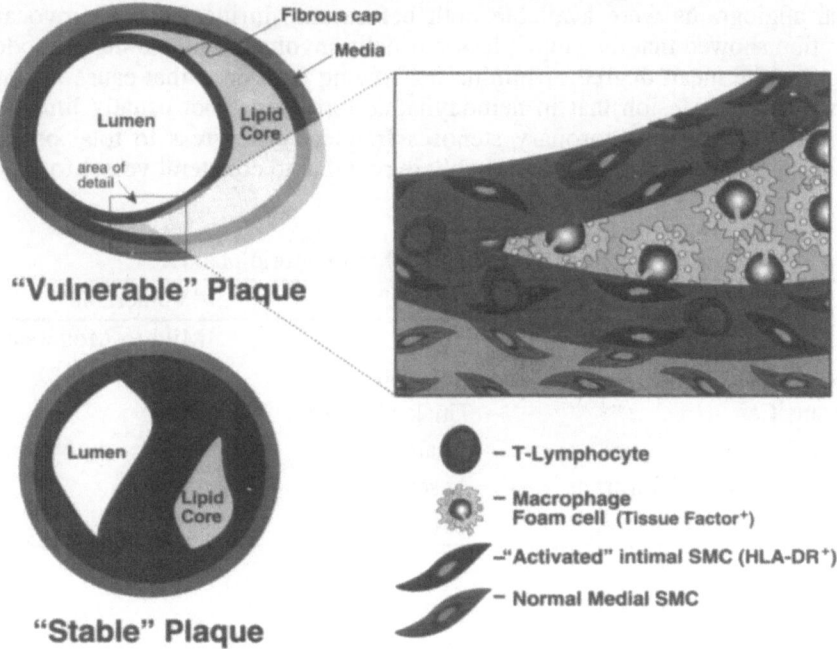

Figure 1. Schematic diagram comparing the features of "vulnerable" and "stable" atherosclerotic plaques. The vulnerable plaque typically has a large lipid core with a thin fibrous cap separating the tissue-factor-rich macrophages from the blood. The "shoulder" region is a common site of plaque rupture, with infiltration of T-lymphocytes and activation of smooth muscle cells (SMCs), as detected by expression of HLA-DR antigen. In contrast, the stable plaque has a relative thick fibrous cap and smaller lipid core. Reproduced with permission *Circulation* (Reference 11). Copyright 1995 American Heart Association.

macrophage foam cells derived from blood monocytes. These cells consume lipid and can produce large amounts of tissue factor, a powerful procoagulant. Rupture of the atherosclerotic plaque can precipitate the formation of an occlusive thrombus which causes acute myocardial infarction. Indeed, recurrent subclinical episodes of plaque disruption, with local thrombin formation and subsequent healing, may also represent one of the major pathways for progression of atherosclerotic lesions in addition to causing acute coronary syndromes.

The integrity of the fibrous cap overlying the lipid core is fundamental to the stability of the atherosclerotic plaque. "Vulnerable" plaques, i.e., those prone to rupture, tend to have thin, friable fibrous caps. Biomechanical analyses demonstrate high circumferential stress at the shoulder region of such plaques, which are frequently the sites of plaque rupture [26-28]. In contrast, "stable" plaques tend to have a smaller lipid core and thicker fibrous caps, enabling them to resist mechanical disruption (Table 1).

Counterintuitively, the degree of angiographic stenosis appears inversely related to plaque vulnerability. Thrombolytic trials, in which angiography was performed after thrombolysis in acute myocardial infarction, found that culprit atherosclerotic lesions frequently did not involve a high-grade stenosis. Trials in which angiograms were available both before and during an acute myocardial infarction showed that the culprit lesion usually involved only a mild-to-moderate stenosis. The mean degree of luminal narrowing of lesions that cause an infarct is about 50%, a lesion that in hemodynamic terms does not usually limit blood flow [3-5,27]. Severe coronary stenoses frequently progress to total occlusion without myocardial infarction, probably in part due to collateral vessel formation.

Table 1. Features of stable vs. vulnerable atherosclerotic plaque.

	"Stable"	"Vulnerable"
Degree of Luminal Stenosis	High	Mild-to-Moderate
Lesion Geometry	Concentric	Eccentric
Fibrous Cap	Thick	Thin
Lipid Pool	Small	Large
Inflammatory Cell Infiltrate	Absent	Present
Matrix Degrading Activity	Low	High

Plaque biology

Recent studies also demonstrate that local biologic factors modulate lesion vulnerability [10,11]. The ability of any tissue to withstand an imposed force depends not only on the magnitude of the force, but also on the inherent strength of the tissue. The stress-laden fibrous cap is all that stands between the blood and the thrombogenic lipid core of the plaque. The fibrous cap, as its name implies, is composed of a dense, fibrous extracellular matrix with interstitial collagens and elastin as its major components. The vascular smooth muscle cell provides the bulk of these extracellular matrix proteins. The integrity of the fibrous cap can be impaired due to decreased production and/or increased degradation of the extracellular matrix (Figure 2).

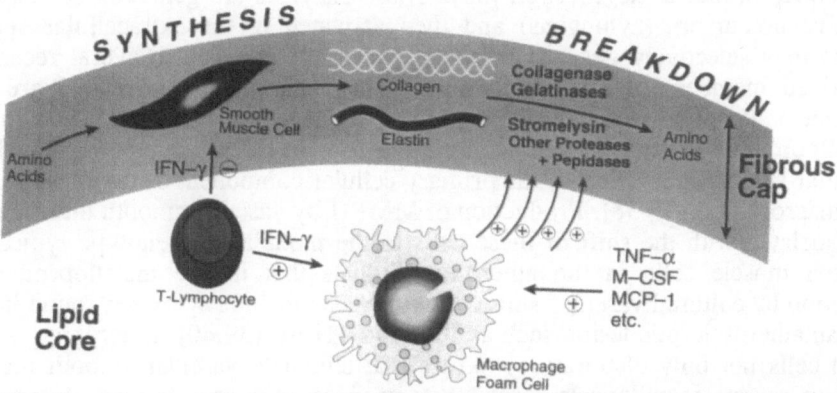

Figure 2. Schematic diagram of collagen and elastin metabolism in the fibrous cap of the atherosclerotic plaque. The extracellular matrix is synthesized by vascular smooth muscle cells from amino acids. In the vulnerable plaque, collagen synthesis can be inhibited by interferon-γ (IFN-γ) secreted by activated T-cells. In addition, activated macrophages secrete proteases that can break down collagen and elastin. Together, these effects weaken the structural integrity of the fibrous cap and make it prone to disruption and precipitation of acute coronary syndromes. Plaque macrophages can be activated by IFN-γ, secreted by the T-cells, and by tumor-necrosis factor-α (TNF-α), macrophage colony stimulating factor (M-CSF), and macrophage chemoattractant protein-1 (MCP-1), among others. Reproduced with permission *Circulation* (Reference 11). Copyright 1995 American Heart Association.

Studying the role of inflammation in vascular pathobiology, we have tested the effects of cytokines and growth factors on smooth muscle cell production of interstitial collagens. While TGF-β and PDGF increase gene expression and protein synthesis of interstitial collagen precursors, IFN-γ potently inhibits this effect [30]. Interestingly, among the cells found in human plaque, only T-lymphocytes can produce IFN-γ. Studies have shown activated T-cells in human atheroma [31], predominantly at sites of plaque rupture [32]. As evidence that these T-cells are likely producing IFN-γ, neighboring smooth muscle cells were shown to express high levels of HLA-DR, a cell surface protein characteristically induced by IFN-γ [32]. Thus, the rupture-prone shoulder region of the cap appears to be the site of active inflammation, with activated T-cells producing IFN-γ which in turn inhibits smooth muscle cell production of extracellular matrix. In addition, IFN-γ has been shown to not only inhibit smooth muscle cell proliferation, but to also promote the loss of smooth muscle cells through apoptosis, further compromising the production of extracellular matrix [33,34]. While smooth muscle cell proliferation has had a prominent role in our thinking about atherosclerosis progression, and it may indeed contribute importantly to early lesion progression, acute clinical manifestations may depend more on impaired smooth muscle cell proliferation and matrix elaboration.

Another important mechanism in reduced fibrous cap integrity is degradation of the extracellular matrix. The matrix metalloproteinase family members likely participate in matrix degradation [35]. These enzymes are generally secreted as inactive precursors (zymogens) and then activated in the extracellular space, where they selectively degrade extracellular matrix proteins. (Several recently-described members of this family have transmembrane domains and are not secreted.) Potential sources of interstitial collagenase (MMP-1) and other metalloproteinases such as stromelysin (MMP-3) in the stable atheroma include vascular smooth muscle cells, the primary cellular component of the fibrous cap, and macrophages [36-38]. Production of MMP-1 by vascular smooth muscle cells is associated with the shift of these cells to the modulated phenotype typical of smooth muscle cells in the atheroma. Signals that induce metalloproteinase secretion by cultured vascular smooth muscle cells include cytokines found in the human atherosclerotic lesion such as IL-1 and TNF-α [39,40]. Macrophages and foam cells not only elaborate cytokines that stimulate vascular smooth muscle cells to secrete metalloproteinases, they produce proteases as well. Interstitial collagenase is also contained in endothelial cells overlying human atheroma, but not in normal vessels. Directly testing human atheroma for the presence of active matrix-degrading enzymes (using in situ zymography) demonstrates that such enzyme activity is present, particularly at the vulnerable shoulder region of the plaque [41].

Thus, we now know that the fibrous cap is a dynamic connective tissue, probably with asymptomatic rupture, episodic inflammation, cell death, and ongoing synthesis and degradation of extracellular matrix components [30,32,34,42]. Biochemical, molecular, and cellular biology studies of human atheroma point to compromized structural integrity of the fibrous cap, with active inflammation and excess matrix degradation, at lethal coronary rupture sites.

Potential mechanisms for atherosclerosis "regression"

Lipid-lowering trials, as mentioned above, have shown marked reductions in clinical events. In both patients with and without clinical evidence of coronary artery disease, treatment with HMG CoA reductase inhibitors dramatically reduced cardiovascular mortality, overall mortality, and lessened the severity of myocardial ischemia [43,44]. In contrast, angiographically-monitored studies of the effect of lipid lowering on coronary luminal diameter have revealed minimal regression in stenosis severity [45,46]. This apparent paradox suggests that the small changes in lesions visualized by angiography are accompanied by much more substantial reductions in clinical events.

The results of these lipid-lowering trials raise an essential question. By what mechanism(s) does lipid-lowering produce the profound improvement in clinical outcomes in the absence of major angiographic changes? One contributing factor may be the reduction of coronary endothelial dysfunction seen with lipid-lowering (with or without antioxidant) therapy [17,18,47,48]. Increased bioavailability of NO may reduce vasoconstriction, improve coronary blood flow, and reduce the thrombotic milieu of the plaque. Another potential mechanism is that there is regression of plaque, but with reverse compensatory enlargement so that the luminal size does not change.

The most widely postulated mechanism is that lipid-lowering therapy "stabilizes" the atherosclerotic plaque. Structural changes, such as an increase in fibrous cap thickness and/or a reduction in lipid pool size, would improve the biomechanical stability of the plaque and reduce its propensity for rupture. Lipid-lowering therapy may also improve the biologic milieu within the plaque [49] by altering the lipid content, reducing oxidation, and/or decreasing the inflammatory cell infiltrate and associated matrix degradation activity.

To delineate these mechanisms of plaque "remodeling" and stabilization by "regression" therapy, we require tools to assess characteristics of atherosclerotic lesions distinct from our traditional focus on luminal caliber as revealed by contrast angiography. This will be important not only to assess patients with coronary artery disease, but also to understand more fully the mechanisms of atherosclerosis progression and regression and to aid in the development and evaluation of novel therapeutic strategies aimed at stabilization of the vulnerable atherosclerotic plaque.

Imaging the atherosclerotic lesion

No imaging technique currently has the capability to characterize fully the multiple structural and cellular components of the coronary atherosclerotic plaque (Table 2). Ultrasound is the most widely applied clinical imaging modality capable of directly imaging the arterial wall. Peripheral ultrasound has become a standard clinical tool in the evaluation of carotid artery stenosis, primarily through the use of Doppler to measure blood flow velocity rather than directly characterizing atherosclerotic plaque burden. Peripheral ultrasound has also been actively used as a research tool for measuring surrogate markers for atherosclerosis, including loss of flow-dependent vasodilation (primarily in the brachial artery) and intima-media thickening (primarily in the carotid artery) [50,51]. These methods have considerable appeal as potential noninvasive screening tests, but their direct correlation to atherosclerotic plaque vulnerability has not been demonstrated.

Intravascular ultrasound (IVUS) directly images coronary atherosclerotic plaque, providing high resolution cross-sectional views of the vessel lumen and wall for quantitative measurement of lumen area, plaque area, and vessel area [52-57]. Studies with IVUS provided an *in vivo* validation of the capacity for compensatory enlargement in atherosclerotic coronary arteries in humans [58-61]. While capable of detecting lesion geometry and calcification [62], current IVUS imaging cannot adequately distinguish features of the vulnerable plaque, such as fibrous cap thickness and lipid pool size. However, IVUS technology continues to evolve rapidly (higher resolution 40 MHz transducers, enhanced signal processing), and may in the future permit more comprehensive imaging of plaque structural components.

Nuclear scintigraphy has been used to noninvasively identify atherosclerotic plaque. Radio-labeling LDL particles or antibodies to proliferating smooth muscle

Table 2. Comparison of current *in vivo* modalities for imaging atherosclerotic plaque.

	Luminal Stenosis	Wall Thickness	Fibrous vs. Lipid	Calcification	Plaque Rupture	Notes
X-ray Angiography	+	-	-	+/-	+/-	Invasive; Iodinated contrast agent
Ultrasound/IVUS	+	+	-	+	+/-	Peripheral: noninvasive; Coronary: invasive
Nuclear Scintigraphy	-	-	*	-	-	Noninvasive; *Target based on radio-labeling
Computed Tomography	+	+/-	-	+	-	Noninvasive; Iodinated contrast agent
Magnetic Resonance	+	+	+	+/-	+	Noninvasive; Coronary imaging limited by motion
Angioscopy	+	-	-	-	+	Invasive; Laser-based method in development

cells, for example, has been used for plaque imaging [63,64]. Unfortunately, the spatial resolution is poor and plaque structure is not elucidated. Ultrafast computed tomography (CT) is capable of noninvasively detecting human coronary artery calcification, one structural component of atherosclerotic plaque [65,66]. Due to its limited soft tissue characterization capability, however, CT is unlikely to be able to image other plaque components, such as fibrous and lipid regions, which are crucial to plaque stability.

Recent improvements in magnetic resonance (MR) technology now allow for noninvasive high-resolution structural imaging, termed MR microscopy. The tissue characterization properties of MR imaging give it the capability to distinguish plaque components, such as fibrous vs. lipid regions, and to detect plaque disruption [67-69]. To date, in vivo plaque imaging has been applied in both animal models of aortic and carotid atherosclerosis and in human carotid artery disease [69-71]. Further improvements in structural resolution and tissue characterization can be expected with technical advances, including higher magnetic field strength, stronger and faster gradient coils, and specialized radiofrequency receiver coils. For noninvasive MR imaging of coronary plaque, however, significant additional improvements in methods to limit respiratory and cardiac motion artifacts will be needed. Another MR approach to vascular plaque imaging (with potential application to the coronaries) is the use of an intravascular MR receiver coil. Initial prototypes suffer from inadequate methods for minimizing catheter motion within the vessel [72], which degrades image quality.

Angioscopy, as a light-based imaging modality, has been used to directly image coronary plaques [73,74]. However, it visualizes the plaque surface and thus has limited ability to characterize plaque structure. The use of reflected laser light, so-called optical coherence tomography, is capable of *in vitro* imaging of coronary plaque features at a depth of 1-2 mm with a spatial resolution of 10-20 microns [75]. While promising, technical challenges remain for the implementation of this technique *in vivo*.

Future directions

Imaging plaque biology

While imaging plaque structure would be a significant advance, assessing the biologic state of the plaque may be of equal or greater importance to determining its vulnerability. Nuclear scintigraphy has potential through the use of monoclonal antibodies to active plaque markers (e.g., adhesion molecules, oxidized LDL, activated T-cells or smooth muscle cells) [74], but has been limited by spatial resolution. The use of labeled monoclonal antibodies for MR imaging is another potential approach [76], but is currently limited by low signal-to-noise ratio.

Even more detailed biologic information could be obtained with spectroscopic techniques. MR spectroscopy of atheroma lipids *in vitro* has been used to quantify cholesterol ester content between obstructive and nonobstructive plaques [77]. Raman spectroscopy, using reflected laser light, has been shown to discern aortic plaque collagen, elastin, and cholesterol esters [78]. These techniques are far from practical *in vivo* use today, but offer the future promise of imaging plaque biology.

Cost-effective clinical application

There is clearly a need to identify better which patients will develop clinically-significant coronary artery disease. Clinical risk factors alone are not adequate and the initial symptoms can include myocardial infarction or sudden death. In addition, despite the marked reduction in clinical events with lipid-lowering therapy, coronary artery disease is still the primary cause of death in many clinical trails. Methods are needed to determine a patient's response to therapy and to test new therapeutic approaches. Hopefully, cost considerations will not cause the premature abandonment of promising technologies.

However, in the increasingly cost-conscious environment in which medicine now operates, cost-effective approaches to screening and therapy must be developed and tested. One screening approach is to use noninvasive surrogate markers, such as brachial artery vasomotor response or carotid intima-media thickness, to identify patients at risk and offer early, aggressive risk-reduction and lipid-lowering therapy. Catheter-based approaches to coronary plaque imaging (e.g., IVUS, angioscopy) could not be justified as screening tests and would primarily be applied in patients with known disease to further risk stratify. The development of a noninvasive coronary plaque imaging technique, such as MRI, would be ideal. However, it would have to be shown to be both sensitive and specific, and its use to guide therapy would have to be shown to be cost-effective. Clearly, significant advancement needs to occur in order to provide a safe, accurate, and cost-effective imaging technique to characterize coronary atherosclerotic plaque. Observations both on the bench and at the bedside have shown us that our current approach to coronary imaging has not kept pace with our understanding of the mechanisms of plaque progression, regression, and acute events. The current inability to perform detailed plaque imaging *in vivo* is an impediment to improved patient care and further progress in unraveling the complexities of the atherosclerotic process. As coronary imaging shifts its focus from the coronary lumen to the atherosclerotic lesion, both patients and researchers stand to benefit.

References

1. White CW, Wright CB, Doty DB *et al*. Does visual interpretation of the coronary arteriogram predict the physiologic importance of a coronary stenosis? N Engl J Med 1984;310:819-24.
2. Heart and stroke facts: 1996 statistical supplement. Dallas: American Heart Association, 1996.
3. Ambrose JA, Tannenbaum MA, Alexopoulos D *et al*. Angiographic progression of coronary artery disease and the development of myocardial infarction. J Am Coll Cardiol 1988;12:56-62.
4. Little WC, Constantinescu M, Applegate RJ *et al*. Can coronary angiography predict the site of a subsequent myocardial infarction in patients with mild-to-

moderate coronary artery disease? Circulation 1988;78:1157-66.

5.1 Fuster V, Badimon L, Badimon JJ, Chesebro JH. The pathogenesis of coronary artery disease and the acute coronary syndromes (1). N Engl J Med 1992;326:242-50.

5.2 Fuster V, Badimon L, Badimon JJ, Chesebro JH. The pathogenesis of coronary artery disease and the acute coronary syndromes (2). N Engl J Med 1992;326:310-8.

6. Hillis L. Coronary artery bypass surgery. risks and benefits, realise and unrealistic expectations. J Investig Med 1995;43:17-27.

7. Blankenhorn DH, Hodis HN, George Lyman Duff Memorize Lecture. Arterial imaging and atherosclerosis reversal. Arterioscler Thromb 1994;14:177-92.

8. Brown BG, Zhao XQ, Sacco DE, Albers JJ. Lipid lowering and plaque regression. New insights into prevention of plaque disruption and clinical events in coronary disease. Circulation 1993;87:1781-91.

9. Davies MJ, Thomas AC. Plaque fissuring: the cause of acute myocardial infarction, sudden ischeamic death, and crescendo angina. Br Heart J 1985;53:363-73.

10. Falk E, Shah PK, Fuster V. Coronary plaque disruption. Circulation 1995;92:657-71.

11. Libby P. Molecular bases of the acute coronary syndromes. Circulation 1995;91:2844-50.

12. Vita JA, Treasure CB, Nabel EG *et al.* The coronary vasomotor response to acetylcholine relates to risk factors for coronary artery disease. Circulation 1990;81:491-7.

13. Reddy KG, Nair RN, Sheehan HM, Hodgson JM. Evidence that selective endothelial dysfunction may occur in the absence of angiographic or ultrasound atherosclerosis in patients with risk factors for atherosclerosis. J Am Coll Cardiol 1994;23:833-43.

14. McLenachan JM, Vita JA, Fish DR *et al.* Early evidence of endothelial vasodilator dysfunction at coronary branchpoints. Circulation 1990;82:1169-73.

15. Davis SF, Yeung AC, Meredith IT *et al.* Early endothelial dysfunction predicts the development of transplant coronary artery disease at one year post transplant. Circulation 1996;93:457-62.

16. Harrison DG, Ohara Y. Physiologic consequences of increased vascular oxident stresses in hypercholesterolemia and atherosclerosis: implications for impaired vasomotion. Am J Cardiol 1995;75:75B-81B.

17. Anderson TJ, Meredith IT, Yeung AC, Frei B, Selwyn AP, Ganz P. The effect of cholesterol-lowering and antioxidant therapy on endothelium-dependent coronary vasomotion. N Engl J Med 1995;332:488-93.

18. Treasure CB, Klein JL, Weintraub WS *et al.* Beneficial effects of cholesterol-lowering therapy on the coronary endothelium in patients with coronary artery disease. N Engl J Med 1995;332:481-7.

19. Bond MG, Adams MR, Bullock BC. Complicating factors in evaluating coronary artery atherosclerosis. Artery 1981;9:21-9.

20. Armstrong ML, Heistad DD, Marcus ML, Megan MB, Piegors DJ. Structural and hemodynamic responses of peripheral arteries of macaque monkeys to atherogenic diet. Arteriosclerosis 1985;5:336-46.

21. Glagov S, Weisenberg E, Zarins CK, Stankunavicius R, Kolettis GJ. Compensatory enlargement of human atherosclerotic coronary arteries. N Engl J Med 1987;316:1371-5.

22. Stiel GM, Stiel LSG, Schofer J, Donath K, Mathey DG. Impact of compensatory enlargement of atherosclerotic coronary arteries on angiographic assessment of coronary artery disease. Circulation 1989;80:1603-9.

23. Zarins CK, Weisenberg E, Kolettis G, Stankunavicius R, Glagov S. Differential enlargment of artery segments in response to enlarging atherosclerotic plaques. J Vasc Surg 1988;7:386-94.

24. Clarkson TB, Prichard RW, Morgan TM, Petrick GS, Klein PS. Remodeling of coronary arteries in human and nonhuman primates. JAMA 1994;271:289-94.

25. Davies MJ. A macro and micro view of coronary vascular insult in ischemic heart disease. Circulation 1990;823 (Suppl.):II-38-46.

26. Richardson PD, Davies MJ, Born GV. Influence of plaque configuration and stress distribution on fissuring of coronary atherosclerotic plaques. Lancet 1989;2:941-4.

27. Loree HM, Kamm RD, Stringfellow RG, Lee RT. Effects of fibrous cap thickness on peak circumferential stress in model atherosclerotic vessels. Circ Res 1992;71:850-8.

28. Cheng GC, Loree HM, Kamm RD, Fishbein MC, Lee RT. Distribution of circumferential stress in ruptured and stable atherosclerotic lesions. A structural analysis with histopathological correlation. Circulation 1993;87:1179-87.

29. Giroud D, Li JM, Urban P, Meier B, Rutishauser W. Relation of the site of acute myocardial infarction to the most severe coronary arterial stenosis at prior angiography. Am J Cardiol 1992;69:729-32.

30. Amento EP, Ehsani N, Palmer H, Libby P. Cytokines and growth factors positively and negatively regulate interstitial collagen gene expression in human vascular smooth muscle cells. Arterioscler Thromb 1991;11:1223-30.

31. Hansson GK, Holm J, Jonasson L. Detection of activated T lymphocytes in the human atherosclerotic plaque. Am J Pathol 1989;135:169-75.

32. van der Wal AC, Becker AE, Van der Loos CM, Das PK. Site of intimal rupture or erosion of thrombosed coronary atherosclerotic plaques is characterized by an inflammatory process irrespective of the dominant plaque morphology. Circulation 1994;89:36-44.

33. Warner SJC, Friedman GB, Libby P. Immune interferon inhibits proliferation and induces 2'-5' oligoadenylate synthetase gene expression in human vascular smooth muscle cells. J Clin Invest 1989;83:1174-82.

34. Geng YJ, Libby P. Evidence for apoptosis in advanced human atheroma. Colocalization with Interleukin-1 beta-converting enzyme. Am J Pathol 1995;147:251-66.

35. Shah PK, Falk E, Badimon JJ et al. Human monocyte-derived macrophages induce collagen breakdown in fibrous caps of atherosclerotic plaques. Potential role of matrix-degrading metalloproteinases and implications for plaque rupture. Circulation 1995;92:1565-9.

36. Henney AM, Wakeley PR, Davies MJ et al. Localization of stromelysin gene expression in atherosclerotic plaques by in situ hybridization. Proc Natl Acad Sci USA 1991;88:8154-8.

37. Nikkari ST, O'Brien KD, Ferguson M et al. Interstitial collagenase (MMP-1) expression in human carotid atherosclerosis. Circulation 1995;92:1393-8.

38. Galis ZS, Sukhova GK, Kranzhofer R, Clark S, Libby P. Macrophage foam cells from experimental atheroma constitutively produce matrix-degrading proteinases. Proc Natl Acad Sci USA 1995;92:402-6.

39. Barath P, Fishbein MC, Cao J, Berenson J, Helfant RH, Forrester JS. Detection

and localization of tumor necrosis factor in human atheroma. Am J Cardiol 1990;65:297-302.

40. Fleet JC, Clinton SK, Salomon RN, Loppnow H, Libby P. Atherogenic diets enhance endotoxin-stimulated interleukin-1 and tumor necrosis factor gene expression in rabbit aortae. J Nutr 1992;122:294-305.

41. Galis ZS, Sukhova GK, Libby P. Microscopic localization of active proteases by in situ zymography: detection of matrix metalloproteinase activity in vascular tissue. FASEB J 1995;9:974-80.

42. Galis ZS, Sukhova GK, Lark MW, Libby P. Increased expression of matrix metalloproteinases and matrix degrading activity in vulnerable regions of human atherosclerotic plaques. J Clin Invest 1994;94:2493-503.

43. Shepherd J, Cobbe SM, Ford I et al. Prevention of coronary heart disease with pravastatin in men with hypercholesterolemia. West of Scotland Coronary Prevention Study Group. N Engl J Med 1995;333:1301-7.

44. Randomized trial of cholesterol lowering in 4444 patients with coronary heart disease: the Scandinavian Simvastatin Survival Study (4S). Lancet 1994;344:1383-9.

45. Levine GN, Keaney JF Jr, Vita JA. Cholesterol reduction in cardiovascular disease. Clinical benefits and possible mechanisms. N Engl J Med 1995;332:512-21.

46. Vos J, De Feyter PJ, Simoons ML, Tijssen JGP, Deckers JW. Retardation and arrest of progression or regression of coronary artery disease: a review. Prog Cardiovasc Dis 1993;35:435-54.

47. Leung WH, Lau CP, Wong CK. Beneficial effect of cholesterol-lowering therapy on coronary endothelium-depedent relaxation in hypercholesterolaemic patients. Lancet 1993;341:1496-500.

48. Egashira K, Hirooka Y, Kai H et al. Reduction in serum cholesterol with pravastatin improves endothelium-dependent coronary vasomotion in patients with hypercholesterolemia. Circulation 1994;89:2519-24.

49. Harrison DG, Armstrong ML, Freiman PC, Heistad DD. Restoration of endothelium-dependent relaxation by dietary treatment of atherosclerosis. J Clin Invest 1987;80:1808-11.

50. Anderson TJ, Uehata A, Gerhard MD et al. Close relation of endothelial function in the human coronary and peripheral circulations. J Am Coll Cardiol 1995;26:1235-41.

51. Craven TE, Ryu JE, Espeland MA et al. Evaluation of the associations between carotid artery atherosclerosis and coronary artery stenosis. A case-control study. Circulation 1990;82:1230-42.

52. Nishimura RA, Edwards WD, Warner CA et al. Intravascular utrasound imaging: In vitro validation and pathologic correlation. J Am Coll Cardiol 1990;16:145-54.

53. Hodgson JM, Reddy KG, Suneja R, Nair RN, Lesnefsky EJ, Sheehan HM. Intracoronary ultrasound imaging: correlation of plaque morphology with angiography, clinical syndrome and procedural results in patients undergoing coronary angioplasty. J Am Coll Cardiol 1993;21:35-44.

54. Tobis JM, Mallery J, Mahon D et al. Intravascular ultrasound imaging of human coronary arteries in vivo. Analysis of tissue characterizations with comparison to in vitro histological specimens. Circulation 1991;83:913-26.

55. Hausmann D, Lundkvist AJS, Friedrich GJ, Mullen WL, Fitzgerald PJ, Yock PG. Intracoronary ultrasound imaging: intraobserver and interobserver

variability of morphometric measurements. Am Heart J 1994;128:674-80.

56. Nissen SE, Tuzcu EM, DeFranco AC. Coronary intravascular ultrasound: Diagnostic and interventional applications. In: Topol EJ, editor. Textbook of: interventional cardiology. 2nd ed. Philadelphia: Saunders, 1994:207-22.

57. Higano ST, Nishimura RA. Intravascular ultrasonography. Curr Probl Cardiol 1994;19:1-55.

58. Hermiller JB, Tenaglia AN, Kisslo KB et al. In vivo validation of compensatory enlargement of atherosclerotic coronary arteries. Am J Cardiol 1993;71:665-8.

59. Gerber TC, Erbel R, Görge G, Ge J, Rupprecht HJ, Meyer J. Extent of atherosclerosis and remodeling of the left main coronary artery determined by intravascular ultrasound. Am J Cardiol 1994;73:666-71.

60. Ge J, Erbel R, Zamorano J et al. Coronary artery remodeling in atherosclerotic disease: an intravasuclar ultrasonic study in vivo. Coron Artery Dis 1993;4:981-6.

61. Losordo DW, Rosenfield K, Kaufman J, Pieczek A, Isner JM. Focal compensatory enlargement of human arteries in response to progressive atherosclerosis. In vivo documentation using intravascular ultrasound. Circulation 1994;89:2570-7.

62. Kimura BJ, Russo RJ, Bhargava V et al. Atheroma morphology and distribution in proximal left anterior descending coronary artery: in vivo observations. J Am Coll Cardiol 1996;27:825-31.

63. Lees AM, Lees RS, Schoen FJ et al. Imaging human atherosclerosis with 99mTc-labeled low density lipoproteins. Arteriosclerosis 1988;8:461-70.

64. Narula J, Petrov A, Bianchi C et al. Noninvasive localization of experimental atherosclerotic lesions with mouse/human chimeric Z2D3 F(ab')2 specific for the proliferating smooth muscle cells of human atheroma. Imaging with conventional and negative charge-modified antibody fragments. Circulation 1995;92:474-84.

65. Breen JF, Sheedy PF 2nd, Schwartz RS et al. Coronary artery calcification detected with ultrafast CT as an indication of coronary artery disease. Radiology 1992;185:435-9.

66. Budoff MJ, Georgiou D, Brody A et al. Ultrafast computed tomography as a diagnostic modality in the detection of coronary artery disease: a multicenter study. Circulation 1996;93:898-904.

67. Toussaint JF, Southern JF, Fuster V, Kantor HL. T2-weighted contrast for NMR characterization of human atherosclerosis. Arterioscler Thromb Vasc Biol 1995;15:1533-42.

68. Yuan C, Tsuruda JS, Beach KN et al. Techniques for high-resolution MR imaging of atherosclerotic plaque. J Magn Reson Imaging 1994;4:43-9.

69. Skinner MP, Yuan C, Mitsumori L et al. Serial magnetic resonance imaging of experimental atherosclerosis detects lesion fine structure, progression and complications in vivo. Nat Med 1995;1:69-73.

70. Summers RM, Hedlund LW, Cofer GP, Gottsman MB, Manibo JF, Johnson GA. MR microscopy of the rat carotid artery after balloon injury by using an implanted imaging coil. Magn Reson Med 1995;33:785-9.

71. Nelson JA, Yuan C, Hatsukami TS. MR cardiovascular imaging. Nat Med 1995;1:996-7.

72. Martin AJ, Henkelman RM. Intravascular MR imaging in a porcine animal model. Magn Reson Med 1994;32:224-9.

73. Sherman CT, Litvack F, Grundfest W et al. Coronary angioscopy in patients

with unstable angina pectoris. N Engl J Med 1986;315:913-9.

74. Ueda Y, Asakura M, Hirayama A, Komamura K, Hori M, Kodama K. Intracoronary morphology of culprit lesions after reperfusion in acute myocardial infarction: serial angioscopic observations. J Am Coll Cardiol 1996;27:606-10.

75. Brezinski ME, Tearney GJ, Bouma BE *et al.* Optical coherence tomography for optical biopsy. Properties and demonstration of vascular pathology. Circulation 1996;93:1206-13.

76. Sipkins DA, Gijbels K, Tropper FD, Steinman L, Bednarski MD, Li KCP. Antibody-conjugated paramagnetic liposomes: tissue specific contrast agents for disease processes [abstract]. Proc Soc Magn Reson 1995;1139.

77. Toussaint JF, Southern JF, Fuster V, Kantor HL. 13C-NMR spectroscopy of human atherosclerotic lesions. Relation between fatty acid saturation, cholesteryl ester content, and luminal obstruction. Arterioscler Thromb 1994;14:1951-7.

78. Baraga JJ, Feld MS, Rava RP. In situ optical histochemistry of human artery using near infrared Fourier transform Raman spectroscopy. Proc Natl Acad Sci USA 1992;89:3473-7.

8. An overview of fluvastatin clinical trials

AD VAN BOVEN & PASCAL PFISTER

Summary

Cholesterol-lowering therapy has been reported to reduce cardiac morbidity and mortality and has established its place in cardiovascular medicine as secondary prevention. Recent trials using HMG-CoA reductase inhibitors show an effect on clinical events which cannot be attributed to the effect on cholesterol only. Fluvastatin (LESCOL) is a new synthetic HMG-CoA reductase inhibitor with a good tolerability, a cholesterol lowering capacity comparable to other statins and special effects on the vascular wall as well as on platelet function. Retrospective analysis from data files shows an overall reduction in serious events of 25.5% in ± 3000 patients treated with this drug for several years, which is comparable with other studies. Clinical trials with fluvastatin are still ongoing and more results are expected by the end of 1996. Recent study aims are whether fluvastatin reduces restenosis and events peri-PTCA (FLARE, LIPS) and whether fluvastatin reduces progression of coronary atherosclerosis and improvement of perfusion and metabolism assessed by positron emission tomography (LCAS and 4P). Economic analyses performed with fluvastatin suggest that this drug is more cost-effective than other available HMG-CoA reductase inhibitors, which is of interest for the treatment of hypercholesterolemia in primary prevention.

Introduction

The clinical benefits of lowering cholesterol have been accruing over the last 20 years. Prior to the advent of HMG-CoA reductase inhibitors, clofibrate [1], cholestyramine [2], niacin [3], colestipol [4] and gemfibrozil [5] demonstrated a reduction in coronary heart disease (CHD) morbidity and mortality in line with lowering serum cholesterol, especially low-density lipoprotein cholesterol (LDL-C). In addition to the medical management of hypercholesterolemia, studies using surgery (POSCH ileal bypass) [6] and life-style changes [7] have also demonstrated a significant benefit. This indicated that lipid lowering per se was the key factor, not the means by which it was reduced.

The widespread availability of HMG-CoA reductase inhibitors has added considerably to our knowledge of secondary prevention. In patients with existing ischemic heart disease, MAAS [8], MARS [9], CCAIT [10] and REGRESS [11] showed that reduction of cholesterol reduced the progression and enhanced regression of atherosclerosis. However, the data were still not convincing in showing that lowering cholesterol prolongs life, especially as the reduction in CHD deaths was offset by an apparent increase in non-cardiac mortality such as cancer, suicide and violent death [12,13]. The Scandinavian Simvastatin Survival Study (4S) [14] demonstrated a convincing benefit of lipid lowering with an HMG-CoA reductase inhibitor on total mortality, its sole primary endpoint. The

J.H.C. Reiber and E.E. van der Wall (eds.), Cardiovascular Imaging, 109-118.
© 1996 *Kluwer Academic Publishers.*

reduction in total mortality of 30% was highly significant, attributable to a 42% decrease in ischemic heart disease mortality. Moreover, there were no significant differences between the HMG-CoA reductase inhibitor and placebo groups in non-cardiovascular mortality. The clinical benefit of lipid lowering in secondary prevention is further illustrated by a prospectively scheduled meta-analysis of four 2- and 3-year vascular-endpoint clinical trials using another HMG-CoA reductase inhibitor [15]. Although entry criteria differed among the trials, patients had moderate hypercholesterolemia and the majority had evidence of CHD. In the intervention groups, there was a statistically significant reduction in risk of non-fatal myocardial infarction (MI) or CHD death and a large, but not statistically significant reduction in total mortality. The evidence for lowering cholesterol in secondary prevention now appears to be confirmed beyond reasonable doubt, but primary prevention has remained controversial until the results of the West of Scotland Coronary Prevention Study (WOSCOPS) became available recently [16]. In men with hypercholesterolemia but without history of myocardial infarction, a reduction in plasma cholesterol of 20% significantly reduced the incidence of MI and death from cardiovascular causes without adversely affecting the risk of death from non-cardiovascular causes. The key issue within the debate seems to have been resolved by the use of meta-analysis of data from 10 prospective (cohort) studies, three international studies in different communities and 28 randomized controlled trials [17]. The data were from studies using diet, ileal bypass, clofibrate, gemfibrozil, cholestyramine, niacin, probucol, lovastatin or combinations. The meta-analysis showed a "striking consistency between different categories of data". A reduction in cholesterol of 23 mg/dl (approximately 10%) is associated with a decrease in the risk of ischemic heart disease of 40% at 50 years of age and 30% at 60 years of age.

While the meta-analysis was undertaken prior to the 4S results and while the lowering of cholesterol was higher in 4S than in previous studies, the results are consistent with the estimates of Law et al. [16], confirming that the reduction in morbidity and mortality is a function of lowering cholesterol, by whatever means. The existing data also demonstrate that the HMG-CoA reductase inhibitors as a specific class have the capacity to lower cholesterol to a greater extent than previous therapies and that the potential benefit is also greater. This is a directly proportional relationship, not an all-or-nothing response dependent on a fixed percentage reduction.

There is little doubt that the benefits of lowering cholesterol with an HMG-CoA reductase inhibitor are generally considered to be a class effect. The ethical considerations and time requirements of repeating identical cardiovascular event studies prohibit this possibility. New studies addressing the issue in subgroups not yet studied should start (ie, long-term effect of HMG-CoA reductase inhibitors on cardiovascular morbidity in post-PTCA patients). However, retrospective analysis of the fluvastatin database of 2969 patients, representing 4051 patient-years of exposure with an average reduction in LDL-C of 26% add to the consistency seen from all other studies [18]. In total, serious adverse events occurred at a rate of 21/1000 patient-years with fluvastatin against 28.2/1000 patient-years with placebo; a reduction of 25.5% (33.3% in long-term studies). While these data are not truly prospective, the benefits of lowering cholesterol with fluvastatin, and their consistency with results from prospective trials with other HMG-CoA reductase inhibitors, cannot be overlooked.

It is also interesting to observe the levels of serum cholesterol at entry into the recent events studies of HMG-CoA reductase inhibitors and compare the reductions to those achieved in all studies with this class of drug. The serum cholesterol level at entry ranged from 230 mg/dl in MARS to 272 mg/dl in WOSCOPS (Table 1).

Table 1. Average levels of serum cholesterols at entry and completion in recent HMG-CoA reductase inhibitor studies.

	Mean total cholesterol at entry (mg/dl)	Mean total cholesterol at completion (mg/dl)	% change
MARS [9]	230	155	-32%
MAAS [8]	244	190	-22%
CCAIT [10]	250	196	-21%
REGRESS [11]	233	189	-20%
4S [14]	260	194	-25%
WOSCOPS [16]	272	218	-20%

(to convert values for total cholesterol to mmol/l divide by 38.67)

With the exception of MARS, which had the lowest entry level of serum cholesterol and the largest percentage reduction, the other studies show a reasonably consistent pattern. The levels of reduction of total serum cholesterol are certainly within the range of that achieved with fluvastatin in published clinical trials, ranging from -15% with 20 mg daily to -34% with 80 mg fluvastatin. Total serum cholesterol reductions for marketed HMG-CoA reductase inhibitors are shown in Table 2.

Analysis of the fluvastatin database has also shown that the percent change in main lipid and lipoprotein parameters is independent of the baseline level of hypercholesterolemia [17].

These data would support the class effectiveness of the HMG-CoA reductase inhibitor in lowering serum cholesterol and similar figures can be produced for LDL-C as a measure of efficacy. Moreover, data produced in the United States indicate that the majority of hypercholesterolemic patients require a 20% to 25% reduction in LDL-C [19] to meet target levels recommended by the NCEPII guidelines [20]. While the absolute values from the United States differ to those in Europe the percentage reduction requirement is very similar. Prescription data also indicate that 75% of the usage of HMG-CoA reductase inhibitors is in the dosage range producing a 20-30% reduction in LDL-C, ie ≤20 mg for pravastatin and ≤10 mg for simvastatin, and 20-40 mg for fluvastatin. The level of cholesterol reduction appears to be in line also with the recommendations of the European Atherosclerosis Society [21] and give no support to use of different HMG-CoA reductase inhibitors for different levels of hypercholesterolemia. Any variability that may exist between HMG-CoA reductase inhibitors would suggest that, on a mg-for-mg basis, simvastatin should be used in those patients with

Table 2. Range of total cholesterol reduction in clinical trials with HMG-CoA reductase inhibitors.

HMG-COA REDUCTASE INHIBITOR	Dose (mg/day)	Range of total cholesterol reduction (%)
Fluvastatin	20	-15 to -18
	40	-18 to -27
	80	-30 to -37 *
Pravastatin	10	-11 to -19
	20	-16 to -24
	40	-19 to -27
Simvastatin	5	-15 to -22
	10	-18 to -26
	20	-20 to -31
Lovastatin	10	-14 to -21
	20	-17 to -21
	40	-22 to -28
	80	-28 to -32

* Sandoz Data on file

higher levels of serum cholesterol. However, this is not an argument one would support when the majority of patients require 20-25% reduction, as outlined above. Moreover, physicians never compare therapies on the basis of one mg of product vs one mg of another product (eg, antihypertensives). The question is rather, "What dose of this product needs to be prescribed to achieve the desired goal?" For more severe cases, efficacy and safety of fluvastatin in combination with other lipid-lowering drugs have been well established [22-24].

These include long-term (3 years) use with cholestyramine which produced a 30 to 35% reduction in LDL-C which was maintained throughout the study [25]. There were no clinical laboratory abnormalities associated with the long-term administration of the combination. The efficacy and safety of fluvastatin has also been studied in patients with severe familial hypercholesterolemia (FH) using a triple combination [22]. Fluvastatin, bezafibrate and cholestyramine together produced a reduction in LDL-C of 38%, with an HDL-C increase up to 40%. Again, there were no notable abnormalities in liver transaminases or creatine phosphokinase levels.

There are two reported head-to-head comparisons between fluvastatin and pravastatin [26,27]. In a double-blind, placebo-controlled study 134 patients with LDL-C $\geq$ 160 mg/dl and plasma triglyceride $\leq$ 400 mg/dl were randomized to receive either 40 mg daily fluvastatin or 20 mg daily pravastatin for 4 weeks, followed by 12 weeks at double the dose [26]. The reduction in LDL-C was similar (-24%) for both HMG-CoA reductase inhibitors over the first 4 weeks, but the increase in dosage to 80 mg fluvastatin daily produced a further significant (-30.4%; p < 0.001) reduction. Dosage escalation with pravastatin to 40 mg daily did not have a significant effect. In the second study the daily dose of fluvastatin and pravastatin was 40 mg and the entry mean level of total cholesterol was 293 ± 23 mg/dl for fluvastatin and 301 ± 40 mg/dl for pravastatin [27]. The change in mean total cholesterol was -27% with fluvastatin and -23% with pravastatin. Both values were statistically significant compared to baseline $(p < 0.01)$ but not between treatments. However, fluvastatin also reduced triglycerides by 33%, whereas pravastatin resulted in a slight increase in triglycerides (2.7%); the trend was not statistically significant. Fluvastatin also had a greater effect on increasing HDL-C (44%) than pravastatin (7%).

Two other studies [28,29] have directly compared fluvastatin with simvastatin in lowering LDL-C in patients with primary hypercholesterolemia. However, the authors have been unable to provide data on the formulation of fluvastatin used in these studies and whether they are bioequivalent to the marketed form, as is the case with the double-blind, double-dummy pravastatin studies previously mentioned [26,27].

Another study [30] also produced very low rates of cholesterol reduction for 20 mg/day fluvastatin (-12.8%) vs lovastatin (-19.5%). The conclusion of the study is that lovastatin, on a per-mg basis, would be more effective than fluvastatin. Again, the authors have been unable to provide data on formulation or bioequivalence of the fluvastatin used in this study. However, in a study of 120 patients [31], the marketed forms of lovastatin and fluvastatin were compared with an adequate design (double-blind, double-dummy) at a dose of 20 mg/d for 6 weeks. From comparable baseline values in the two groups, fluvastatin and lovastatin caused significant reductions in LDL-C of respectively 20.5 and 19.3%. For none of the parameters the difference between the two treatments was statistically significant. The authors conclude that fluvastatin and lovastatin have equivalent effects on lipid metabolism.

A further important consideration in the efficacy of drugs for chronic disease is patient compliance. This is particularly important when treating patients who are asymptomatic. Patients are unlikely to feel "better" by having their cholesterol reduced or their hypertension controlled. However, they may well be aware of the adverse effects associated with the medicines they are prescribed. The biopharmaceutical profile of fluvastatin provides certain advantages over the other HMG-CoA reductase inhibitors in terms of lack of interaction with other drugs (including antidiabetic, antihypertensive and immunosuppressant drugs). Fluvastatin is also rapidly absorbed and taken up by the liver, has the shortest half-life of all available members of its class and has no active circulating metabolites. A high percentage (98%) of fluvastatin is protein-bound in serum and fluvastatin does not cross the blood-brain barrier. In addition, cost of therapy can have an important effect on compliance and the lower price of fluvastatin should be beneficial in this respect, especially when up to 50% of patients stop treatment after 6 months because of cost.

Much attention is now being given to the mechanisms by which the HMG-CoA reductase inhibitors produce their effects on events, either related to their lipid-lowering ability or to their direct effects on the vasculature. Some of these effects have been put forward as explanations why there appear to be differences in the time-to-effect with different HMG-CoA reductase inhibitors. In the Pravastatin Multinational Study Group for Cardiac Risk Patients [32] there was a rapid (26 weeks) reduction in cardiac events. In WOSCOPS, a divergence appeared in time-to-events curves after 6 months whereas the benefits in 4S began to appear only after 1 year of therapy and increased steadily thereafter. The data from earlier studies indicate that benefit can be realised to a great extent after 2 years but that the full benefit occurs after 5 years of treatment.

As an explanation of the rapid effects of pravastatin on cardiac events, Pearson and Marx [33] suggest mechanisms such as direct endothelial cell inhibitory effects, reduced platelet aggregability, plasma viscosity and fibrinogen could all be important. Considerable work has been undertaken on the effects of HMG-CoA reductase inhibitor on smooth muscle cell proliferation, an early step in atherogenesis [34-37]. A consistent finding in all of this work is the pronounced effect of fluvastatin and simvastatin in inhibiting smooth muscle cells.

The effect of HMG-CoA reductase inhibitors on human arterial myocyte proliferation and migration *in vitro* shows a dose-dependent decrease with fluvastatin and simvastatin. By contrast, pravastatin failed to reduce SMC proliferation, even at the highest nontoxic concentration tested. Similar results were found with in-vivo neointimal formation in rabbit carotid arteries. Adding whole-blood sera from patients with type IIa hypercholesterolemia pretreated with either fluvastatin or pravastatin to cultured human arterial myocytes confirm that these effects are independent of the lipid-lowering ability of the two HMG-CoA reductase inhibitors [38].

Study of 40 mg daily fluvastatin for 24 weeks in 30 hypercholesterolemic patients, revealed a significant reduction in platelet cholesterol/phospholipid ratio by 28% and in platelet aggregation by 33% [39]. Fluvastatin, at low concentration ($1\mu M$) was found also to be a very potent inhibitor of LDL oxidation, both *in vitro* and *ex vivo*, as studied in 10 hypercholesterolemic patients, and may further contribute to the anti-atherogenic effect.

These data are supported by other studies from Rogler [40] and Schmieder [41], the latter study demonstrated that fluvastatin was able to restore endothelial function in hypercholesterolemic patients after 3 months of therapy. Total cholesterol was reduced by 30% ($p < 0.001$) after 12 weeks but the progressive improvement in forearm blood flow over a period of 12 months indicates two separate mechanisms. Another study [42] demonstrated an improvement in myocardial perfusion (using SPECT imaging) with fluvastatin in patients with ischemic heart disease. Again, there was a significant reduction in cholesterol (LDL-C, -30%) accompanied by a restoration of coronary endothelial function as tested by intracoronary acetylcholine infusion. This effect, along with the potential for longer-term regression of stenotic lesions, may lead to a reduction in cardiovascular morbidity and mortality, according to the authors. Myocardial scintigraphy with positron emission tomography (PET) is also being used in the ongoing LCAS (Lipoprotein and Coronary Atherosclerosis Study) study by Herd et al. [43]. A total of 429 subjects with angiographically documented lesions that occluded 30-75% of the diameter of major coronary artery were randomized to receive placebo or fluvastatin 20 mg twice daily for 2.5 years. Of these, 99 patients were also studied by PET at rest and during static exercise (handgrip) with dipyridamole. Approximately 25% of patients (with LDL-C $\geq$ 160 mg/dl) also received cholestyramine, in a dose of 8 g/day. Baseline characteristics show an average age of 59 ± 8 years and the average number of qualified lesions in each subject was 2.8. The results of the study should become available in 1996.

In addition to assessing the progression/regression of atherosclerotic lesions in the coronary arteries, PET studies will provide data on cardiac function and show if this is related to changes in measurable disease.

In Groningen a pilot study has been started to assess the effect of fluvastatin 40 mg twice daily given for 6 months on a PET scan in 20 dyslipidemic non-smoking asymptomatic men. In PET studies, radioactive ammonia ($^{13}NH_3$) is administered to the patient in order to study coronary flow and flow reserve, and in addition cold pressor and dipyridamole stress tests are performed. The study's acronym is 4P= " Pilot Pet in Primary Prevention" and results are expected by the end of 1996.

A study which may support the direct action of fluvastatin on SMCs is the FLuvastatin Angioplasty REstenosis (FLARE) study [44]. FLARE is evaluating the ability of fluvastatin 40 mg twice daily to reduce restenosis after successful PTCA. Treatment of suitable patients commenced 2 weeks before PTCA and continues to follow-up angiography at 26 ± 2 weeks post-PTCA. In addition to measuring restenosis (measured as the loss in minimal luminal diameter), primary clinical endpoints such as death, myocardial infarction, CABG surgery or reintervention up to 40 weeks have been monitored. In this trial more than 1000 patients are included and results are anticipated in 1996.

In another final study LIPS= "Lescol Intervention Prevention Study", which will start in 1996 a longer follow-up of 2 to 2,5 years is included. In this multicentre randomised double-blind placebo controlled trial, the long term effects of fluvastatin on major adverse cardiac events is assessed in patients who already have had a successful first PTCA.

A previous study with lovastatin (Lovastatin Restenosis Trial [45]) showed no difference in restenosis compared with placebo despite a 42% reduction in cholesterol. If the fluvastatin result is positive it will add weight to the existing evidence of a direct effect on the endothelium which is independent of its lipid-lowering action.

The costs of fluvastatin 20 and 40 mg are $\pm$ 40-60% lower than other HMG-CoA reductase inhibitors in the United States. When using these drugs in primary prevention, the reduction of an event like a myocardial infarction in a young patient might cost thousands of dollars. A recent Canadian cost effectiveness analysis [46], which used results of 40 double-blind randomized trials evaluating HMG-CoA reductase inhibitors in patients with hypercholesterolemia and data from the Framingham Heart Study to model changes in serum LDL- and HDL-cholesterol levels and risk of coronary heart disease, demonstrated that fluvastatin 40 mg/day compared favorably with lovastatin 20 mg/day, pravastatin 20 mg/day and simvastatin 10 mg /day as primary prevention. The economic model showed that, among male smokers aged 45 years with a pre-treatment serum LDL cholesterol of 163 mg/dl (4.5 mmol/l), the cost per life-year saved for fluvastatin was Canadian dollars ($Can) 38800 compared with $Can 48300 for simvastatin, $Can 53000 for lovastatin and $Can 56200 for pravastatin.

From the previous data it appears that considering its cost-effectiveness, its excellent overall tolerability and its reported efficacy, therapy with fluvastatin may be the first choice both in primary and secondary prevention.

References

1. A co-operative trial in the primary prevention of ischaemic heart disease using clofibrate. Report from the Committee of Principal Investigators. Br Heart J 1978;40:1069-118.
2. The Lipid Research Clinics Coronary Primary Prevention Trial results I. Reduction in incidence of coronary heart disease. JAMA 1984;251:351-64.
3. Canner PL, Berge KG, Wenger NK *et al*. Fifteen year mortality in Coronary Drug Project Patients: long-term benefit with niacin. J Am Coll Cardiol 1986;8:1245-55.
4. Dorr AE, Gundersen K, Schneider JC Jr, Spencer TW, Martin WB. Colestipol hydrochloride in hypercholesterolemic patients - effect on serum cholesterol and mortality. J Chronic Dis 1978;31:5-14.
5. Frick MH, Elo O, Haapa K *et al*. Helsinki Heart Study: Primary prevention trial with gemfibrozil in middle-aged men with dyslipidemia. Safety of treatment, changes in risk factors, and incidence of coronary heart disease. N Engl J Med 1987;317:1237-45.
6. Buchwald H, Varco RL, Matts JP *et al*. Effect of partial ileal bypass on mortality and morbidity from coronary heart disease in patients with hypercholesterolemia. Report of the Program on the Surgical Control of the Hyperlipidemias (POSCH). N Engl J Med 1990;323:946-55.
7. Ornish D, Brown SE, Scherwitz LW *et al*. Can lifestyle changes reverse coronary heart disease? The Lifestyle Heart Trial. Lancet 1990;336:129-33.
8. Effect of simvastatin on coronary atheroma: the Multicentre Anti-Atheroma Study (MAAS). Lancet 1994;344:633-8.
9. Blankenhorn DH, Azen SP, Kramsch DM *et al*. Coronary angiographic changes with lovastatin therapy. The Monitored Atherosclerosis Regression Study (MARS). The NARS Research Group. Ann Intern Med 1993;119:969-76.
10. Waters D, Higginson L, Gladstone P *et al*. Effects of monotherapy with an HMG-CoA reductase inhibitor on the progression of coronary atherosclerosis as assessed by serial quantitative arteriography. The Canadian Coronary Atherosclerosis Intervention Trial (CCAIT) Circulation 1994;89:959-68.
11. Jukema JW, Bruschke AVG, Van Boven AJ *et al*. Effects of lipid lowering by pravastatin monotherapy on progression and regression of coronary artery disease in symptomatic men with normal to moderately elevated serum cholesterollevels. The Regression Growth Evaluation Statin Study (REGRESS) Circulation 1995;91:2528-40.
12. Oliver MF. Doubts about preventing coronary heart disease. BMJ 1992;304:393-4.
13. Davey Smith G, Pekkanen J. Should there be a moratorium on the use of cholesterol lowering drugs? BMJ 1992;304:431-4.
14. Randomised trial of cholesterol lowering in 4444 patients with coronary heart disease: the Scandinavian Simvastatin Survival Study Group (4S). Lancet 1994;344:1383-9.
15. Byington RP, Jukema JW, Salonen JT *et al*. Reduction in cardiovascular events during pravastatin therapy: pooled analysis of clinical events of the Pravastatin Atherosclerosis Intervention Program. Circulation 1995;92:2419-25.
16. Shepherd J, Cobbe SM, Ford I *et al*. Prevention of coronary heart disease with pravastatin in men with hypercholesterolemia (West of Scotland Coronary Prevention Study Group). N Engl J Med 1995;333:1301-7.

17. Law MR, Wald NJ, Thompson SG. By how much and how quickly does reduction in serum cholesterol concentration lower risk for ischaemic heart disease? BMJ 1994;308:367-72.
18. Peters TK. Fluvastatin in severe hypercholesterolemia: analysis of a clinical trial database. Am J Cardiol 1995;76:71A-75A.
19. Carroll M, Sempos C, Briefel R, Gray S, Johnson C. Serum lipids of adults 20-74 years: United States, 1976-80. Vital Health Stat 1993;11(242):1-107.
20. National Cholesterol Education Program. Second Report of the Expert Panel on Detection, Evaluation, and Treatment of High Blood Cholesterol in Adults (Adult Treatment Panel II). Circulation 1994;89:1333-445.
21. International Task Force for Prevention of Coronary Heart Disease. Prevention of coronary heart disease: scientific background and new clinical guidlines, Nutr Metab Cardiovasc Dis 1992;2:113-56.
22. Leitersdorf E, Muratti EN, Eliav O, Peters TK. Efficacy and safety of triple therapy (fluvastatin-bezafibrate-cholestyramine) for severe familial hypercholesterolemia. Am J Cardiol 1995;76:84A-88A.
23. Eliav O, Schurr D, Pfister P, Friedlander Y, Leitersdorf E. High-dose fluvastatin and bezafibrate combination treatment for heterozygous familial hypercholesterolemia. Am J Cardiol 1995;76:76A-79A.
24. Muratti EN, Peters TK, Leitersdorf E. Fluvastatin in primary hypercholesterolemia: a cohort analysis of the response to combination treatment.Am J Cardiol 1994;73:30D-38D.
25. Jacotot B, Banga J, Waite R, Peters TK. Long-term efficacy with fluvastatin as monotherapy and combined with cholestyramine (a 156-week multicenter study). French-Dutch Fluvastatin Study Group. Am J Cardiol 1995;76:41A-46A.
26. Milani M, Cimminiello C, Merlo B, Loreno M, Arpaia G, Bonfardeci G. Effects of fluvastatin and pravastatin on lipid profiles and thromboxane production in type IIa hypercholesterolemia. Am J Cardiol 1995;76:51A-53A.
27. Jacotot B, Benghozi R, Pfister P, Holmes D. Comparison of fluvastatin versus pravastatin treatment of primary hypercholesterolemia. French-Dutch Fluvastatin Study Group. Am J Cardiol 95;76:54A-56A.
28. Illingworth D R, Stein E A, Knopp R H *et al*. A randomized multicenter trial comparing the efficacy of simvastatin and fluvastatin. J Cardiovasc Pharmacol Ther 1996;1:23-30.
29. Ose L, Scott R, Brusco O *et al*. Double blind comparison of the efficacy, safety and tolerability of simvastatin and fluvastatin in patients with primary hypercholesterolaemia. Clin Drug Invest 1995;10:127-38.
30. Berger M L, Wilson H M, Liss C L. A comparison of the safety and efficacy of lovastatin and fluvastatin [abstract]. Atherosclerosis 1995;115 Suppl:S96.
31. Haasis R, Berger J. Fluvastatin versus lovastatin: eine randomisierte, doppelblinde, multizentrische parrallel-gruppen studie zur effektivität und sicherheit einer lipidsenkung. Herz Kreislauf 1995;27:375-80.
32. Effects of pravastatin in patients with serum total cholesterol levels from 5.2 to 7.8 mmol/liter (200 to 300mg/dl) plus two additional atherosclerotic risk factors. The Pravastatin Multinational Study Group for Cardiac Risk Patients. Am J Cardiol 1993;72:1031-7.
33. Pearson TA, Marx HJ. The rapid reduction in cardiac events with lipid-lowering therapy: mechanisms and implications. Am J Cardiol 1993;72:1072-3.
34. Soma MR, Corsini A, Paoletti R. Cholesterol and mevalonic acid modulation in cell metabolism and multiplication. Toxicol Lett 1992;64-65 Spec No:1-15.

35. Soma, MR, Donetti E, Parolini C et al. HMG-CoA reductase inhibitors. In-vivo effects on carotid intimal thickening in normocholesterolemic rabbits. Arterioscler Thromb 1993;13:571-8.

36. Corsini A, Mazzotti M, Raiteri M et al. Relationship between mevalonate pathway and arterial myocyte proliferation: in vitro studies with inhibitors of HMG-CoA reductase. Atherosclerosis 1993;101:117.

37. Corsini A, Raiteri M, Soma MR, Bernini F, Fumagalli R, Paoletti R. Pathogenesis of atherosclerosis and the role of 3-hydroxy-3-methylglutaryl coenzyme A reductase inhibitors. Am J Cardiol 1995;76:21A-28A.

38. Corsini A, Bernini F, Quarato P et al. Non-lipid-related effects of 3-hydroxyl-3-methylglutaryl coenzyme A reductase inhibitors. Cardiology 1996. In press.

39. Aviram M. Interrelationships among platelet activation, LDL oxidation and foam cell formation in hypercholesterolemic patients; antiatherogenic effects of statin therapy [abstract]. Asian-Pacific Congress on Vascular Disease Prevention 1996.

40. Rogler G, Lackner KJ, Schmitz G. Effects of fluvastatin on growth of porcine and human vascular smooth muscle cells in vitro. Am J Cardiol 1995;76:114A-116A.

41. Schmieder RE, Schobel HP. Is endothelial dysfunction reversible? Am J Cardiol 1995;76:117A-121A.

42. Eichstädt HW, Eskötter H, Hoffman I, Amthauer HW, Weidinger G. Improvement of myocardial perfusion by short-term fluvastatin therapy in coronary artery disease. Am J Cardiol 1995;76:122A-125A.

43. Herd JA, West MS, Ballentyne C, Farmer J, Gotto AM Jr. Baseline characteristics of subjects in the Lipoprotein and Coronary Atherosclerosis Study (LCAS) with fluvastatin. Am J Cardiol 1994;73:42D-49D.

44. Foley DP, Bonnier H, Jackson G et al. Prevention of restenosis after coronary balloon angioplasty: rationale and design of the Fluvastatin Angioplasty Restenosis (FLARE) Trial. The FLARE Study Group. Am J Cardiol 1994;73:50D-61D.

45. Weintraub WS, Boccuzzi SJ, Klein JL et al. Lack of effect of lovastatin on restenosis after coronary angioplasty. Lovastatin Restenosis Trial Study Group. N Engl J Med 1994;331:1331-7.

46. Martens LL, Guibert R. Cost- effectiveness analysis of lipid-modifying therapy in Canada: comparison of HMG-CoA reductase inhibitors in the primary prevention of coronary heart disease. Clin Ther 1994;16:1052-62, discussion 1036.

9. Lessons learned from angiographic coronary atherosclerosis trials

J. WOUTER JUKEMA, ALBERT V.G. BRUSCHKE & JOHAN H.C. REIBER

Summary

From observational studies, we may conclude that progression and regression of coronary atherosclerosis is still a highly unpredictable process. Medical intervention studies have demonstrated that lipid lowering in general, and administration of HMG-CoA reductase inhibitors in particular, retards progression and promotes regression of coronary atherosclerosis and diminishes subsequent clinical events, even when cholesterol levels are not strongly elevated. Risk factor modification-changes in lifestyle, ileal bypass surgery and low-density-cholesterol apheresis also have their merits in reducing progression, whereas the definite place of calcium channel blockers in retarding established coronary atherosclerosis yet has to be determined.

Introduction

Coronary atherosclerosis is a chronic and usually progressive disease. In patients with coronary atherosclerosis, progression of the disease is one of the major factors that determine clinical prognosis [1-3]. The dynamics of this process, that is, progression and regression of atherosclerotic lesions, the healing of lesions and development of new ones, has intrigued cardiologists since the time that this process could be followed by repeated coronary arteriographic examinations. Ideally, studies on the dynamics of coronary atherosclerosis should comprise patients in whom repetitive coronary arteriographic examinations are performed at regular intervals, e.g. every one or two years. However, such studies are neither feasible nor ethically justifiable and therefore practically all progression studies are limited to patients who underwent coronary arteriography twice. This makes angiographic studies subject to several biases. First, there are strong indications that progression of coronary atherosclerosis is a nonlinear process which occurs in bouts rather than as a continuous process [4]. Therefore, the evolution of atherosclerotic lesions over a certain period of time cannot be automatically extrapolated to longer time intervals. In the second place, if the interval between the two studies is short, progression (or regression), although perhaps present, may not be marked enough to be detectable by angiography, whereas, if the interval between the studies is very long, the incidence of ischemic events such as cardiac death or increasing angina pectoris making coronary bypass surgery or PTCA necessary, may easily influence the outcome. Another problem concerns the nature of the information obtained by angiography. Angiography demonstrates the outlines of the arterial lumen, however, it does not provide direct information about the structure of the vessel wall or the

J.H.C. Reiber and E.E. van der Wall (eds.), Cardiovascular Imaging, 119-132.
© *1996 Kluwer Academic Publishers.*

composition of narrowing lesions. In this respect intravascular ultrasound studies may provide valuable additional information. However, at present it is not feasible to study the entire coronary arterial tree by intravascular ultrasound in a standardized and reproducible manner as may be achieved by computer assisted analysis of coronary angiograms. Furthermore, also ultrasound studies do not allow the assessment of the microscopical structure of the vessel wall.

In spite of the inherent limitations, the results of angiographic progression studies are fairly consistent and these studies have provided important information about the dynamics of coronary atherosclerosis and the factors which may influence this process.

Progression and regression of atherosclerotic lesions. General considerations

Obviously, mechanical interventions such as PTCA and other catheter interventions and coronary bypass surgery, have a profound influence on atherosclerotic lesions which has little relation to the evolution of the disease process itself. Therefore, we will exclude from this discussion lesions that are or may be influenced by mechanical intervention.

Observational studies

Observational studies may be defined as studies based on observations in regular patient populations. Typically, the patients have not been subjected to a specific type of treatment and usually these studies are of a retrospective nature. Sometimes the term "natural history" is used which is only appropriate if "natural history" is defined as the evolution of the disease under usual treatment and, in the case of coronary artery disease, excluding mechanical interventions. Particularly in view of the development of new effective therapeutic modalities it is becoming increasingly difficult to study the natural history because: "it is the function of the physician to make the history as desirably unnatural as possible" [5]. Therefore, to obtain data about some aspects of the dynamics of coronary atherosclerosis we have to resort to older observational studies. Unfortunately, none of these studies was carried out in accordance with the strict rules for quality assurance that are currently recommended for angiographic trials [6], which also makes these angiographic data unsuitable for quantitative analysis. These problems may in part be overcome by analyzing the data as categorical variables using fairly large steps (e.g. 20% or 25% increase or decrease of luminal narrowing) to define progression and regression. An overview of the largest observational studies is presented in Table 1. It appears that in all studies the percentages of patients showing progression and regression are remarkably similar. The major determinant of progression appears to be the time interval between the angiograms. This corroborates the common notion that coronary atherosclerosis is essentially a progressive disease process. Nevertheless, the process may remain inactive for a certain period of time. This inactivity may last

Table 1. Observational studies comprising 100 or more patients.

First Author	No. of patients	Mean interval (months)	% Prog.	Correlation with time	Correlation with other riskfactors
Kramer [7,8]	317	30	49	+	none
Bruschke [9]	286	39	56	+	none
Moise [10]	313	39	44	+	young age
Visser [11]	300	30	56	+	none
Ishikawa [12]	227	36	32	-	not reported
Sainsous [13]	122	34	57	+	none
Vanhaecke [14]	100	35	60	+	diabetes mellitus

several years to be followed by episodes of progression [4], however, in some cases the disease appears to be "burnt out", which is also observed in longterm clinical follow-up studies [15]. Most observational studies have shown no or only a weak correlation between progression and commonly recognized non-angiographic risk factors. This finding should be interpreted cautiously. In the first place, in the majority of the observational studies no attempt was made to reduce risk factors drastically as may be necessary to influence progression. In the second place, because of the rather crude angiographic analysis small changes, or differences in changes, over time may have escaped recognition.

There is some controversy as to the type of lesions which are most likely to progress. Some investigators found a positive correlation between severity of narrowing and chance of progression [8,9], whereas others did not find such a correlation [10,12,14]. There is also uncertainty about the significance of the morphology of lesions.

The situation is even more complex if not separate lesions but patients are considered. As was demonstrated in several studies [4,9,11], in most patients the presence of a relatively large number of slight or moderate narrowings (with a low chance of progression) and a small number of severe narrowings (with a high chance of progression) makes the prediction of progression in individual cases very uncertain. This is recently reconfirmed in studies dealing with the basic mechanisms of the evolution of atherosclerotic plaques [16].

Many angiographers intuitively feel that progression itself is of predictive significance. If, for example, in two years an obstruction progresses from 25% to 60% diameter narrowing, it is often assumed that in the near future this will result in a critical stenosis and frequently this is interpreted as an indication for mechanical intervention. However, in a study on patients who had more than one follow-up angiogram it was demonstrated that frequently progression of individual lesions does not continue, at least not in a more or less linear fashion (Figure 1) [4]. Conversely, if a lesion showed no progression over a certain period of time, this did not mean that the lesion has become inactive because significant progression was often noted afterwards. These inconsistencies were of great importance if the results were analyzed in patient groups. Patients who showed progression during the first interval (from angiogram 1 to angiogram 2) often had no progression during the second interval (from angiogram 2 to angiogram 3) and vice versa. Likewise, if there was progression during both intervals this more often than not involved different lesions. This behavior has become more understandable in the light of recent knowledge about the pathogenesis of atherosclerotic lesions.

Practically all observational studies have also shown regression of atherosclerotic lesions although this occurs less frequently than progression. Regression appears to be just as unpredictable as progression.

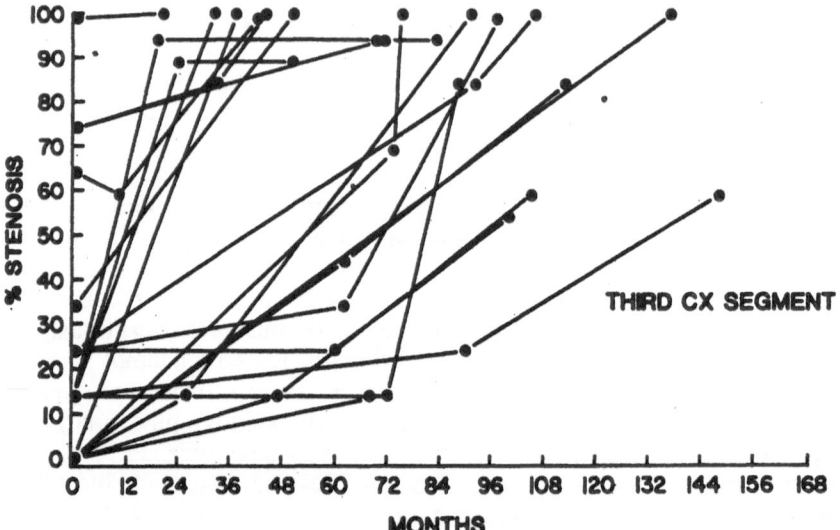

Figure 1. Progression in one coronary segment in a study on patients who underwent two follow-up coronary angiographies [4]. Progression is clearly a nonlinear process.

Intervention studies

Methodological considerations concerning intervention studies

Most intervention studies have been designed as prospective (placebo-controlled) studies which makes it possible to define in advance strict criteria for end point definition [17], and quality control [6], which are of particular importance for the angiographic part. If these criteria are fulfilled, then automated quantitative analysis of the coronary angiograms is warranted. Quality control involves two aspects of major importance, that is: 1) the projections in which the coronary arteries are visualized at baseline and follow up should be absolutely identical and the influence of vasomotor tone must be reduced to a minimum; and 2) because quantitative analysis uses not only relative (percentage) but also absolute measures, a reliable calibration object must be present.

Examples of intervention studies

Types of interventions used to reduce progression of coronary atherosclerosis or to stimulate regression and the placebo controlled trials in these specific fields are listed in Table 2. Of the lipid lowering intervention trials the number of included patients, study duration and intervention medication are listed in Table 3. Of the lipid intervention trials, inclusion criteria and entry serum lipids are listed in Table 4. These tables show that, although all studies are placebo controlled intervention trials, large differences in design exist between these trials, resulting in different clinical implications of their outcomes. Over a period of 15 years a large number of intervention studies has been published, of which we will discuss only the, in our opinion, most important placebo controlled trials.

Table 2. Lipid intervention trials - placebo controlled angiographic trials with (expected) year of publication.

Drug intervention			
+NHLBI-II [18]	1984	* MARS [24]	1993
+CLAS I [19]	1987	* CCAIT [25]	1994
+CLAS II [20]	1990	* MAAS [26]	1994
*SCOR [21]	1990	* HARP [27]	1994
*FATS [22]	1990	* REGRESS [28]	1995
*STARS [23]	1992	* PLAC I [29]	1995

Risk factor modification	
*Lifestyle Heart [30]	1990
*Heidelberg [31]	1992
*SCRIP [32]	1994

Ileal bypass	
#POSCH [33]	1990

Low-density-lipoprotein cholesterol apheresis	
*FHRS [34]	1995
*LAARS [35]	1995

+ = partly analyzed by quantitative coronary analysis; * = designed for quantitative coronary analysis; # = angiographic analysis not primary endpoint

Lipid intervention trials

Drug intervention trials

CLAS (Cholesterol Lowering Atherosclerosis Study), initiated by Blankenhorn et al. [19] is one of the first well designed placebo controlled studies that was published. For this study 162 nonsmoking men were selected who had previously undergone coronary artery bypass surgery. Two years of treatment with a combination of colestipol and niacin resulted in a 26 % reduction of serum cholesterol and a 37 % elevation in HDL cholesterol. Progression was somewhat less in the treated group but, more remarkable, regression was present in 16.2 %

Table 3. Drug intervention trials: number of included patients, study duration and intervention medication.

Trial	Number of Patients (finished)	Study Duration in Months (extension)	Study Medication
NHBLI-II	143 (116)	60	Cholestyramine
CLAS I	188 (162)	24 (48)	Colestipol + niacin
SCOR	97 (72)	26	Colestipol + niacin/ lovastatin
FATS	146 (120)	30	Lovastatin/ colestipol/niacin
STARS	90 (74)	39	Diet/diet + cholestyramine
MARS	270 (246)	26	Lovastatin
CCAIT	331 (299)	24	Lovastatin
MAAS	381 (345)	24 (48)	Simvastatin
HARP	91 (79)	29	Pravastatin/niacin/ cholestyramine/gemfibrozil
REGRESS	885 (778)	24	Pravastatin
PLAC I	408 (320)	36	Pravastatin

For trial references, see Table 2.

of the drug treated vs 3.6% in the placebo group. Initially no quantitative analysis was performed; however, the investigators used a sophisticated method of panel assessments. This may be an appropriate way to evaluate changes in patients with previous bypass surgery [36]; however, it makes comparison with other studies, analyzed by quantitative coronary analysis difficult. Furthermore, the final angiographic classification contains a significant degree of subjectivity, especially in those patients who showed a combination of progression and regression. A subgroup of the patients included in CLAS later underwent a third coronary arteriography. The results of the latter study appeared to corroborate the initial findings and indicated that therapy had a beneficial effect for at least 4 years [20]. FATS (Familial Atherosclerosis Treatment Study) showed that in patients with a high apolipoprotein B level ($\geq$ 125 mg per deciliter) and a family history of vascular disease, treatment with lovastatin and colestipol, or niacin and colestipol, reduced the frequency of progression and increased the frequency of regression of coronary lesions [22]. Clinical events (death, myocardial infarction, or revascularization for

Table 4. Lipid intervention trials: inclusion criteria and entry serum lipids.

Trial	Inclusion Criteria	Entry Serum Lipids
NHBLI-II	Type II hypercholesterolemia	LDL-chol >95 percentile
CLAS I	Previous coronary bypass surgery	Total chol 4.8-9.1 mmol/l
SCOR	Heterozygous familial hypercholesterolemia	LDL-chol >5.17 mmol/l
FATS	Family history of vascular disease	Apolipoprotein-B >125 mg/dl
STARS	Coronary artery disease	Total-chol 6.0-10.0 mmol/l
MARS	Coronary artery disease	Total-chol 4.9-7.6 mmol/l
CCAIT	Coronary artery disease	Total-chol 5.7-7.6 mmol/l
MAAS	Coronary artery disease	Total-chol 5.5-8.0 mmol/l
HARP	Coronary artery disease	Total-chol 4.6-6.4 mmol/l
REGRESS	Coronary artery disease	Total-chol 4.0-8.0 mmol/l
PLAC I	Coronary artery disease	LDL-chol 3.4-4.9 mmol/l

For trial references, see Table 2.
NB. The definition of coronary artery disease differs between studies ranging from vessels (only minimally) visibly involved with atherosclerosis to at least one segment with ≥50% diameter stenosis.
LDL = low density lipoprotein, chol = cholesterol

worsening symptoms) occurred significantly less in the treatment groups than in the placebo group. Concerning the analysis of the coronary angiograms it must be noted that the quantitative assessment/edge detection algorithm was not fully automated.

The SCOR (Specialized Center of Research) Intervention Trial, randomized 72 patients with heterozygous familial hypercholesterolemia to test whether reducing plasma low-density lipoprotein levels by diet and combined drug regimens (see Table 3) could reduce progression of coronary lesions [21]. For the analysis of the coronary angiograms, they used in part the same (semi)quantitative analysis method as in the FATS study [22]. The mean change in percent area stenosis among controls was +0.80, indicating progression, while the mean change for the treatment group was -1.53 indicating regression. Noteworthy was that regression among women, analyzed separately, was also significant, which had not been convincingly demonstrated before.

STARS (St. Thomas' Atherosclerosis Regression Study) randomized 90 men with coronary artery disease to receive usual care (controls), dietary intervention, or diet plus cholestyramine [23]. Angiography was performed at baseline and after a mean of 39 months. The investigators used change of mean absolute width of segments (MAWS) as principal angiographic end point. For each patient an overall MAWS change, averaged from all changes of measurable segments, was calculated. MAWS decreased by 0.201 mm in controls, increased by 0.003 mm in the dietary group and increased by 0.103 mm in the diet plus drug treated group. Although only a relatively small number of segments was analyzed the results of this study appear to warrant intensive lipid lowering therapy as part of secondary prevention. It should be noted, however, that a minimum plasma cholesterol concentration of 6.0 mmol/l was an inclusion criterion and the mean plasma cholesterol was 7.23 mmol/l, and that vasomotor tone was not standardized.

In the late 1980's a new powerful class of lipid lowering drugs became available, with only few side effects, the 3-hydroxy-3-methylglutaryl-coenzyme A (HMG-CoA) reductase inhibitors. Five angiographic progression trials using an HMG-CoA reductase inhibitor as monotherapy have been reported, namely the Monitored Atherosclerosis Regression Study (MARS) [24], the Canadian Coronary Atherosclerosis Intervention Trial (CCAIT) [25], the Multicentre Anti-Atheroma Study (MAAS) [26], the Regression Growth Evaluation Statin Study (REGRESS) [28], and the Pravastatin to Limit Atherosclerosis in the Coronary Arteries (PLAC I) study [29]. The first two studies used lovastatin, the MAAS study used simvastatin and the REGRESS and PLAC I studies used pravastatin. In MARS the primary endpoint (change in mean percent diameter stenosis assessed by quantitative arteriography) was not statistically different between treatment groups, however, a subdivision showed a significant beneficial effect on stenoses narrowing the lumen diameter more than 50%. These results are not entirely comparable with studies using absolute diameters provided by quantitative coronary analysis. Percentage stenosis may underestimate progression if diffuse luminal narrowing occurs which also reduces the reference diameter. In MARS, mean global change score, used as a secondary endpoint, showed a significant difference between the treatment groups [24].

In CCAIT the primary endpoint was change in minimal lumen diameter (MLD) [25]. In this study, which excluded many patients, possibly leading to a selection bias, a mean difference between treatment groups of 0.04 mm in MLD was noted and this was statistically significant.

In MAAS two arteriographic endpoints were used; in a period of four years (the study was extended after an interim analysis at two years, which was the initially planned study duration) the treatment effects were 0.06 and 0.08 mm for mean (reflecting diffuse atherosclerosis) and minimum lumen diameter (reflecting focal atherosclerosis), respectively [26]. In spite of the important information obtained from the above mentioned trials, until recently little was known about the potential benefit of serum cholesterol reduction in the broader range of patients with coronary atherosclerosis who have normal to moderately elevated serum cholesterol levels (4-8 mmol/l) and are scheduled to undergo various forms of primary treatment, in particular medical management, PTCA or CABG. The Regression Growth Evaluation Statin Study (REGRESS) specifically addressed this large group of patients which represents the majority of patients seen in clinical practice [28]. Of the 885 patients included, 778 patients (88%) had an evaluable final angiogram. The mean segment diameter (mainly reflecting diffuse atherosclerosis) decreased 0.10 mm in the placebo group versus 0.06 mm in the pravastatin group (p= 0.019). The median minimum obstruction diameter (mainly reflecting focal atherosclerosis) decreased 0.09 mm in the placebo group versus 0.03 mm in the pravastatin group (p=0.001). Thus, in symptomatic men with significant coronary atherosclerosis and normal to moderately elevated serum cholesterol, in the group of patients treated with pravastatin significantly less progression of coronary atherosclerosis was observed than in the placebo group. The beneficial effect of pravastatin did not differ significantly between the four subgroups (quartiles) with regard to baseline cholesterol levels. This raises the question whether cholesterol lowering should be an integral part in the management of patients with coronary atherosclerosis, regardless of initial serum cholesterol level. It seems justified to at least consider this option seriously.

In PLAC I minimal lumen diameter was significantly less reduced in the pravastatin group, compared to the placebo group, whereas there was no statistically significant effect on the mean lumen diameter.

All five studies (MARS, CCAIT, MAAS, REGRESS and PLAC I) showed some reduction of cardiac events during the study period, however this did reach statistical significance in the REGRESS and PLAC I studies only.

The only other angiographic regression study other than REGRESS evaluating the controversy about the effect of cholesterol lowering in patients with a plasma cholesterol level generally considered normal in Western Countries, the HARP trial, in our view suffered from some methodological problems and was a relatively small study (91 patients) [27]. HARP did not demonstrate any beneficial effect of cholesterol lowering in symptomatic patients with a (near) normal entry serum cholesterol level.

Risk factor modification - Changes in lifestyle

A study on the effect of changes in lifestyle on progression of coronary artery disease was published by Ornish et al. [30] in 1990. This study is open to criticism on many points (e.g. unequal numbers of patients in experimental and control group, large number of drop outs for reasons which may easily have influenced the angiographic results, and most strikingly a difference of more than 10 kg in weight at baseline which had reverted to less than 1 kg at the end of the study) and therefore the conclusions are unreliable.

A more convincing study was published by Schuler et al. [31] who showed increased regression of lesions on a strict regimen of diet and exercising.

Another study designed as a risk factor reduction trial was the Standford Coronary Risk Intervention Project (SCRIP) [32]. In the Risk Reduction group of SCRIP total cholesterol was lowered intentionally by diet and exercise from 6.03 mmol/l to 5.03 mmol/l (16.4% reduction) and per year there was 0.021 mm less decrease of minimal diameter than in the usual care group. There were also less cardiac events in the risk reduction group than in the usual care group (25 vs 44). However, this may not be interpreted as a beneficial effect of simple risk reduction because at the end of the study 90% of the patients in the risk reduction group and 23% of the patients in the usual care group used lipid lowering drugs. It seems that the gain by a combination of measures was not greater than may be achieved by cholesterol lowering only.

Ileal bypass surgery

In POSCH (Program on the Surgical Control of the Hyperlipidemias) 838 patients who had survived a first myocardial infarction were randomized to a control group and a group of patients who underwent partial ileal bypass surgery to lower plasma cholesterol [33]. Overall mortality and mortality due to coronary artery disease were not significantly reduced in the surgical group; however, comparison of baseline coronary angiograms with those obtained at 3,5,7 and 10 years consistently showed less disease progression in the surgical group. No quantitative arteriographic analysis method was used; the changes between the two films were graded by two-member teams using a simple 8 point scale. Follow-up angiograms were not performed in all patients and, although the angiographic assessments were made with the reader blinded to the patient's assigned treatment, there obviously could not be a double blind study design. Despite these limitations, also POSCH appears to substantiate a beneficial effect of cholesterol lowering on progression.

Low-density-lipoprotein cholesterol apheresis

Extracorporeal removal of cholesterol by long-term plasma exchange, latterly by the more selective procedure of low-density-lipoprotein cholesterol apheresis, may also retard the rate of progression of coronary atherosclerosis, in general in addition to lipid lowering drugs [34,35]. In light of extensive procedures associated with apheresis, low-density-lipoprotein cholesterol apheresis mainly seems suitable as alternative means of treating those people with severe hypercholesterolemia, who are intolerant of, or insufficiently responsive to, combination drug therapy [34]. Because of this restricted indication, low-density-lipoprotein cholesterol apheresis will not be discussed in more detail.

Calcium channel blockers

Results with regard to experimental atherosclerosis, gave rise to the expectation that calcium channel blockers are able to retard progression of coronary atherosclerosis in man [37]. However, the results of the large randomized placebo controlled clinical trials such as INTACT (International Nifedipine trial on Antiatherosclerotic Therapy [38] and a study performed in Canada [39] on close scrutiny are not very convincing. These studies claim that calcium channel blockers retard progression of minor lesions and inhibit development of new lesions, but it is doubtful whether the methods used allow such conclusions. In any case, calcium channel blockers appear to have no effect on the evolution of significant coronary artery narrowings. A recent publication suggests that there may be a synergistic anti-atherosclerotic effect of lipid lowering together with calcium channel blocker administration [40].

Conclusions

From observational studies, we may conclude that progression and regression of coronary atherosclerosis is still a highly unpredictable process. Interventions aimed at lowering of plasma cholesterol, even if the level is not strongly elevated, appear to have a beneficial effect on progression of coronary atherosclerosis as well as on clinical events. This beneficial effect of lipid lowering therapy may be due to other factors than retarding angiographic progression and inducing regression of coronary atherosclerosis as well. Plaque stabilization, preventing a plaque from rupturing with acute occlusive thrombosis, which is thought to result from a decrease in the lipid content of plaques consequent to sustained reductions in LDL cholesterol is probably of importance in the effectiveness of various lipid-lowering regimens in decreasing ischemic events [41-45].

Since it has been demonstrated that there is a good correlation between coronary artery lesion progression and risk of future clinical coronary events [1-3], it can be concluded that angiographic trials, apart from having value in their own right, may also serve to assess the clinical efficacy of antiatherosclerotic agents.

References

1. Buchwald H, Matts JP, Fitch LL *et al*. Changes in sequential coronary arteriograms and subsequent coronary events. Surgical Control of the Hyperlipidemias (POSCH) Group. JAMA 1992;268:1429-33.
2. Waters D, Craven TE, Lesperance J. Prognostic significance of progression of coronary atherosclerosis. Circulation 1993;87:1067-75.
3. Azen SP, Mack WJ, Cashin-Hemphill L *et al*. Progression of coronary artery disease predicts clinical coronary events: long-term follow-up from the Cholesterol Lowering Atherosclerosis Study. Circulation 1996;93:34-41.
4. Bruschke AVG, Kramer JR Jr, Bal ET, Haque IU, Detrano RC, Goormastic M. The dynamics of progression of coronary atherosclerosis studied in 168 medically treated patients who underwent coronary arteriography three times. Am Heart J 1989;117:296-305.
5. Proudfit WL, Bruschke AVG, Sones FM Jr. Natural history of obstructive coronary artery disease: ten year study of 601 nonsurgical cases. Prog Cardiovasc Dis 1978:21:53-78.
6. Reiber JHC, Jukema JW, Koning G, Bruschke AVG. Quality controle in quantitative coronary arteriography. In: Bruschke AVG, et al., editors. Lipid-lowering therapy and progression of coronary atherosclerosis. Dordrecht: Kluwer Academic Publishers, 1996:45-63.
7. Kramer JR, Matsuda Y, Mulligan JC, Aronow M, Proudfit WL. Progression of coronary atherosclerosis. Circulation 1981;63:519-26.
8. Kramer JR, Kitazume H, Proudfit WL *et al*. Segmental analysis of the rate of progression in patients with progressive coronary atherosclerosis. Am Heart J 1983;106:1427-31.
9. Bruschke AVG, Wijers TS, Kolsters W, Landmann J. The anatomic evolution of coronary artery disease demonstrated by coronary arteriography in 256 non-operated patients. Circulation 1981;63:527-36.
10. Moise A, Theroux P, Taymans Y *et al*. Clinical and angiographic factors

associated with progression of coronary artery disease. J Am Coll Cardiol 1984;3:659-67.

11. Visser RF, van der Werf T, Ascoop CAPL, Bruschke AVG. The influence of anatomic evolution of coronary artery disease on left ventricular contraction: an angiographic follow-up study of 300 nonoperated patients. Am Heart J 1986;112:963-72.

12. Ishikawa H, Uwatoko M, Watabe S *et al*. Analysis of the evolution of coronary artery disease: evaluation of 227 cases by restudy of coronary arteriography. Jpn Circ J 1986;50:575-86.

13. Sainsous J, Baragan P, Benichou M, Bory M, Serradimigni A. Coronarographies iteratives chez 122 patients traités medicalement. Arch Mal Coeur Vaiss 1985;78:184-90.

14. Vanhaecke J, Piessens J, van de Werf F, Willems JL, De Geest H. Angiographic evolution of coronary atherosclerosis in non-operated patients. Eur Heart J 1983;4:547-56.

15. Proudfit WL, Bruschke AVG, MacMillan IP, Williams GW, Sones FM Jr. Fifteen year survival study of patients with obstructive coronary artery disease. Circulation 1983;68:986-97.

16. Libby P. Molecular bases of the acute coronary syndromes. Circulation 1995;91:2844-50.

17. Jukema JW, van Boven AJ, Zwinderman AH, Bal ET, Reiber JHC, Bruschke AVG. The influence of angiographic endpoints on the outcome of lipid intervention studies. A proposal for standardization. Angiology 1995. In press.

18. Brensike JF, Levy RI, Kelsey SF *et al*. Effects of therapy with cholestyramine on progression of coronary arteriosclerosis: results of the NHLBI type II Coronary Intervention Study. Circulation 1984;69:313-24.

19. Blankenhorn DH, Nessim SA, Johnson RL, Sanmarco ME, Azen SP, Cashin-Hemphill L. Beneficial effects of combined colestipol-niacin therapy on coronary atherosclerosis and coronary venous bypass grafts. JAMA 1987;257:3233-40.

20. Cashin-Hemphill L, Mack WJ, Pogoda JM, Sanmarco ME, Azen SP, Blankenhorn DH. Beneficial effects of colestipol-niacin on coronary atherosclerosis. A 4 -year follow up. JAMA 1990;264:3013-7.

21. Kane JP, Malloy MJ, Ports TA, Phillips NR, Diehl JC, Havel RJ. Regression of coronary atherosclerosis during treatment of familial hypercholesterolemia with combined drug regimens. JAMA 1990;264:3007-12.

22. Brown G, Albers JJ, Fisher LD *et al*. Regression of coronary artery disease as a result of intensive lipid-lowering therapy in men with high levels of apolipoprotein B. N Engl J Med 1990;323:1289-98.

23. Watts GF, Lewis B, Brunt JNH *et al*. Effects on coronary artery disease of lipid-lowering diet or diet plus cholestyramine in the St Thomas' Atherosclerosis Regression Study (STARS). Lancet 1992;339:563-9.

24. Blankenhorn DH, Azen SP, Kramsch DM *et al*. Coronary angiographic changes with lovastatin therapy. The Monitored Atherosclerosis Regression Study (MARS) The MARS Research Group. Ann Intern Med 1993;119:969-76.

25. Waters D, Higginson L, Gladstone P *et al*. Effect of monotherapy with an HMG-CoA reductase inhibitor on the progression of coronary atherosclerosis as assessed by serial quantitative arteriography. The Canadian Coronary Atherosclerosis Intervention Trial. Circulation 1994;89:959-68.

26. Effect of simvastatin on coronary atheroma: the Multicentre Anti-Atheroma

Study (MAAS). Lancet 1994;344:633-8.

27. Sacks FM, Pasternak RC, Gibson CM, Rosner B, Stone PH. Effect on coronary atherosclerosis of decrease in plasma cholesterol concentrations in normocholesterolaemic patients. Harvard Atherosclerosis Reversibility Project (HARP) Group. Lancet 1994;344:1182-6.

28. Jukema JW, Bruschke AVG, van Boven AJ *et al*. Effects of lipid lowering by pravastatin on progression and regression of coronary artery disease in symptomatic men with normal to moderately elevated serum cholesterol levels. The Regression Growth Evaluation Statin Study (REGRESS). Circulation 1995;91:2528-40.

29. Pitt B, Mancini GBJ, Ellis SG, Rosman HS, Park JS, McGovern ME Pravastatin limitation of atherosclerosis in the coronary arteries (PLAC I): reduction in atheroslcerosis progression and clinical events PLAC I investigators. J Am Coll Cardiol 1995;26:1133-9.

30. Ornish D, Brown SE, Scherwitz LW *et al*. Can lifestyle changes reverse coronary heart disease? The Lifestyle Heart Trial. Lancet 1990;336:129-33.

31. Schuler G, Hambrecht R, Schlierf G *et al*. Regular physical exercise and low-fat diet. Effects on progression of coronary artery disease. Circulation 1992;86:1-11.

32. Haskell WL, Alderman EL, Fair JM *et al*. Effects of intensive multiple risk factor reduction on coronary atherosclerosis and clinical cardiac events in men and women with coronary artery disease. The Stanford Coronary Risk Intervention Project (SCRIP). Circulation 1994;89:975-90.

33. Buchwald H, Varco RL, Matts JP *et al*. Effect of partial ileal bypass surgery on mortality and morbidity from coronary heart disease in patients with hypercholesterolemia. Report on the Program on the Surgical Control of the Hyperlipidemias (POSCH). N Engl J Med 1990;323:946-55.

34. Thompson GR, Maher VMG, Matthews S *et al*. Familial Hypercholesterolaemia Regression Study: a randomised trial of low-density-lipoprotein apheresis. Lancet 1995;345:811-6.

35. Kroon AA, Ajubi N, van Asten P, Stalenhoef AFH. The prevalence of peripheral vascular disease in familial hypercholesterolemia. J Intern Med 1995;238:451-9.

36. Azen SP, Cashin-Hemphill L, Pogoda J *et al*. Evaluation of human panelists in assessing coronary atherosclerosis. Arterioscler Thromb 1991;11:385-94.

37. Schneider W, Kober G, Roebruck P *et al*. Retardation of development and progression of coronary atherosclerosis: a new indication for calcium antagonists? Eur J Clin Pharmacol 1990;39(Suppl.1):S17-23.

38. Lichtlen PR, Hugenholtz PG, Rafflenbeul W, Hecker H, Jost S, Deckers JW. Retardation of angiographic progression of coronary artery disease by nifedipine. Results of the International Nifedipine Trial on Antiatherosclerotic Therapy (INTACT). INTACT Group Investigators. Lancet 1990;335:1109-13.

39. Waters D, Lespérance J, Francetich M *et al*. A controlled clinical trial to assess the effect of calcium channel blocker on the progression of coronary atherosclerosis. Circulation 1990;82:1940-53.

40. Jukema JW, Zwinderman AH, van Boven AJ *et al*. Evidence for a synergistic effect of calcium channel blockers with lipid lowering therapy in retarding progression of coronary atherosclerosis in symptomatic patients with normal to moderately raised cholesterol levels. Arterioscler Thromb Vasc Biol. In press.

41. Zeiher AM, Drexler H, Saurbier B, Just H. Endothelium-mediated coronary

blood flow modulation in humans. Effects of age, atherosclerosis, hypercholesterolemia, and hypertension. J Clin Invest 1993;92:652-62.

42. Treasure CB, Klein JL, Weintraub WS *et al*. Beneficial effects of cholesterol-lowering therapy on the coronary endothelium in patients with coronary artery disease. N Engl J Med 1995;332:481-7.

43. Galis ZS, Sukhova GK, Kranzhover R, Clark S, Libby P. Macrophage foam cells from experimental atheroma constitutively produce matrix-degrading proteinases. Proc Natl Acad Sci USA 1995;92:402-6.

44. Fuster V, Lewis A. Connor Memorial Lecture. Mechanisms leading to myocardial infarction: insights from studies of vascular biology. Circulation 1994;90:2126-46.

45. Falk E, Shah PK, Fuster V. Coronary plaque disruption. Circulation 1995;92:657-71.

10. Regression/progression in women: the estrogen angiographic trials

DAVID M. HERRINGTON

Summary

Observational studies in women and clinical trials in non-human primates suggest that estrogen has favorable effects on both structural and functional manifestations of coronary atherosclerosis. Two new angiographic endpoint trials, the Estrogen Replacement and Atherosclerosis (ERA) Trial and the Women's Estrogen/Progestin Lipid Lowering Hormone Atherosclerosis Regression Trial (WELL-HART) have been initiated to determine the effects of estrogen replacement, with or without progestin, on the progression or possible regression of coronary atherosclerosis in postmenopausal women. These trials will also provide important information on progression of disease in other vascular territories and changes in coronary endothelial function. Together with the currently ongoing clinical endpoint trials, those angiographic trials will provide a comprehensive assessment of the effects of estrogen on structural functional and clinical coronary disease.

Introduction

Estrogen replacement therapy shows great promise as a new intervention for the prevention and treatment of coronary atherosclerosis in postmenopausal women. Clinical and epidemiologic studies, as well as studies in animal models of atherosclerosis, all suggest that estrogen plays a fundamentally important role in the prevention of coronary artery disease. Furthermore, estrogen is known to have favorable effects on several cardiovascular risk factors including plasma lipids. Several large primary and secondary prevention trials are underway to test the efficacy of estrogen replacement therapy in preventing clinical cardiovascular events.

Recently, two new angiographic endpoint trials have been initiated to determine the effect of estrogen replacement therapy on the progression of coronary atherosclerosis. In addition to directly measuring the effects of estrogen on the anatomic manifestations of coronary atherosclerosis, these studies will also provide important information about the progression of disease in other vascular territories such as the carotid arteries as well as the effects of estrogen on the functional health of the coronary arteries by examining changes in endothelial-dependent vasodilator capacity. These angiographic endpoint trials will complement the clinical endpoint trials, providing a comprehensive assessment of the effects of estrogen on cardiovascular disease and the potential mechanisms through which estrogen exerts its effects. This chapter will review the rationale and methodology for these angiographic endpoint trials in detail.

J.H.C. Reiber and E.E. van der Wall (eds.), Cardiovascular Imaging, 133-143.
© 1996 *Kluwer Academic Publishers.*

Estrogen and cardiovascular disease in postmenopausal women

Cardiovascular disease is the most common cause of morbidity and mortality in postmenopausal women [1]. Epidemiologic studies have demonstrated that risks for cardiovascular disease in postmenopausal women is greater than similar-aged pre-menopausal women [2,3] suggesting that endogenous estrogen has a protective effect on the development of cardiovascular disease. A large number of case-control and cohort studies have subsequently demonstrated that postmenopausal estrogen users have a lower risk for cardiovascular disease than similar women who do not use estrogen replacement therapy [4-6]. The favorable effects of estrogen may be even more striking in postmenopausal women who already have established cardiovascular disease. In a cohort of 1822 women with angiographically-demonstrated coronary disease, women on estrogen replacement therapy had a death rate of 4% in 10 years compared to 33% among those who did not take estrogen (relative risk=0.16, $p < 0.05$) [7].

The effects of estrogen on anatomically-defined atherosclerosis

Despite the abundance of data on the relationship between estrogen replacement therapy and clinical cardiovascular events, there are relatively few data examining the relationship between estrogen and directly measured atherosclerosis (Figure 1). Three cross-sectional angiographic studies have demonstrated less severe coronary atherosclerosis as measured by angiography in estrogen replacement users than non-users. Sullivan et al. [7] compared 1444 postmenopausal women

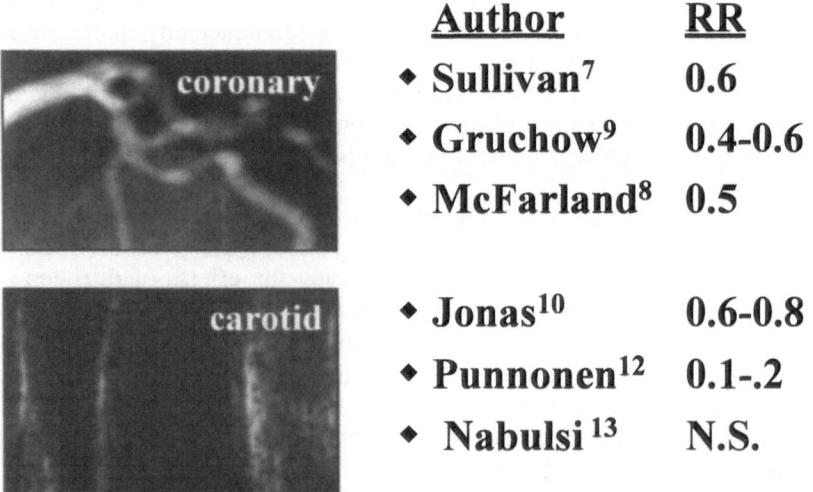

Author	RR
◆ Sullivan[7]	0.6
◆ Gruchow[9]	0.4-0.6
◆ McFarland[8]	0.5
◆ Jonas[10]	0.6-0.8
◆ Punnonen[12]	0.1-.2
◆ Nabulsi[13]	N.S.

Figure 1. Cross sectional studies of estrogen use and risk of coronary or carotid atherosclerotic lesions. RR = relative risk of disease among users vs. non-users. All RR's are significantly less than 1.0 ($p < 0.05$) except for Nabulsi et al. Reproduced with permission. Circulation; 1996 American Heart Association (in press)

with at least one $\geq$ 70% coronary stenosis by angiography with 744 women who had no angiographic evidence of disease. Only 2.7% of the women with significant coronary disease were current users of estrogen replacement therapy compared with 7.7% of the women with normal angiograms. This statistically significant difference remained even after adjustment for age and other cardiovascular risk factors (odds ratio=0.44, p=0.04). Similarly, McFarland et al. [8] also reported that women with a 70% or greater coronary stenosis (N=137) were significantly less likely to be using hormone therapy than a group of similar-aged women (N=208) with angiographically normal coronary arteries (odds ratio=0.50, p<0.01). Gruchow et al. [9] reported age-adjusted odds ratios of 0.59 and 0.37 for use of postmenopausal estrogen in 933 women with moderate and severe coronary occlusion, respectively. This association was independent of type of menopause and conventional cardiovascular risk factors except HDL cholesterol levels. It was suggested that changes in HDL may be one of the mechanisms through which estrogen could effect the development of stenotic coronary disease.

The favorable effects of estrogen do not appear to be limited to the coronary arteries. Several large cross-sectional studies of estrogen use and carotid wall thickness have demonstrated significantly lower internal and common carotid artery wall thickness among users of estrogen replacement therapy compared to non-users. In the Cardiovascular Health Study, Jonas et al. [10,11] examined carotid artery wall thickness in 2962 women over the age of 65. Both internal and common carotid artery wall thickness were significantly smaller among current users of estrogen replacement therapy compared to non-users (p<0.01), and the risk of any wall thickening of $\geq$ 1% stenosis was significantly lower among estrogen users (p<0.05). Punnonen et al. [12] also demonstrated that the total number of fibrous and calcific plaques in the abdominal aorta and the femoral and carotid arteries was significantly less in women who were current users of estradiol valerate when compared to similar aged women who were not hormone users (p<0.01). In the Atherosclerosis Risk in Communities (ARIC) study, no association between estrogen and carotid wall thickness was found [13].

There are even fewer prospective data examining the relationship between hormone replacement therapy and development or progression of atherosclerosis. Recently O'Brien et al. [14] described the relationship between estrogen replacement therapy and restenosis in a subset of the women participating in the Coronary Angioplasty vs. Excisional Atherectomy Trial (CAVEAT I). At six months following either PTCA or directional atherectomy, the 39 postmenopausal women who were taking estrogen replacement therapy had significantly less restenosis measured by quantitative angiography than the women who were not on estrogen therapy (p<0.01). This apparent protective effect was most pronounced in the women undergoing directional atherectomy, suggesting that estrogen made an important role in modulating the inflammatory component of the pathogenesis of restenosis.

Similar differences between users and non-users of estrogen were also demonstrated in a subset of participants in the Asymptomatic Carotid Atherosclerosis Progression Study (ACAPS) - a clinical trial testing the effects of lovastatin or placebo on progression of carotid intimal-medial wall thickness [15]. Among the postmenopausal women randomized to placebo, non-users of estrogen had significant progression of their carotid intimal medial wall thickness over three years, whereas similar women who were current users of estrogen had regression of their carotid intimal medial wall thickness ($p < 0.05$). The differences in progression rates between users and non-users of estrogen remained significant even after adjustment for other cardiovascular risk factors.

These observations are consistent with an extensive body of data demonstrating the protective effect of estrogen in the development of coronary atherosclerosis in non-human primate models. Early studies demonstrated that loss of endogenous estrogen through ovariectomy or low social status yielded rates of coronary atherosclerosis in female non-human primates that was comparable to their male counterparts [16]. On the other hand, elevated levels of estradiol associated with pregnancy resulted in almost complete protection from atherosclerosis in monkeys [17]. Subsequently, several clinical trials in non-human primates have demonstrated that ovariectomized cynomolgus monkeys on atherogenic diets had less coronary atherosclerosis when treated with estrogen replacement therapy when compared to placebo-treated animals [18-20].

Estrogen and functional manifestations of atherosclerosis

Typically angiographic endpoint trials, as well as trials using carotid ultrasound, focus on anatomic manifestations of atherosclerosis as the primary outcome of interest. While thickening of the vascular wall and luminal encroachment are critically important manifestations of atherosclerosis with direct clinical implications, atherosclerosis is also associated with abnormalities in the functional integrity of the vessel wall. One such functional abnormality is impaired endothelial-dependent vasodilator capacity. Studies in humans [21,22], animals [23,24], and in vitro [25,26], have established that atherosclerotic vascular disease is accompanied by, and perhaps preceded by [27,28], significant impairment in endothelium-mediated vasodilation. Many lines of evidence suggest that this occurs from an abnormality in endothelial synthesis or release of nitric oxide [25,26,29]; however, abnormalities in the diffusion of nitric oxide to the vascular smooth muscle cells, or the response of the vascular smooth muscle cells to nitric oxide, are also possible. Impaired endothelium-mediated vasodilation can be demonstrated in both the coronary [21,30,31] and peripheral arterial circulation [22,32] and is present in both conduit (macrovascular) [21,30-32] and resistance (microvascular) [32-34] arteries of individuals with coronary artery disease. Changes in coronary artery luminal diameter in response to vasodilator stimuli are ideally suited to measurement by quantitative coronary angiography. Thus, angiography can be used to assess both the anatomic and functional extent of coronary atherosclerosis.

In-vivo angiographic studies in both human and non-human primates document chronic and acute estrogen administration can attenuate or even reverse the abnormal coronary vasomotor response to acetylcholine that occurs as a consequence of atherosclerosis. In angiographic studies of ovariectomized cynomolgus monkeys, chronic estrogen replacement therapy resulted in normal endothelium-dependent vasodilation to acetylcholine despite the presence of atherosclerosis [35]. Virtually identical observations were subsequently made in postmenopausal women undergoing coronary angiography (Figure 2) [21,32,36]. This effect does not appear to be limited to the coronary arteries. Several investigators have also demonstrated beneficial effects of estrogen on endothelial-dependent vasodilator capacity in the brachial arteries of postmenopausal women with and without coronary artery disease [22,34,37]. Furthermore, estrogen administration has been shown to improve treadmill times in women with chronic stable angina [38], an effect that is presumably mediated, in part, through an influence on endothelial-dependent vasodilator capacity. If estrogen reduces or reverses the vasoconstrictor response associated with impaired endothelial function in atherosclerotic arteries in women, it may help protect against atherosclerotic-associated syndromes that are caused or complicated by vasospasm. These effects of estrogen on coronary and brachial artery endothelial function are ideally suited for clinical trials using quantitative coronary angiography or brachial artery ultrasound as the primary outcome of interest.

Thus, there are compelling observational data, secondary analyses from clinical trials of other interventions, and data from clinical trials in non-human primates all suggesting that estrogen may indeed play an important role in the pathogenesis and prevention of anatomically-defined coronary atherosclerosis. In addition, it appears that estrogen may also play a fundamentally important role in maintaining the functional integrity of the coronary arteries. Specifically, estrogen appears to maintain or restore endothelial-dependent vasodilator capacity that is typically impaired in the face of coronary atherosclerosis. Nonetheless, appropriately designed angiographic endpoint trials are required to prove that estrogen does impart these favorable effects on coronary arteries in postmenopausal women. Furthermore, angiographic endpoint trials will provide the opportunity to clarify the mechanisms through which estrogen may impart its favorable effects. A clearer understanding of the mechanisms of estrogen's cardioprotective effect may provide new directions for basic and clinical research concerning the pathogenesis and prevention of atherosclerosis.

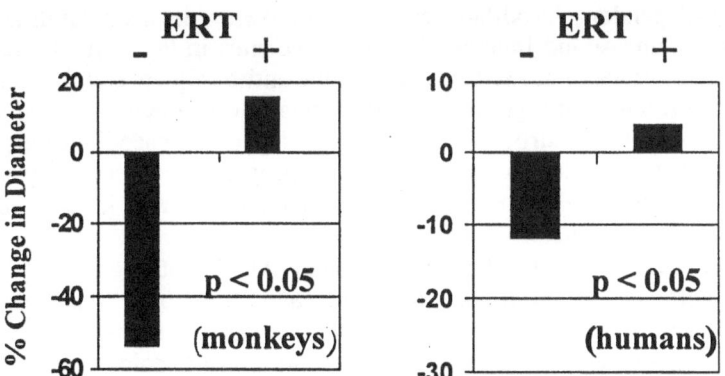

Figure 2. Percent change in coronary artery diameter in response to $10^{-6}M$ acetylcholine in ovariectomized monkeys (A) and postmenopausal women (B) according to estrogen replacement status. + = chronic estrogen replacement therapy, - = no estrogen replacement. Reproduced with permission. Circulation;1996 American Heart Association (in press)

Angiographic endpoint trials of estrogen replacement therapy

Currently there are two angiographic endpoint trials testing hypotheses regarding estrogen replacement therapy and progression of coronary atherosclerosis. The first trial is the Estrogen Replacement and Atherosclerosis (ERA) trial. This is three-arm trial comparing the effects of conjugated oral estrogen (0.625 mg. p.o. qd.) with or without low continuous dose medroxyprogesterone acetate (2.5 mg. p.o. qd.) and placebo on progression of coronary stenoses in women with established coronary artery disease. The primary outcome of interest will be minimum diameter of coronary stenotic lesions before and after three years of study drug. A number of other angiographic parameters will also be quantified including percent diameter stenosis and average diameter of all lesions, minimum diameter, percent diameter stenosis and average diameter of all segments irrespective of presence or absence of disease, proportion of segments with new lesions > 20% diameter stenosis, and the minimum diameter of segments following PTCA or atherectomy. These other angiographic endpoints will be considered secondary endpoints.

In addition to the assessment of progression of coronary atherosclerosis as measured by angiography, the ERA trial will evaluate the effects of estrogen on coronary artery wall thickness as measured by intracoronary ultrasound and the functional integrity of the coronary endothelium by measuring endothelial-dependent vasodilator capacity. In the subset of participants eligible for the endothelial function study, an intracoronary ultrasound catheter is placed in the proximal LAD through which intracoronary acetylcholine infusions with estimated final concentrations of 10^{-8}, 10^{-7}, and 10^{-6} M are administered for two minutes each. Quantitative coronary angiography is used to measure the average diameter in the mid and distal LAD and large diagonals at baseline and following each of the acetylcholine infusions. The women then receive an IV infusion of conjugated estrogens which is allowed to circulate for 10 minutes. After 10 minutes, the entire procedure is repeated in order to document the acute effects of estrogen on endothelial-dependent vasodilator capacity. Following the acetylcholine infusion, intracoronary ultrasound images of four to five sites in the LAD are obtained at specific anatomic landmarks. By repeating the entire sequence at the baseline and follow-up coronary angiograms, it will be possible to document both the acute and chronic effects of estrogen on endothelial-dependent vasodilator capacity and the effects of chronic estrogen replacement on progression of coronary artery wall thickness measured by quantitative intracoronary ultrasound [39,40] in a subset of the ERA participants.

To further clarify the mechanisms through which estrogen may impart its favorable effects on both the anatomic and functional manifestations of atherosclerosis, a number of important mediators and/or confounders of estrogen's effects will be measured including: plasma lipids and lipoproteins, regulators of blood pressure and glucose metabolism, plasma hemostatic factors and measures of antioxidant capacity (Table 1). Finally, although the study is not powered to detect significant differences in clinical events, the incidence of fatal and non-fatal MI, sudden death, coronary revascularization procedures and admissions for unstable angina or CHF will be compared between the three treatment groups.

Table 1. Plasma factors to be measured in the ERA trial.

Lipids	Blood pressure
lipid profile	renin
LDL/VLDL beta quant	angiotensin II [1-7]
HDL subfractions	
Apo-A$_1$, B, E,	Hemostasis
Apo-E isoforms	fibrinogen
Lp(a)	factor VII
	PAI-1
Carbohydrate metabolism	Antioxidants
Insulin/glucose during	plasma antioxidant
2 hr OGTT	capacity
Estrogen(s)	
estradiol, estrone, SHBG	

The other angiographic endpoint trial currently underway is the Women's Estrogen/Progestin Lipid Lowering Hormone Atherosclerosis Regression Trial (WELL-HART). This is a randomized placebo-controlled, double-blind serial coronary angiographic and carotid ultrasonographic trial of hormone replacement therapy and lipid lowering in postmenopausal women with established coronary artery disease. Two hundred forty (240) women will be randomized to receive micronized 17-ϐ estradiol (1.0 mg p.o. qd.), micronized 17-ϐ estradiol (1.0 mg p.o. qd.) plus cyclic medroxyprogesterone acetate (5.0 mg p.o. qd. for 12 days out of 30) or placebo. In addition, all women will receive instruction in a low-fat diet and pravastatin, if required, in order to achieve LDL of $\leq$ 100 mg/dl consistent with the NCEP ATP II guidelines. The primary outcome will be mean per patient change in percent diameter stenosis determined by quantitative coronary angiography. The change in global extent score based on a panel of expert angiographers will serve as a secondary outcome. In addition, the rate of change of intimal-medial thickness of the far wall of the distal common carotid artery will be treated as another secondary endpoint. As in the ERA trial, a number of other potentially important risk factors and/or mediators of the effect of estrogen on atherosclerosis will also be measured including measures of plasma, lipids and lipoproteins, carbohydrate metabolism and hemostasis factors.

The ERA and WELL-HART trials bear important similarities as well as important differences (Table 2). Both trials will help confirm or refute the hypothesis that estrogen replacement therapy slows the progression or induces regression of coronary atherosclerosis as measured by coronary angiography. In addition, both trials will examine the impact of the addition of progestin on the relationship between estrogen replacement therapy and progression of coronary disease. The ERA trial will extend these observations to the functional integrity of the coronary arteries by measuring the effect of estrogen on endothelial function. The WELL-HART study, on the other hand, will extend the anatomic observations to the carotid arteries.

Table 2. Comparison of the ERA and WELL-HART angiographic endpoint trials of estrogen replacement therapy.

	ERA	WELL-HART
Sample size (N)	375	240
Interventions	CEE CEE & continuous MPA Placebo	E_2 E_2 + cyclic MPA Placebo
Follow-up	3 years	3 years
1^0 angiographic outcome	minimum diameter - QCA	% diameter stenosis - QCA
2^0 outcomes[*]	coronary endothelial function intracoronary ultrasound	carotid wall thickness

[*] Selected 2^0 outcomes
CEE = conjugated equine estrogen 0.625 mg; MPA = medroxyprogesterone acetate

The two trials will also make unique contributions to our understanding of the relationship between estrogen and atherosclerosis through differences in the study design and treatment interventions. For example, the ERA trial will examine the effect of estrogen replacement therapy in addition to usual care. The WELL-HART study, on the other hand, will examine the incremental effect of estrogen therapy above and beyond what can be achieved by aggressive lipid lowering therapy alone. This will help to tease apart the portion of the effect of estrogen that can be attributed to lipid lowering and that which can be attributed to other effects of estrogen. Furthermore, significant controversy exists concerning the potential attenuating effects of progestins on the beneficial effects of estrogen. In animal models, continuous administration of progesterone significantly diminished the effects of estrogen on coronary plaque extent and vasomotor function, whereas cyclic progestin administration had no adverse effect [18,41]. Comparing the effects of continuous progestin administration (ERA) with cyclic administration (WELL-HART) in the human angiographic trials will provide additional data on this important aspect of hormone replacement.

ERA and WELL-HART in the context of other cardiovascular trials of estrogen replacement therapy

The ERA and WELL-HART trials will measure anatomic and functional atherosclerosis in both the coronary and carotid arteries of postmenopausal women. These trials will complement other estrogen replacement trials that have been completed or which are currently underway. These trials include the Postmenopausal Estrogen/Progestin Intervention study (PEPI) which was a large multi-center trial of various hormone replacement regimens and their effects on cardiovascular disease risk factors and the Heart and Estrogen/Progestin Replacement Study (HERS) and the Women's Health Initiative (WHI) which are secondary and primary prevention trials to examine the effect of estrogen on clinical cardiovascular events. The ERA and WELL-HART trials will provide an anatomic and functional link between the information already available from PEPI on cardiovascular risk factors and the information that will become available from the clinical outcome trials on clinical events. Taken together these trials will provide a comprehensive assessment of the effect of estrogen replacement therapy on the pathogenesis of atherosclerosis and provide important additional data on progression and regression of both anatomic and functional coronary disease in women.

References

1. Heart and stroke facts. Dallas: American Heart Association, 1992.
2. Lerner DJ, Kannel WB. Patterns of coronary heart disease morbidity and mortality in the sexes: a 26-year follow-up of the Framingham population. Am Heart J 1986;111:383-90.
3. Gordon T, Kannel WB, Hjortland MC, McNamara PM. Menopause and coronary heart disease. The Framingham Study. Ann Intern Med 1978;89:157-61.
4. Stampfer MJ, Colditz GA. Estrogen replacement therapy and coronary heart disease: a quantitative assessment of the epidemiologic evidence. Prev Med 1991;20:47-63.
5. Grady D, Rubin SM, Petitti DB *et al*. Hormone therapy to prevent disease and prolong life in postmenopausal women [see comments]. [Review]. Ann Intern Med 1992;117:1016-37.
6. Bush TL. Noncontraceptive estrogen use and risk of cardiovascular disease: an overview and critique of the literature. In: Korenman SG, editor. The menopause: biological and clinical consequences of ovarian failure: evaluation and management. Norwell, MA: Serono Symposia, 1990:211-3.
7. Sullivan JM, vander Zwaag R, Lemp GF *et al*. Postmenopausal estrogen use and coronary atherosclerosis. Ann Intern Med 1988;108:358-63.
8. McFarland KF, Boniface ME, Hornung CA, Earnhardt W, Humphries JO. Risk factors and noncontraceptive estrogen use in women with and without coronary disease. Am Heart J 1989;117:1209-14.
9. Gruchow HW, Anderson AJ, Barboriak JJ, Sobocinski KA. Postmenopausal use of estrogen and occlusion of coronary arteries. Am Heart J 1988;115:954-63.
10. Jonas HA, Kronmal RA, Psaty BM *et al*. Current estrogen-progestin and estrogen replacement therapy in elderly women: association with carotid atherosclerosis [abstract]. Am J Epidemiol 1995;41(SUppl.):S56.
11. Manolio TA, Furberg CD, Shemanski L *et al*. Associations of postmenopausal estrogen use with cardiovascular disease and its risk factors in older women. The CHS Collaborative Research Group. Circulation 1993;88:2163-71.

12. Punnonen RH, Jokela HA, Dastidar PS, Nevala M, Laippala PJ. Combined oestrogen-progestin replacement therapy prevents atherosclerosis in postmenopausal women. Maturitas 1995;21:179-87.

13. Nabulsi A, Folsom A, Szklo M, White A, Higgins M, Heiss G. Is menopausal status or hormone replacement therapy associated with carotid intimal-medial wall thickness? [abstract]. Am J Epidemiol 1992;136:1003-4.

14. O'Brien JE, Peterson ED, Keeler GP, Berdan E, Ohman M, Faxon DP. Impact of estrogen replacement therapy on restenosis following percutaneous coronary interventions [abstract]. Circulation 1995;92(Suppl.I):I-345.

15. Espeland MA, Applegate W, Furberg CD, Lefkowitz D, Rice L, Hunninghake D. Estrogen replacement therapy and progression of intimal-medial thickness in the carotid arteries of postmenopausal women. ACAPS Investigators. Asymptomatic Carotid Atherosclerosis Progression Study. Am J Epidemiol 1995;142:1011-9.

16. Adams MR, Kaplan JR, Clarkson TB, Koritnik DR. Ovariectomy, social status, and atherosclerosis in cynomolgus monkeys. Arteriosclerosis 1985;5:192-200.

17. Adams MR, Kaplan JR, Koritnik DR, Clarkson TB. Pregnancy-associated inhibition of coronary artery atherosclerosis in monkeys. Evidence of a relationship with endogenous estrogen. Arteriosclerosis 1987;7:378-84.

18. Adams MR, Kaplan JR, Manuck SB *et al.* Inhibition of coronary artery atherosclerosis by 17-beta estradiol in ovariectomized monkeys. Lack of an effect of added progesterone. Arteriosclerosis 1990;10:1051-7.

19. Adams MR, Golden DL. Atheroprotective effects of estrogen replacement therapy are antagonized by medroxyprogesterone acetate in monkeys [abstract]. Circulation 1995;92(Suppl.I):I-627.

20. Williams JK, Anthony MS, Honore EK *et al.* Regression of atherosclerosis in female monkeys. Arterioscler Thromb Vasc Biol 1995;15:827-36.

21. Herrington DM, Braden GA, Williams JK, Morgan TM. Endothelial-dependent coronary vasomotor responsiveness in postmenopausal women with and without estrogen replacement therapy. Am J Cardiol 1994;73:951-2.

22. Lieberman EH, Gerhard MD, Uehata A *et al.* Estrogen improves endothelium-dependent, flow-mediated vasodilation in postmenopausal women. Ann Intern Med 1994;121:936-41.

23. Williams JK, Adams MR, Herrington DM, Clarkson TB. Short-term administration of estrogen and vascular responses of atherosclerotic coronary arteries. J Am Coll Cardiol 1992;20:452-7.

24. Williams JK, Honore EK, Washburn SA, Clarkson TB. Effects of hormone replacement therapy on reactivity of atherosclerotic coronary arteries in cynomolgus monkeys. J Am Coll Cardiol 1994;24:1757-61.

25. Vanhoutte PM. Endothelium and control of vascular function. State of the Art lecture [Review]. Hypertension 1989;13:658-67.

26. Luscher TF, Richard V, Tschudi M, Yang Z. Serotonin and the endothelium [Review]. Clin Physiol Biochem 1990;8(Suppl.3):108-19.

27. Celermajer DS, Adams MR, Clarkson P *et al.* Passive smoking and impaired endothelium-dependent arterial dilatation in health young adults. N Engl J Med 1996;334:150-4.

28. Vita JA, Treasure CB, Nabel EG *et al.* Coronary vasomotor response to acetylcholine relates to risk factors for coronary artery disease. Circulation 1990;81:491-7.

29. Moncada S, Palmer RM, Higgs EA. The discovery of nitric oxide as the

endogenous nitrovasodilator. [Review]. Hypertension 1988;12:365-72.

30. Treasure CB, Klein JL, Weintraub WS *et al*. Beneficial effects of cholesterol-lowering therapy on the coronary endothelium in patients with coronary artery disease. N Engl J Med 1995;332:481-7.

31. Anderson TJ, Meredith IT, Yeung AC, Frei B, Selwyn AP, Ganz P. The effect of cholesterol-lowering and antioxidant therapy on endothelium-dependent coronary vasomotion. N Engl J Med 1995;332:488-93.

32. Gilligan DM, Quyyumi AA, Cannon RO 3rd. Effects of physiological levels of estrogen on coronary vasomotor function in postmenopausal women. Circulation 1994;89:2545-51.

33. Reis SE. Oestrogens attenuate abnormal coronary vasoreactivity in postmenopausal women [editorial]. Ann Med 1994;26:387-8.

34. Gilligan DM, Badar DM, Panza JA, Quyyumi AA, Cannon RO, 3rd. Effects of estrogen replacement therapy on peripheral vasomotor function in postmenopausal women. Am J Cardiol 1995;75:264-8.

35. Williams JK, Adams MR, Klopfenstein HS. Estrogen modulates responses of atherosclerotic coronary arteries. Circulation 1990;81:1680-7.

36. Collins P, Rosano GM, Sarrel PM *et al*. 17 beta-Estradiol attenuates acetylcholine-induced coronary arterial constriction in women but not men with coronary heart disease. Circulation 1995;92:24-30.

37. Gilligan DM, Badar DM, Panza JA, Quyyumi AA, Cannon RO 3rd. Acute vascular effects of estrogen in postmenopausal women. Circulation 1994;90:786-91.

38. Rosano GM, Sarrel PM, Poole-Wilson PA, Collins P. Beneficial effect of oestrogen on exercise-induced myocardial ischaemia in women with coronary artery disease. Lancet 1993;342:133-6.

39. Van Horn MH, Snyder WE, Braden GA, Herrington DM. Intracoronary ultrasound catheter motion compensation using the generalized Hough transform. Comput Cardiol 1994:293-6.

40. Zhu Y, Snyder WE, Herrington DM. A gradient field metric for quality control of automated intracoronary ultrasound boundaries. Comput Cardiol 1994:285-8.

41. Adams MR, Williams JK, Kaplan JR. Effects of androgens on coronary artery atherosclerosis and atherosclerosis-related impairment of vascular responsiveness. Arterioscler Thromb Vasc Biol 1995;15:562-70.

11. Is peripheral B-mode ultrasound a substitute for coronary arteriography?

ERIC DE GROOT, J. WOUTER JUKEMA, ALEXANDER D. MONTAUBAN VAN SWIJNDREGT, AD J. VAN BOVEN, AEILKO H. ZWINDERMAN, ROB G.A. ACKERSTAFF, ANTON F.W. VAN DER STEEN, NICOLAAS BOM, KONG I. LIE & ALBERT V.G. BRUSCHKE, on behalf of the REGRESS Study Group, Interuniversity Cardiology Institute The Netherlands, Utrecht, The Netherlands

Summary

The Regression Growth Evaluation Statin Study (REGRESS) is a double blind, placebo controlled, 2 year atherosclerosis regression study in 885 men with angiographically proven coronary artery disease. The effect of treatment with pravastatin was investigated. In addition to repeated quantitative arteriography, repeated peripheral B-mode ultrasound intima-media thickness measurements were performed in 255 patients.

In the peripheral arteries and the coronary arteries highly significant pravastatin treatment effects were observed. To deal with the question whether carotid and femoral intima-media thickness measurements can predict the state and progression of atherosclerosis in the coronary arteries, the data of both vascular imaging modalities were compared.

In individuals, the baseline correlations between peripheral intima-media thickness as measured with B-mode ultrasound, and the coronary artery stenosis as measured with quantitative arteriography, were low to moderate. No correlations in treatment effect between the two vascular beds could be demonstrated. Peripheral B-mode ultrasound measurements are therefore unable to describe the state of the coronary arteries in the individual, but are well suited to non-invasively assess anti-atherosclerotic properties of agents.

Introduction

B-mode ultrasound imaging of the arterial walls of the large peripheral arteries allows the recognition of the early stages of atherosclerosis [1-3]. Unlike angiography, which visualizes the vascular contours and lumen, B-mode ultrasound depicts the structural morphology of the arterial wall itself. As shown by Pignoli et al. [1] for the common carotid arterial far wall, the leading edges of the B-mode ultrasound double line pattern represent the lumen-intima interface and the media-adventitia interface of the intima-media complex. Consequently, the distance between these edges is called intima-media thickness (IMT) (Figure 1). IMT is influenced by cardiovascular risk factors such as age, serum LDL-cholesterol, hypertension, and smoking [4-16]. As demonstrated by a number of lipid intervention studies, a reduction of risk factors may inhibit the increase of IMT [17-23].

J.H.C. Reiber and E.E. van der Wall (eds.), Cardiovascular Imaging, 145-156.
© 1996 *Kluwer Academic Publishers.*

The noninvasive patient-friendly nature of the B-mode ultrasound examination allows repeated measurements in large populations. The method has therefore become a powerful tool in epidemiological studies and medical intervention trials designed to study the progression of atherosclerosis. In the Regression Growth Evaluation Statin Study (REGRESS) the effect of two-year treatment with pravastatin on the evolution of coronary atherosclerosis was studied in a randomized fashion. The primary endpoints of the study concerned the changes in the coronary arteries as assessed by quantitative coronary arteriography [24]. In a subgroup of the REGRESS patients, B-mode ultrasound studies of the carotid and femoral arterial walls were performed to determine the treatment effect of pravastatin on the large peripheral arteries. Contrary to other studies, which either investigated the treatment effects of agents in the coronary arteries [25-27] or in the peripheral arteries [17,20,22,23], in REGRESS both vascular beds were assessed [21,24]. Our study therefore allowed us to compare the changes over time in the peripheral arteries to the changes occurring in the coronary arteries.

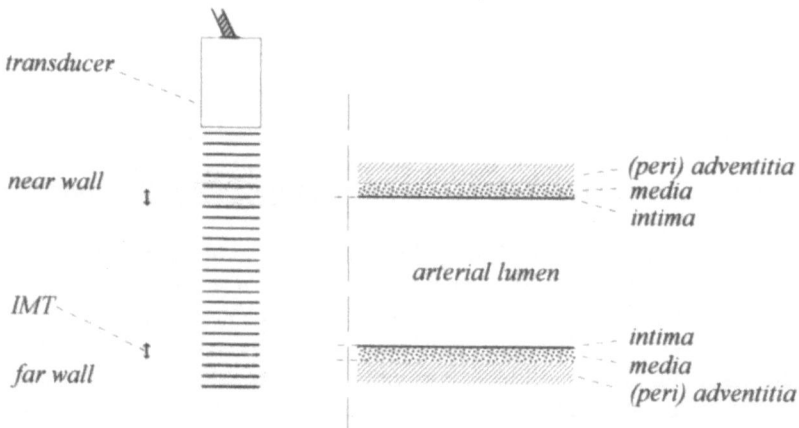

Figure 1. Diagram of a B-mode ultrasound image of the near and far arterial wall (left), and its morphological counterpart (right).

Methods

REGRESS study design and patient selection

REGRESS is a double blind, placebo controlled, multicenter study to assess the effect of two-year treatment with a fixed daily dosage of 40 mg of the 3-hydroxy-3-methyl-glutaryl HMG-CoA reductase inhibitor pravastatin on the progression of coronary atherosclerosis as determined by quantitative coronary arteriography (QCA). Eligible were symptomatic males, <70 years of age, with a serum cholesterol between 4.0 and 8.0 mmol/l (155 and 310 mg/dl), and a serum triglyceride level of ≤ 4.0 mmol/l. The coronary angiogram had to show a visually assessed ≥ 50% diameter reduction in at least one major coronary artery and had to be of sufficient quality for QCA assessment. A total of 885 patients from 11 participating hospitals were included [24].

Quantitative Coronary Arteriography

QCA procedures have been described in extenso previously [24]. In short: following a standardized protocol, coronary arteriography was performed at the start of the study and after two years. The coronary tree was divided into 13 segments, according to the American Heart Association classification, excluding the posterolateral branches [28]. In a single core QCA laboratory all REGRESS arteriograms were analyzed with the Cardiovascular Measurement System (CMS-MEDIS, Medical Imaging Systems, Nuenen, the Netherlands). This system converts selected arteriographic cine-frames into digitized images. It enables automated lumen contour detection and consecutive diameter measurements of user-specified coronary vessel segments [29].

B-mode ultrasound imaging and image analysis

In three of the centers participating in REGRESS (St. Antonius Hospital, Nieuwegein, and the University Hospitals of Groningen and Nijmegen) B-mode ultrasound studies of the carotid and femoral arterial walls were performed. Patients of these centers underwent five B-mode ultrasound scans: at baseline and after 6, 12, 18 and 24 months. In our B-mode imaging studies we used two ultrasound instruments (ACUSON 128 and ACUSON 128 XP systems. ACUSON Corporation; Mountain View, CA). Both instruments were equipped with L7384 7.0 MHz linear array transducers. The scanning protocol was standardized for all subjects. The patients lay in the supine position and the carotid arteries were imaged from a fixed lateral transducer angle. The femoral arteries were imaged from a fixed anterior transducer angle. The carotid and femoral arterial segments were defined by landmarks as represented in the B-mode image. The arterial segment comprising one centimeter proximal to the carotid dilation was defined as the common carotid arterial segment (CCA). The carotid bulb (BUL) was defined as the arterial segment between the carotid dilation and carotid flow divider. A one centimeter long arterial segment distal to the flow divider was defined as the internal carotid arterial segment (ICA) (Figure 2). A one centimeter long arterial segment proximal to the femoral dilation was defined as the common femoral arterial segment (CFA). The one centimeter arterial segment distal to the femoral flow divider was defined as the superficial femoral arterial segment (SFA) (Figure 3). Of each arterial segment, the near and far walls were imaged and acoustically focused upon independently. The visualization of the arterial wall image was improved by using the Regional Expansion Selection (RES) mode of the ultrasound instruments [30]. In this mode, effectively an area of 2 by 2 cm is imaged (Figure 4). Real-time B-mode image sequences of the wall segments were stored on S-VHS video tape for off-line analysis.
For video image processing we used S-VHS video-cassette recorders (Panasonic NV-FS 100 HQ), multisync monitors (Sony GVM-1400 QM), time base correctors (IDEN IVT-7P), and personal computers (IPC, 80386 processor). The personal computers were equipped with frame grabbers (DT2861 and DT2862. Data Translation Inc., Marlboro, MA.). The Data Translation board converts a

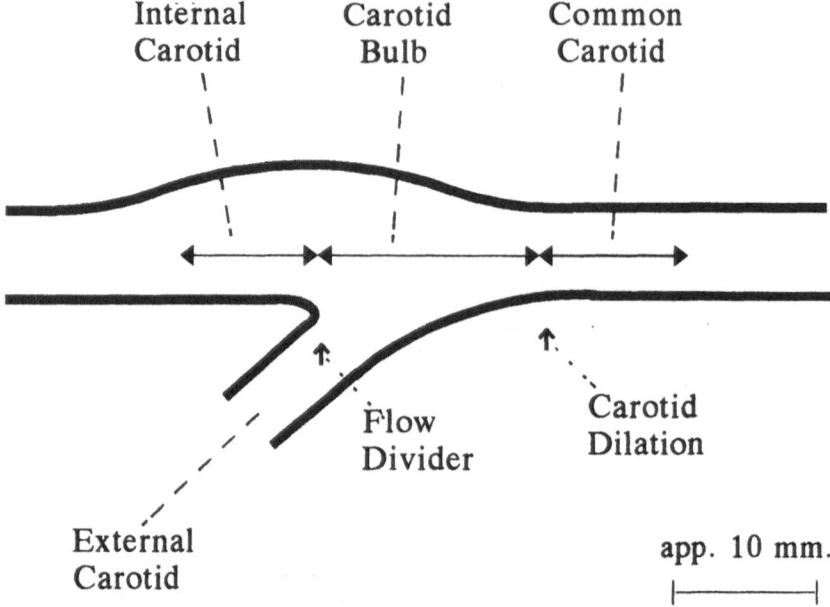

Figure 2. Carotid arterial segments. In the carotid artery, the sonographer identifies the anatomical landmarks, carotid dilation and flow divider, with vertical arrows.

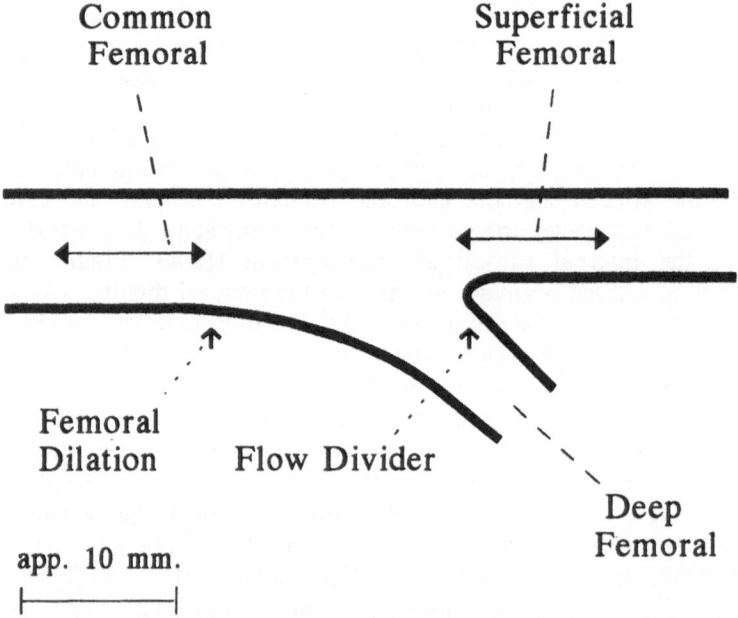

Figure 3. Femoral arterial segments. In the femoral artery, the sonographer identifies the anatomical landmarks, the femoral dilation and flow divider, with vertical arrows.

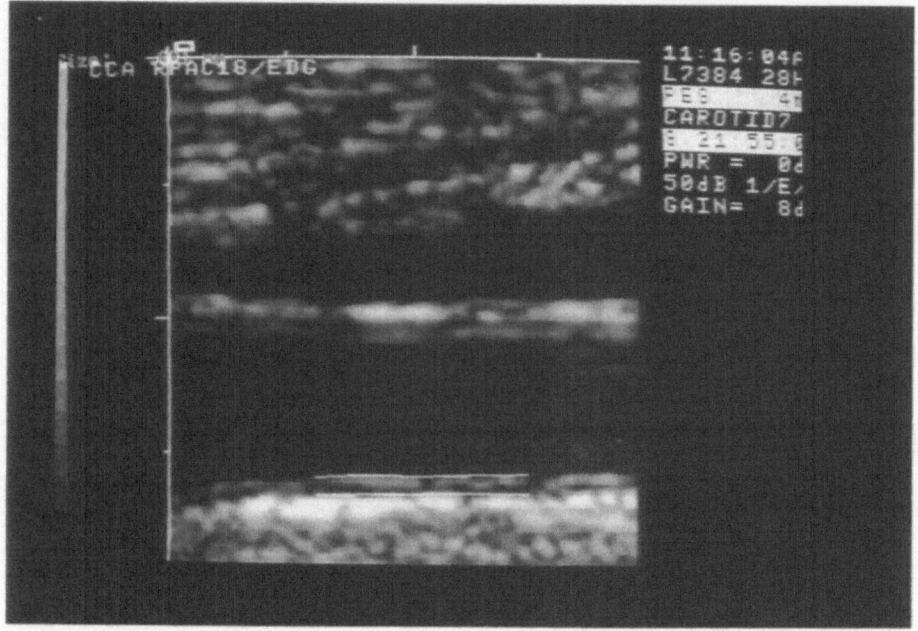

Figure 4. RES 2 x 2 cm. B-mode ultrasound image of the common carotid arterial segment. In the far wall, a measurement of approximately 10 mm along the arterial wall has been performed. The MEAN thickness of this specific segment was denoted as 0.681 mm. (For colour plate of figure 4 see page 559)

video image into a 512 by 480 digital array with 256 gray levels per picture element [31]. IMT measurements were carried out with computer software developed in cooperation with R.S. Selzer, Ph.D. [31]. The image analysis procedure was as follows. A single videoframe of the real-time B-mode image sequence of each of the arterial wall segments was selected and digitized. The selected image was to show a double line pattern. The frame selection was non ECG-triggered. To prevent observer bias, analysts were blinded to prior B-mode images or IMT data of the patient when selecting the frames. The IMT measurements on the digitized videoframes were done by positioning several crosshair markers along predefined edges of the near and far wall double line patterns. The computer program drew lines through the crosshairs. The maximum and mean distances between the lines were calculated (measurements defined as MAX IMT and MEAN IMT, respectively) (Figure 5).

Angiographic endpoints

Primary endpoints of the REGRESS study were: (1) change in average mean segment diameter (MSD) per patient, and (2) change in average minimum obstruction diameter (MOD) per patient [24]. Figure 6 shows a diagram of a coronary vessel segment indicating the area encompassing the MSD and the MOD. To make baseline correlations between coronary arteriographic and ultrasound data possible, baseline and follow-up mean percentage obstruction

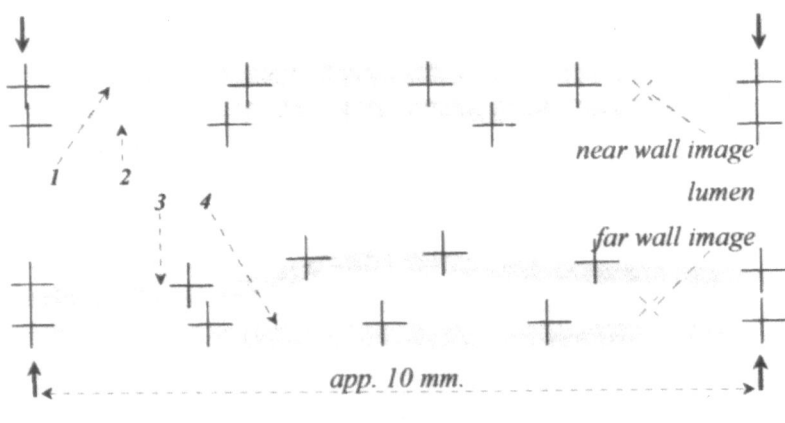

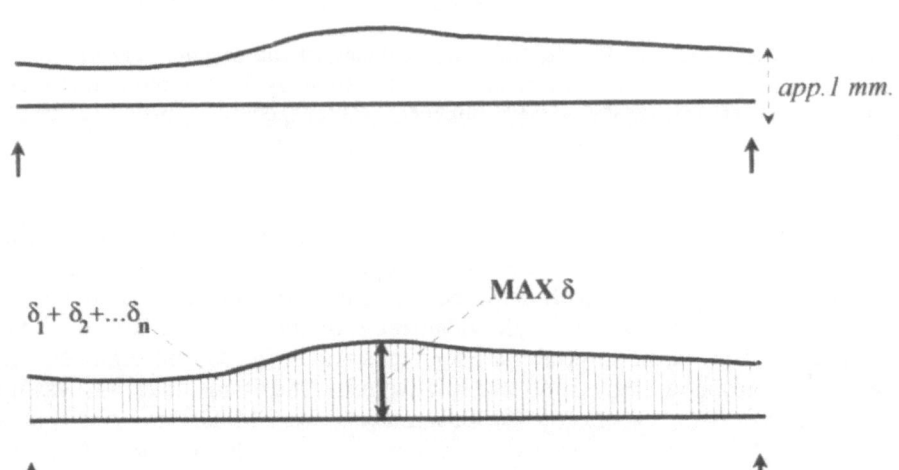

Figure 5. Off-line MAX and MEAN intima-media thickness (IMT) measurements. A) B-mode ultrasound image of the near and far wall. Predefined edges are identified with cross-marks. In the near wall, cross-marks identify the trailing edge of the undefined (peri)adventitial-media (1) and gain-dependent trailing edge of the intima-lumen interfaces (2). In the far wall, the crossmarks identify the well-defined leading edges of the lumen-intima (3) and media-adventitia interfaces(4). B) Image analysis software draws lines through the crossmarks (far wall measurement shown only). C) A MEAN IMT measurement is defined as $\delta_{MEAN} = \delta_1 + \delta_2 + ..\delta_n/n$ between the two lines. A MAX IMT measurement is defined as the maximum δ between the two lines. The MAX IMT is automatically selected by the computer software.

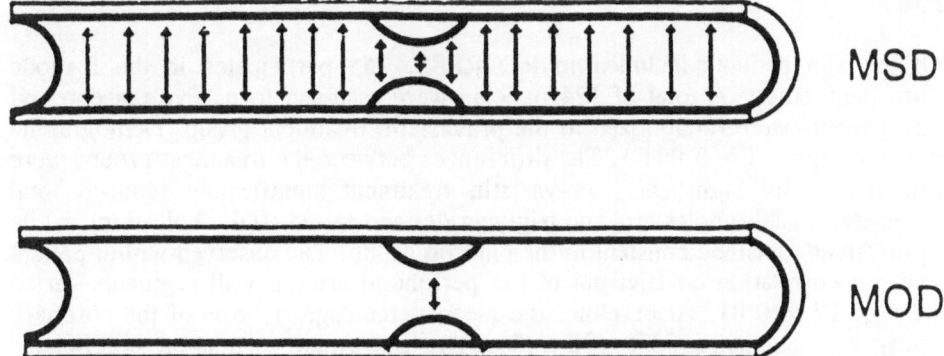

Figure 6. Diagram of a coronary vessel segment indicating the Mean Segment Diameter (MSD), and the Minimum Obstruction Diameter (MOD). MSD $= \Sigma_1^N \updownarrow /N$.

scores were determined as follows: for each patient the most severe narrowing, expressed as % lumen diameter reduction, was determined for each analyzable coronary segment (as previously defined); the percentages were summed and the total was divided by the number of contributing segments [24].

Endpoints of the ultrasound study

Primary endpoint of the B-mode ultrasound study was the differential change over time of the means of the combined segment MAX(imum) IMT's [21]. Secondary endpoints included the use of the MEAN IMT data, and the separate analyses of the combined arterial far wall segments. The baseline and treatment effect correlations between peripheral and coronary parameters were assessed.

Statistical Analysis

The angiographic effect of treatment on mean segment diameter was assessed using analysis of covariance with baseline levels as covariates. The treatment effect on the median of the minimum obstruction diameter was analyzed with non-parametric methods (Mann-Whitney test and rank ANOVA), because of the extremely skewed distribution. Therefore the median and the median change of the minimum obstruction diameter was presented to illustrate treatment effects [24]. For the ultrasound study, the IMT analyses were modelled using ANOVA with a random patient factor, fixed segment and therapy factors. Time since start of therapy was modelled as a (linear) covariate [32]. Relationships between peripheral arterial segment IMT's were described by Pearson correlation coefficients. Relationships between peripheral arterial segment IMT's and mean % coronary stenosis were described by Spearman correlation coefficients. A p-value of ≤ 0.05 was considered to be significant.

Results

Of the 885 patients included in REGRESS, 255 participated in the B-mode ultrasound study. A total of 124 patients were assigned to receive placebo and 131 patients were randomized to the pravastatin treatment group. Demographic data are reported in Table 1. The differences between the treatment groups were not statistically significant. Pravastatin treatment significantly reduced total cholesterol, LDL-cholesterol and triglycerides and raised HDL-cholesterol, while lipid values remained constant in the placebo group. The observed within-patient Pearson correlation coefficients of the peripheral arterial wall segments varied from -0.17 to 0.81. At baseline, the mean percentage stenosis of the coronary artery segments was 35% (SD=12). The Spearman correlation coefficients between baseline IMT measurements of each of the arterial wall segments and baseline % stenosis in the coronary vessels varied from -0.30 to 0.36. Repeated QCA data showed significant pravastatin treatment effects in the coronary arteries (δMSD=0.04 mm, p=0.02; δMOD=0.06 mm, p=0.001) [24]. The treatment effects on the peripheral arterial walls were highly significant (p=0.0024 for the combined MAX IMT and p=0.0085 for the combined MEAN IMT). This result was mainly due to the differential change over time in the combined far wall IMT's: p<0.0001. No significant correlations were found between the change in the mean percentage coronary stenosis (or in any of the other parameters of coronary diameter change), and the change in IMT of any of the arterial wall segments (all p>0.30) [21].

Discussion

In agreement with clinical practice and autopsy studies [18], our data reflect the great variability in the manifestation of atherosclerosis within and between vascular beds. The correlations between the peripheral arterial wall segments within the individual were low to moderate. Low correlations were found between peripheral IMT and the mean % coronary stenosis. No correlations in treatment effect between the two vascular beds were observed. Several reasons may be given to explain the lack of correlation between peripheral B-mode ultrasound and coronary arteriography. In the first place, the reason for the relatively poor correlation may be a biological one [18,34]. It is conceivable that in the short 2 year period of the REGRESS study, individual changes in the coronary and the peripheral arteries did not run parallel [33], whereas there would have been a better agreement if the patients were followed over longer periods of time. Secondly, B-mode imaging is characterized by a relatively low resolution (0.2-0.4 mm) [30,31] if compared to the structures of the intima-media complex (the mean of MAX IMT in REGRESS during the study was 1.08 (0.42) mm), and treatment effect (in the order of 0.01-0.1 mm) [20-23]. Thirdly, ultrasound and arteriography have different approaches to the observation of atherosclerosis: B-mode ultrasound imaging investigates the structures of the arterial wall itself, and coronary arteriography investigates the contours of the arterial lumen.

Table 1.

Baseline Characteristics[*]		Placebo (N=124)	Pravastatin (N=131)	p[**]
Age in years(SD)		55.2 (7.7)	56.8 (8.1)	0.10
Body Mass Index in kg/m²(SD)		26.4 (2.8)	26.1 (2.7)	0.27
SBP in mmHg(SD)		137.1(17.7)	133.8(17.3)	0.13
DBP in mmHg(SD)		82.2(11.3)	79.6(10.0)	0.06
Ejection Fraction(%)		70.5(12.7)	69.5(12.2)	0.55
Initial treatment (number(%))				
	M	61(49)	59(45)	0.79
	C	29(23)	34(26)	
	P	34(27)	38(29)	
Hypertension (number(%))		39(32)	28(21)	0.07
Familial Heart Disease		65(52)	63(48)	0.49
Smoking History		111(90)	119(91)	0.72
Smoking at randomisation		37(30)	43(33)	0.61
Smoking during study		39(32)	43(33)	0.81
Previous Myocardial Infarction		58(47)	73(56)	0.15
Previous PTCA		15(12)	10 (8)	0.23
Anginaclass(NYHA):number(%)				
	I	25(20)	18(14)	0.35
	II	50(40)	61(47)	
	III	42(34)	48(37)	
	IV	7 (6)	4 (3)	
Number of coronary	1	60(49)	60(46)	0.26
arteries with > 50%	2	41(33)	36(28)	
stenosis:number(%)	3	22(18)	34(26)	
Baseline lipid levels				
TC (mmol/L)(SD)		6.12(0.88)	6.18(0.88)	0.58
HDL (mmol/L)		0.97(0.22)	0.99(0.25)	0.41
LDL (mmol/L)		4.33(0.79)	4.36(0.77)	0.77
Triglycerides (mmol/L)		1.82(1.02)	1.85(0.78)	0.78

[*]SBP=Systolic Blood Pressure; DBP=Diastolic Blood Pressure; M=Medication, C=CABG=Coronary Artery Bypass Grafting; P=PTCA=Percutaneous Transluminal Coronary Angioplasty; NYHA=New York Heart Association; TC=Total Cholesterol; HDL=High Density Lipoprotein; LDL=Low Density Lipoprotein.
[**]significance level of Student's unpaired t-test or the chi-squared test, where appropriate.

In conclusion, within the individual an IMT measurement of a given peripheral arterial wall segment cannot be used as a surrogate endpoint to predict the state of atherosclerosis in the coronary arteries [34], let alone the prediction of, even smaller, individual treatment effects. This makes peripheral IMT measurements unsuitable as a screening method for coronary artery disease, or as a test for individual medication treatment effects on the coronary arteries. However, in the entire population treatment effects in the peripheral and coronary arteries showed parallel trends. The peripheral IMT measurements showed highly significant treatment effects, and are therefore suitable to investigate the anti-atherosclerotic properties of pharmaceutical agents.

Acknowledgements

The REGRESS study was sponsored by Bristol-Myers Squibb Company, Princeton, N.J., U.S.A.

References

1. Pignoli P, Tremoli E, Poli A, Oreste P, Paoletti R. Intimal plus medial thickness of the arterial wall: a direct measurement with ultrasound imaging. Circulation 1986;74:1399-406.
2. Poli A, Tremoli E, Colombo A, Sirtori M, Pignoli P, Paoletti R. Ultrasonographic measurement of the common carotid artery wall thickness in hypercholesterolemic patients. A new model for the quantitation and follow up of preclinial atherosclerosisin living human subjects. Atherosclerosis 1988;70:253-61.
3. Linssen FMJ. Non-invasive arterial wall tissue characterization: developement and evaluation of narrowband ultrasound techniques [dissertation]. Maastricht: University of Limburg, 1992.
4. Bots ML, Mulder PGH, Hofman A, van Es GA, Grobbee DE. Assessment of early atherosclerosis: a new perspective. J Drug Res 1991;16:150-4.
5. Howard G, Sharrett AR, Heiss G et al. Carotid artery intimal-medial thickness distribution in general populations as evaluated by B-mode ultrasound. ARIC Investigators. Stroke 1993;24:1297-304.
6. Bots ML, Brestan PJ, Briet E et al. Cardiovascular determinants of carotid artery disease. The Rotterdam Elderly Study. Hypertension 1992;19:717-20.
7. Bots ML, van Swieten JC, Breteler MM et al. Cerebral white matter lesions and atherosclerosis in the Rotterdam Study. Lancet 1993;341:1232-7.
8. Heiss G, Sharrett AR, Barnes R, Chambless LE, Szklo M, Alzola C. Carotid atherosclerosis measured by B-mode ultrasound in populations: associations with cardiovascular risk factors in the ARIC study. Am J Epidemiol 1991;134:250-6.
9. O'Leary DH, Polak JF, Wolfson SK et al. Use of sonography to evaluate carotid atherosclerosis in the elderly. The Cardiovascular Health Study CHS Colloborative Research Group. Stroke 1991;22:1155-63.
10. Salonen R, Salonen JT. Determinants of carotid intima-media thickness. A population based ultrasonography study in Eastern Finnish men. J Intern Med 1991;229:225-31.

11. Salonen R, Salonen JT. Progression of carotid atherosclerosis and its determinants: a population based ultrasonography study. Atherosclerosis 1990;81:33-40.

12. Salonen R, Salonen JT. Ultrasonographically assessed carotid morphology and the risk of coronary heart disease. Arterioscler Tromb 1991;11:1245-9.

13. Wendelhag I, Wiklund O, Wikstrand J. Arterial wall thickness in familial hypercholesterolemia. Ultrasound measurement of intima-media thickness in the common carotid artery. Arterioscler Thromb 1992;12:70-7.

14. Wendelhag I, Wiklund O, Wikstrand J. Ultrasonographic assessment of intima-media thickness and plaque accurance. Atherosclerotic changes in the femoral and the carotid arteries in familial hypercholesterolemia. Arterioscler Thromb 1993;13:1404-11.

15. Tell GS, Howard G, McKinney WM, Toole JF. Cigarette smoking cessation and extracranial carotid atherosclerosis. JAMA 1989;261:1178-80.

16. Gnasso A, Pujia A, Irace C, Mattioli PL. Increased carotid arterial wall thickness in common hyperlipidemia. Coron Artery Dis 1995;6:57-63.

17. Furberg CD, Adams HP Jr, Applegate WB *et al.* Effect of lovaststatin on early atherosclerosis and cardiovascular events. Asymptomatic Carotid Artery Progression Study (ACAPS) Research Group. Circulation 1994;90:1679-87.

18. Blankenhorn DH, Nodis HN. George Lyman Duff Memorial Lecture. Arterial imaging and atherosclerosis reversal. Arterioscler Thromb 1994;14:177-92.

19. Blankenhorn DH, Selzer RS, Crawford DW *et al.* Beneficial effects of colestipol-niacin therapy on the common carotid artery. Two- and four-year reduction of intima-media thickness measured by ultrasound. Circulation 1993;88:20-8.

20. Salonen R, Nyyssonen K, Porkkala E *et al.* Kuopio Atherosclerosis Prevention Study (KAPS). A population-based primary preventive trial of the effect of LDL lowering on atherosclerotic progression in carotid and femoral arteries. Circulation 1995;92:1758-64.

21. De Groot E, Jukema JW, van Boven AJ *et al.* The effect of pravastatin on progression and regression of coronary atherosclerosis and vessel wall changes in carotid and femoral arteries: a report from the Regression Growth Evaluation Statin Study (REGRESS). Am J Cardiol 1995;76:40C-46C.

22. Crouse JR, Byington RP, Bond MG *et al.* Pravastatin, Lipids, and Atherosclerosis in the carotid arteries (PLAC II). Am J Cardiol 1995;75:455-9.

23. Byington RP, Furberg CD, Crouse JR, Espeland MA, Bond MG. Pravastatin, Lipids, and Atherosclerosis in the carotid arteries (PLAC-II). Am J Cardiol 1995;76:54C-59C.

24. Jukema JW, Bruschke AVG, van Boven AJ *et al.* Effects of lipid lowering by pravastatin on progression and regression of coronary artery disease in symptomatic men with normal to moderately elevated serum cholesterol levels. The Regression Growth Evaluation Statin Study (REGRESS). Circulation 1995;91:2528-40.

25. Blankenhorn DH, Azen SP, Kramsch DM *et al.* Coronary angiographic changes with lovastatin therapy. The Monitored Atherosclerosis Regression Study (MARS). Ann Intern Med 1993;119:969-76.

26. Waters D, Higginson L, Gladstone P *et al.* Effect of monotherapy with an HMG CoA reductase inhibitor on the progression of coronary atherosclerosis as assessed by serial quantitative arteriography. The Canadian Coronary Atherosclerosis Intervention Trial. Circulation 1994;89:959-68.

27. Effect of simvastatin on coronary atheroma: the Multi-Centre Anti-Atheroma Study (MAAS). Lancet 1994;344:633-8

28. Austen WG, Edwards JE, Frye RL *et al.* A reporting system on patients evaluated for coronary artery disease. Report of the Ad Hoc Committee for Grading of Coronary Artery Disease, Council on Cardiovascular Surgery, American Heart Association. Circulation 1975;51(Suppl.4):5-40.

29. Reiber JHC, van der Zwet PMJ, von Land CD, Koning G, van Meurs B, van Voorthuizen AE. Quantitative coronary arteriography: equipment and technical requirements. In Reiber JHC, Serruys PW, editors. Advances in quantitative coronary arteriography. Dordrecht: Kluwer Academic Publishers, 1992:75-111.

30. Montauban van Swijndregt AD, Salem HK The, Gussenhoven EJ *et al.* An in vitro evaluation of the line pattern of the near and the far walls of carotid arteries using B-mode ultrasound (unpublished data, 1996).

31. Selzer RH, Hodis HN, Kwong-Fu H *et al.* Evaluation of computerized edge tracking for quantifying intima-media thickness of the common carotid artery from B-mode ultrasound images. Atherosclerosis 1994;111:1-11.

32. Espeland MA, Byington RP, Hire D, Davis VG, Hartwell T, Probstfield J. Analysis strategies for serial multivariate ultrasonographic data that are incomplete. Stat Med 1992;11:1041-56.

33. Bruschke AVG, Kramer JR Jr, Bal ET, Haque IU, Detrano RC, Goormastic M. The dynamics of progression of coronary atherosclerosis studied in 168 medically treated patients who underwent coronary arteriography three times. Am Heart J 1989;117:296-305.

34. Adams MR, Nakagomi A, Keech A *et al.* Carotid intima-media thickness is only weakly correlated with the extent and severity of coronary artery disease. Circulation 1995;92:2127-34.

12. The digital catheterization laboratory - is it practical today?

JACK T. CUSMA & THOMAS M. BASHORE

Summary

The rapid pace of change in information technologies - computer hardware, software, and networking - has led to expectations among many in the cardiology community that these advances now make it a simple matter to replace 35mm cinefilm with digital techniques. This objective has been delayed, however, due to the difficulty of replacing *all* the roles played by cinefilm using digital alternatives. Recent developments in technology and in the implementation of standard methods for communicating information among cardiac laboratories and imaging systems demonstrate sufficient promise that it is now realistic to speak of an all-digital catheterization laboratory. It is even, in fact, now feasible to produce a patient and exam record in a digital format containing multiple imaging modalities: x-ray angiography, echocardiography, and nuclear cardiology. In addition to the digital acquisition and review systems which have become commonplace in today's cardiac catheterization laboratory, it is now possible to exchange patient exams in a digital format using the internationally accepted DICOM standard. Development and acceptance of this standard, implemented using either portable exchange media or over a digital network, has served to overcome one of the most significant obstacles to the transition from cinefilm to an all-digital environment. In addition, the multiple options available for the long-term storage of digital x-ray angiograms make it possible for laboratories with varying needs to move to a cine-less practice. As these laboratories better define their local requirements and balance these needs against the cost and technical capabilities of available options, they will demonstrate that there is no single way to function without cinefilm but, rather, multiple paths that can be taken to the all digital catheterization laboratory.

Introduction

The rapid pace of developments in information technologies - digital computers and networks - has led to significant changes in all aspects of society including the healthcare community. In the specific area of cardiac x-ray angiography - the principle means for the diagnosis of cardiac disease - the long awaited replacement of 35 mm cinefilm as the procedure record using digital methods has remained a seemingly unattainable goal [1,2]. There are a number of factors which have been responsible for the *delay* in achieving this goal, but recent developments have demonstrated significant promise for cardiac catheterization laboratories which are considering the move to an operating environment without cinefilm.

While the introduction of digital technology in the cardiac catheterization

157

J.H.C. Reiber and E.E. van der Wall (eds.), Cardiovascular Imaging, 157-170.

laboratory took place in the mid-1980's, the complete replacement of cinefilm with digital technologies remained difficult to achieve. The advantages provided by digital angiographic methods for acquisition of the x-ray images formed during the catheterization procedure compared to cinefilm were significant [3,4]. These included immediate access to high quality image data and the capability for image processing and quantitative analysis of angiographic frames while the patient procedure was still underway [5]. Many of these capabilities - not available with cinefilm - led to the rapid embrace of the digital acquisition of cardiac x-ray images *in parallel with 35 mm cinefilm*, especially for interventional procedures such as PTCA.

Acquisition of angiographic images, however, is only one of the roles provided by cinefilm and it is the delivery of these additional functions *at an economical cost* which has been difficult to achieve. In most laboratories in the world, cinefilm is the *archival* record for the procedure; it is consulted repeatedly following the initial encounter and diagnosis in order to evaluate subsequent therapies and progress of a patient. While not very elegant, it is easily accessed from a storeroom or a warehouse and can be displayed with little technical training. When it is reviewed, it provides a display of the heart of a patient at real-time rates, i.e. the cardiac function and dynamic processes are shown at the *same* rate at which they occurred while the patient was on the examination table. While apparently straightforward, the effective digital rate required to perform the same function is well beyond those required for more familiar digital computing applications and networks which one encounters on a routine basis. In addition, cinefilm has become by far the universal means for *exchange* of data between hospitals and medical centers, for example, when a patient is referred to a second site for surgery or interventional procedures.

Achieving a cine-less environment in the cardiac catheterization laboratory requires the delivery of all the imaging functions currently utilized, plus new capabilities which will certainly arise once their potential implementation becomes practical. The incentives for replacement of cinefilm have led, for example, approximately 300 laboratories in the U.S. to install a cine-less system which may or may not be an *all-digital* archive and display system [6]. As has been pointed out recently, the lack of standard methods for such systems - whether they are analog or digital systems - can lead to significant difficulties [7]. In the remainder of this paper, the specific requirements of an all-digital replacement for cinefilm will be described in greater detail and an assessment will be provided of how close the technology and, possibly more importantly, the market is to delivering these capabilities at a cost that is within reach of the typical cardiac catheterization laboratories.

Acquisition of cardiac x-ray angiographic procedures

Digital acquisition of cardiac x-ray images has become commonly accepted in modern laboratories despite its relatively high additional cost in the purchase of an x-ray system for cardiac angiography. This is due to the unquestioned advantages such technology provides in the modern catheterization laboratory: immediate access to high quality images; real-time image processing and manipulation; capability for performing quantitative analysis [8]. The cost of providing such capabilities is high due to the demanding technical requirements; in digital terms, the need to deliver dynamic images of the heart translates into very large amounts of data and very high acquisition and display rates. For example, a typical exam consisting of 3000 frames of x-ray images in a 512 x 512 format acquired at a rate of 30 frames/sec results in 750 Megabytes (MB) of data and a transfer rate of 7.5 MB/sec. These parameters remain significantly difficult to achieve using the widely available "consumer" oriented computer systems and networks and, thus, their delivery is relatively expensive. Nonetheless, the perceived *necessity* of digital image acquisition has led to the situation where digital acquisition is an *accepted* part of the catheterization routine. In other words, digital acquisition has become a *practical* reality in today's catheterization laboratories if not an inexpensive option.

Review and display of digital angiographic procedures

The diagnostic review of cardiac x-ray images requires dynamic display at the same rate at which the images were originally acquired (or faster). Sampling rates sufficient to detect abnormalities in cardiac function can routinely be as high as 60 frames/sec and, accordingly, review must be provided at similar rates. Again, assuming a typical digital image matrix of 512 x 512 x 8 bits, this leads to a display requirement of 7.5 MB/sec at a rate of 30 frames/sec and twice that at 60 frames/sec. Until recently such display rates were only possible on the same high-performance equipment used for image acquisition; only the parallel transfer disks, proprietary bus technologies, and dedicated image processors provided in the digital acquisition system could provide these required data rates. The state-of-the-art computers available today can deliver the required display rates once the exam data is accessible, i.e. stored on local disk and/or written to local random access memory (RAM) from which the cardiac sequences can be displayed. A typical injection, for example, lasting 10 seconds results in some 300 frames of digital data (at the matrix size and rate assumed above) or 75 MB. Computers in a hospital environment are rarely found equipped with this large amount of RAM; the alternative is high-speed network and disk access to deliver the data at the required rate. Such capabilities remain beyond the reach of commonly available computers and networks; for the time being, it is a fair assumption that they can be delivered only using the same equipment employed for image acquisition.

Network and disk technology is resulting in performance which is approaching the required specifications but, even then, the distribution of dynamic review stations beyond the acquisition laboratory is limited by a lack of means for exporting the acquired digital exam data from the acquisition system. While development efforts by medical imaging equipment vendors were successful in delivering the required clinical functions, in general, they led to proprietary formats for data and its communication. This means that, even if "off-the-shelf" computers and networks could provide diagnostically useful display, there remains no *standard* way to access the acquired exam data. Work on standards for medical imaging described below demonstrates promise for overcoming this obstacle but these standards are not yet at the point where the exam data is easily accessible.

To summarize the issues relating to display and review, such capabilities are possible on a limited basis within the catheterization laboratory and, possibly, on review stations that can interface to the usually proprietary acquisition systems. While the technical capabilities of commonly available equipment is approaching the required parameters, for such capabilities to become truly widespread and practical, further work on the development and establishment of standards for image exchange must be done.

Interchange of digital angiographic data

One of the most important functions of cardiac image data is the interchange between institutions of a patient's data for routine referral purposes, for example, when a patient is referred to a second medical center for surgery or an interventional procedure. In addition, the exchange of image data in clinical trials of drug or other therapies has become commonplace in order to perform quantitative analysis at a central core laboratory. Cinefilm has served well as a truly universal exchange medium and any digital replacement for it must meet this vitally important function.

As manufacturers of imaging equipment and potential suppliers of archival systems (more of which will be discussed below) have considered the available options for delivering all the capabilities of digital images, the issue of interchange and the uncertainty around the digital means for achieving it, has served to potentially delay further developments. For that reason, the American College of Cardiology began working with manufacturers to develop a protocol and media options for exchanging patient exams between institutions regardless of the type of equipment used to acquire or display the exam data at either institution. This effort, begun in 1993 with the cooperation of the National Electronic Manufacturer's Association (NEMA) , has resulted in an extension of the DICOM (Digital Imaging and Communication in Medicine) standard to include image data found in cardiac exams [9,10]. These image modalities include digital x-ray angiography, digital echocardiography, and nuclear cardiology exam data. The extension, labeled DISC - DICOM Interchange Standard for Cardiology - specifies the data format to be used and the media options which are acceptable for the various modalities. As a result, clinical laboratories are assured that digital data acquired in their laboratory can be displayed at another institution in the same manner and with the same quality present in the originating laboratory. While the focus of the ACC/NEMA effort was initially on portable media, the same standard has been employed for network or telecommunication implementations of exam interchange.

The media choice adopted by the ACC/NEMA process for digital x-ray cardiac exams was the Compact Disc - Recordable (CD-R); since then, other standards committees for echocardiography and nuclear cardiology have designated other media as well but all have endorsed the use of CD-R as an approved exchange medium. As of early 1996, a number of vendors have offered products which incorporate the CD-R with the DICOM standard for the exchange of x-ray cardiac data. The feasibility of the DICOM standard has been demonstrated at a number of international meetings over the last several years and a number of sites in Europe and the U.S. have installed commercial systems (Figure 1). The flexibility, low cost, and universal acceptance and compatibility of CD-R demonstrates promise that the necessary means for exchanging digital exam data will be in place as archival and communications systems continue in development and eventual deployment.

As a result of the successful standards development in the U.S. and Europe, the exchange of digital cardiac data is becoming much more of a certainty. This, in turn, leads to an increasing likelihood that more laboratories will take the step of adopting digital-only systems, assured that a practical and reliable means for exchange of patient data is in place.

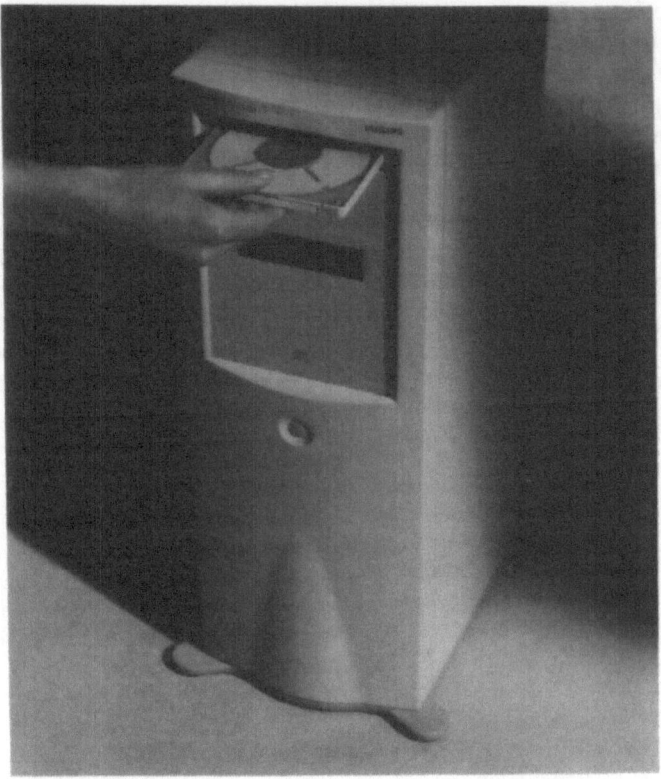

Figure 1. An example of an early commercial version of the digital exchange medium which meets the DICOM standard for cardiology. The single patient record Compact Disc - Recordable (CD-R) stores angiographic data in a format which can be interpreted by multiple vendors. (Courtesy of Philips Medical Systems)

Archival Systems

One of the more difficult tasks which must be addressed in order to replace cinefilm with digital alternatives is the development of suitable means for archiving, i.e. long-term storage, of patient exam data. Among the reasons that this task is made more complex is the fact that few in the clinical cardiology community are in agreement on what constitutes a sufficient amount of time that an archive must be maintained and what degree of reliability must be provided by the archive. These issues - not truly technical in nature - make it more difficult for manufacturers to justify extensive development efforts for long-term archives.

The length of time required for maintenance of an archive of cardiac catheterization records ranges from as few as three years to as long as fifteen years. This range has obvious impact on the type of archival system selected by a laboratory. Other questions that must be resolved by the laboratory personnel is the means by which stored data will be retrieved, i.e. manually or in an automated fashion. The goal of achieving automated access to unlimited amounts of data has been implicit in the thinking of many who have considered digital archiving in the cardiac imaging application - this, even though the existing method using cinefilm is a very manual and unsatisfactory method. The remaining issue that impacts upon the selection of an archival medium and method is whether a *single-patient record* is considered a desirable objective. This last term refers to the fact that a single piece of media contains only one exam record; this is more reassuring to those who are concerned with potential damage to the archived records. A comparison of media which could be used for the two approaches is shown in Figure 2.

The way that the above issues are decided for a given laboratory impacts significantly upon the cost of an archival system and, in turn, on whether a given solution is considered to be a practical one. In the discussion that follows, several levels of complexity and concordant cost are examined.

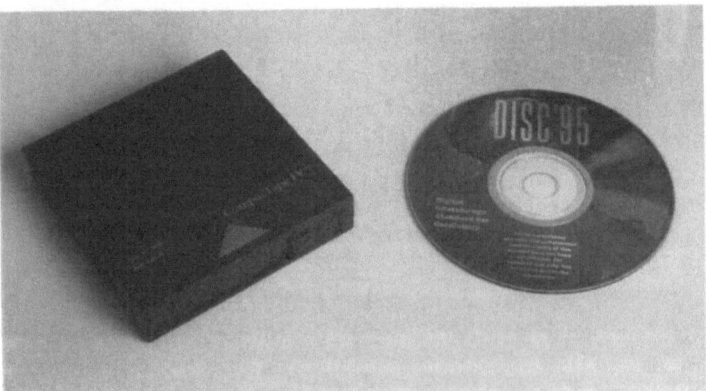

Figure 2. A comparison of a single exam record CD-R and a multiple exam Digital Linear Tape (DLT) which can be used to archive digital cardiac angiographic images. The DLT can hold from 40 to 80 patient exams - depending on the acquisition rate and image matrix - at a cost 5-6 times that of the CD-R.

Small-volume laboratory with non-automated archive

A laboratory that performs a relatively small number of procedures, e.g. less than 1,000 annually may find it difficult to justify the relatively large capital expenditure of an automated archival system. The acceptance of the DICOM exchange standard means that a laboratory can, if it chooses, generate single exam records for all of its patient procedures which will serve as the internal archive as well as an exchange medium between institutions when necessary. This type of system is illustrated schematically in Figure 3.

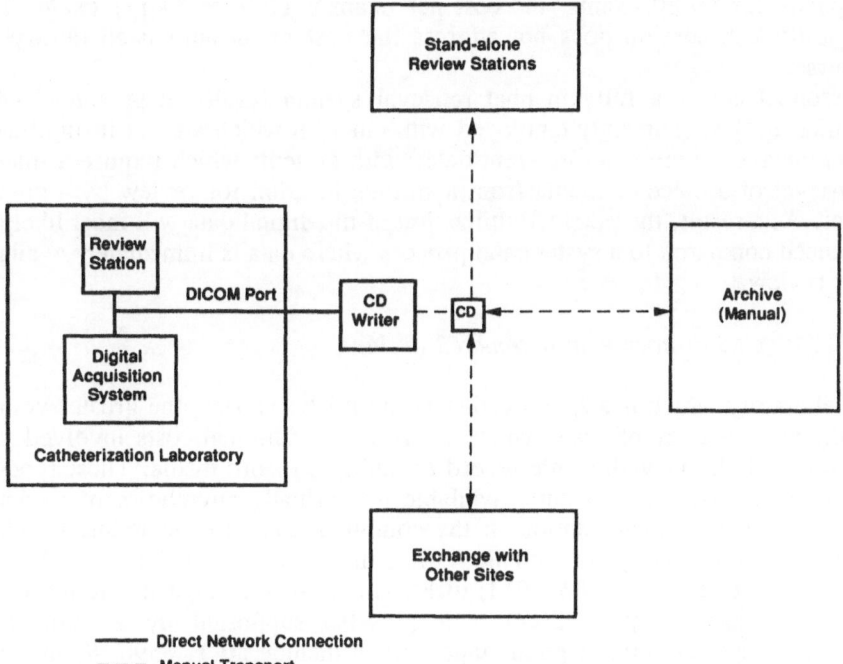

Figure 3. A schematic diagram of an archive system for a small laboratory which utilizes single exam media (such as CD-R) as both the exchange medium and the archive medium. No automation is employed and networking is not included but it does provide for the complete replacement of cinefilm.

The advantages compared to film:
* reduced costs - the cost of the media and the initial investment for a media writer, e.g. CD-R writer, become lower at some point than the cost of maintaining a cinefilm developing capability and the cost of the cinefilm itself.
* digital reproducibility - storage of the data in a digital format means that exact copies can be made with no degradation in quality and, in turn, avoiding the potential loss of the only existing exam record.
* potential for upgrade - storage in a standard digital format (including DICOM) assures a laboratory of the option for upgrading their archive in the future as

needed and, in addition, provides the implicit compatibility with other digital information systems and networks as applications become available.

There are also disadvantages to pursuing this option which should be noted:

* cost per exam - the strategy which focuses on a single piece of media per each exam results in a higher media cost per exam than would be possible with a high capacity medium which can hold multiple exams. For example, a CD-R with a single exam results in a media cost of $10-20/exam (at 1996 prices) not including the cost of equipment required to take images from the acquisition system, write a CD record, and reverse the process for review. If a high capacity streamer tape such as the Digital Linear Tape (DLT) is used with a capacity for 40-80 exams, the cost per exam is close to $1 per exam. This simplified discussion does not address the cost of an automated library, of course.

* personnel cost - a fully manual retrieval system results in personnel costs similar to those currently employed with cinefilm which are not insignificant.

* time delays - there is an inherent delay with systems which require a manual retrieval of a piece of media from a storage location for review by a clinical user. As a result, the potential utilization of the digital data will most likely be reduced compared to a system and process where data is immediately available for review.

Medium-size laboratory with automated archive

In a laboratory which has 2 to 3 catheterization laboratories, the greater volume permits an efficiency of scale which justifies the additional costs involved with an automated library with single-record or multiple-record media. These types of automated libraries are currently available for virtually any choice of media as a result of their implementation in the computer data storage industry. These include digital optical media such as CD-R's, magneto-optical (read/write) disks, and write-once-read-many (WORM) disks which range in capacity from a single exam up to as many as 20-40 exams. Also supported by a number of manufacturers are digital magnetic tapes which include DLT, 3590, 8mm, 4mm DAT, and digital video tapes such as D2 and D1. The capacity of these tapes ranges from 4 exams per piece of media up to 40 or more. Library capacities range from as low as 200 pieces of media (CD-R) to the equivalent of 25,000 exams or more and costs range from $25,000 to greater than $1,000,000.

While a broad variety of applications have been developed in the computer storage industry addressing different levels of access frequency and multiple media systems, their implementation in the medical imaging industry is preliminary at this time. The multiplicity of options available are one of the reasons that vendors have not rushed to offer these types of systems; manufacturers of imaging equipment have not had the advantage possessed in the computer industry of large customer bases which make it cost-effective to pursue multiple development efforts. The lack of standards for storing and exchanging images, described above, has also been a major factor in the incorporation of these relatively complex systems.

Large-volume laboratory with automated archive and secondary access

As an institution's archival needs increase to, for example, 5000 exams annually or more, the incentive for a large automated archive becomes greater. Along with the additional numbers of acquisition labs required to generate this number of exams, there are also significantly more potential reviewers of the stored images - both recent acquisitions and archived exams. In addition to the large archive, this type of institution requires a distributed network which can deliver image data from a number of acquisition labs, display old exams at a large number - as many as 10 - review stations [11]. In addition, a larger institution generally has the need to integrate the image data from the cardiac catheterization laboratory with other image data as well as with other information systems [12] as shown in Figure 4. An automated archive along with a system manager which is responsible for migration of exam data from the long-term (deep) archive onto a near-line or short-term storage where it is available for review and diagnosis becomes a desirable objective. An example of a high capacity automated archive is shown in Figure 5.

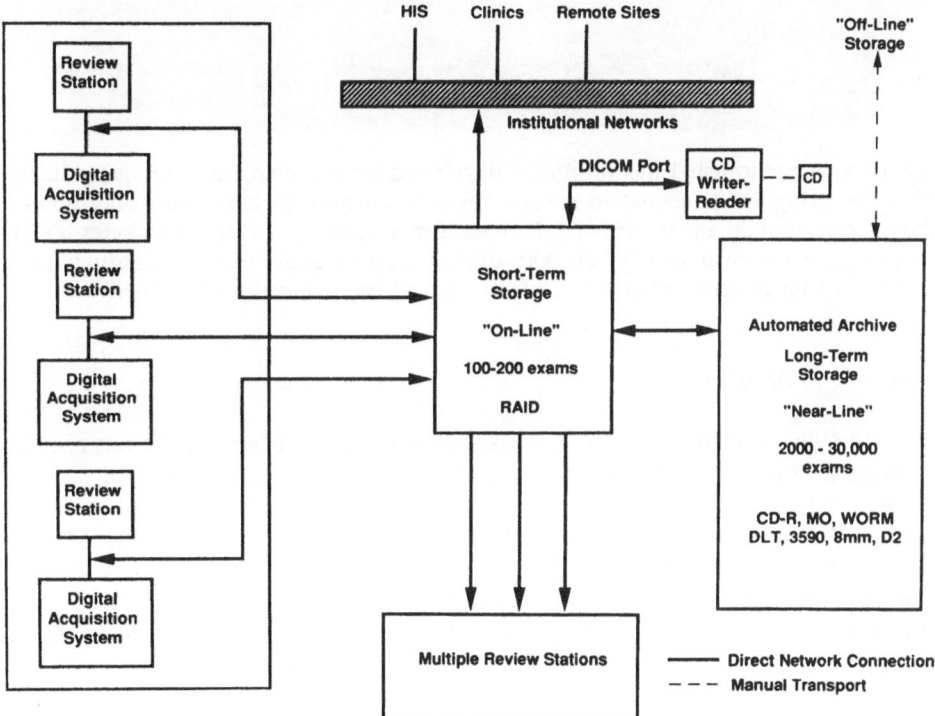

Figure 4. A schematic diagram of an archive and review system which includes multiple levels of storage, automated management of many patient exams, and interfaces with institutional information networks.

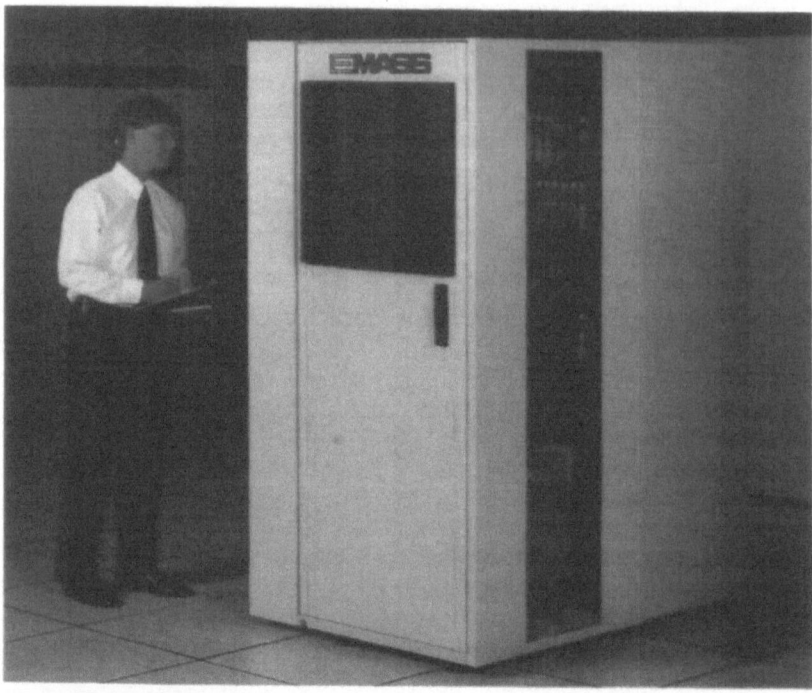

Figure 5. An automated media library developed for the computer storage industry which is being implemented in several medical imaging installations. The module shown can contain up to 450 DLT tapes for a capacity of 18 Terrabytes (TB), equivalent to approximately 24,000 digital angiographic exams acquired in a 512x512x8 bit matrix and at a rate of 30 frames/sec. (Courtesy of EMASS Corp.)

Summary of archiving

In early 1996, systems which can work for small laboratories that do not require automated libraries are being delivered for use. Automated systems for smaller installations are available as well where some 1000 to 2000 exams are available on line. A few sites in the U.S. currently possess large automated libraries which keep some 15,000 exams available for review within 40-60 seconds. Media employed included optical media such as CD-R, MO, and WORM disks as well as tape libraries. As the DICOM standard becomes accepted, it could be expected that more laboratories will make the move to digital archive systems.

The role of image compression in the digital cath lab

In all the discussion above of capacity, rates, and corresponding costs, it has been assumed that the image data acquired, transmitted, and stored is the same data acquired in the x-ray laboratory. One issue in the cath lab environment is whether data compression methods can be employed to lower the costs associated with digital cath image data. For example, if the amount of data can be reduced sufficiently, multiple exams can be stored and displayed on the equivalent of today's personal computers at a fraction of the cost of the equipment currently required for uncompressed data. Similarly, a reduction in the rates required to support real-time display and transmission reduces the type of network required to achieve these capabilities, reduces the cost, and improves the potential for widespread application of distribution systems.

The types of data compression which do not result in a loss of data, i.e. the original information can be reproduced exactly, are known as *lossless* data compression techniques and have been employed for some time in digital acquisition systems. One of these methods - lossless JPEG - has been designated for use in the CD-R implementation of the DICOM standard for x-ray angiograms. In general, these reversible methods result in at best reductions in the size of angiographic files to approximately one-third of their original size which, while helpful, does not provide the efficiencies referred to above.

A number of data compression methods can achieve much higher reductions in the amount of data but they result in files which can no longer be converted back to precisely the same data which was acquired in the x-ray procedure [13,14]. These are known as *lossy* or irreversible compression methods. Figure 6 shows the result of lossy compression used to reduce the size of a digital angiographic frame by a factor of approximately 15. Evaluations of the effects of lossy compression on the diagnostic content of cardiac x-ray images are currently underway [15,16] and, depending upon the results, the use of lossy compression may become an accepted part of the digital cath lab environment.

How to determine if a system is practical ?

It may appear as if the situation regarding whether a cine-less cath lab is practical remains confusing despite significant efforts over the past decade. The confusion today, however, arises not due to a lack of possibilities but, rather, the existence of multiple options - all of which could work for some lab to one degree or another. In determining what the *best* solution is for a given situation, a laboratory should first set the assumptions for their environment. This requires the answers to a number of questions:

1. Is a multiple exam medium acceptable or will there be a single exam per piece of media?
2. Are there requirements regarding the type of media, e.g. tape vs. disk?
3. Is a manual retrieval system acceptable?
4. Will exams have to be retrieved into the acquisition systems for display?
5. How often will old exams be accessed?
6. How many access points to the archived data are required?
7. How long must exams be archived?
8. Will it be necessary to import or export exams to other institutions?
9. Will it be necessary to transmit exams over computer or telecommunications networks?
10. Are there applications where lossy data compression can be utilized?

Once the requirements are determined, the available options can be compared on the basis of performance and cost. There are currently systems available or under development that can answer many of the above requirements.

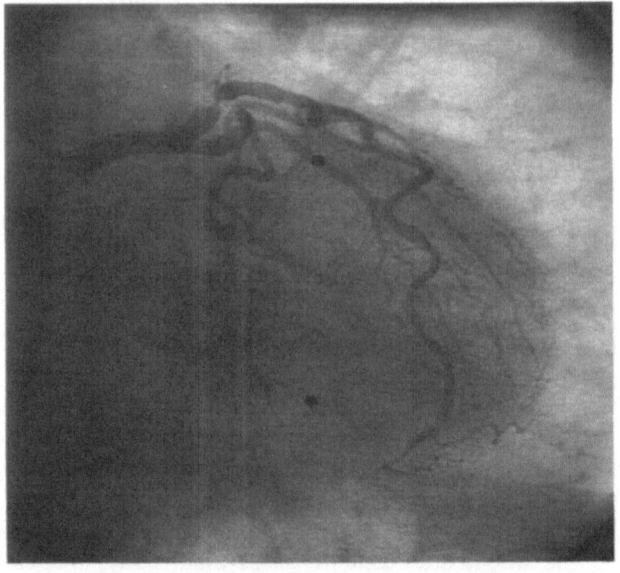

a

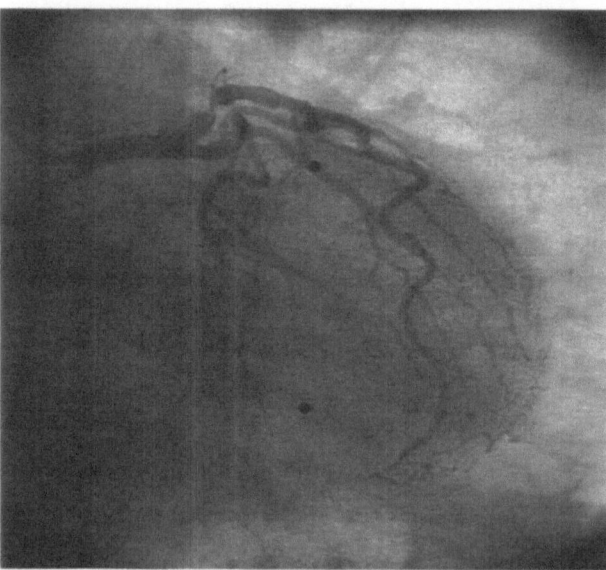

b

Figure 6. A digital angiographic frame before and after the application of lossy JPEG compression. A) The original frame which requires 240 kB of storage space. B) The compressed file which has a size of approximately 16 kB.

Conclusion

In mid-1996, it is now technically possible to assemble all the components of an all-digital catheterization laboratory. From acquisition and review to archive and exchange, there are practical methods available for taking advantage of digital angiographic technology. There may be some delay for all of the above types of systems to be made available by manufacturers of medical imaging equipment but market demand is moving all in that direction. While all options will not generally be available from every system, there are enough alternatives available such that an informed decision can be made regarding the inevitable move to a cineless environment.

References

1. Cusma JT, Fortin DF, Spero LA, Groshong BR, Bashore TM. Which media are most likely to solve the archival problem? Int J Card Imaging 1994;10:165-75.
2. Morris KG. A perspective: designing the all digital cardiac catheterization laboratory. Am J Card Imaging 1988;2:251-8.
3. Mistretta CA, Peppler WW. Digital cardiac x-ray imaging: fundamental principles. Am J Card Imaging 1988;2:26-39.
4. Whiting JS. Physical principles and instrumentation in digital angiography. In: Marcus ML, Skorton DJ, Schelbert HR, Wolf GL, editors. Cardiac imaging. Philadelphia: Saunders, 1991:281-94.
5. Van Lysel MS, Ergun DL, Miller WP *et al*. Cardiac digital angiography and dual-energy subtraction imaging: current and future trends. Am J Card Imaging 1987;1:254-66.
6. Cardiac archive and review systems for cardiac catheterization laboratories -- a post 1995 American College of Cardiology Meeting update. S.l.: Systems Techniques, Inc. 1995.
7. Cardiac angiography without cine film: erecting a "Tower of Babel" in the cardiac catheterization laboratory. American College of Cardiology Cardiac Catheterization Committee. J Am Coll Cardiol 1994;24:834-7.
8. Reiber JHC, Serruys PW. Quantitative coronary angiography. In: Marcus ML, Skorton DJ, Schelbert HR, Wolf GL, editors. Cardiac imaging. Philadelphia: Saunders, 1991:211-80.
9. Bidgood WD Jr, Horii SC. Introduction to the ACR-NEMA DICOM standard. Radiographics 1992;12:345-55.
10. American College of Cardiology, American College of Radiology and industry develop standard for digital transfer of angiographic images. ACC/ACR/NEMA Ad Hoc Group. J Am Coll Cardiol 1995;25:800-2.
11. Condit PB. Requirements for cardiac interchange media and the role of recordable CD. Int J Card Imaging 1995:11(Suppl.3):153-7.
12. Cusma JT, Spero LA, Groshong BR, Cho T, Bashore TM. Design and evaluation of a high capacity digital image archival library and high speed network for the replacement of cinefilm in the cardiac angiography environment. Proc SPIE 1993;1899:413-22.
13. Brennecke R, Lang M, Fritsch JP, Erbel R, Meyer J. A framework for PACS development in cardiology. Comput Cardiol 1992:259-61.

14. Rabbani M, Jones PW. Image compression techniques for medical diagnostic imaging systems. J Digit Imaging 1991;4:65-78.
15. Rigolin VH, Robiolio PA, Spero LA *et al*. Compression of digital coronary angiograms does not affect visual or quantitative assessment of coronary artery stenosis severity. Am J Cardiol. In press.
16. Whiting J, Eckstein M, Honig D, Gu S, Einav S, Eigler N. Effect of lossy image compression on observer performance in dynamically displayed digital coronary angiograms [abstract]. Circulation 1992;86(Suppl.I):I444.

13. The role of DICOM in the digital catheterization laboratory

BOB GOEDHART & JOHAN H.C. REIBER

Summary

Over the last decade, the specification of a standard format for digital (medical) images has received a great deal of attention. The yearly meetings of the ACC (95 and 96) and ESC (95) were used to promote the DICOM (Digital Imaging and Communications in Medicine) format, the result of a joined effort by the ACC, ACR, NEMA and ESC. At the moment, one of the most interesting questions is: how will the introduction of the DICOM standard affect the daily practice in the catheterization laboratory (cath lab) in the near future?

In this chapter, the position of the cath lab (and especially the digital image acquisition system) is described in a digital networked environment. An abstract scheme of such an environment is used to illustrate the place of and connection between the different components. The requirements for these components are formulated and discussed and will be related to the current and future developments of the major manufacturers. It will be shown that the use of the DICOM format is crucial in such an environment.

Introduction

The use of cinefilm as the major image review, exchange and archival medium has decreased significantly over the years. During the late eighties and early nineties, a large number of non-standard, non-compatible cineless acquisition systems were installed world-wide. The media used to record the images were either non-standard, non-interchangeable or could not retain adequate image resolution for diagnosis. The lack of a standard for digital image exchange resulted in what has been called by Nissen et al. [1] a *Tower of Babel* in the cath lab: the use of proprietary file formats by each vendor or manufacturer of digital image acquisition systems.

Fortunately, this trend was recognized and responded to by the American College of Cardiology (ACC), the American College of Radiology (ACR) and the National Electrical Manufacturers Association (NEMA). Over the last several years, the development of a standard for the exchange of medical images has been studied by a committee initiated by the ACC, the ACR and NEMA [2]. Not long thereafter, a Task Force was formed by the European Society of Cardiology (ESC) to support these activities [3].

Currently, this work has been finalized to a large extent. As a result, the DICOM (Digital Imaging and Communications in Medicine) standard has been introduced. The standard guarantees the smooth exchange of medical images between the equipment of different manufacturers. In addition, other cardiac societies (Echocardiology, Nuclear Cardiology, Magnetic Resonance) have committed to

171

the DICOM standard at a later stage. In this chapter, a brief overview of the standard will be provided.

With the DICOM standard now accepted, we were curious how and when the major manufacturers are going to conform to the standard. Therefore, we developed an abstract scheme of a digital cath lab environment, which will be presented in this chapter. Based on the schematic cath lab environment, a questionnaire was developed and presented to the major manufacturers. The main topics that were distinguished in the questionnaire were acquisition, review and analysis, exchange and archiving of cardiovascular images. The answers to the questions have been summarized and will be discussed.

The chapter is concluded with a discussion on the applicability of DICOM and its role in the (future) setting of medical imaging. Clearly, the results of the questionnaire form the input for this discussion.

DICOM

The DICOM standard consists of a set of rules that allow the exchange of digital medical images and information between different pieces of equipment within an institution or with equipment used outside of the institution. The standard serves as a common language that guarantees that digital images produced on one vendor's equipment can be displayed or printed on the equipment of another one. For a detailed description of the DICOM format we refer to [4].

The current generation of digital image acquisition systems supports the acquisition and the display/review of angiographic image series. However, there is a wide variety of solutions for the exchange and archiving of the digital images. For instance, S-VHS video tape is one of the media that is currently used for exchange and archiving. However, this medium has been proven of insufficient quality for this purpose [5].

The choice for CD-R as the storage medium

The replacement of cinefilm by a digital equivalent not only requires the specification of a digital storage *format* but the choice of a digital storage *medium* as well. Both storage medium and format need to be standardized to guarantee the universal archiving and exchange of digital images.

A number of criteria was formulated for the choice of a digital storage medium; only the most important ones will be briefly discussed here. In [6-8], the full range of criteria and the media that have been tested against these have been clearly described. The capacity of the medium must allow the storage of one patient study (about 4800 images). The quality of the images should be sufficient for subsequent quantitative analysis. The medium should show almost no degradation over time and the cost of a patient study must be significantly lower than the cost of cinefilm. From [6], it was concluded that the CD-R is the most suitable candidate for the storage medium. The CD-R technology has some clear advantages: it is used in other large industrial branches (consumer electronics, computer industry), it is cheap (currently about $5-10 per CD-R), it has a long lifetime and (from a technical viewpoint) it has an enormous growth potential.

Characteristics of the DICOM format

The description of the DICOM standard (the DICOM documents) consists of a number of parts and supplements. In the parts, the basic information (Information Object Definition, Data Dictionary, Network Communication, etc.) is described. The supplements describe the use of DICOM with different imaging modalities (X-ray Angiography, Ultrasound, MRI, etc.).

The data in a DICOM file is ordered hierarchically starting with a patient object, that may have several study objects. Each study object may contain one or more image series and each series contains a number of image objects. Each object contains information that is specific for that object.

Information on the image size and pixel representation are stored within the image object. Further, image compression may be used to reduce the amount of space that is consumed by image data. In the DICOM format, only one image compression technique is allowed: Lossless JPEG. The use of lossless JPEG guarantees that the decompressed image exactly equals the original image. Other compression algorithms or other variants (lossy) of JPEG cannot guarantee this.

The DICOM format is very flexible in the way the files are filled. All data fields have their specific identification *tag*. This tag contains the field length as well, which enables an application to ignore a field when it is not used in that application. Furthermore, a number of fields have been marked to indicate that they must be present in each individual DICOM file.

Conformance and acceptance

In the description of new products, it is often claimed by the manufacturer that the product is DICOM compatible. In general, the following is meant by this term:

*"A product is DICOM **compatible** when it supports (a part of) the DICOM image file description."*

However, due to the size of the standard, it is possible that the products of two different vendors are both DICOM compatible, but are still unable to communicate. In such a case, both pieces of equipment support a different part of the standard. Therefore, it is of utmost importance that each vendor declares which part of the standard is supported by its equipment. This is described in the so-called conformance statement. Part 2 of the DICOM documents describes the ins and outs of conformance statements and as such is of special interest for potential buyers of any system (either acquisition or review/analysis). In brief, the definition of a conformance statement is:

*"Each vendor should work out a statement that declares the **conformance** of its implementation to the DICOM standard."*

When purchasing digital image archiving or review equipment, one should request the vendor's DICOM conformance statement.

An important requirement for the acceptance of a standard is the approval by national standardization institutes. Currently, the DICOM standard has been approved by the American (ANSI), the European (CEN) and the Japanese (JIRA) standardization committees.

The digital cath lab in a networked environment

Currently, the image acquisition system in a cath lab is a stand alone system. Image series are generated, reviewed and analyzed on the same system. Exchange of images is primarily done through the exchange of cinefilm. In the (near) future, image acquisition systems will be connected to local and wide area networks (LANs and WANs). As a result, the exchange of data and sharing of resources will increase and the interaction between pieces of equipment connected to the network is made much more comfortable. For example, a direct link to the hospital information system (HIS) can easily be realized and printers and other resources connected to the LAN can be shared. Further, a (digital) review system can be connected to the network. Such a review system need not necessarily be located in or near the cath lab, but can be located at the cardiologists' desk as well. When needed, the connection to the WAN can be used to exchange images and information between institutions.

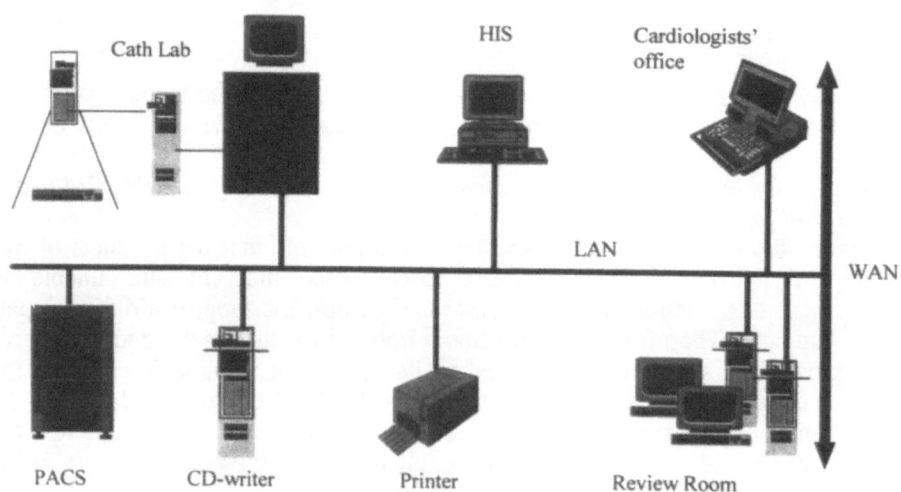

Figure 1. A networked cath lab environment.

An abstract scheme of such a networked environment is depicted in Figure 1. The following components are distinguished: the image acquisition system, the picture archiving and communication system (PACS), a hospital information system (HIS), a review and analysis system (which can be situated in a separate review room or simply in the cardiologists' office), a CD-writer and a network printer.

Image acquisition system

Obviously, the image acquisition system can be of any brand as long as it outputs digital images. The internal representation and storage medium of the images may be vendor-specific (for reasons of real-time acquisition and display). However, the external representation must be in a standardized format, preferably DICOM.

Picture archiving and communication system

For long term storage and communication purposes within one or more departments in the hospital, a picture archiving and communication system (PACS) is used. The choice for a specific brand or storage medium is again left open here, the only demand is that it can handle image files in DICOM format.

Hospital information system

Information on patients and other administrative data can be stored in a central hospital information system (HIS). In stead of storing these data locally again (in the cardiology or radiology department), these data can be retrieved from the HIS over the LAN (or a WAN if necessary).

CD-R writer

A CD-R writer must be used for the writing of patient studies (in DICOM format) onto a CD-R. Such a CD-R writer can be part of the image acquisition system; in the scheme presented in Figure 1, the CD-R writer is connected to the network. This allows other connected pieces of equipment to use it as well.

Review and analysis station

A review and analysis station can be used to review a patient study off-line. This can be done in a special viewing room, but in a networked environment this can be done in other places as well. For instance, when the cardiologist has a network connection in his/her office, viewing and analyzing patient studies can be done from behind the desk. The patient study can be imported over the network (preferably in DICOM format) or from CD-R (when the review station has a built-in CD-R reader).

Hardcopy unit

In networked environments, hardcopy units are usually shared. The output can be generated from each device connected to the network. Special purpose hardcopy units, like video printers, are in most cases used by just one device (the acquisition system or the review station) and should preferably be connected directly to that device.

An inventory of current developments in the market

A small scale investigation was carried out in order to obtain an overview of the current developments in industrial products. Part of the investigation was a questionnaire that was sent to 6 major vendors of X-ray angiographic equipment: Camtronics Medical Systems, GE Medical Systems, Eastman Kodak Company, Philips Medical Systems, Siemens Medical and Toshiba Medical Systems.

The questionnaire consisted of a set of questions related to the different components that were introduced in the schematic networked environment (see Figure 1). The responses were ordered around the topics that are described in the following subsections: acquisition, review and analysis, exchange, archiving, CD-R writer, hard copy unit and networking. The questionnaire was meant for a typical cath lab department with 2-3 rooms. If the situation is different for large departments (> 5 rooms), the differences are indicated.

Acquisition

As has been argued in the previous section, with respect to the acquisition, we are mainly interested in the external representation of the images. Therefore, on this subject the questionnaire was restricted to one question

Q.1. What is the storage format that is going to be used for the output of the digital image acquisition system?

The answers are presented in Table 1. Note: DICOM+ is used as a shortcut for *DICOM plus specific vendor information.*

Table 1. Response to the acquisition question.

Question	Camtronics	GE	Kodak	Philips	Siemens	Toshiba
Q.1	DICOM+	DICOM	DICOM+	DICOM+	DICOM+	DICOM

Clearly, all vendors claim to support the DICOM format. Further, the majority of them plans to add specific vendor information into the files. As explained earlier, the flexibility of the DICOM format in terms of adding user-defined fields allows the storage of this information in a way that it can be ignored by other implementations. This vendor specific information that is added should be described in the conformance statement. In practice this means that minimally a dual path approach is followed, whereby lossy compressed data for rapid review purposes has been added to the lossless 2:1 JPEG data. Philips Medical Systems has even included MPEG compressed data for CD-I applications.

Exchange

As explained, for exchange purposes both the storage medium and the storage format are important in the replacement of cinefilm.

Q.2. What is the storage medium that is going to be used for exchange purposes?

Q.3. What is the storage format that is going to be used for exchange purposes?

Further, the used image sizes and the supported compression ratios are important aspects of the storage format.

Q.4. Which matrix sizes are allowed?

Q.5. What is the compression ratio that is going to be used?

Finally, an estimation of the costs per patient is of interest.

Q.6. What are the estimated expenses per patient study?

The answers to questions Q.2 to Q.6 are presented in Tables 2A and 2B. Again, DICOM+ is used as a shortcut for *DICOM plus specific vendor information*.
From the answers, it can be concluded that although CD-R will be supported by all vendors, other media will be supported as well. One of the reasons for this will probably be the fact that a CD-R can contain only one or a few patient studies, while the tape and optical disc media can contain large quantities. Clearly, all vendors claim to support the DICOM format for exchange as well. Again, the majority of them plan to add specific vendor information to the files. A variety of matrix sizes will be supported; the 512x512x8 size is supported by each vendor. Clearly, the costs of the new medium will be much lower than the expenses of cinefilm.
Apart from lossless JPEG, all vendors plan to use a lossy image compression schemes as well. Currently, task groups of the ACC and ESC cooperate in a large Image Compression Viability study (ICV) that is focused on the lossy JPEG 6:1, 10:1 and 14:1 compression ratios. The results of this study will be crucial in the decision to be made about the acceptance of lossy image compression in the DICOM format.

Archiving

Let us distinguish 3 archiving time periods: short-term or on-line storage (not longer than 1 week), medium-term or near-line storage (between 1 week and 1 month) and long-term or off-line storage (longer than 1 month). For each storage period, the following 3 questions were posed:

Q.7. What is the hardware technology used?

Q.8. What is the access time per patient study?

Q.9. What are the estimated expenses per patient study?

From Table 3 it is clear that RAID technology will be used by the majority of the vendors for short- and even medium-term storage. For long-term storage, the answers are almost similar to the exchange media: CD-R is supported by all vendors, while tape and optical disc technology is supported only by a minority. The access times for studies from the long-term storage ranges from 30 seconds to 10 minutes, which is acceptable in most cases. The costs of long-term storage are based on the expenses of writing a CD-R (both medium and CD-R writer).

The DICOM standard was developed as the standard for the exchange of digital images, not for archiving. However, it is clear that archiving systems that support the DICOM standard are preferred.

Table 2A. Response to the exchange questions.

Question	Camtronics	GE	Kodak
Q.2	CD-R, 12'' DOD	CD-R	CD-R
Q.3	DICOM+	DICOM+	DICOM+
Q.4	512x512x8 1024x512x8 1024x1024x(8-10-12)	512x512x8	512x512x8
Q.5	Lossless JPEG 2:1 Lossy JPEG 8:1	Lossless JPEG 2:1	Lossless JPEG 2:1 Lossy JPEG 8:1
Q.6	US$ 15	Cost 0f CD-R	US$ 15

Table 2B. Response to the exchange questions (continued).

Question	Philips	Siemens	Toshiba
Q.2	CD-R	CD-R	CD-R, D2 tape
Q.3	DICOM+	DICOM+	DICOM
Q.4	512x512x8	512x512x8	512x512x8 (CD-R) 1024x512x(8-10) (D2 tape)
Q.5	Lossless JPEG 2:1 Lossy JPEG 6:1 MPEG	Lossless JPEG 2:1 Lossy JPEG 6-14:1	Lossless JPEG 2:1 (CD-R) No compression (D2 tape)
Q.6	Cost of CD-R	US$ 8	US$ 8-10 (CD-R) US$ 3-6 (D2 tape)

CD-R writer

With respect to the CD-R writer to be used, 4 practical questions were posed.

Q.10. When will a CD-R writer be commercially available?

Q.11. Can you give a list price indication for the CD-R writer?

Q.12. How long will it take to write a CD-R for a typical patient study of approximately 4000 frames (512x512x8)?

Q.13. Is the X-ray image acquisition blocked during the writing of the CD-R?

Table 3. Response to the archiving questions.

Question	Camtronics	GE	Kodak	Philips	Siemens	Toshiba
Q.7 (short)	RAID	Int disc ===		CD-R/RAID	RAID	RAID
(medium)	RAID	CD-R ===		CD-R/RAID	RAID	RAID
(long)	CD-R, DOD	CD-R ===		CD-R	CD-R, Opt tape	CD-R D2 tape
Q.8 (short)	0	<5 sec	===	30 sec	10 sec	1 sec
(medium)	===	10-30 min	===	30 sec	45 sec	1 sec
(long)	===	10-30 min	===	30 sec	3 min	30 sec
Q.9 (short)	US$ 15	===	===	CD cost	===	===
(medium)	===	CD costs	===	CD cost	===	US$ 8-10
(long)	===	CD costs	===	CD cost	US$ 4	US$ 3-6

=== No answer specified.

Table 4. Response to the CD-R writer questions.

Question	Camtronics	GE	Kodak	Philips	Siemens	Toshiba
Q.10	Now	Now	Now (6x)	Now	Now	Sept '96
Q.11	US$ 15,000	===	US$ 20,000	===	***	===
Q.12	30 min	22 min	15 min	20 min	22 min	15 min
Q.13	No	No	No	No	No	No

=== No answer specified.
*** Built into the acquisition and review system.

From Table 4 it can be concluded that all vendors have their CD-R writer now available. There are only small differences with respect to the price of the CD-R writer and the time required to actually write a CD-R. Writing a CD-R can be done without blocking the image acquisition process, which is an almost inevitable requirement. Clearly, all vendors acknowledge this fact.

Review and analysis station

The use of stand alone review and analysis stations will increase in networked environments. The computer hardware (PC based or workstations) that is going to be used will probably be standard of-the-shelf computer hardware. Similar to the hardware question, the question of which operating system (DOS, Windows, UNIX, etc.) is used is an important one.

Q.14. What is the hardware configuration of the review station?

Q.15. What is the operating system used by the review station?

An important feature of such a review station is the fact whether or not it can view the image runs in real-time. If it does, what can be said about the speed of the viewing process and quality of the images that are displayed. Further, the networked environment allows the simultaneous access of files and resources. It was asked whether the review station allows simultaneous access of patient studies.

Q.16. Is the review of image runs done in real-time?

Q.16a. If so, what is the maximal frame rate?

Q.16b. If so, are the images displayed at the original image quality?

Q.17. Can the same patient study be reviewed simultaneously?

Image filtering is used to enhance the visual interpretation of the image runs. If filtering is supported, the control of the filters can be given to the user or it can be automated. Further, it is of importance whether the filtering can be carried out in real-time, i.e. at the maximal frame rate specified above.

Q.18. Is image filtering supported?

Q.18a. If so, what kind of image filtering is supported?

Q.18b. If so, what are the control possibilities?

Q.18c. If so, can it be used in real-time?

The availability of a QCA package is of major importance for a number of potential buyers of the review station. If such a package is available, it was asked to specify the name of the package.

Q.19. Is there a QCA package available?

Finally, two practical questions were posed with respect to price and availability of the review station.

Q.20. When will the review station be commercially available?

Q.21. Can you give a list price indication for the review station?

A number of different hardware and software configurations is supported. For the PC based configurations, a tendency towards Windows-NT as the operating system can be noticed. As may be expected, all review stations support the real-time (at least 30 frames/sec) viewing of images at diagnostic quality. The method of image filtering that is used differs from station to station. If necessary, the filtering can be disabled on most systems. The QCA package that is implemented also differs between the review stations.

Hardcopy unit

With respect to the hardcopy unit, three practical questions were asked. The questions concentrate on the type, connection and price of the hardcopy unit.

Q.22. What type of hardcopy unit is advised?

Q.23. What is the device to which the hardcopy unit is connected to?

Q.24. Can you give a list price indication for the hardcopy unit?

From Tables 6A and 6B it can be seen that both video and laser printer output will be supported. The control of the device can vary between acquisition system, review station and LAN. Video printers will probably be connected to acquisition systems and review stations. Laser printers will probably be connected to review stations and the LAN.

Networking and communications

One (technical) question was asked with respect to the supported network protocols.

Q.25. What are the network protocols that are supported?

Table 5. Response to the review station questions.

Question	Camtronics	GE	Kodak	Philips	Siemens	Toshiba
Q.14	PC based UNIX	PC based UNIX	PC based	PC and spec HW	PC and spec HW	PC based
Q.15	Win-NT Solaris 2.4	= = =	Win-NT	MS-Win	MS-Win	Win-95 Win-NT
Q.16	Yes	Yes	Yes	Yes	Yes	Yes
Q.16a	30 f/s	30 f/s	30 f/s	30 f/s	60 f/s	30 f/s
Q.16b	Yes	Yes	Yes	Yes	Yes	Yes
Q.17	Yes	= = =	No	Yes	Yes	Yes
Q.18	Yes	Yes	Yes	Yes	Yes	Yes
Q.18a	30x30 mask	= = =	Edge enh.	Edge enh.	Edge enh.	= = =
Q.18b	Dynamic	= = =	Dynamic	Dynamic	Dynamic	= = =
Q.18c	Yes	Yes	Yes	Yes	Yes	= = =
Q.19	***	= = =	***	ACA	***	= = =
Q.20	Now	Now	Now	Now	Now	Now
Q.21	US$ 40,000	= = =	US$ 40 - 50,000	= = =	= = =	= = =

= = = No answer specified.
*** Available but package name not specified.

Table 6A. Response to the hard copy unit questions.

Question	Camtronics	GE	Kodak
Q.22	Video printer	Video printer	Laser printer Video printer Film laser camera
Q.23	Review station, LAN	Acquisition system, Review station	Review station
Q.24	US$ 10,000	= = =	= = =

= = = No answer specified.

Table 6B. Response to the hard copy unit questions (continued).

Question	Philips	Siemens	Toshiba
Q.22	Laser printer	Laser printer Video printer	Laser printer Video printer Film laser camera
Q.23	Review station	Acquisition system, Review station, LAN	Acquisition system, Review station, LAN
Q.24	= = =	US$ 1,000-15,000	= = =

= = = No answer specified.

Table 7. Response to the networking question.

Question	Camtronics	GE	Kodak	Philips	Siemens	Toshiba
Q.25	TCP/IP,NFS	TCP/IP	TCP/IP	TCP/IP	TCP/IP	TCP/IP (ATM)

As expected, all vendors support the TCP/IP protocol. This protocol is a de facto standard in network communication nowadays. Although the DICOM format allows the use of other network protocols, TCP/IP will most likely be implemented in the majority of the applications.

Conclusions

Without any doubt, the future of cardiac imaging is digital. The advantages of digital imaging clearly outperform the current (analog) alternatives. However, some work has still to be done to reach a sufficient level of standardization in the exchange and the archiving. Both from the literature (see for instance [9,10]) and from industrial developments, it is clear that DICOM will be the standard file format.

Three remarks are to be made with respect to the questionnaire: 1) the lifetime of this information will be limited as technology nowadays develops very rapidly; 2) although the responses to this questionnaire as printed in this chapter have been checked by the company representatives, it is still possible that some questions / answers will lead or have led to some confusion; and 3) it was apparent that during the iterative editing process, in which the complete responses were made available to the different company representatives, a slight converging process occurred.

Further, from our questionnaire it has become clear that the major manufacturers support the reading and writing of image files in DICOM format. Although much work in this direction has been done already, far more work still needs to be carried out in the coming years. As explained, DICOM compatibility of equipment is described in the conformance statement. It is of utmost importance for potential buyers of medical imaging equipment that the conformance statement is read carefully before buying.

A subject that has not been given any attention here is the subject of data security. Although this is an important topic when discussing the use of networking (especially WANs), it is judged to fall outside the scope of this chapter. Before putting the technical possibilities described in this chapter into practice, the security aspects of the used hard- and software should be studied carefully.

Acknowledgments

The authors wish to thank the participating company representatives for their rapid and adequate response to the questionnaire.

References

1. Cardiac angiography without cinefilm: erecting a "Tower of Babel" in the catheterization laboratory. American College of Cardiology Cardiac Catheterization Committee. J Am Coll Cardiol 1994;24:834-7.
2. American College of Cardiology, American College of Radiology and industry develop standard for digital transfer of angiographic images. ACC/ACR/NEMA Ad Hoc Group. J Am Coll Cardiol 1995;25:800-2.
3. Simon R, Brennecke R, Heiss O, Meier B, Reiber H, Zeelenberg C. Report of the ESC Task Force on Digital Imaging in Cardiology. Recommendations for digital imaging in angiocardiography. Eur Heart J 1994;15:1332-4.
4. Parisot C. The DICOM standard. A breakthrough for digital information exchange in cardiology. Int J Card Imaging 1995;11(Suppl.3):171-7.
5. Reiber JHC, Koning G, van der Zwet PMJ, Schiemanck L. Inaccuracy of quantitative coronary arteriography when analyzed from S-VHS videotape. Cathet Cardiovasc Diagn 1996;37:32-8.
6. Condit PB. Requirements for cardiac interchange media and the role of recordable CD", Int J Card Imaging 1995;11(Suppl.3):153-7.
7. Cusma JT, Fortin DF, Sparo LA, Groshong BR, Bashore TM. Which media are most likely to solve the archival problem? Int J Card Imaging 1994;10:165-75.
8. Bronkalla M, Kennedy T, "Holding out for a digital solution", J Cardiovasc Management 1993; 11/12: 21-4.
9. Bjerde KW. IPI, MEDICOM and DICOM: relations and possible future. Int J Card Imaging 1995;11(Suppl.3):165-70.

14. Philips CD-Medical - A new era in digital cardiac review, exchange and archiving

KITTY VREESWIJK

Summary

A major cost component in cardiac angiography is the use of cinefilm. In addition, cinefilm is very inefficient to develop and to store and also difficult to reproduce. There is one unique archival copy, and if it becomes torn, or lost, it cannot be replaced. Consequently, physicians and administrators looking to save time, increase efficiency and cut costs are also looking to eliminate cinefilm use. The increase in digital cardiac procedures has led to a desire for a compatible, effective digital archiving and communication system. The challenge in cardiology is to find a digital solution for cardiac archiving that meets three basic requirements:
1. Cost effectiveness
2. Ability to perform the basic clinical functions: Review, Exchange and Archive
3. Standard format for exchange
CD-Medical is a single-medium solution, based on CD technology, that fully conforms to the DICOM standard for exchange as defined by the ACC/NEMA Committee. By extending the functionality to review and archive, Philips has created a cost-effective solution to cardiac image management.
CD-Medical is based on a scalable, natural growth path. As advanced technology becomes available, further efficiency improvement can be achieved as extensions to the digital cine replacement based on CD-Medical. Such networked, multimedia solutions will offer short term on-line storage of images, information integration and communication over larger distances.

Introduction

The increase in digital cardiac procedures has led to a desire for a compatible, effective digital archiving and communication system. This chapter presents an analysis of the clinical needs and explains the philosophy behind different digital archiving and communication solutions.

Today, almost 100% of the new cardiac cath labs have digital acquisition systems. With most cardiac images being generated digitally, it is logical that the exchange and storage standard should also be digital. New emerging technologies contribute to solutions with improved performance and lower cost. Communication both within and outside the department and hospital requires a compatible digital approach.

Cardiology's challenge is to find a digital solution for cardiac archiving that meets three basic requirements without compromising image quality, diagnostic capability and departmental efficiency. These requirements are:
- Cost effectiveness

J.H.C. Reiber and E.E. van der Wall (eds.), Cardiovascular Imaging, 185-192.
© 1996 *Kluwer Academic Publishers.*

- Basic clinical functionality
- Standard format for exchange

Requirements for cinefilm replacement

Cost-effectiveness

The primary impetus to replace cinefilm is to save money. It is estimated that the current per patient cost for cinefilm to archive a typical cardiac angiographic procedure is about $70. The medium itself is expensive, as are the associated costs of processing, storage and personnel time.

Ability to perform basic clinical functions

To be viable, a digital archiving system must be capable, at minimum, of the following basic functions.

> **Review**: Following an examination, the images must be available to the cardiologist for analysis and reporting. General requirements for review are: immediate access to all images, dynamic review and original image quality.

> **Exchange**: The need to share cardiac images with another clinical site usually arises in situations where a diagnostic hospital refers a patient to an interventional institute or when a hospital participates in a multi-center research study in which images are analyzed at a central location. Especially for exchange, a standard format must exist to prevent that different vendors offer digital solutions that are incompatible. Until recently, cinefilm was the gold standard.

> **Archive**: Images need to be stored safely for approximately ten years or more, and be conveniently available for future consultancy. Digital archive represents a quantum improvement over cinefilm storage. With cine, the department has only a single unique archival copy; if it becomes torn, fogged or lost, it cannot be replaced. And, because it is film, any reproduction of the original will automatically be at least one generation away in terms of image quality.

Standardized Format

For institutions to freely exchange information such as cardiac angiograms, a standardized exchange format must exist. A joint committee of the American College of Cardiology and the National Electrical Manufacturers Association (ACC/NEMA) has developed such a standard based on the use of CD-Recordable. This standardization activity is supported by the European Society of Cardiology.

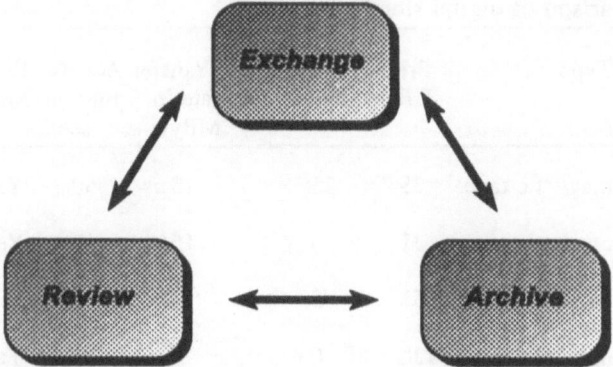

Figure 1. A digital communications system should enable review, exchange and archival at full diagnostic quality within a flexible, cost-effective framework.

The DICOM standard

In 1983, NEMA formed a joint committee with the American College of Radiology to develop a standard to facilitate the communication of digital image information, regardless of device manufacturer, both within a hospital and among institutions. This committee specified the DICOM (Digital Imaging and Communications in Medicine) format which was initially focused on the ability to communicate between vendors over ethernet networks.

The DICOM effort in cardiology has been focused on the ability to interchange data between institutions. A joint committee from the ACC/NEMA has chosen CD-Recordable as the standard exchange medium within the DICOM standard. The specified DICOM format for cardiology is 512^2, 8 bit resolution. The images are compressed with JPEG factor 2 (Joint Photographic Expert Group). This compression is lossless, enabling to reconstruct the original images.

The ACC/NEMA standard defines DICOM as the digital interchange format and CD-Recordable as the digital medium for exchange. An overview of the available media from which one had to choose is given in Table 1. There are no similar standards for review and archive. The ACC/NEMA avoided any attempt to standardize review and archive, leaving to industry the development of creative and cost-effective solutions and equipment. Medical centers will remain free to continue making their own choices among the products offered.

DICOM on CD-R does not provide a complete replacement for cinefilm. Although CD-R can be used as an archive medium by everybody, there are serious limitations when DICOM on CD-R is used for review. Because the retrieval speed of current CD technology is limited, one can show DICOM images only as still images or in slow motion or one has to download the images to a hard disk which is very time-consuming. Both situations seem unacceptable for diagnostic review.

Table 1. Comparison of digital storage media.

	Type	Price GByte	Capacity in GByte	Transfer rate in MByte/sec	Access time in secs	Erasable Medium	Growth potential
D2 small cass	magnetic tape	3$	25	15	50	Yes	low
D3 comp cass	magnetic tape	3$	10	15	12	Yes	low
Exabyte	magnetic tape	5$	5	0.5	66	Yes	low
IBM 3490	magnetic tape	13$	0.4	7	28	Yes	low
Creo tape	optical tape	0.2$	1000	3	65	No	low
12" WORM	optical disc	60$	6	<1	<1	No	low
5$^{1}/_{4}$" MOD	optical disc	100$	0.65 per side	<1	<1	Yes	medium
3$^{1}/_{2}$" MOD	optical disc	250$	0.23	<1	<1	Yes	medium
CD-R	optical disc	17$	0.7	<1	<1	No	high

Although Philips Medical Systems Nederland BV is confident that the information provided above is correct, it may be subject to change beyond its control, and therefore no responsibility can be accepted for such information.

Hybrid approaches

Since CD-Recordable has been established as the ACC/NEMA standard for exchange only, systems may use other media for review and archive. This "partial" solution means that digital information can be transferred from one medium to another with no loss in quality, but each transfer will involve separate hardware and require personnel time for handling. Thus, the process of intra-media communication will probably be expensive.

Several digital archiving approaches have surfaced recently that offer a combination of different media. Some of these systems employ a hierarchical storage management approach that requires the use of RAID (Redundant Array of Independent Discs) technology for review and analysis on short term. Images are copied to a tape or optical disc for long-term storage. Many of these systems must then copy the images a third time to a DICOM compatible CD-Recordable medium, for exchange.

RAID systems offer on-line availability of images in the cath lab for a few days following the procedure. The images are accessible at workstations which must be electronically connected to the RAID system. RAID systems can increase the efficiency of short-term storage and image review for multiple cath lab departments with high volumes. Advantage of the RAID concept is that examinations remain on-line for the time that the patient is still on the department. This frees the cath lab, while real time digital reviewing can be done at a departmental level. For the majority of cath labs, however, the RAID approach at the present state of technology is still unnecessarily expensive without significantly improving the efficiency of the lab.

Since RAID systems are not designed for long-term image storage, additional archiving equipment must be added, such as a digital tape system. Such digital tape systems typically use D2 or D3/D5 tape. These tapes are fast enough for real-time recording. Disadvantage, however, is that magnetic media are subject to degradation over time. Digital tape is relatively inexpensive; however, the "jukebox" mechanism required to retrieve selected patient studies is not. With this medium, only one user can access the array system at a time unless multiple recorders are employed. Even then, only one station can access a recorder at a time. In addition, because many patients' images must be stored on a single tape, that tape cannot be used for exchange.

Originally developed for the broadcast industry, most digital tape media have no apparent future applications in consumer electronics. Because the broadcast industry changes standards fairly often, there is a strong chance that this medium will soon become obsolete. And, there is little hope that prices for digital tape will drop since there have been no new applications for the technology.

The primary disadvantages of RAID systems are their expense and inflexibility. Rapid changes in technology are also making their future uncertain, so obsolescence is a major concern.

CD-Medical, the single medium solution

A single medium approach that can fulfill all the requirements for review, exchange and long term archive while enabling cardiac studies to be easily and inexpensively reproduced, with no loss in image quality, would be the most logical and cost-effective solution.

The ability to adapt to current cath lab operational protocols would be another advantage. Today, the cath lab has its review, exchange, and archive systems set up to accommodate cinefilm as a single patient unit medium (each film contains a single patient exam). Restructuring the normal operation of the lab just to accommodate new archiving technology is not only expensive, but counterproductive.

Based on the above analysis, Philips Medical Systems has developed CD-Medical as the optimum single-medium solution for replacing cinefilm. Compact Disc technology was invented by Philips, and its application to cardiology is the logical extension of Philips Medical Systems' experience in cardiac imaging.

CD-Medical is fully DICOM compatible and meets all the recommendations from the ACC/NEMA standardization committee for exchange using CD-R within the DICOM standard. By extending the DICOM format with dynamic review possibilities, the CD-Medical discs can be used for dynamic review as well. Furthermore, CD technology provides a good solution for long-term archive since CD's are compact, use a caddy for optimal data security and do not deteriorate in time.

The CD-Medical concept comprises a recording system, viewstations and a duplication system, all of which employ CD technology (Figure 2). The digital imaging system transfers images to the recording system which records these on CD's. A single CD-Medical disc can hold sufficient image data for one complete patient exam. These discs can be viewed dynamically in real time at viewstations throughout the hospital, providing quick access to images of equal quality to those in the lab. In addition, the viewstations may offer quantitative analysis and reporting functions. These viewstations are the primary diagnostic workplace for reporting a cardiac exam, and will thus supersede the function of the cinefilm projector.

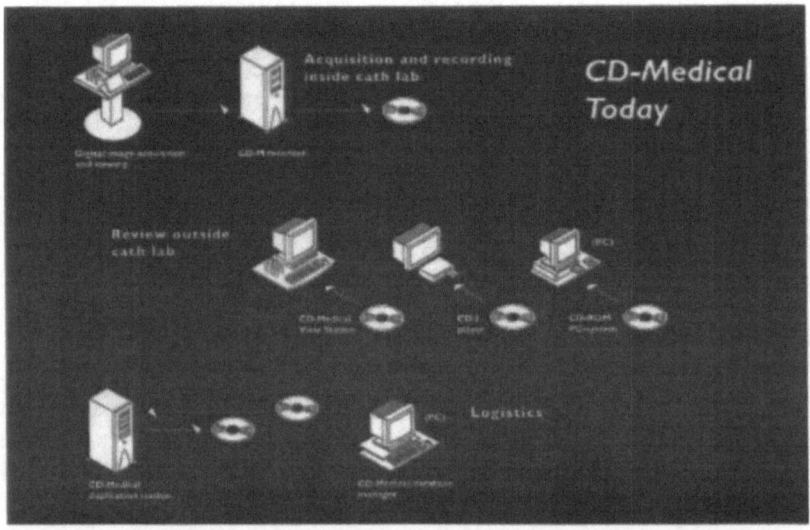

Figure 2. CD-Medical is a DICOM compatible, single-medium solution for dynamic review, exchange and archive and a true digital replacement of cinefilm.

Philips CD-Medical discs are also compatible with standard consumer CD-Interactive (CD-i) players. This offers the ability for dynamic review of cases with very inexpensive 'viewers'. This can be of great value in places where no primary diagnosis and reporting functionality is needed, e.g. conferencing, consultation with surgery, patient family demonstration, etc. This concept offers a very cost-effective approach to suit the different viewing needs of the cardiology department.

CD technology is already a consumer standard in such devices as CD-digital audio, CD-Interactive (CD-I) and CD-ROM. Because it has so many consumer applications, the cost of the medium is driven by a broader market than just medical. This affords economies of production that will continue to lead toward lower costs. It is expected that the price of CD-Recordable media will decline to approximately five dollars per unit.

Because CD's are consumer-oriented, it is unlikely that the technology will be quickly abandoned without an appropriate upgrade path. Further, the application is independent from the device. Since the software is written on the individual disc, advances in software will not make older discs incompatible with CD players.

CD-Medical fits the traditional work flow of the lab. Because each CD-Medical contains a single exam, the logistics of use are the same as with cinefilm. Thus, there is no need to restructure the operation or organization of the cath lab. CD-Medical also offers immediate access to each run/image, plus dynamic viewing.

As a single medium solution, CD-Medical does not require images to be copied onto different media to accomplish different functions. In addition, backup and maintenance procedures, common with larger systems, are not needed. As a result, CD-Medical involves much less handling than other systems.

CD-Medical is compatible with all Philips digital cardiac systems. All new and existing Philips digital labs can easily and economically be upgraded to this system, ensuring departmental compatibility and procedural efficiency.

Today's challenge: the future

Further developments of archiving technology must give careful consideration to the full range of clinical, communication, and economic needs represented by diverse clinical requirements. This means that present configurations must enable institutions to "phase-in" a system as time and budget dictate. Whether the cath lab is looking for a review mechanism, an exchange medium, an archive system – or a combination of all of these – CD-Medical will allow the transition to occur in a timely and affordable fashion.

Some large institutions will best be served in the future by a network solution that employs mixed media and an intermediate short-term archive, as described in the previous section. However those institutions that will benefit the most from a network may have problems with current options because present technology is still expensive without significantly improving the efficiency of the cath lab. Often these solutions are not based on firm standards and rapid changes in technology are making their future uncertain, so obsolescence is a major concern. Consistent with its approach in all aspects of managing the flow of information, CD-Medical is based on a scalable, natural growth path (Figure 3). It offers a practical solution now, without asking the institution to invest in an expensive infrastructure that may become obsolete in the future.

As advanced technologies become available, further efficiency improvements can be achieved as extensions to the digital cine replacement based on CD-Medical. Networked multi-media solutions will be based on a standard open platform, be backwards compatible with the installed base and have a modular and scalable set-up to customize to different needs of various hospitals. These solutions will offer short term on-line storage of images to enable immediate on-line viewing from multiple locations. With the images being generated and stored digitally, it is possible to combine them with all other information available in digital format. When both the images and related information are available on-line, an integrated workplace evolves where clinicians can access images and other information at the same time and create for example an integrated patient report.

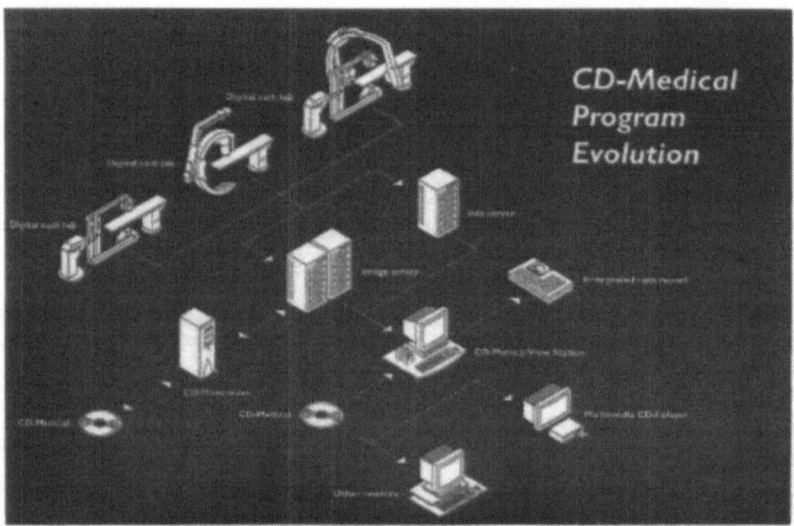

Figure 3. CD-Medical is based on scalable, natural growth path and can easily be incorporated into network systems, enabling flexible review throughout the hospital and exchange with other institutions as well.

Conclusion

CD-Medical is a digital cardiac communication system for dynamic review, exchange and archival of cardiac images at full diagnostic quality within a flexible, cost-effective framework. As such, it is a true digital replacement of cinefilm.

Meeting the requirements of cost-effectiveness, clinical functionality and standard format, CD-Medical offers a practical solution for now and a safe step into the future of cardiac information management.

15. Status of the GE approach to the digital catheterization laboratory

JOHN F. NEALON

Summary

At the 1995 American College of Cardiology (ACC) meeting in New Orleans, a major advancement in the effort to replace cinefilm was achieved with the DISC '95 (Digital Interchange Standard for Cardiology) demonstration. The digital interchange medium to replace cinefilm, CD-R, and the digital interchange format, DICOM (Digital Imaging and Communications in Medicine), were introduced. A DICOM CD-R was created by the ACC with images from various equipment manufacturers. Cardiologists were allowed to take a CD-R around the exhibit floor at the ACC and view the images in the booths of manufacturers supporting DISC '95. This demonstration was successfully repeated at the 1995 European Congress of Cardiology (ECC) meeting in Amsterdam. These two demonstrations proved that a digital standard now exists to address the need to exchange cinefilm between two cardiology centers [1]. Thus, the cineless cath lab can now become a reality.

This chapter will explore the key roles of cinefilm in today's cath labs and the applicable digital technologies. Standards and technologies applicable to cine replacement will be explored. Finally, the status of GE's cineless cath lab product, GEMnet, will be discussed.

Replacement of cinefilm: what is required?

Cinefilm serves the following four key roles in today's cath labs: acquisition, display, interchange and archive. Replacing cinefilm with digital technology requires addressing each of these roles of cinefilm:

	Today	Future
- Acquisition	Cinefilm + Digital	Digital
- Interchange	Cinefilm	DICOM CD-R
- Display/Review	Cine projector	Workstation and PC technology
- Archive	Cinefilm	DICOM media

In the area of acquisition, almost 100% of today's cath labs have digital systems and almost all of the digital systems operate in parallel with cinefilm [2]. It is expected that cinefilm will completely disappear from all cath labs in 10 years and digital will be the only method of acquisition. For interchange between hospitals, the DICOM CD-R (recordable optical compact disk) will replace cinefilm. This means that the "image record and film" going from one hospital to another will now be a CD-R instead of cinefilm. For display of the image data from the CD-R, workstations and PC technology using DICOM software for cardiology image review will replace cine projectors. For long term archive

J.H.C. Reiber and E.E. van der Wall (eds.), Cardiovascular Imaging, 193-200.
© 1996 *Kluwer Academic Publishers.*

within an institution, cardiologists will find solutions ranging from CD-R to digital optical disk to high performance digital tape options. Cardiologists will choose the archive solution which best meets the price and performance needs of their institution.

In addition, we need to look critically at the method of transport for cinefilm within a hospital: sneaker-net. Cinefilm has always been transported by hand, because there was no other choice -- it was an analog medium and not easily duplicated. With digital technology, distributing images via an image network will be possible. Networking will produce significant labor and time savings for the hospital by eliminating the time and cost of carrying cinefilm around the hospital by the "sneaker-net method".

Standards and cine replacement

Standards are critical in the development of new technologies because they protect the consumer by reducing the risk of obsolescence, lowering costs, providing upgrade paths and improving performance. A variety of standards are going to be critical in the development of cine replacement technology. These include DICOM, CD-R, Workstation and PC technology, ATM fiber optic networks, JPEG compression and mass digital storage technology. Let us explore each of these standards and why they are important:

DICOM

The Digital Imaging and Communications in Medicine (DICOM) Standard is the most important standard enabling cine replacement. DICOM defines a common format for digital image data which enables communication between different manufacturers' equipment. The DICOM effort began in radiology and it was initially focused on the ability to communicate between vendors over ethernet networks. The goal was to develop a standard that allowed different imaging equipment to communicate with different image management archive systems, printers and workstations without the need for custom interfaces at each device. The DICOM effort in radiology has been a success. Conformance to the DICOM standard is now required in the radiology field. The DICOM effort in cardiology has been focused on the ability to interchange data between institutions. This was the critical issue for cardiology in order to replace cinefilm. At the 1995 ACC and ECC meetings, we demonstrated that using DICOM formatted data on a CD-R we can solve the interchange issue. However, should cath lab manufacturers apply their support of DICOM to include DICOM networking? Many manufacturers will claim to be DICOM compliant because they can create a DICOM CD-R, while using proprietary interfaces between their cardiac cath lab equipment and review and archive stations. While technically complying with the new ACC and European Society of Cardiology (ESC) DICOM standard for media interchange using CD-R, these systems do not address the customer need for DICOM network output from the cath lab. The benefits of a DICOM network output from the cath lab digital system are:
- Allows customer to purchase a cath lab from one vendor and a review station

or archive system from another. It creates additional options reducing system acquisition and future upgrade costs.
- Allows networking of cath labs from different manufacturers without custom interfaces.
- Creates future possibilities with HIS/RIS and hemodynamic equipment.
- Opens the institution to multi-modality possibilities.

CD-R

Recordable optical compact disk (CD-R) is a new standard coming from the computer and multimedia industry. CD-R has been selected by the ACC/ACR-NEMA Committee and the ESC DIGICARE Task Force as the digital interchange media for angiography. CD-R is an excellent choice because it can store 650 MB of data (one patient) at 2:1 lossless compression, it will be available from multiple vendors which will keep prices low and it will benefit from significant investment to improve performance for the multimedia application [3]. However, CD-R has two major limitations: First, reading and writing lossless data for one patient operation will take about 20 minutes. If CD-R is used only as an interchange medium, this 20 minutes may not be a critical issue as the data can be transferred in the background. Second, one CD-R can store only one patient. Thus, digital technology duplicates the cinefilm process of one patient/one film. The ACC and ESC committees recognized this in their evaluation of media and did not attempt to define the digital archive media for cardiology due to the lack of "a perfect technology" to replace cinefilm and serve as both the interchange and archive standard [4]. This statement means that CD-R is the new digital interchange medium and institutions may choose to use CD-R as an archive medium if they wish, but the committees recognize that CD-R does not have adequate speed or storage capacity to make it an acceptable choice for an archive for every institution.

Workstations and PC technology

A new development today is the availability of high performance computer graphics workstations which are able to store and review 512^2 images at 30 frames/sec with upscan and edge enhancement. Companies such as SUN, HP, Silicon Graphics and DEC are major players in this market. The expectation is that computer hardware technology will advance rapidly to yield significant cost reduction and performance improvements on a yearly basis. In the near future, high performance PC-based systems will be able to store and review 512^2 images at 30 frames/sec.

ATM fiber optic networks

ATM fiber optic networks allow for high speed data transmission and are being installed by telephone and cable companies throughout the world. Uncompressed cardiac images require the high speed data transmission rates that ATM networks provide. ATM networks will allow transfer of cardiac images within and outside the hospital. Networking will benefit cardiology and the hospital by:

- Eliminating sneaker-net cinefilm approach and saving employee and physician time by allowing multiple cath labs and multiple review stations to be connected in a digital image network.
- Allowing remote viewing of cardiology images and consultation by telephone between institutions through the use of Wide Area Networks.

JPEG compression

The JPEG (Joint Photographic Experts Group) standard was originally defined for compression of continuous-tone color images and was later applied to grayscale images. JPEG compression was adopted for medical imaging by the ACC/NEMA DICOM committee as a compression format because it is a widely used standard. Digital image compression comes in two forms: lossless and lossy. Lossless data compression is a standard of every x-ray cardiac digital system sold today. Lossless data compression allows the original digital images to be reproduced exactly as acquired in the lab (bit for bit). It ensures that image data will not be lost or altered -- an essential component to accurate diagnosis. Lossy data compression can cause artifacts or defects in the image data when used in conjunction with edge enhancement and upscan 1024 display -- standard features on today's x-ray cardiac digital systems. Scientific investigation has proven the existence of these artifacts. Lossy data compression can greatly improve the performance and reduce the cost of our systems, but at a potential sacrifice to image quality [5].
The standard adopted by the ACC and the ESC uses JPEG lossless data compression (2:1) in the DICOM standard. The committees chose lossless data compression, because lossy data compression can not guarantee reproducibility of the data and its clinical impact must be thoroughly studied and validated by cardiologists in a clinical environment before being institutionalized. Some manufacturers have adopted the "lossy" dual path approach which utilizes both lossy and lossless images. The lossy images will allow for direct viewing of images from the CD-R at 30 frames/sec but how much will image quality suffer? At the present time, major cardiology centers in Europe and the US are trying to validate a clinically acceptable level of lossy compression to use in a clinical setting. This study is being supported by all of the major imaging manufacturers. Once this study is complete, it is expected the DICOM standard will be updated.

Digital image storage technology

For multi-lab facilities, the cardiac archiving systems of the future will be digitally networked to provide high speed transmission from multiple acquisition systems to multiple review stations. A networked system will use a hierarchical storage strategy permitting immediate on-line access whenever necessary, while providing the option of going to lower-cost near- and off-line storage media for long-term archival [6]. For multi-lab facilities, that means utilizing High Speed Disk Arrays (RAIDS) for on-line high speed access, and high-capacity, high-reliability digital storage media for long-term storage and retrieval.
Digital storage technology is rapidly evolving. The most cost effective technology for the mass storage of digital data is computer digital tape. It has been validated

by the banking and insurance industries for database storage. These tapes have extremely high performance capability and with automatic tape libraries, systems can be configured to store up to 10,000 patients.

Hierarchical storage and media options allow a facility to match performance, capacity and operating costs to their case loads, clinical requirements and capital budgets. The majority of single cath lab facilities and some multi-lab facilities will purchase their first cineless systems using CD-R for long-term archive. The majority of multi cath lab facilities will prefer systems with centralized storage using digital tape for mass archive. As digital technology evolves over the next five to ten years, most cardiac facilities are expected to adopt some type of centralized image management system.

GE status/key features

GE Medical Systems first cineless product is called GEMnet and it was recently introduced into the market. The GEMnet DCR-500 is designed for a single cath lab setting. The key features of the product and the status is as follows:

DICOM transfer from the cath lab

GE is the first x-ray cardiology cath lab manufacturer supporting the transfer DICOM 3.0 formatted images directly out of the cath lab digital system. This will allow any vendor with a review station or image archive system supporting DICOM networking via ATM to connect directly to our digital output. For the DCR-500 product, the DICOM formatted images are transferred directly to GE's off-line Advantage CRS (Cardiac Review Station) to allow image review and archival on CD-R.

As proof of our DICOM network compliance and support of open communication, we recently established the world's first DICOM network interface between separate imaging vendors in the cardiac cath lab market with Kodak. The interface was made possible by an industry standard DICOM ATM output from GE's Advantx LC DLX cath lab and a cardiac archiving station, under development by Kodak, which supports the DICOM ATM protocol. The alpha clinical trials validate that a customer can purchase a digital cath lab with an industry standard DICOM output and a review station or image archive system from any vendor that supports the DICOM ATM protocol.

GE recognizes the business risk inherent with providing an industry standard output. Competitors will be able to connect directly to the DICOM output from the Advantx cath lab. However, we believe the DICOM cath lab output is the right choice for our customers as this open system will provide customers more options, increased competitive offerings and better upgrade paths. We believe this will result in improved health care at lower costs.

Background transfer from the cath lab

Image transfer from our lab will be in background mode, which means the digital system in the cath lab can transfer images (in the background), while the user is using the digital system for its primary task of acquiring patient data in the cath lab. This means that the digital system is never locked up (or in a wait mode) during image transfer. This is a critical feature for cardiology cath lab customer. With pressure to reduce costs and increase cath lab patient throughput, access to the cath lab digital is required at all times.

Image quality

Image quality was a key criteria in the design of the DCR-500. The image quality in the cath lab must be equal to the image quality on cardiac review station outside the cath lab. To ensure outstanding image quality, GE decided to use no lossy compression and selected the highest quality monitor available. When and if the DICOM standard is revised to include lossy compression, GE will adopt that approach.

Immediate off-line review after the case

GE's cardiac review station will be connected to the cath lab to allow the cardiologist to review images outside of the lab immediately after the case. The images can be transferred from the digital system in the background as they are acquired (while the patient is on the table in the lab). This allows the cardiologist to walk directly to the review station immediately after the case and begin reviewing the patient, eliminating the traditional 20 minute cinefilm development time. The review station is networked to the cath lab, but off-line, which allows the next case to begin in the cath lab without any impact on the review immediately after the case.

Multitasking review station

In addition, our cardiac review station is designed for the multitasking capabilities demanded by the cardiology departments. The Advantage CRS will allow the customer to simultaneously review images, receive images from the cath lab and write or read a CD-R. During this multitasking capability, 30 frames/sec review capability is maintained at all times.

Image archival and exchange on CD-R

From the cath lab perspective, our CD-R archiving system is similar to the cinefilm process in that it requires a technician to create one CD-R for each patient. The CD-R can then be stored on a shelf, but with much less storage space than the cinefilm.
Similar to cinefilm, the DICOM CD-R can be exported to other institutions. However in a major improvement over cinefilm, the DICOM CD-R can be copied before export eliminates the cinefilm loss problem. Data on the CD-R will be stored in lossless JPEG 2:1 compression with a 512^2 matrix as defined by the ACC and ESC DICOM committees. Based on potential legal liability and FDA issues, no lossy data will be utilized on our CD-R until clinical studies show evidence that compression is acceptable in x-ray angiography imaging and the

standard is updated to reflect that fact.

The major issue at this time with image exchange via CD-R is that cardiology centers do not have cardiac review stations capable of reading the CD-R. While we expect these cardiac review stations to become available in 1996, we expect the lack of these cardiac review stations to delay some cardiology centers from going cineless today.

Reliability and serviceability

GE believes that reliability and serviceability of the cine replacement solution is the most critical aspect. If the digital system goes down, there will be no cinefilm for backup. Therefore, GE has integrated its exclusive InSite technology into the GEMnet system. It allows us to remotely service our cath lab equipment via modem. During our clinical testing, we utilized our InSite technology to remotely troubleshoot a problem with the CD-R media that the customer was not aware of. We were able to call the customer and inform them about the problem without a service engineer on site.

Cost savings and productivity

In addition to reducing the media cost from $40-75 US per case to $15 per case, the CD-R solution is saving technician labor time by eliminating the need to load and store cinefilm and saving cardiologist time by allowing them the ability to review and complete reports immediately after the case.

Conclusions

Cardiology is entering a new era with the replacement of cinefilm. Digital technology is a rapidly evolving field in both performance and cost. Avoid the urge to purchase a system based on proprietary, in-house designs. While these solutions may look good today, you may compromise future upgradeability and performance enhancements. When selecting a cineless solution for your cath labs, the following criteria should be considered:

- The cath lab digital system should provide a DICOM network output open to all suppliers
- The cath lab digital system should allow background image transfer (no lock up during transfer)
- The cine replacement system should allow off-line image review immediately after the case without the need to create a CD-R
- Until lossy compression is clinically validated, the cine replacement system should not use any form of lossy compression
- The cine replacement system should have some type of remote service capability to allow rapid system repair

By following the above guidelines, you should have success as you enter the cineless future.

References

1. Parisot C. The DICOM standard. A breakthrough for digital inormation exchange in cardiology. Int J Card Imaging 1995;11(Suppl.3):171-7.
2. American College of Cardiology, American College of Radiology and industry develop standard for digital transfer of angiographic images. ACC/ACR/NEMA Ad Hoc Group. J Am Coll Cardiol 1995;25:800-2.
3. Condit PB. Requirements for cardiac interchange media and the role of recordable CD. Int J Card Imaging 1995;11(Suppl.3):153-7.
4. Cardiac angiography without cine film: erecting a "Tower of Babel" in the cardiac catheterization laboratory. American College of Cardiology Cardiac Catheterization Committee. J Am Coll Cardiol 1994;24:834-7.
5. Brennecke R, Reiber JH. The future of image storage, analysis and communication in the cauterization laboratory [editorial]. Int J Card Imaging 1994;11(Suppl.3):145-6.
6. Bronkalla M, Kennedy TE. Holding our for a digital solution. J Cardiolvasc Management 1993;11/12:21-4.

16. Requirements for cardiac interchange media and the adoption of recordable CD

PAUL B. CONDIT, GERRY PELANEK & TERENCE ROURKE

Summary

Over the past four years, representatives of the American College of Cardiology (ACC) have collaborated with the x-ray equipment industry through the National Electrical Manufacturers Association (NEMA) to develop a digital standard for the exchange of x-ray angiographic images. These efforts have resulted in an extension of the Digital Imaging and Communications in Medicine (DICOM) Standard and the selection of recordable CD (CD-R) as the medium for interchange. This report is based on an INCIS '94 presentation by Paul B. Condit, PhD in Mainz, Germany and provides an update on the progress made since then. Included is a discussion of the distinction between archiving and interchange of digital image data, a review of the medium selection criteria, a mapping of CD-R against these criteria, and a discussion of the future of this medium.

Background

In early 1992 the Cardiac Catheterization Committee of the American College of Cardiology (ACC) formed a subcommittee to facilitate efforts to standardize digital image archiving in the cardiac catheterization laboratory. The committee was concerned about the proliferation of non-standard, non-compatible "cineless" systems being installed, and particularly about the image quality associated with certain media being used to exchange patient studies between health care institutions. In March, and later in October of that year, this group called together cardiac catheterization lab imaging suppliers, all members of the National Electrical Manufacturers Association (NEMA), to call attention to this issue. Their objective was to facilitate the selection of a standardized medium and development of formats for the storage of digital images obtained during cardiac catheterization. Participants in those meetings were provided the list of requirements outlined in Table 1 and were asked to work together on this standards activity. The result of these meetings was general agreement that a standards effort was warranted. Furthermore, the group agreed to build on the standards work that had been going on for a number of years under the auspices of the American College of Radiology (ACR) and NEMA. This latter activity had resulted in an agreed upon format for the network communication of digital radiographic images among vendors; referred to as the Digital Imaging and Communications in Medicine (DICOM) Standard.

J.H.C. Reiber and E.E. van der Wall (eds.), Cardiovascular Imaging, 201-209.
© 1996 *Kluwer Academic Publishers.*

Table 1. ACC requirements for a digital storage alternative to cinefilm.

- Image quality must be equal to or better than cinefilm.
- Capable of real-time motion reproduction 30 frames/sec or faster.
- Ability to archive entire image run without time delay requirements for editing (e.g., device should store all frames rather than selected).
- Ability to provide single patient unit record.
- Patient unit needs to be viewable off-line outside the cath lab with random access type of viewing as opposed to only sequential access.
- Need to retain capability to handle both cinefilm and digital technologies during transition period.
- Components, wherever possible, should be modular so they can be replaced as technology advances during the transition period.
- Archiving process for patient unit record should not slow down acquisition.
- Downloading process should be both time- and cost-efficient.
- Ability to play back with no time delay.
- Should have relatively long (i.e., years) shelf life.
- Simultaneously record from two planes.
- Should have equipment compatible for playing back images used from other diagnostic tests (e.g., MRI, echocardiography, etc.).

Formation of the ACC-NEMA committees

As a result of these early discussions, two ACC-NEMA ad hoc subcommittees were formed. One focused on the angiographic "information object" or data format, and the other focused on the selection of an appropriate digital medium. These groups have met monthly since early 1993. This report, which is based on an INCIS '94 presentation in Mainz, Germany, is specifically focused on the results of the medium selection. Included will be discussions about:
-   the distinction between digital image data *archiving* and image data *interchange,*
-   an outline of the selection criteria for an interchange medium,
-   mapping of the selected medium, CD-R, against these criteria,
-   a discussion of the future of CD-R, and
-   a report of the ongoing ACC-NEMA activities.

Image archiving versus interchange

The committees recognized early in their work the distinction between *archiving* of cardiac cath lab image data within a facility, and the *interchange* of image data between facilities. It was recognized that within a facility unique requirements might exist for how information is stored, archived and retrieved. However, one barrier preventing a facility from converting from cinefilm to a non-film alternative was the lack of a standard for providing the digital image data to another facility.

At that time, a number of approaches were being developed to store images within the facility. However, Super VHS tape was the only convenient technology used by "cineless" labs for image interchange. The American College of Cardiology was concerned about the use of Super VHS tape for this application, not only because it is an analog format, but in many cases the resolution was deemed inadequate, requiring the patient to be re-catheterized at the receiving facility [1]. Recognizing, therefore, that interchange of digital data was most important, the committee focused on this issue.

Criteria for selection of an interchange medium

Discussions during the early meetings resulted in identifying a number of important criteria for selection of an interchange medium. These can be divided into two categories: quantitative and qualitative.

The quantitative measures defined were:
- data capacity (the amount of data that can be stored),
- read speed (the speed at which data can be read from the medium), and
- access time (the time required to find and access a single record, or group of records, on the medium).

Although not specifically discussed due to legal requirements under which NEMA operates, the cost of the media and system components were also important.

The qualitative criteria defined were:
- multiple vendors for components,
- standard equipment interfaces,
- standards for the medium itself,
- high probability of non-obsolescence of the hardware and media, and
- the growth potential for the medium selected.

Table 2 summarizes these two categories of criteria. The next few sections of this article will provide detail for the quantitative criteria.

Table 2. Criteria for the selection of an interchange medium.

Quantitative	Qualitative
Data Capacity	Multiple Vendors
Read Speed	Equipment Interface
Access Time	Media Standards
Cost	Non-Obsolescence
	Potential for Growth

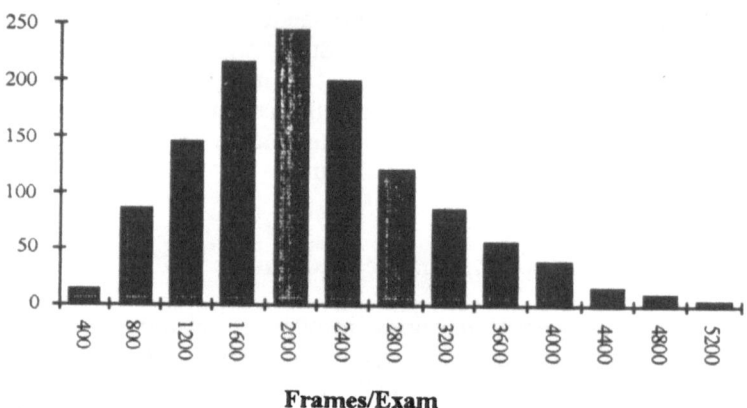

Frames/Exam

Figure 1. Distribution of number of frames per exam.

Discussion of quantitative criteria for selection of an interchange medium

Data Capacity

A simple experiment was done to understand the capacity required to accommodate typical cardiac cath studies. A random selection was made of 1,500 rolls of cinefilm in 100 U. S. labs. The diameters of these rolls were measured and converted to equivalent frames. As Figure 1 shows, the number of frames per exam fell within a roughly normal distribution, with an average of about 2,000 frames. This is equivalent to a little over one minute of cinerecording. Ninety-five percent of all the exams contained 4,800 frames or less (almost three minutes of cinefilming). Similar data gathered in Europe yielded comparable results. Based upon this information, the assumption was made that the media considered as candidates should be capable of storing the equivalent of 4,800 frames of cinefilm.

Examination of digital equipment matrix sizes available today, and discussion of the resolution that was acceptable for digital images in the lab, resulted in the minimum requirement of a pixel matrix of 512 x 512 x 8 bits deep. There was also general agreement that lossless compression, which generally results in a reduction of the data by about two to one, would be acceptable for this application. (Lossless data compression is completely reversible; i.e., the original data can be reproduced bit by bit.)

The 512 x 512 x 8 bits per frame yields a quarter of a megabyte of data per frame. A 4,800 frame study thus results in 1,200 megabytes. When reduced by one half through lossless compression the result is that the media candidates must have storage capacities of at least 600 megabytes to handle a single patient record (Table 3).

Table 3. Quantitative criteria for selection of an interchange medium.

Characteristic	Requirement
Pixel matrix	512 x 512
Bit depth	8 bits
Number of frames	4,800
Compression	2:1 lossless
Data capacity	600 MB
Retrieval speed	7.5 fps
Read speed	900 KB/sec
Access time	10 seconds

Read Speed

There was general agreement that the rate at which the data can be read *directly* from the medium need not be at 30 frames per second for the interchange application. This was based on the assumption that in a review/workstation the data could be uploaded onto some other device (for example, a hard disk) with a real-time (30 frames per second) display capability. However, it was agreed that a *reasonable* read speed must be possible as the clinician will probably not be comfortable waiting very long before being able to review the case at 30 frames per second. For these reasons, the criterion for retrieval speed was set at a "nice-to-have" one-quarter rate so that potentially at least 7 1/2 frames per second could be viewed during the uploading process.

Again, the 512 x 512 x 8-bit frame yields a quarter of a megabyte of data. With two to one lossless compression, this reduces to 1/8 of a megabyte of data per frame. This multiplied by the 7 1/2 frames per second requirement results in an "acceptable" read rate of 0.9 megabytes (900 kilobytes) per second (Table 3).

Access Time

In a discussion similar to that of read speed, it was suggested that any time in excess of 10 seconds to access any frame sequence would be unacceptable to the practitioner. This became the requirement shown in Table 3.

Cost

Due to the NEMA rules there was not much discussion of cost, but there was general feeling that the acceptable media candidates be less expensive than cinefilm.

Selection of an interchange medium and mapping against the criteria

The quantitative and qualitative requirements just reviewed were used to evaluate over 15 potential media candidates. The candidates ranged from tape formats such as DD2, Exabyte, and 3490E; optical disk formats such as 5 1/4-inch WORMs, magneto-optical, and CD-R; and the evolving formats of optical credit cards and optical tape. Evaluation against the criteria led to the conclusion that the medium that best met the defined requirements was CD-R. At its meeting in March of 1994, the ACC published the following statement: "We have concluded the first phase of this report and have chosen for the interchange of data an optical medium based on the standard called CD-R or recordable CD."

Table 4 compares the performance of CD-R against the quantitative criteria outlined previously. The data capacity requirement of 600 megabytes is met by the current CD-R capacity of 682 megabytes. While the read speed of CD-R was, at best, only 300 kilobytes per second when this committee started its work, read speeds have continued to increase, with many currently meeting and a few exceeding the 900 kilobyte per second requirement. The random access capability of CD-R allows for access times of much less than the 10-second requirement. Finally, because the cost of CD-R has been falling rapidly since its introduction, it is projected to be less expensive than cinefilm.

Table 4. Quantitative criteria compared to performance of recordable CD.

Characteristic	Requirement	Recordable CD
Pixel matrix	512 x 512	
Bit depth	8 bits	
Number of frames	4,800	
Compression	2:1 lossless	
Data capacity	600 MB	682 MB
Retrieval speed	7.5 fps	
Read speed	900 KB/sec	900 KB/sec
Access time	10 seconds	<0.7 seconds

Table 5 compares CD-R against the qualitative criteria. The first three of these were easily handled. There are numerous vendors of hardware and media. These vendors have all developed equipment to read and record CDs utilizing the Small Computer Systems Interface (SCSI) standard. From the beginning, very strict

Table 5. Qualitative criteria compared to performance of recordable CD.

Requirement	Recordable CD
Multiple Vendors	Yes
Equipment Interface	SCSI
Media Standards	ISO 9660 & Orange Book
Non-Obsolescence	Computer/Consumer Driven
Potential for Growth	Numerous Developing Applications

standards were developed for the hardware-to-media interfaces. This allows for the desired total interchangeability of disks and drives. It was concluded that the CD standard was least likely to become obsolete as it is driven by computer and consumer applications with new offerings appearing daily.

The Freeman Report [2] on the history and projection for CD-ROM drive growth supports this latter conclusion. The forecast plotted in Figure 2 suggests a growth rate over the next five years of greater than 30 percent per year. This growth rate is for CD-ROM drives alone and does not include the demand for other CD products, such as audio CD hardware. To put this in perspective, the number of CD-ROM drives sold in the first few years of their existence eclipsed the total of all other optical drives ever sold. These growth rates drive tremendous economies of scale.

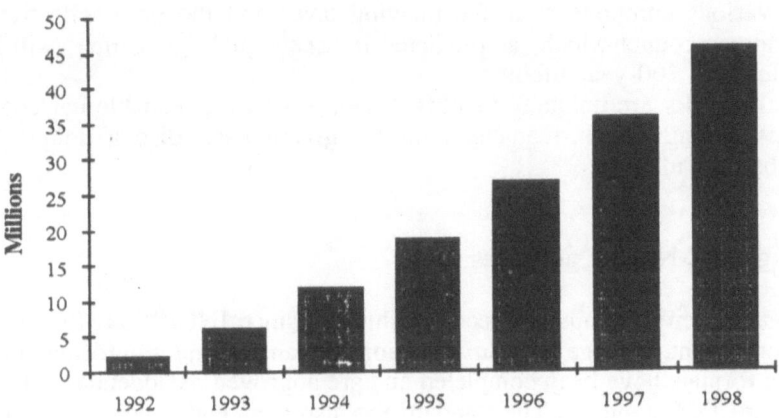

Figure 2. CD-ROM Drive Growth Rate.

Fueling the future growth in the CD industry are a number of developing consumer applications. Three of the most important are:
- the interest in extending the audio CD concept to putting movies on CDs
- the requirement to use CD in all sorts of multimedia applications, and
- productivity requirements in CD desktop publishing applications.

All of these create the need for higher capacities and faster read/write rates. To satisfy the need, research and development is focused on:
- the creation of blue lasers providing for more data to be put on the CD due to their higher-powered, more focused output, and
- physical modifications to the media and hardware, which will support the higher capacity DVD (digital video disc) formats. (Presently these DVD formats are being defined for the mass-produced CD-ROMs and are read only. Standards for recordable formats are likely to follow with the goal of being backward compatible with today's products.)

Additional benefits of CD-R

There are a number of characteristics of CD-R that were not requirements of selection but provide additional value in this application. Some of these characteristics exist with all recordable CDs and some are unique to the Kodak products.

All recordable CDs have these features:
- random access or retrieval of data,
- ability to write only once, precluding the data from being altered, and
- multi-session writing, allowing the capability to append additional data later.

Features that are specific to the Kodak product have been incorporated as a result of the need for this product to archive traditional photographic images.
- A durability overcoat to protect the data layer from scratches and fingerprints.
- The various components in the imaging layer and the gold reflective layer provide a product which, as predicted in accelerated age testing, will have a greater-than 100-year lifetime.
- Kodak CD-Rs are uniquely identified with a machine-readable bar code, and corresponding human-readable number, giving each disc a unique "serial number" or identity.

Ongoing ACC-NEMA activities

There have been a number of accomplishments since INCIS '94. In addition to finalizing the interchange medium selection, the angiographic information object and data formats have been completed and are approved as addenda to the ACR-NEMA DICOM standard. The standard has also been endorsed by the European Society of Cardiology. By way of a process similar to the above, the American Society of Echocardiography has also recommended CD-R as the medium of choice for exchange of echo images. Finally, active development is taking place on higher-resolution profiles (up to 1024 x 1014 x 10 bit), and also on profiles and information objects for nuclear cardiology images.

At the March 1995 ACC convention, over 20 vendors exhibited prototype review stations demonstrating implementation of the standard. Each vendor read a common DICOM interchange CD and displayed the x-ray angiography and echocardiography images contained therein for the clinician. This was a "read-only" feasibility demonstration to show the progress of this group and the capability of the CD-R standard.

It is expected at the March 1996 ACC meeting that there will be broader demonstrations. A common CD, similar to that used in 1995, will contain not only angiography and echo images, but also nuclear cardiology images. In addition, educational materials will be included on the CD along with a basic software utility to view the materials on a simple computer.

Lossy compression study

After the 1995 ACC demonstration, there was a proposal to extend the present standard to include the data, written a second time, in a lossy compressed form. This would allow the data to be read directly from the CD and the images to be displayed at real-time rates without the time-consuming process of uploading image data to a hard drive prior to review. Since lossy compression is not reversible and the process can introduce artifacts into the image, the ACC, ESC, and NEMA are currently fielding a study in the U.S. and Europe to determine the clinical effects of various levels of lossy compression. This study should be complete in 1996, and pending the outcome, the standard may be extended to include lossy compression.

Conclusion

CD-R has been selected as the digital interchange medium standard. The ACC-NEMA Committee, and its European counterpart, continue to move forward with the definition of additional application formats, extensions of the standard, and demonstrations of the feasibility of this medium for digital data interchange from a variety of modalities. Kodak is participating not only in the design of these standards, but will also utilize its digital imaging technology to bring customer-focused products to the marketplace.

Acknowledgement
This chapter is an update of an earlier publication [3].

References

1. Cardiac angiography without cine film: erecting a "Tower of Babel" in the cardiac catheterization laboratory. American College of Cardiology Cardiac Catheterization Committee. J Am Coll Cardiol 1994;24:834-7.
2. Freeman Reports: Optical data storage outlook. July 1993.
3. Condit PB. Requirements for cardiac interchange media and the role of recordable CD. Int J Card Imaging 1995;11(Suppl.3):153-7.

17. Status of the Camtronics approach to the digital catheterization laboratory

THOMAS E. KENNEDY & EUGENE W. BERGHOLZ

Summary

The Archium™ Cardiac Digital Archive System is a high performance network-based system that provides a digital solution for filmless operation in the cardiac catheterization environment. With the primary goal of maintaining image fidelity outside of the cardiac cath lab, the Archium system meets the clinical requirements for access and review of x-ray cardiographic images. Based on an open architecture, the Archium system can be incorporated as a component of an integrated patient information management system within a health-care institution. The Archium system is scaleable to address the requirements of a wide spectrum of cath department sizes and patient volume. The Archium system is modular, and key components of the system can be upgraded as technology advances warrant. The Archium system is DICOM-compliant and media independent.

Introduction

The maturity of digital x-ray acquisition and image processing systems means digital cine images are now generally regarded as diagnostically equivalent to film-recorded cine images [1-3]. This makes it possible for the cardiac cath lab to eliminate cineangiographic film use completely. The demand for filmless operation in the cardiac catheterization environment has been driven by the promises of decreased operating costs and improved department efficiency.

There are immediate cost savings to be gained through cinefilm replacement. These include the labor and expense of cinefilm processing, a significant reduction in film storage and retrieval costs, and elimination of the expenses associated with the handling and disposal of film processor chemicals. The degree of savings that can be realized vary from one facility to the next. In many cases, however, it is very difficult for a cardiac catheterization department to justify the investment in a digital archive and review system based on film savings alone. While the *per* patient media costs for a digital archive system are substantially less than for 35 mm film, the media savings can be quickly eroded by the investment costs in the digital equipment and service.

In the era of health-care cost containment, health-care providers are looking for operating expense reductions on a broad scale; strategies that increase department productivity, patient throughput, and physician efficiency are of great interest. Beyond this, however, the operation of the cardiac catheterization is nearly always viewed in the context of the operation of the entire health-care facility. Technology decisions for the cardiac catheterization department must be synergistic with the overall patient information management goals of the institution. Digital cardiac archive and review systems, integrated into campus-

J.H.C. Reiber and E.E. van der Wall (eds.), Cardiovascular Imaging, 211-219.
© 1996 *Kluwer Academic Publishers.*

wide information systems, offer the potential of decreasing departmental and institutional operating expenses while enhancing patient management. Decreased review delays, remote consultation, access to relevant patient information, and elimination of redundant entry of patient demographics all combine to yield efficiencies that justify conversion of the cardiac catheterization department to filmless operation.

Designed to satisfy both the specific requirements of the cardiac catheterization environment and the broader information management requirements of the health-care institution, Camtronics Medical Systems introduced the Archium Cardiac Archive System. Archium is a network-based system that allows a cardiac catheterization department to convert to filmless operation while expanding access to all information relevant to the cardiac patient. Camtronics is a major supplier of digital video image processors in the cardiac catheterization laboratory with a world-wide installed base of over 500 Video Plus™ systems. Archium is a natural extension of the company's expertise and commitment to x-ray cardiographic image acquisition and management.

Archium requirements

Many of the functional requirements for the Archium Cardiac Archive and Review System reflect input provided by a number of cardiologists, cath lab technicians, and department administrators. These specifications relate primarily to work flow, image access, and user interface design. Additional specifications relate to good design practices that reflect technology trends, standards development, and the economics of current health-care delivery. The more important design specifications include:

1. Network-based
   The archive solution should be digitally networked, meaning that the acquisition and review stations have the ability to access and send all patient images at full speed to other remote locations. All transactions must be done electronically to eliminate the need for manual tracking of stored information. The network must also interface with other information systems to permit integration of multi-modality images and patient information at the review stations.
2. Image Quality
   The digital archive and review system must provide a direct digital transfer of unprocessed images from the lab with no loss of resolution or gray scale data. All images acquired in the lab must be automatically archived. Accessing the original images without re-digitization ensures that the images viewed outside the lab are exactly the same as those acquired in the lab. This is necessary for appropriate off-line processing or analysis.
3. Image Storage and Access
   The digital archive and review system must support two levels of image storage and access. The first level of image storage must be "on-line" such that the archive system provides access to full speed review of any study in one second or less. Longer waiting times fall into the category of "near-line"

storage and access. All near-line studies must be accessible from anywhere on the network, and the near-line image data must be promotable to on-line status.

4. Concurrent Review

The digital archive and review system must support simultaneous access and concurrent review of the stored data. The technology should allow multiple users to access the same patient study, as well as provide individuals with access to multiple patient studies - without locking one or all parties out of the system or creating unpredictable delays.

5. Dynamic Post-Processing

The archive system must provide dynamic post-processing of the image data at the review station. This allows physicians to enhance images on-the-fly using edge sharpening, window and leveling, and other manipulations - identical to the capabilities available to them in the cath lab.

6. Media Independent

The archive system must be media independent. The archive component of the system must be sufficiently modularized so that the core system architecture is not designed around the archive medium. This important requirement is recognition of the fact that the capacities and the form factors of large capacity digital recording medium are in a constant state of flux. Systems designed around the performance characteristics of a particular medium risk obsolescence as a function of the life of the recording medium. Analog optical disk-based cardiac archival systems present such a precedent.

The Archium system

Based on the requirements outlined, a central server network topology was selected for the Archium system as shown in Figure 1. This architecture is modular in nature and permits any component of the system to be modified or enhanced without impacting the rest of the system. This approach allows the Archium system to follow a favorable price/performance curve while protecting against obsolescence. The system architecture is best described by tracing the data flow beginning in the cath lab.

With the ultimate goal of preserving all of the original image data so that what is seen on the review stations is exactly what was seen on the digital system in the cath lab, the Archium system employs direct digital interfaces to the x-ray acquisition system. The direct digital interfaces require specialized hardware designed to the proprietary specifications of the digital image processor subsystem of the x-ray acquisition system. In cases where such interfaces cannot be developed, an acceptable alternative is to place a Video Plus processor in parallel to the installed image processor. The Video Plus is an 8-bit processor that can support interlaced or progressive scan inputs at resolutions of 512×512 (60 frames/sec max) or the default 1024x512 (30 frames/sec max). These interface options allow the Archium system to be installed in a mixed vendor cardiac catheterization department.

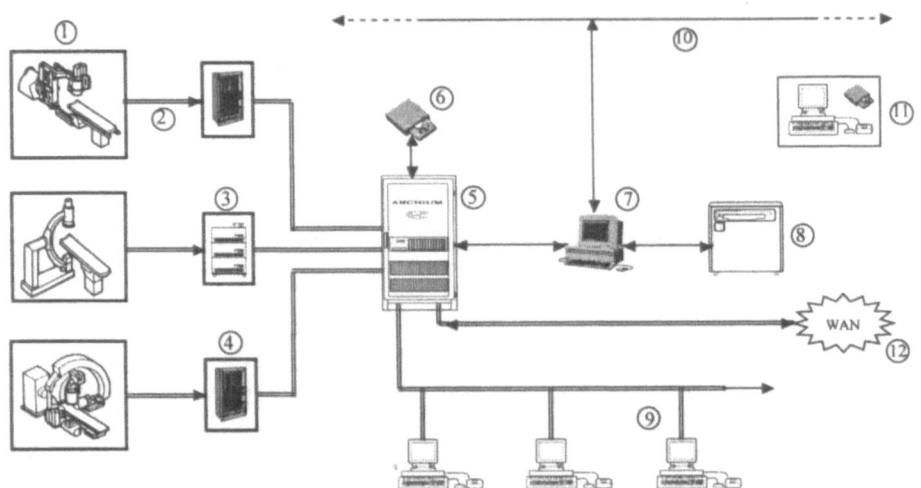

Figure 1. Archium ™ Cardiac Digital Archive System: 1) X-ray Acquisition System; 2) STL (Storage Transfer Link); 3) Video Plus™ Image Processor; 4) Direct Digital Interface; 5) WSC (Working Storage Controller); 6) DICOM Exchange CD-R Reader-Writer; 7) AM (Archive Manager); 8) Digital Archive Device; 9) Diagnostic Review Stations; 10) HIS/Hemodynamic Interfaces; 11) DICOM Independent Review Station; 12) WAN (Wide Area Network) Interface.

Frame grabbers do not provide an acceptable acquisition interface solution for the Archium system. Re-digitization of the output video signal introduces unacceptable levels of noise, and the captured image data precludes post-processing at the review station.

Image data generated in the cath lab is transferred at real-time rates to the Working Storage Controller (WSC) over the Storage Transfer Link (STL) - a high speed fibre optic network using the TAXI (Transparent Asynchronous Xmitter-Receiver Interface) protocol. At the Working Storage Controller, the images are lossless compressed using first-order DPCM with Huffman encoding in compliance with the JPEG standard [4]. For x-ray angiographic images, an average compression ratio of 2:1 is realized.

Based on RAID technology, the Working Storage Controller acts as a high performance digital image server for the networked review stations, and the WSC supports the on-line image storage and access requirements previously described. The storage and bandwidth capacity of the WSC is configurable by the number of RAIDs. The RAIDS (8+1, level 3) each provide 32 GB of storage and 20 MB/sec of input/output bandwidth. The WSC can support 3 RAIDS for a total capacity of 96 GB and an aggregate bandwidth of 60 MB/sec. Additional WSCs can be daisy-chained to increase capacity.

With an average exam size of 2,000 frames [5], a single-RAID WSC can store 128 patients (512×512, 8-bit image matrix). A fully configured WSC can therefore provide an on-line storage capacity of about 380 studies; this represents two weeks to three months of on-line image access, depending on the departmental patient volume.

After a study has been transferred out of the cath lab to the WSC, it is automatically archived to the archive device. To prevent accidental loss of data, a study cannot be deleted from the WSC until it has been fully archived. Further, a study only becomes a candidate for removal from the WSC after it has been reviewed by a physician. As the capacity of the WSC is reached, the oldest studies are removed to accommodate new studies.

The WSC fulfils the requirement for multiple, simultaneous review stations. The WSC can serve each review station, over the STL network, at a data rate equal to the image acquisition rate (30 frames/sec, max) for the study. As mentioned the max aggregate bandwidth of the WSC is 60 MB/sec, and a $512 \times 512 \times 30$ frames/sec study requires a bandwidth of 3.75 MB/sec. The server allows multiple users to simultaneously access different patients; the WSC also permits concurrent review of the same patient. The later feature facilitates remote consultation on a case, although the image play at each workstation is currently not synchronized.

The Archium diagnostic review stations are based on SUN™ Sparc 5 platforms running Solaris™. The review station also consists of an external image processor that permits real-time enhancement of images delivered from the WSC. The image processor is a minimally configured Video Plus processor that features a 30×30 filter kernel for edge enhancement. Real-time window/level and $2 \times$ zoom/roam are also supported. Processed images are transferred directly from the external image processor to a dual-plane, 8-bit frame buffer in the Sparc computer for image display. Images are never written to the Sparc internal hard disk.

To ensure optimal diagnostic image quality, all images, regardless of their native matrix resolution, are upscanned to 1024×1024 for display using bicubic interpolation. Images are displayed on either a 17" or 20" monochrome monitor. Initial tests revealed that color monitors do not provide image quality adequate for clinical use.

The user-interface for the diagnostic review station is based on OSF Motif. The user-interface is very simple and designed to minimize required interaction with the work station during a review session. Image motion control is provided through an external jog-wheel connected to the serial port of the SUN. This interface device emulates the motion control of a cinefilm projector; playback speed and direction are controlled with the jog-wheel. Additional buttons allow the user to toggle between images or access the patient directory. The review station provides optional QCA and LV analysis packages.

The Archive Manager (AM), based on a SUN Sparc 5 platform, is the controller for the Archium system. The AM maintains the patient database, regulates transfers between devices on the network, and serves as a remote service port. The AM also serves as the gateway to hospital information systems, cardiac information systems, and multi-modality imaging systems for campus-wide information integration.

The Archium system, as shown in Figure 1, is media independent. No system architectural details are dependent on the specific characteristics of a particular digital medium and drive. Currently, the Archium system supports the SONY™ 30 cm Digital Optical Disk (DOD). The 30 cm DOD is provided in capacities of

6.5 GB and 15 GB, with 12 platter and 77 platter jukeboxes, respectively.

Current Archium issues

Information systems integration

The Archium system currently has some integration with hospital information systems (HIS), cardiac information systems, and in-lab hemodynamic patient monitoring instruments. The level of integration and the complexity of implementation is highly variable from one institution to the next. A lack of standards on the hemodynamic monitoring side, and uneven implementation of HIS standards (HL7) often forces a high degree of customization.

Select still images can be exported form the Archium diagnostic review station to an external system, and image transfers are currently initiated at the review station. Summary hemodynamic reports can be imported and archived into the Archium system. In the cath lab, HIS or hemodynamic interfaces to the Archive Manager eliminates the problem of redundant entry of patient demographic data.

DICOM

The DICOM (Digital Imaging and Communications in Medicine) standard for medical images was developed jointly by the American College of Radiology (ACR) and the National Electrical Manufacturers Association to facilitate the exchange of multi-modality diagnostic images between mixed vendor acquisition devices, review stations, and printers [6].

Recent additions to the DICOM standard have incorporated x-ray angiography applications , including cardiac and vascular imaging. These additions, made with input from the American College of Cardiology (ACC), were motivated by the need for a suitable digital medium for the inter-hospital exchange of cine images as a replacement for cineangiographic film [7].

The performance characteristics of a number of different media were compared, and recordable (write-once) 120 mm optical disc (CD-R) was selected for the DICOM interchange standard. While the criteria used to select CD-R were developed to address specific problems associated with inter-hospital exchange of patient records, no effort was made to formulate requirements for long-term, on-site archival of the cineangiographic record. This distinction reflects the fundamental difference between image interchange and image archival. The interchange medium must be well defined to ensure universal compatibility for inter-facility exchange. The archive medium, however, must be matched to the unique operating practices of each catheterization department.

The Archium system supports the currently defined DICOM x-ray angiographic application profiles. The applications profiles are a means to narrowly define the choices of parts of the DICOM standard relative to the media format. For example, the Basic Cardiac application profile restricts the images to $512 \times 512 \times 8$ bits and bi-plane acquisitions are encoded as two single plane acquisitions.

The DICOM exchange discs can be loaded onto the Archium system via a PC-based DICOM CD-R connected directly to the working storage controller via a SCSI link; exchange discs can also be created from the same device (see Figure 1). DICOM compliant CD-R writers are used in the cath lab as a backup for the Archium system. While used infrequently, a digital backup capability is required in the cineless environment to ensure data integrity in the event of a network failure.

Independent DICOM review station

In recognition of the fact that some low patient-volume cardiac cath departments do not require a network-based archive and review system, Camtronics has introduced a stand-alone DICOM review station that can be used in conjunction with the in-lab DICOM CD-R writer just described. The combination of the CD-R writer and review station provides a cath department with the ability to transition to cineless operation in a relatively inexpensive way. In this scenario, a CD-R is created for every study at the end of the exam, and the CD-R serves as the archive media.

The Independent Review Station is based on a Intel Pentium™ platform with the Microsoft Windows™ NT operating system. A high performance image processor and graphics/video display card has been developed that interface directly to the PC via the platform's PCI bus. Images (512×512, 8-bit) loaded from the CD-R to the internal hard disk of the computer can be enhanced, upscanned, and displayed at 30 frames/per second. As with the Archium review station, an external jog-wheel is provided for motion control.

With a network connection to the working storage controller, the Independent Review Station can be used to replace the SUN/Video Plus image workstation. Once connected to the Working Storage Controller, the PC-based review station is capable of supporting full dynamic replay of higher resolution images. Forward production of all Archium systems will feature the PC-based review stations. Customers who purchase the "sneaker-net" option today will be in a position to upgrade to the network-based solutions without loss of their initial investment. The PC-based review station also has the advantage that standard desk-top applications can be run from the review station. The dual-use functionality of the review station is attractive to most users.

Future Archium directions

As with any large and complex system, there are numerous evolutionary changes and enhancements that will be made to the Archium system. A desire to reduce the system cost drives some changes, and the transition to a PC-based review station reflects, in part, that ongoing effort. More importantly, however, clinical experience and changes in technology drive most planned Archium enhancements. Engineering design efforts are directed towards finding ways of making the Archium system even more scaleable across the spectrum of department sizes and patient volumes. On-line, near-line, and network bandwidth requirements scale as a function of department volume. Designs that satisfy low-volume departments do not necessarily scale in a cost effective way to very high volume departments.

For example, while CD-R may be an acceptable archive media for low volume cath departments, the same medium represents a challenge for the large department environment. In this case, CD-R presents the same media handling problems as the cinefilm it is intended to replace. Likewise, a very large capacity tape or optical disk jukebox system may be required for the large department but is excessively expensive for the smaller department. Similar arguments apply to networks and image servers. A balance must be found that does not require large amounts of site customization.

The Archium system will evolve to support greater levels of DICOM services, and additional exchange application profiles will be supported as they become available. Of particular interest is the proposed "Dynamic Cardio Review" application profile. This application profile specifies that two tracks of image data be written to the CD-R. The format of the first track is identical to the format specified by the basic application profile. The first track is produced with lossless JPEG compression and is always available for review. The second data track is a lossy compressed version of the original data. This track of images permits dynamic review of the exam directly from the CD-R and is a way to ameliorate the transfer rate limitations of CD-R. Archium system can support the lossy data already but will not make lossy compression available until the dual-mode application profile is incorporated into the DICOM standard.

Of great interest to many cath departments and hospitals is the ability to transmit cine exams over a wide area network for remote consultation. The Archium system supports interfaces to high speed commercial networks, but the carrier costs are prohibitively high for most institutions. Alternative solutions may be available pending approval of the Dynamic Cardio Review application profile.

In addition to expanding the capabilities of the Archium System, Camtronics has introduced significant changes to the Video Plus image processor. The new product, Video-Plus Cardiac (VPC) , is a high resolution 10-bit processor with multi-patient storage capability. The VPC features an adaptive spatial filter for edge enhancement, a two-pole temporal filter with motion detection, and a number of other advanced features to support emerging x-ray cardiographic procedures.

Conclusions

Camtronics Medical Systems is committed providing innovative solutions for the digital cath lab. The DICOM exchange standard has provoked interest in the health-care community for filmless operation, but adoption has been paced by the availability and cost of the technologies required for developing high performance digital archive and review systems. Camtronics offers cost effective solutions for in-lab digital acquisition and department-wide digital archive and review. The Archium system, in particular, addresses the requirements of current health-care economics.

References

1. Gurley JC, Nissen SE, Booth DC *et al*. Comparison of simultaneously performed digital and film-based angiography in assessment of coronary artery disease. Circulation 1988;78:1411-20.
2. Vogel RA, LeFree MT, Mancini GBJ. Comparison of 35 mm cine film and digital radiographic image imaging for quantitative coronary arteriography. In: Heintzen PH, Bürsch JH, editors, Progress in digital angiocardiography. Dordrecht: Kluwer Academic Publishers, 1988:159-71.
3. Mancini GBJ. Digital coronary angiography: advantages and limitations. In: Reiber JHC, Serruys PW, editors, Quantitative coronary arteriography. Dordrecht: Kluwer Academic Publishers 1991:23-42.
4. Pennebaker WB, Mitchell JL. JPEG still image compression standard. New York: Van Nostrand Reinhold, 1993.
5. Condit PB, Requirements for cardiac interchange media and the role of the recordable CD. Int J Card Imaging 1995;11(Suppl.3):153-7.
6. Digital Imaging and Communications in Medicine (DICOM), Parts 1-13, 1993-1996.
7. Charter: The Digital Angiographic Media Selection Ad Hoc Group. MED-PACS Section. ACC/NEMA, 1993.

18. The approach at the German Heart Institute in Berlin - the BERMED - System

ECKART FLECK & HELMUT OSWALD

Summary

Integration and communication of medical patient data play a key role in improving medical care and providing intelligent systems support for diagnosis and therapy. Medicine is traditionally associated with the two aspects of documentation and communication of patient data and findings. In this respect, documentation and communication not only serve the scientific aims, but also help to ensure the rationality, consistency and continuity of medical care itself. Nowadays, much of the medical patient data already exists in digital form, for example x-ray images, angiographic images and patient data of heart catheterization, ECG curves, findings, medical reports and intensive care monitor data. Other data may exist in analog form, in writing or even only orally. In order to provide efficient and, above all, high-quality support for the work of the nursing staff and the physicians, the various types of data and the way in which they are managed and used must be related to the intended applications. There must be a logical integration of the data and the related functionality. Traditionally, this is a task for the physician. However, the vast amount of information contained in the data, and the fact that automatic digital processing often yields more information than can be obtained by unaided human perception, as in the case of digital image processing, leads to the conclusion that the integration of medical patient data and the related functionality, including the logical interpretation, should be supported by computer. The electronical medical record is not only the complete and gapeless documentation of an even extremely complex situation, such as a hospital stay, but the utilization of all patient related information which during the complete course of the disease has been acquired regardless of where, when and of which data structure. (Multimedia in the true sense.) Any centralized solution, such as a general database, smart card etc., will be inappropriate since it cannot cope with the demands for the integration of existing distributed subsystems nor for the demands of future systems.

Introduction

Integration and communication of medical patient data play a key role in improving medical care and providing intelligent systems support for diagnosis and therapy. Medicine, seen both as a science and as the provision of medical care, is traditionally associated with the two aspects of documentation and communication of patient data and findings. In this respect, documentation and communication not only serve the scientific aims, but also help to ensure the rationality, consistency and continuity of medical care itself.

Many diseases have a relatively long course, during which the patient is cared for

J.H.C. Reiber and E.E. van der Wall (eds.), Cardiovascular Imaging, 221-232.
© 1996 *Kluwer Academic Publishers.*

at different locations and passes through various stages of treatment. Consequently, a natural need arises to have access to the data obtained at each step, in order to use it for diagnostic and therapeutic purposes. To provide appropriate care, and to avoid the expense and stress of repeated examination procedures, it is therefore necessary to make the data available not only within the clinic or for a individual physician caring for the patient, but also to allow access for external institutions involved in the care of patient. In addition, consultation of specialists, or the use of advanced information using analysis and evaluation techniques which are not generally available, also require communication of the relevant patient data.

This situation is exemplified in the case of coronary heart disease which may have a course of more than fifteen or twenty years. The medical institutions involved during this period can include the family doctor, the specialist, a local hospital providing a higher level of care, a specialized clinic (e.g. a heart institute with various departments for diagnostics, treatment and surgery), a rehabilitation clinic and, finally, a return to the specialist or family doctor. Subsequently, there may be an emergency admission elsewhere, again involving the same types of institutions. Such a cycle is not unusual. In fact, in the Federal Republic of Germany, this or a similar cycle occurs in considerably more than hundred thousand cases of heart disease every year. In the case, large quantities of data are obtained at every stage of care, with a wide variation in quality and type: text data on the clinical history and clinical examination, graphic data from the ECG, ultrasound or other noninvasive examinations, numerical data from laboratory examinations, intensive care or specialized diagnostic techniques and, finally, stationary and moving images from x-ray equipment or other imaging techniques. In addition to the integration and communication of such data, it is also necessary to store the information it contains to allow for its later use. In view of the large quantity of data involved, this requires appropriate selection, compression and editing, so that the data necessary for ensuring the quality of medical care and for supporting diagnosis and therapy are accessible and manageable.

Nowadays, much of the medical patient data already exists in digital form, for example x-ray images, angiographic images and patient data of heart catheterization, ECG curves, findings, medical reports and intensive care monitor data. Other data may exist in analogue form, in writing or even only orally. In order to provide efficient and, above all, high-quality support for the work of the nursing staff and the physicians, the various types of data and the way in which they are managed and used must be related to the intended applications. In other words, there must be a logical integration of the data and the related functionality. Traditionally, this is a task for the physician. However, the vast amount of information contained in the data, and the fact that automatic digital processing often yields more information than can be obtained by unaided human perception, as in the case of digital image processing, leads to the conclusion that the integration of medical patient data and the related functionality, including the logical interpretation, should be supported by computer.

When a system for the integration and communication of patient data and findings has been brought into use, questions arise with respect to data security and responsibility. This question is rooted in a long-standing medical tradition, and the answer is based on medical confidentiality and ethics. Consequently, the transfer of medical information to a computer requires a new approach, and the development of both adequate security measures and acceptable working methods. As a result of the new techniques for data processing and communication, many of the current methods for archival and transmission of patient data must be reconsidered, and answers must be found to newly arising problems of data protection and security. For example, traditional methods of identifying patient data, such as adding the patient's name and other personal data to chest radiographs or examination records, is not acceptable in an open communication network with the possibility of external access. Also, although unrestricted access to the data might be desirable on medical grounds, social and legal reasons make it impossible for it to be fully realized in practice.

Some difficult questions are encountered with respect to copying, communication and access, as well as determining the status of medical documentation, the selection of information and archival. As yet, many of these questions do not have a general answer, and not all of the problems will have a technical solution. Nevertheless, it appears that precisely the fact that the information is distributed, and the distribution can be maintained by integration and communication, will to a great extent prevent the possibility of misuse and falsification.

Taking all these arguments in consideration, the electronical medical record is not only the complete and gapeless documentation of an even extremely complex situation, such as a hospital stay, but the utilization of all patient related information which during the complete course of the disease has been acquired regardless of where, when and of which data structure. (Multimedia in the true sense.) Any centralized solution, such as a general database, smart card etc., will be inappropriate, since it cannot cope with the demands for the integration of existing distributed subsystems nor for the demands of future systems.

Several arguments can be found against any centralization. There is definite demand for documentation, archiving and quality control for each workplace generating and handling medical data. Distribution avoids the need to guarantee the data quality from outside systems. It provides better security against the misuse of patient data by maintaining it into the responsibility of the involved physician. The often used term "gläserner patient" can be seen as an inappropriate apprehension for the system approach. The responsibility and responses are left in the hand of responsible persons and institutions.

The result is a complex and complete medical documentation which serve for further requirements. These are given by demands from administration, economics and health care politics. The increasing costs for health care have worldwide brought about considerations and measures to limit or even reduce the cost explosion. Since part of a medical record in the given sense are information, management and communication components, the electronical medical record can serve as the basis for all needs, additional to the medical, in terms of overall administration, accounting, stock and store control, personal planning and payroll as well as management and controlling.

This enables a more rational approach to the discussion of the difficult and costly problems by avoiding flat budget restrictions as steering instrument.

Distributed systems in patient care

The trend in computing in general is away from the monolithic centralized mainframe systems prevalent of the 1970s and which still exist in many hospitals, towards what has been termed decentralized or distributed computing. This trend, called downsizing, has been enabled by networking technologies and the continual decrease in hardware costs. Today's PC has far more system resources and processing power than a mainframe of twenty years ago and brings attractive functionality to the desktop, such as word processing, spreadsheets, and e-mail. Distribution and sharing of resources such as file systems and databases brings improved performance and availability, but also introduces many technical and administrative problems that were not present or were easily controlled with the centralized systems. For example, naming and translation issues resulting from component heterogeneity; accounting, security, and resource management issues created by component autonomy; and synchronization, consistency, and error recovery problems resulting from component distribution. In most cases proprietary and closed solutions are adopted to tackle the problems generated by distribution. Hence, it would seem that we have not progressed much further than the closed centralized systems. Nowadays we have distributed systems with closed heterogeneous components and minimal integration. In many cases the possible advantages of a distributed system are far outweighed by the administrative, security, and integration problems they bring. The aim of the BERMED open distributed management system has been to provide the architecture and the infrastructure components to help overcome these problems.

Open systems

In conjunction with the current trend towards decentralized, or distributed computing systems, the term Open Systems has been receiving increased attention. In most cases, this term is taken in the general sense to mean exactly what it says - open as opposed to closed - it is possible to communicate with and integrate the components of the system. The term open does not imply public domain. Proprietary systems can be considered open if interfaces are publicly declared, allowing true communication and integration. An Open Systems Environment has been defined by the IEEE Technical Committee on Open Systems as: "a comprehensive and consistent set of international information technology standards that specify interfaces, services and supporting formats to accomplish interoperability and portability of applications, data and people..." Following most authors (for example see [2]) we consider the concerns of open systems to include not only portability and interoperability, but also integration. Portability refers to the ability to allow the system components to be used in various environments or hardware platforms. Interoperability to the ability for components to communicate, to exchange information. Although the aspects of portability and interoperability are essential for achieving an open system, they are in most part concerned with the use of de-facto or de-jure standards. Here we shall concentrate here on what we consider to be the most challenging and needed aspect of openness which is integration.

Information Management

There is an important difference between data and information. Data being the bits stored by the computer, information is something that is meaningful to the end-user. In the technical world, the two terms are often confused. In many cases data processing is taken to be synonymous with information processing, and data management with information management. Whilst we attempt to make consistent use of the terms, it is clear, that in some cases a strict differentiation is cumbersome.

The term information management is widely used but often with different meanings. Many of the activities of health professionals may be considered to relate to information management in the true sense of the term [3] - obtaining and recording information about patients, consulting colleagues, reading scientific literature, planning diagnostic procedures, devising strategies for patient care, interpreting results of laboratory and radiological studies, or conducting case-based and population-based research. From the business informatic perspective, the term has more to do with the provision of computer support, and has been applied to cover a very broad range of activities [4] - management of the information infrastructure; the management of the application systems, that is the activities involved in the planning, design, development, maintenance, and support of these systems; and the management of the information use, that is the activities for the requirements analysis, the user schooling, the organizational aspects etc. Whilst all aspects of both perspectives should be considered, most of these must remain outside the scope of this book. Here we concentrate on the issues concerning the management of distributed data, ensuring the reliable long term storage, the ease of retrieval, the consistency, and the security of data, and the issues concerning the management of information for the end-user, the support for the integration, processing and presentation of information.

Hence, the requirements for information management in patient care come from both the perspective of the end-user (the medical perspective) and the perspective of system developer and administrator (technical perspective). From the end-user perspective, the demand is for the management of the ever increasing volume of patient related, scientific, administrative and accounting information. Computer-based information management brings support for the health professional, providing the transparent access to all components of the computerized patient record from local and remote sources, the generation of multimedia documents, the true integration of medical applications, the support for administrative tasks such as appointment scheduling or bed planning, the automatic transfer of information for administrative purposes, the integration of medical databases, and the support for research related access. From the technical perspective, information management is required to ensure the achievement of the consistency, availability, and security of distributed data, and provide services that support the administration of accounts, resources, configuration, performance, security, and faults. In BERMED, we have aimed to realize some, but not all, of these requirements. Some have been realized through the infrastructure which we term the open distributed management system (ODMS), some through the use of existing system services, databases, archives and medical applications, and some by what we have termed the integrated medical application (IMA).

Integration in BERMED

Many of the requirements of information management relate to the task of integration, particularly the integration of patient data and application functionality. In BERMED we have aimed to provide what has been termed logical-functional integration. The first part is the logical integration of patient data, providing the transparent access to local and remote patient data. For the end system to have any chance of acceptance, the integration of all patient data is essential. This means the integration of the demographic data, medical history, all text based documentation such as reports and protocols, scanned documents, image data from all modalities, ECG results, laboratory results, etc. This integration forms the basis of the computer-based patient record (CPR). Significant amount of research is being carried out in Europe and America on the aims and requirements for a CPR. These are reported elsewhere [5-7]. The simplest method of realizing the CPR is to provide a central repository which contains all patient data. In contrast to this centralized approach we aim for the logical integration of distributed data. The original data remains in the archive or database at its place of origination. The data is integrated logically rather than physically.

We aim for the functional integration of applications. Integration is required of medical applications (image processing, medical documentation, access to medical databases,...), of administrative programs, and of standard desktop applications (statistics packages, word processing, and e-mail). Functional integration usually implies that the output of one program can be taken as the input of another [2]. In the BERMED context, we also mean the transparent sharing of certain context information between application components, for example the selected patient or selected document is shared between application components. Experience has shown the extreme practical difficulties in achieving the functional integration of applications that were never designed for this purpose.

A future aim of BERMED concerns not only the integration of patient data and related applications, but also the integration of administrative and management related information, for example the automatic extraction of billing and stores information from the documentation of medical procedures, the integration of tools for organizational tasks such as appointment or bed planning.

Key issues for information management in patient care

Certain issues must be considered in a patient care setting that are not found in other application environments. Our work on the integration of data and functionality has highlighted certain issues which have proven to be critical in achieving the desired aims:

Patient Identification over distributed local and remote archives and databases.
This would not be a problem if each person were assigned a unique global identifier. However, in many countries, constitutional laws prohibit the assignment of global identifiers. It is necessary to provide support that enables a patient to be uniquely identified even in the presence of data entry errors. In most cases this can be achieved through the combined use of information such as

name, date of birth, and insurance number, together with heuristics to deal with common entry inconsistencies.

User identification and authentication over distributed local and remote archives and databases.

It is essential to protect patient data against unauthorized disclosure. A distributed computing environment covering not only a single hospital raises issues that need careful attention. Adequate mechanisms for ensuring the protection of data in distributed systems are well-known. The problems lie not with the technology, but on the organizational and administrative side such as the difficulties of introducing new mechanisms in parallel with established facilities.

Use of controlled vocabularies to code information.

The problematic of coding data in medicine has not been satisfactorily solved. Coding is essential for the achievement of complete integration and the truly open management of medical information. This topic is discussed in a later chapter in detail.

The work in BERMED has also highlighted certain technical, organizational, and administrative aspects which must be given adequate attention. These aspects are not necessarily unique to the patient care setting:

Data consistency over distributed databases.

Distribution brings many advantages over the centralized solution. However, distribution implies that certain patient data will be duplicated in several databases. It is essential to ensure that the complete system is always kept in a consistent state. This may require the use of distributed transaction facilities which ensure consistency even in the event of abort actions or failure to update in subsystems.

Provide adequate robustness, reliability, and performance.

Hospital information systems are required to operate 24 hours a day. Minimal down-time can be tolerated. Adequate experience shows that a system that is unreliable, requires continuous attention, or is slow to respond will be ignored.

The system should not increase the burden on administrative activities.

All software requires administrative attention: e.g. configuration, updates, error tracing, and user-administration. Support must be given for the automation of all these activities.

The system should be open.

It should be scalable and portable, providing features that allow evolutionary growth and dynamic reconfiguration. It must operate over the wide range of computer platforms that are typical for a patient care environment. Consideration must be made of the impact that PC desktop computers are making in patient care. Where appropriate, relevant de-facto or international standards should be adopted, such as DICOM for access to image archives, HL7 for messages between hospital information system components, and the OSF DCE services for RPC communications, naming, and security. Self defined standards add flexibility, but inhibit the adoption of available software components. Interfaces to the system must be fully declared to allow others to access and extend the services.

The provision of new services must be evolutionary. Existing computer systems do support health professionals. Any change must provide enhancements to the familiar and valuable functionality.

An architectural approach for information management

An architecture is generally understood as the art of construction [8]. Applied to an information system, the architecture must specify the individual building blocks, their functional properties, their interactions, the details of the interfaces. In addition, the architecture is not just restricted to the description of the components, but may also be taken to include the description of how the system is to be built, it should provide the clear construction rules for all persons concerned (e.g. the end users and administrators, the software system developers, external advisors, external developers, hardware manufacturers, etc.) to ensure the logical consistency of the entire project.

Standard architectures have been developed to cover certain specific application areas such as transport industries, finance, manufacturing, and airlines. The trend is to consider an enterprise wide architecture. That is, rather than focusing interest on isolated parts of the complete business and building autonomous information systems for each, it has been recognized that truly integrated information systems and businesses can only be achieved if an enterprise wide architecture has been developed. The European effort for the standardization of healthcare informatics, CEN technical committee [9] is developing a framework for future standardization. This framework is "a logical mapping between the real world, in particular the healthcare environment, and its Healthcare Information Systems Architecture. This framework - representing main healthcare subsystems, their connections, rules etc. - is the basis for an evolutionary development of heterogeneous computer supported healthcare and communication system."

Although this standardization effort is still in very early stages, it is encouraging to note the positive influence of enterprise modelling from, in particular, the area of CIM (computer integrated manufacturing), the ANSA (advanced network systems architecture) project [10], and the ISO ODP (open distributed processing) standardization effort, all of which have also greatly influenced the development of the BERMED architecture. The general agreement is that the analysis and design of information systems in complex environments such as healthcare requires the consideration of many different aspects from several viewpoints. The ANSA work has led to the formalization of the treatment of the complexity in enterprise wide architectures. Both ANSA and ODP introduce the idea of five viewpoints (enterprise, information, computational, engineering, and technology) from which the information systems and business concerns must be considered. In an interim report the CEN PT010 committee has put forward a more complex framework than ODP, adding ideas resulting from the CIM world. The framework also considers the dimensions of the software evolution process. In our experiences, the inclusion of such considerations in the framework is essential for healthcare. In many instances little regard is taken for evolutionary strategies and the possible effects that new systems will have on existing work processes. Failure to consider these dimensions can result in much wasted effort. However, the CEN PT010 framework would appear to be relatively complex. It is questionable as to whether the outcome of such a complex framework could be applied in a healthcare environment that in many respects lacks the resources and expertise. In [11] a far simpler, and pragmatic, architectural approach for healthcare information systems is put forward. The approach detailed follows the current trends of concentrating on business processes and business process re-engineering [12], and again considers the system and business from different viewpoints: "Any hospital is a collection of business processes. These business processes use data and are supported by technology. The business processes need to be organized effectively (Business Architecture); the data needs to be organized effectively (Data Architecture); and the technology needs to be organized effectively (Technology Architecture). Furthermore, there must be an alignment among these three elements. The degree of alignment is determined by the control systems of the hospital." However, in the BERMED project we have not concentrated on the business processes or business process re-engineering. These aspects must be given more consideration.

ODP and object-oriented approach

Structuring mechanisms are required to deal with the complexity of distributed, heterogeneous, and autonomous systems. The object-oriented approach has proven to be the natural model. An object encapsulates. Access to the services provided by an object can only be made by sending messages to a well-defined interface. This model brings the means to cope with autonomy and heterogeneity. The architectural approach adopted in BERMED follows that outlined in the ISO ODP standards. ODP provides the groundwork for a common structuring to enable different distributed system technologies to be integrated. This has been achieved through the creation of the Reference Model, and the identification or definition of specifications governing the implementation and use of the functions to realise the systems. The reference model specifies a common language and structure for describing distributed systems. Central to this are the five viewpoints, the enterprise, the information, the computational, the engineering, and the technology viewpoints, and the use of common concepts and the consistent use of object modelling techniques for each viewpoint.

The enterprise and information viewpoints "abstract away from issues of distribution, leaving only statements of requirements which are independent of the distribution process. The enterprise viewpoint is concerned with business policies, management policies and human user roles with respect to the systems and the environment with which they interact... The information viewpoint is concerned with information modelling..."

The computational viewpoint "is concerned with the description of the system as a set of interacting objects, without considering the details of how they interact. It describes the algorithms and data flows which provide the distributed system function..."

The engineering and technology viewpoints "are concerned with the provision of an environment in which the computational description of a system can be interpreted... The engineering viewpoint is concerned with the distribution mechanisms and the provision of the various transparencies needed to support distribution; the technology viewpoint is concerned with the detail of the components and links from which the distributed system is constructed."

In BERMED we have used object-oriented approaches in all stages of the project, for analysis, design and implementation. We have found it necessary to identify two distinct categories or types of object. These correspond to the difference between the information and the computational viewpoint. Those objects in the information viewpoint represent real entities, things that are of interest to the end-user. Those in the computational viewpoint encapsulate units of computation, units that provide specific well-defined computational services. These may be application services, that is application functionality for the end-user which may process objects that represent real entities such as images or text documents. They may be databases that store objects that represent real entities. They may be infrastructure or management objects that provide services transparent to the end-user, but are required to enable the secure, integrated, and transparent access to distributed data. In the future, with the introduction of truly distributed object management systems [13], these differences may disappear. It may then be possible to consider information and computational objects at the same level of granularity.

Object-oriented analysis and design [14,15] are methods that examine requirements from the perspective of the classes and objects that are found in the vocabulary of the problem domain. We have found these techniques extremely advantageous over older techniques such as structured analysis and design. Objects are abstractions of real-life things. Hence they are identifiable by both the analysists and the domain experts (the physicians and other healthcare personnel) leading to far improved understanding and communication in all stages of the project. Since these real-life things, or entities, are unlikely to change rapidly in character, the resulting specifications are likely to be relatively stable with a long lifetime. Object-oriented techniques are ideal for modelling the multimedia types of data occurring in healthcare. Objects encapsulate, providing information hiding. Classes allow the grouping together of objects with similar properties. Inheritance and aggregation are powerful tools for abstraction, for coping with complexity. The consistent use of object-oriented methods provides very close coupling between analysis, design, and implementation. The models may vary in details and structure, but the key concepts and relationships remain constant.

The BERMED architecture

We consider the complete BERMED system architecture in three logical parts. This is illustrated in figure 1 from the computational viewpoint.

The first part covers the services needed for the integration of data within a self contained patient care provider, such as a hospital or general practice, and the provision of various common facilities such as advanced image processing, medical thesaurus, or access to medical literature databases. The services of this provider are made available to local and remote clients through established interfaces. The next part of the architecture covers the integrated medical application. This provides the functional integration of the applications that directly support the work of the physician. These applications may be clients of the local and remote services described in the first part. Examples for the medical applications are facilities for the access, processing, and visualization of all types of patient data (e.g. image, text, and graphic), or facilities to support cooperation, such as asynchronous (e.g. email) and synchronous communications

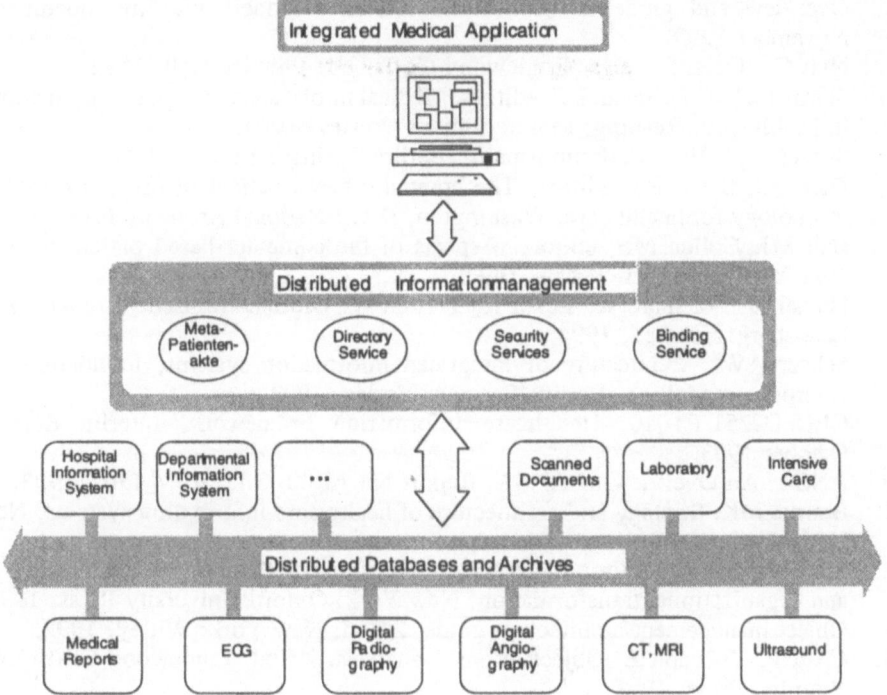

Figure 1. BERMED Architecture.

services (e.g. desktop conferencing). The last part of the architecture covers the wide area integration of patient data and the infrastructure to enable communications between health professionals. It provides components such as the telemedicine directory which is used to obtain the address and interface description of available services, and the component to enable the global identification and authentication of end-users. The BERMED open distributed management system is concerned with the first and last parts.

It is important to note that these three parts represent a logical and not necessarily a physical division. For example, components indicated in the integrated medical application may execute on more than one computer, they themselves may be distributed and shared. In addition, it is also important to note that the computational objects themselves represent logical and not necessarily physical encapsulation. Several components may be implemented within one software process. Similarly one computational object may be realized through several software components. This abstraction provided in the computational viewpoint, away from the actual software realization and physical distribution, has proven essential for a stable and reusable design. The resulting specification can be utilized independent of the underlying infrastructure and technology.

References

1.   ISO 10746-1, Basic reference model open distributed processing part 1

Overview and guide to use of the reference model: Working document, November 1993.

2.   Nutt GJ. Open Systems. Englewood Cliffs, NJ: Prentice-Hall, 1992.
3.   Shortliffe EH, Perreault LE, editors. Medical informatics: computer applications in health care. Reading, Mass: Addison-Wesley, 1990.
4.   Scheer AW. Wirtschaftsinformatik, Berlin: Springer-Verlag, 1994.
5.   Dick RS, Steen EB, editors. The computer-based patient record: an essential technology for health care. Washington, D.C.: National Academy Press, 1991.
6.   Ball MJ, Collen MF, editors. Aspects of the computer-based patient record. New York: Springer-Verlag, 1992.
7.   Hölzel D, Adelhard K, Eckel R, Tretter W. Die elektronische Krankenakte. Landsberg: Ecomed, 1994.
8.   Scheer AW. Architecture of integrated information systems, foundations of enterprise modelling. Berlin: Springer-Verlag, 1992.
9.   CEN/TC251/PT010, Healthcare Information Framework, Interim Report, October 1993.
10.   ANSA, An Overview of ANSA, Report No.AR00. S.l.: APM Ltd., 1993.
11.   Bourke MK. Strategy and architecture of health care information systems. New York: Springer-Verlag, 1994.
12.   Scott Morton MS, editor. The corporation of the 1990s: information technology and organizational transformation. New York: Oxford University Press, 1991.
13.   Object management architecture guide. 2nd ed. New York: Willey, 1992.
14.   Coad P, Yourdon E. Object-oriented analysis. 2nd ed. Englewood Cliffs, NJ: Yourdon Press, 1991.
15.   Rumbaugh J. Object-oriented modelling and design. London: Prentice-Hall, 1991.

19. Archival systems for cineangiographic film replacement

DAVID R. HOLMES Jr., MERRILL A. WONDROW, KIRK N. GARRATT & MALCOLM R. BELL

Summary

Replacement of coronary cineangiographic film should become a reality within 2 to 3 years. This process has been accelerated by the American College of Cardiology, American College of Radiology, and the National Electrical Manufacturers Association Joint Committee, which has established a logical format (Digital Imaging and Communications in Medicine 3.0) and physical format (CD-R) as the standard media for the transport of cardiac catheterization images in place of cineangiographic film. Another integral part of the process is identification of the archival media. Standardization of this archival media has not been undertaken. The requirements for archival systems are as stringent as for the transport media. Several archival systems are described which meet these requirements, including capacity, read/write speed, access time, and backward/forward compatibility without the need for data compression. They are promising solutions to storage of large data sets.

Introduction

Replacement of coronary cineangiographic film has become an achievable goal. Current digital systems provide image quality equal to or superior to that of cineangiographic film. The rationale for replacement of the film has been discussed previously and relates to the multiple problems of cineangiographic film, including, among others, cost, lack of post-processing digital enhancements, delays for film development, and storage requirements (Table 1) [1]. In the past, a major impediment to film replacement has been the plethora of potential vehicles that make standardization, compatibility, and transportability of data extremely difficult [2]. Through the intense effort of the American College of Cardiology, American College of Radiology, and the National Electrical Manufacturers Association (ACC/ACR/NEMA) Joint Committee, which has now been joined by the European Society of Cardiology (ESC), a logical format (DICOM 3.0; Digital Imaging and Communications in Medicine) [3] and a physical format (CD-R) have been established as the standard media for the transport of cardiac angiographic images in place of cineangiographic film [1].

The DICOM standard is the most important standard enabling replacement of cineangiographic film. DICOM defines a common format for digital image data which enables communication between equipment from different manufacturers. The DICOM effort began in radiology and was initially focused on the ability to communicate between different vendors over Ethernet networks. The goal was to develop a standard that allowed different imaging equipment to communicate

J.H.C. Reiber and E.E. van der Wall (eds.), Cardiovascular Imaging, 233-241.
© 1996 *Kluwer Academic Publishers.*

Table 1. Cineangiographic film technology.

Advantages	Disadvantages
Industry standard	Static technology
Worldwide compatibility	Processing delays
Unit record	No post-processing capability
Fulfills archive and transport requirements	Radiation dose levels
Longevity and stability	Cost
	Storage space requirement

with different archival systems, printers, and workstations without the need for custom interfaces at each device. The DICOM method in cardiology has been focused on the ability to interchange data between institutions. This remains a critical issue for cardiology in order to replace cineangiographic film. The benefits of a DICOM conformance from the catheterization laboratory digital system are: 1) it allows the customer to purchase a catheterization laboratory from one vendor and a workstation from another; 2) DICOM will allow multimodality interfaces; 3) DICOM will allow catheterization laboratories from different manufacturers to be networked together without custom interfaces; and 4) DICOM will create the possibility for interface with hospital information systems, radiology information systems, and hemodynamic data.

Interchange media

In choosing the interchange media, the ACC/ACR/NEMA considered cost, availability, capacity, read/write speed, access time, and forward/backward compatibility. CD-R was selected because it best met the stringent requirements (Table 2). With current CD-R systems, lossless compression of the digital image data will be required because of the relatively limited streaming rates and capacity. This, however, is not thought to be a significant concern for image integrity for interchange media.

Archival media

An equally important part of the process of replacement of cineangiographic film involves the archival system. Several issues are involved (Table 3). An initial potential goal of the ACC/ACR/NEMA deliberations was to identify a physical format that could be used not only for transport but also for archival purposes. This goal was not achieved; whether it will be readdressed in the future is not clear. The ACC/ESC/ACR/NEMA committee did not attempt to define the digital archive media for cardiology because of the lack of "a perfect technology" to replace cineangiographic film and serve as both the interchange and the archive

Table 2. Description of CD-R.

Media size (inches)	4.75 x 1/4 inches
Maximal capacity	650 Mbytes
Data transfer rate	Write 2.4 Mbit/sec, read 4.8 Mbit/sec*
Media life	> 30 years
Equipment interface	SCSI
Media standard	ISO 9660 and orange book
Access time	< 0.7 seconds
Compression	2:1 lossless
Source	Multiple vendors

* Forecasted to read/write at 7.5 Mbit/sec

Table 3. Issues affecting catheterization laboratory archival design.

Number of procedure rooms

Single or multiple vendors

Number of cases
    Requirement for on-line, near-line, and off-line access

Interconnections
    Central tape library
    Number of work and review stations
    Location of work and review stations
        In laboratory
        In hospital (CCU, ER, cardiovascular surgery)
        Remote (satellite facilities)
        Cineangiographic film digitization

Relationship between hospital information system, radiology information system, cardiology database
    Echocardiography
    Computed tomography
    Magnetic resonance imaging

Abbreviations: CCU = coronary care unit; ER = emergency room

standard. The most important considerations were logical format and then the physical format for transport media. Accordingly, each laboratory or vendor will need to develop its own archival system. This will not have an impact on the ability of any laboratory to export images on the CD-R format, but it may have an impact on laboratories with more than one vendor system. In the latter case, transfer and analysis of archival data (digital) between the different x-ray systems may be difficult or even impossible.

Requirements for the archival system

Requirements for the archival system are as stringent as those for the transport system. If anything, the speed requirements and the need for compressionless capacity are more important. Similar requirement considerations must be kept in mind for transfer rates, capacity, and cost. Modern cardiac systems use a matrix of 512 x 512 pixels with 8 bits/pixel providing 2^8 (256) gray levels. One 512 x 512 x 8 bit image consists of 256,000 bytes. At conventional speeds of 30 frames/sec, coronary angiography requires a transfer rate of > 7.5 Mbytes/sec. Matrix sizes of 1,024 x 1,024 will demand transfer rates that are four times faster than 512 x 512 systems. The data storage requirements per case depend on the typical number of frames per study. An assessment of 960 cases by the ACC/ACR/NEMA determined that an average cineangiogram contains 2,400 frames. A safety factor of two has been used for selection of interchange media requirements. Similarly, a capacity requirement of 4,800 frames is reasonable for the archival unit record.

The absence of an industry media standard for archival systems will foster the development of multiple vendor-driven approaches (Table 4). Over time, one or another may dominate as the advantages and disadvantages of each become better understood. At some time, a similar archival media standard may become possible which will greatly simplify data handling in laboratories with procedure rooms from multiple vendors. The lack of standardization of the media for archival systems, however, does not preclude adoption of the DICOM logical format. Adoption of the DICOM logical format for archiving provides the necessary header and image data formatting to enable the communication of images across any media or network infrastructure and allows the archival storage media to be compatible with the interchange media.

Table 4. Potential digital archival systems.

D-2 video tape

CD-R

Magneto-optical disk

Exabyte 8 mm

Metrum RSP 2150

Martin Marietta compact tape archive (Digital D-3)

IBM new technology (3590)

Sony Digital Tape Format (DTF)

DEC Digital Linear Tape (DLT)

Each laboratory may well have different and unique requirements (Table 3). These specific considerations may have an impact on the system selected. Optimal systems should be modular and upgradable. These features will allow for growth in the system and for continuous upgrades as new technology becomes available. The typical "lifetime" of a new x-ray system is approximately 5 years; thus, new equipment will be required frequently.

There are several different potential archival media (Table 4). Some of these are currently in use, such as Super VHS tape, but this approach has limited resolution and should not be used. Digital videotape (D-2) also has been studied, but its disadvantages are that it does not use the DICOM standard and it is not computer digital. Two other media, CD-R and magneto-optical disk, are slow for archiving and will require lossy compression. A goal for any archival system should be lossless compression to preserve all the data. Whether lossy compression would result in clinically important degradation of data is not clear. Archival systems that require lossy compression do so because of inherent media limitations, not because of inherent advantages to lossy compression.

Lossless data compression is a standard of every x-ray cardiac digital system available today. Lossless data compression allows the original digital images to be reproduced exactly as acquired in the laboratory (bit for bit). It ensures that image data will not be lost or altered--an essential component to accurate diagnosis. Lossy data compression can greatly improve the performance and reduce the cost of systems but at a potential sacrifice to image quality. Although lossy data compression is used successfully in the multimedia industry, scientific investigation has shown it can cause artifacts or defects in the image data when used in conjunction with edge enhancement and upscan of 1,024 display, both of which are standard features on today's x-ray cardiac digital systems.

Cost and storage are also issues related to CD-R because each CD-R will be used as a single unit record. Data for multiple patients will not be put on a single CD-R.

Potential newer alternatives have strikingly improved performance (Table 5), and several manufacturers are involved in their development. At the high end, transfer rates from 9 to 12 Mbytes/sec are available, whereas the rate is 0.9 Mbytes/sec for CD-R. Media capacity ranges from 10 to 55 Gbytes and the capacity of CD-R is 650 Mbytes. Perhaps the most striking difference is in the library available with the new types, in which capacity is up to 576 Terabytes (TB) (in excess of 40,000 patients).

The digital image sensor in the catheterization laboratory digitizes x-ray video, stores the images, and transfers the images and also processes and displays them on the control and review console. The review console provides the cardiologist with a platform capable of performing image review as well as off-line cardiac quantitative analysis while the patient is still in the catheterization laboratory. This function has become increasingly important as emphasis grows on matching the specific coronary lesion with the specific size of the device to be used for interventional cardiology procedures. Patient angiographic sequences can be transferred instantaneously from the acquisition module to the review station, a feature allowing peak performance. As an option, the review station can also interface to an archival device so that images and patient records can be exported to the central archival library (Figure 1). This archival capability can be provided

Table 5. Advanced archival systems.

	System			
	Digital D-3	IBM 3590	Sony DTF*	DEC DLT*
Drive type	D3 Helical	Linear Serpentine	Digi Beta Helical	Linear Serpentine
Transfer rate, Mbytes/sec	10.8	9	12	1.25
Media capacity, Gbytes	55	10	42	10
Library, Terabytes	3.8-26	2-576	30	2.6

*DLT = Digital Linear Tape; DTF = Digital Tape Format

on an open-architecture network with fiberoptic cable so that a channel network switching device can provide connectivity of the digital images to a central archival library.

These new media will be accommodated in a central automatic tape library (Figure 2). This will be an essential component of the archival system when media loading and unloading are accomplished automatically. Such a library will need to be modular so that depending upon the specific configuration, smaller or larger modules can be used. If the capacity of the central archive library is exceeded, the entire library can be downloaded and taken to off-line storage. If a tape that has been taken to off-line storage is needed, it can be retrieved and brought back, just as old cineangiographic films are transported today and replayed into the archive if the patient is referred back into the system; thus, there is access to previous image data and to image data being acquired in the catheterization laboratory.

Components of network system

The channel network switching device is a device that connects all the various modules, the catheterization laboratory, the remote viewing stations, and the quantitative analysis workstations with fiberoptics to wide-band data gateways (Figure 1). The gateway allows for the communication of digital images from other networks and other satellite communication systems and land line terrestial networks provided they conform to the DICOM format. This also allows other remote laboratories to transmit on-line data during procedures to facilitate optimal triage and management.

A medical database manager provides for the management of both the network switching and the central archival facility (Figure 1). From a single terminal, one can access a specific patient's image data, whether stored on the archival device or the redundant array of inexpensive disks (RAID) short-term storage, to provide

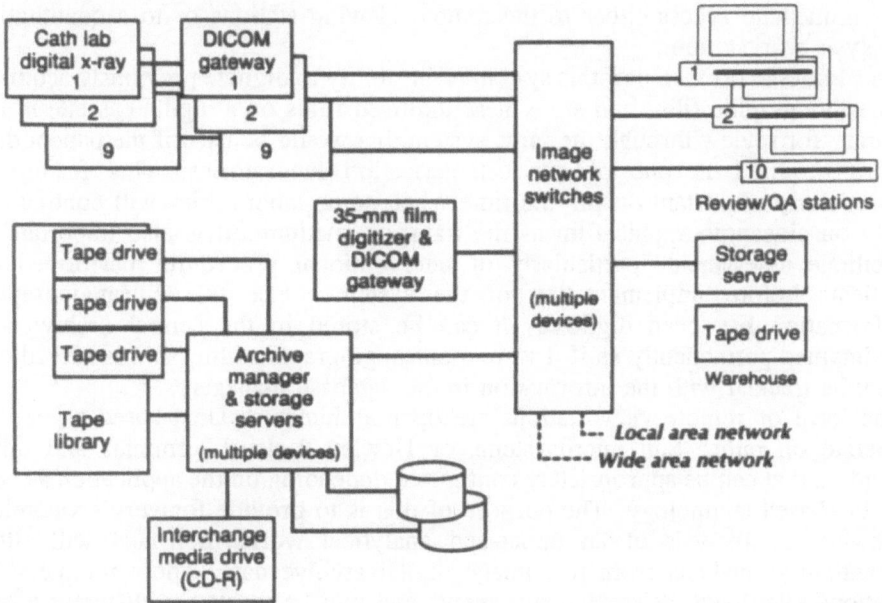

Figure 1. A digital image acquisition network for archiving and reviewing cardiac images.

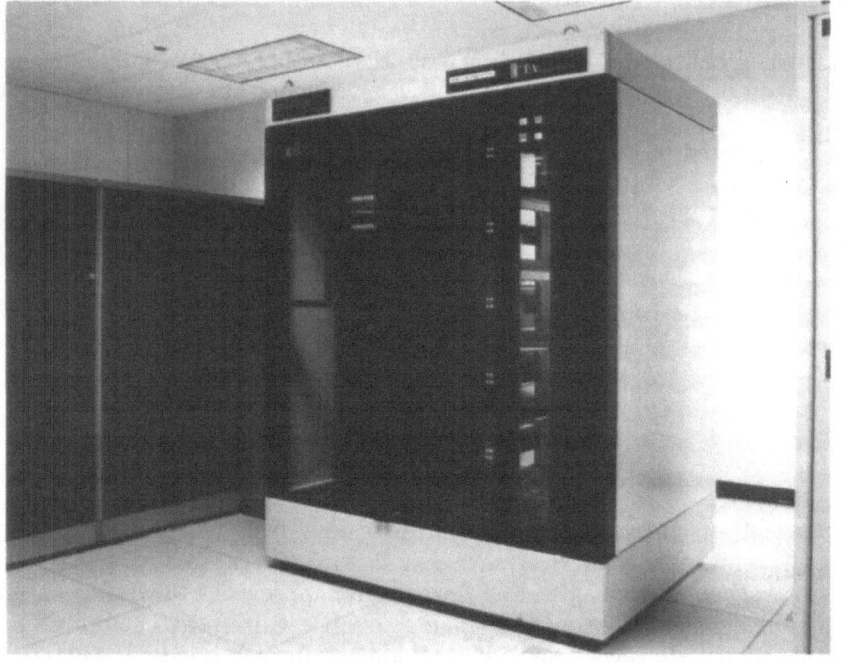

Figure 2. Automatic tape library capable of storing 2.6 to 576 Terabytes of data, depending on specific configuration chosen.

for immediate access either to the remote viewing stations or to a quantitative analysis workstation.

An additional provision of this system is the ability to digitize previously acquired cineangiographic films and store these digitized films on a digital cassette in the library for review through the same system that would be used if the patient data were acquired in one of our catheterization laboratories. This feature is particularly important during the time when some laboratories will continue to rely on cineangiographic film as the transport medium. It is also important to facilitate assessment, particularly of interventional procedures performed on patients before implementation of the system. Once this cineangiographic information has been digitized, it can be stored in the central archive and maintained permanently as if it were a cineangiographic film, so this record can now be tracked with the information in the database manager.

The local or remote view stations are open-architecture Unix-based types that operate on either Sun microsystems or Hewlett-Packard terminals and other vendors that can be appropriately configured depending on the application as well as PC-based technology. The purpose of this is to provide for very economical viewing or analysis of an upper-end analytical workstation that will allow quantitative analysis from this image digital archive data. These remote view stations may have different requirements and will be located in different areas, for example, cardiac surgery or coronary care units to allow for better, more efficient management of patients.

Economics of replacement of cineangiographic film

An important consideration of archival systems is cost. One of the rationales for replacement of cineangiographic film was reduction in cost as a result of elimination of cineangiographic processors, development, and storage. The cost has been assessed in the configuration of our film replacement (Table 6). Cost reduction will be substantial. Cineangiographic film in our institution currently costs $107.82 per patient. With the digital archival system, this cost will dramatically decrease to $19.32 per patient. The automatic tape library adds additional cost, but even with the library, which will decrease storage and the need for personnel for record keeping, the cost reduction per year will be $229,840. Harder to quantitate but just as important is the potential for clinical cost reduction by expediting decision making and patient care.

Conclusions

Replacement of cineangiographic film has now been widely accepted as a practical, achievable goal over the next 2 to 3 years. Industry, users, and regulatory agencies have agreed on formats and approaches for transport media. Archival media and architecture continue to evolve. Currently, no archival media standard exists. However, the DICOM logical format standard will facilitate interchange between vendors and networks. Any system must allow for upward growth and economics of scale and must foster the ability for networking multiple

Table 6. Mayo Clinic Cardiac Imaging Center: cost analysis of digital cineangiographic film replacement.

	Cineangiographic		Digital	
	Per patient	Yearly	Per patient	Yearly
Total system cost				
Cost without library	$107.82	$733,200	$19.32	$131,400
Cost with library	$107.82	$733,200	$61.08	$503,360
Total savings				
Savings without library	$0.00	$0.00	$88.50	$601,800
Savings with library			$46.74	$229,840

interfaces. The current system fulfills these requirements and should play an important role in various catheterization environments.

References

1. Holmes DR Jr, Wondrow MA, Gray JE. Isn't it time to abandon cine film? Cathet Cardiovasc Diagn 1990;20:1-4.
2. Cardiac angiography without cine film: erecting a "Tower of Babel" in the cardiac catheterization laboratory. American College of Cardiology Cardiac Catheterization Committee. J Am Coll Cardiol 1994;24:834-7.
3. Digital Imaging and Communications in Medicine (DICOM) Version 3.0 Standard. Washington, DC: National Electrical Manufacturers Assocation, 1994.

20. What are the advantages and limitations of three-dimensional intracoronary ultrasound imaging?

ERIC MAURINCOMME & GÉRARD FINET

Summary

Intracoronary ultrasound imaging is able to provide real-time high resolution images of sections of the arterial wall. It is particularly interesting for analyzing, both qualitatively and quantitatively, features of vascular pathology that are inaccessible to other modalities. However, this analysis is still based on two-dimensional images, whereas the structure and the extent of atherosclerotic lesions are three-dimensional.

In fact, three-dimensional reconstructions of arteries through stacking up a series of images have appeared shortly after the introduction of intravascular ultrasonography. Thanks to the sophistication of acquisition procedures and the speed improvement in image reconstruction and display, three-dimensional images are more and more readily available, during the intervention. Nevertheless, the real question is to know whether three-dimensional intracoronary ultrasound has anything new to contribute in comparison with standard in-vivo real-time two-dimensional images.

Because of limitations in the knowledge of the acquisition geometry, the three-dimensional reconstructed image may not correspond to the reality. Moreover, 3D display only offers a more pleasant way to look at images, but all three-dimensional information actually comes from the original two-dimensional images. This three-dimensional rendering is still, and information that can be inferred from the sequence of moving images, such as the detection and understanding of image artifacts, may be lost. This paper analyzes all limitations of current three-dimensional reconstruction techniques for intravascular ultrasound, proposes different ways to solve them, and concludes on the clinical interest of three-dimensional intracoronary ultrasound reconstructions.

Introduction

Three-dimensional intravascular ultrasound (IVUS) imaging is a natural extension to standard intravascular ultrasonography. Its purpose is to display three-dimensional images, or volumes, reconstructed from a stack of 2D cross-sectional images, in the same way as what can be seen in other modalities (computed tomography or magnetic resonance imaging).

Although all 3D information is already present in the original images (only smoothing occurs, through interpolation between slices), a three-dimensional reconstructed image brings longitudinal information that may have passed undetected.

The medical usefulness of 3D intravascular or intracoronary ultrasound (ICUS) has been confirmed recently [1-5]. However, there are still many limitations

J.H.C. Reiber and E.E. van der Wall (eds.), Cardiovascular Imaging, 243-255.
© 1996 *Kluwer Academic Publishers.*

associated with 3D ICUS. The aim of this chapter is to first review briefly the main 3D reconstruction techniques, then to detail all limitations and to discuss possible solutions, and finally to conclude on what really the 3D ICUS added value could be.

When dealing with ICUS images, one should always try to solve the two fundamental questions:

- what do we see ?
- where are we ?

Answers to the first question have been brought in almost all cases, after a systematic analysis of the physics of image formation [6-9]. The second question is the most limiting factor to ICUS; unfortunately, no suitable answer has been found yet.

3D reconstruction techniques

The 3D extension to intravascular ultrasound imaging is so natural that the first three-dimensional images appeared very shortly after the introduction of intravascular ultrasound imaging. First, peripheral arteries were concerned [10-14], and then all arteries could be reconstructed [1,2,5,15]. Three-dimensional intracoronary ultrasound currently consists of two parts: (i) acquisition and (ii) display. The 3D reconstruction process itself being very primitive, it is considered as part of image acquisition.

Image acquisition and reconstruction

Just like with CT or MR images, a series of cross-sections is necessary to start with. In order to acquire a correctly sampled set of images, a number of pullback techniques have been developed. The principle is either to continuously pull the catheter from its distal position back to a more proximal one [1,13,15], or to sense the displacement of the catheter being maneuvered manually [16]. Generally, a slow pullback speed of .5 mm/sec permits the acquisition of slices corresponding to the same instant of the cardiac cycle every half-millimeter. The acquisition is or is not synchronized to the ECG, and a number of images are recorded. In most cases, images are not available in digital format, but only in video format. Therefore, an additional step is to digitize the video output through a frame grabber.

Digital images are then stacked one above the other. Essentially, it is the same process as what is being done in CT or MR imaging. The three-dimensional reconstructed vessel thus contains all structures present in the cross-sections, but the reality is distorted [17].

The main assumptions are that the explored vessel is straight, and that the cross-sections are parallel. These assumptions are very fragile, and a few methods try to improve the stacking-up. The theoretical spatial orientation of each slice can be taken into account:

- either by detecting the curvilinearity of the vessel from an x-ray image [15],
- or by first reconstructing the arterial tree in three dimensions from two x-ray projections of the vessel [18,19].

Another recent 3D reconstruction method uses more exotic forward-viewing catheters [20,21], but will not be further described.

Display and segmentation

The computer that displays this stack of slices, is a substitute to the physician's brain, which unconsciously performs 3D reconstruction from a series of images. The display mode should then pinpoint details that have not been seen in the original cross-sections, such as longitudinal or oblique information. As for any other three-dimensional image, two different display modes can be used:
- volume rendering, where the vessel is usually cut along its longitudinal axis,
- surface rendering, that requires the segmentation of the image.
Volume rendering is clearly more interesting, but it may lead to uninterpretable volumes. It is indeed sometimes difficult to distinguish blood from intima, let alone other arterial structures. The loss of dynamic information, such as blood flow, appears as an intrinsic limitation of any 3D rendering. To enhance the lumen contour, several protocols have been designed, either by flushing the imaged vessel with a saline solution or with iodine, or by injecting echogenic contrast agents [22]. These flushing techniques add complexity to the image acquisition protocol. And simple image processing can help to *clean up* the image, by averaging a number of acquired images for example [23].
Quantifying features of interest is a promising goal of 3D intracoronary ultrasound imaging. Manual tracing is possible [24], but because of the large number of images being processed, automatic quantification is preferable. This involves segmentation, either with simple thresholds (bound to poor results), or with more complex algorithms [25,26]. Taking into account three-dimensional information should allow a better segmentation [27,28], hence a better quantification.

Limitations

Limitations of 3D reconstruction techniques follow the two fundamental questions asked earlier. They include respectively:
- segmentation, *(What do we see ?)*,
- the knowledge of the geometry of acquisition with respect to the vessel central axis *(Where are we ?)*.
In fact, the most limiting factor for a correct 3D reconstruction is the geometry of acquisition. With pullback techniques, the catheter movement is sensed at its proximal site, but it is the distal tip that produces the images. While the catheter is being pulled back, the questions to answer about its position are:
- is the catheter axis centered and parallel to the longitudinal axis of the vessel?
- is the catheter axis eccentric and parallel to the longitudinal axis of the vessel?
- is the catheter axis centered but angulated with respect to the longitudinal axis of the vessel ?
- is the catheter axis eccentric and angulated with respect to the longitudinal axis of the vessel ?
An answer to these questions is necessary for understanding possible artifacts in

the image. Furthermore, the ultimate question to answer for 3D reconstruction is:
- which three-dimensional movement of the catheter tip did occur between this cross-sectional image and the previous one ?

Most studies make assumptions on the geometry of acquisition, generally without being certain it is correct. In this section, the complex possible movements of the catheter tip are artificially separated for the sake of simplicity. But the geometry of acquisition is not the cause of all limitations. Other possible limitations include the artery itself, whose shape may be dependent on the cardiac cycle, and the interpretation of the image, which may lead to non-coherent segmentations.

Synchronization of image acquisition

Image acquisition is or is not synchronized to the ECG signal. Two limiting factors may intervene in the case where there is no synchronization.

Arterial deformation
During the four phases of the cardiac cycle, the artery is deformed due to the pressure variation. Although coronary, i.e. muscular, arteries are more rigid than elastic arteries because of the absence of elastic fibers in their media, they are subject to some distension. The *distensibility* of an artery, which is defined as the percent change in lumen cross-sectional area during a cardiac cycle, can be measured with intravascular ultrasound imaging [29,30]. It has been shown to be around 14% ($\pm$5%) for normal coronary arteries and as low as 4% ($\pm$2%) for pathological segments. It does therefore play a non-negligible role when measurements are to be made, especially on normal cross-sections.
The solution for accurate three-dimensional reconstruction and analysis is then to synchronize the image acquisition to the ECG signal. If the ECG is not taken into account, the three-dimensional reconstruction is likely to look like a pipe of fluctuating diameter.

Cardiac movement
Movements of the heart may also change the position of the catheter tip within the arterial cross-section. For some sinuous coronary arteries, such as the left anterior descending artery, the tip of the catheter may also move longitudinally during the cardiac cycle. Consequently, another reason for synchronizing the image acquisition on the ECG is that the catheter is more likely to be at the same position within each slice for similar instants of the cardiac cycle.

Catheter movement within one slice

During the acquisition of a series of images using the pullback technique, the catheter undergoes two basic movements, **translation** and **rotation**, as is being illustrated in Figure 1. Indeed, as it is being pulled back, the catheter can move in the radial direction within the vessel and it can rotate. The only stable reference between two subsequent images is in fact the catheter itself.

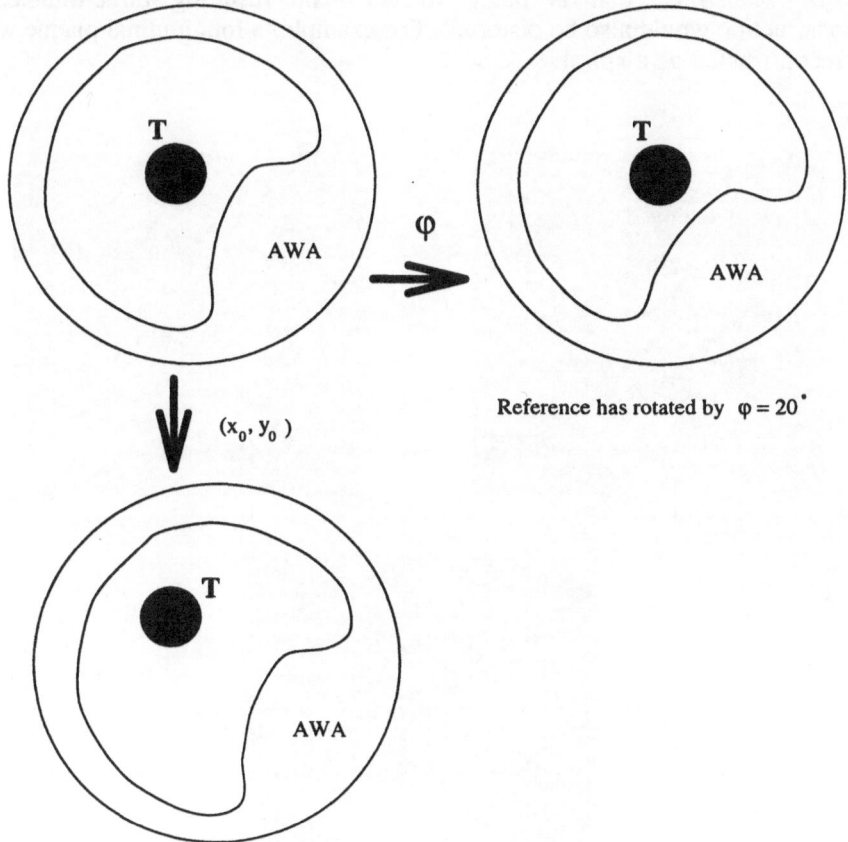

Reference has rotated by $\varphi = 20°$

(x_0, y_0)

Transducer has been translated by (x_0, y_0)

Figure 1. Rotation and translation of the transducer **T**. The Arterial Wall Area (AWA), defined as the area delimited by the lumen contour and the media-adventitia border, exhibits a small plaque between 3 and 6 o'clock. The first frame, on the upper left may yield a combination of two basic movements: rotation, as is seen on the right, where the reference of the image has rotated by $\varphi = 20°$; and translation, as is shown below, where the catheter has translated by (x_0, y_0). Both images would look different, although they represent the same arterial cross-section.

An example with in-vivo images of a coronary artery is shown in Figure 2. Translation of the catheter is easily detected, as the whole artery moves within the image. Rotation is noticeable thanks to the guidewire shadow.

As a result of catheter translation, the reconstructed three-dimensional image looks like a nice cylinder in its center, corresponding to the catheter, and a winding vessel around it, as may be seen in most studies. However, it clearly should be the other way around. These movements are currently not taken into account, and the stacked slices therefore do not depict the exact reality.

The rotation is less discernible than the translation, since it is the reference, say the 0° scan line, that is being rotated. The resulting three-dimensional reconstruction would also be distorted. For example, a longitudinal plaque would be reconstructed as a spiral.

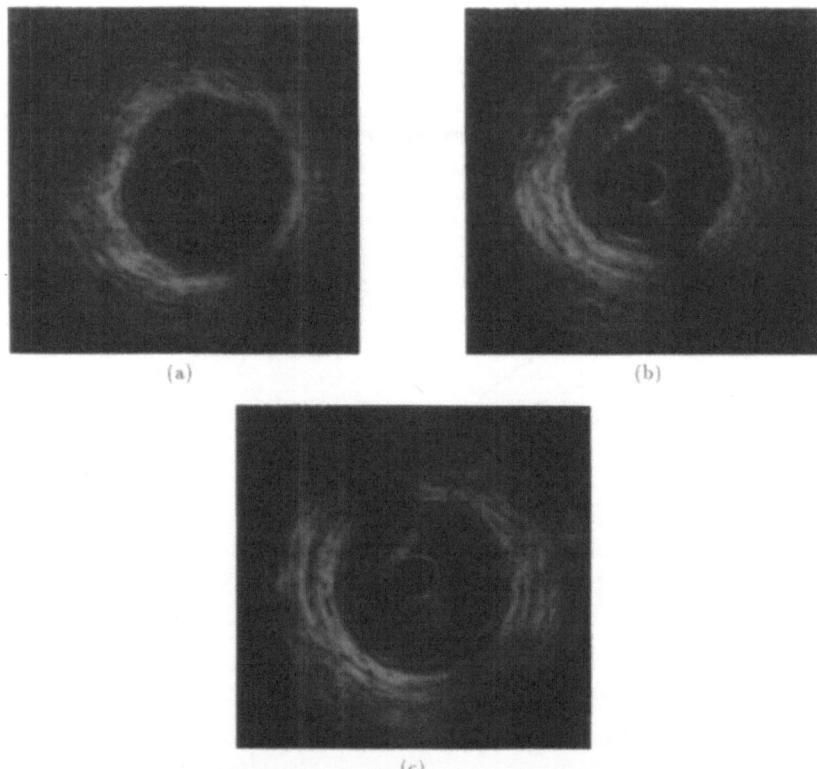

Figure 2. Slices from a pullback acquisition in a coronary artery. (A) First image: the guidewire shadow may be seen at 5 o'clock. (B) Second image: the catheter has rotated (guidewire closer to 6 o'clock) and has been translated (artery is now centered further up-and-left in the image). (C) Third image: the catheter has translated again (against the plaque at 11 o'clock) and has slightly rotated (guidewire closer to 5 o'clock again).

Acquisition planes are not parallel

No artery is perfectly straight. However, they are generally considered as straight tubes. In fact, this assumption is similar to considering all imaging planes being parallel. The effect is depicted in Figure 3. The 3D reconstruction would suffer from the similar problems exposed previously, related to the catheter tip movement, of a straight catheter and a winding vessel around it.

Therefore, these two limitations combined together are likely to aggravate the distortions between the histological reality and its three-dimensional rendering.

The way to correct this irregular acquisition of images would be to have *a priori* information about the shape of the vessel, from its x-ray lumenogram for example [15,18]. But the three-dimensional position of the catheter and the orientation of its imaging plane would still be unknown.

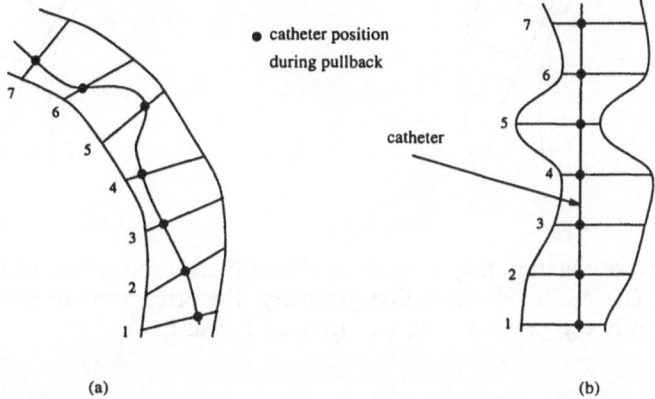

Figure 3. Imaging planes are not parallel. (A) Seven images are acquired. (B) Reconstructed geometry: all slices are considered parallel. Both morphology and lumen dimensions may be wrong. The vessel is rendered tortuous around image 5, which does not correspond to any histological curvilinearity.

Slice orientation

Even if the vessel curvature is known, and if the imaging planes are not considered parallel, another limitation is the orientation of the imaging plane with respect to the vessel longitudinal axis. It is always assumed that the imaging plane is perfectly perpendicular to the vessel long axis.

For example, the acquisition symbolized in Figure 4A is assumed to be like in Figure 4B. In this figure, the reconstructed three-dimensional size of the lumen and of the artery would vary between slices 1, 2, and 3, which is incorrect. In fact, the catheter orientation can only be given by an outside imaging source, such as x-ray fluoroscopy for example. Before stacking up slices, the 3D coordinates of every imaging plane should be transmitted to the 3D reconstruction process, that would then interpolate according to this three-dimensional information. Getting this spatial 3D information is also a prerequisite for any study on the progression or regression of atherosclerosis. If an intravascular ultrasound exam is being conducted every 6 months, the interventional cardiologist must know precisely which area had been imaged previously.

Segmentation

Both quantification and surface rendering require segmentation of the image. The first common pitfall is to segment features that clinically and ultrasonically do not make sense. It can be avoided by keeping in mind the physics of image formation

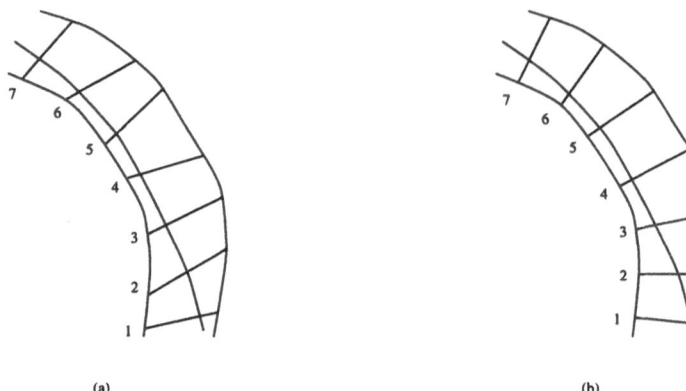

Figure 4. Slice orientation may vary along the pullback acquisition. (A) Seven slices are acquired. (B) Assumed acquisition geometry: the orientation of each slice is not the real one; it is especially wrong for slices 1, 2, and 6.

and the basics of echography [31]. For example, only measurements from one leading edge to another leading edge can be performed [9]. A leading edge is defined as the inner border of an edge. Electronically, it corresponds to the beginning of the pulsed echo. Trailing edges should never be delineated, since the point spread function (PSF) of the system is convolved with the pulsed echo. The position of this trailing edge is therefore dependent upon the characteristics of the PSF. When measuring layer thicknesses, it is the radial component of the PSF which is convolved. Therefore, any layer of thickness of the order of the wavelength (either 75 or 50 μm for 20 and 30 MHz transducers, respectively) is rendered as thick as the radial resolution, which is three to four times larger. This thickening of any distinct interface is sometimes called ''blooming effect'', but is rarely well interpreted.

Because of this artifact, the intima is presented by overestimated thicknesses; and consequently, the media is rendered with a lower thickness than corresponding histopathologic data. For this reason, measuring the thickness of the intima or the media alone is not correct acoustically.

For a three-layer coronary artery, the only contours that can be drawn are:
- the lumen contour, located at the leading edge of the blood-intima interface,
- the leading edge of the media-adventitia border.

Therefore, the only quantifiable entities, shown in Figure 5, are:
- the lumen area, delineated by the leading edge of the lumen contour,
- the arterial wall area, which represents the cross-sectional area of the plaque plus the intima plus the media, and which is defined as the area between the two leading edges of the intra-luminal and the media-adventitia borders.

An automatic segmentation scheme of the lumen contour, based on active contour models, and called ADDER, has been evaluated recently on a database of in-vitro images, and compared to manual contours drawn by cardiologists [32]. For the second contour (media-adventitia border), an automatic method seems more difficult. Because of imaging artifacts, this contour may not be present in the image. Therefore, a semi-automatic approach is probably more efficient, with a proposed initial solution that could be a circle.

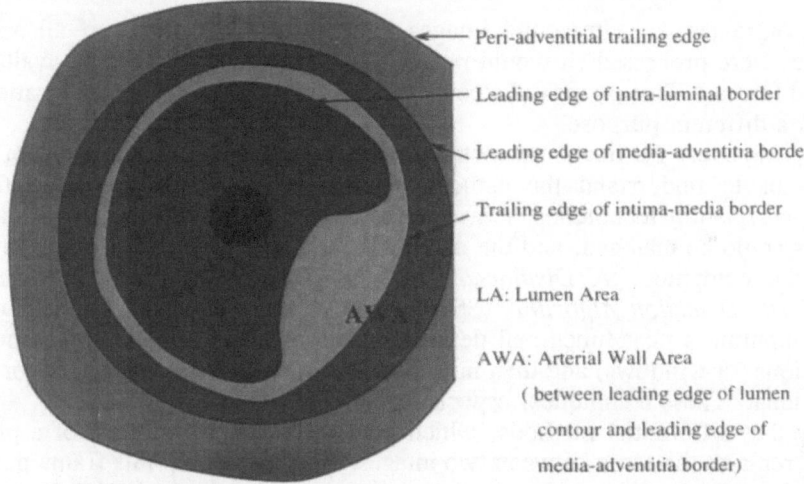

Figure 5. Relevant quantities for intracoronary ultrasound. The only quantifiable features are the *lumen area* (LA) delineated by the leading edge of the lumen contour and the *arterial wall area* (AWA) corresponding to the plaque + intima + media, and located between the two leading edges of the lumen contour and the media-adventitia contour.

Other possible limitations

For mechanically rotated transducers (or mirrors), expansion or compression of one part of the image may occur, due to the non-uniform rotation speed of the catheter. However, this artifact is well-known and easily recognizable. It happens for example when trying to pass a tight stenosis. But this artifact is less likely to be present when performing a pullback acquisition, since the catheter and its guidewire have already passed the entire explored site to be reconstructed.

Possible solutions

In the list of all exposed limitations, some could be solved and others require much more effort. Some solutions, such as ECG gating, are already present in some 3D reconstruction systems, and are essential. The most limiting problem for 3D intracoronary ultrasound is clearly the poor knowledge of the geometry of acquisition. Some solutions can be found, and they are divided into two categories:
- extracting more information about the geometry of acquisition from the intracoronary ultrasound images themselves,

- obtaining information on the geometry of acquisition through external sources, i.e., other imaging modalities.

Intravascular ultrasound images can say more !

First, intravascular ultrasound images could indeed say more, if all acquired images were processed (it would naturally be easier if they were all available in digital format). This seems to be contradictory with the ECG synchronization, but it has a different purpose.

Analyzing every 2D image reconstructed from the rotated ultrasound beam would allow us to understand the catheter movement. Through the application of cross-correlation techniques between two or more subsequent images, arterial layers could be matched, and the displacement and rotation of the catheter could then be computed. A *Displaced Frame Difference* (DFD) or a *Sequential Similarity Detection Algorithm* (SSDA) may be applied. These methods consist in computing a cost functional defined by the distance between two luminance functions (or windows) and then in finding a minimum for this distance (or error) functional. These techniques, especially the DFD, are time consuming, and it is likely that differential methods, which assume that the brightness of a physical point remains the same between two images, would speed up this frame matching procedure. In that case, the displacement would be determined iteratively by minimizing the distance between the image at time t and the image at time $(t-1)$ corrected by an estimated movement. Indeed, when this distance is null, the displacement has been estimated correctly. Furthermore, more sophisticated approaches, such as gain-compensated DFD may also be used, as they take into account a variation in brightness of the structures due to displacement. It would be the case for example, when the catheter goes from a normal segment to a calcific plaque.

These methods have been used in many applications for coding displacements between two images, and are closely related to the computation of optical flow. The correction for rotation is however a risky procedure. It may actually correct for plaques that indeed follow a spiral path along the wall, thus creating another artifact. Image segmentation could also improve the efficacy of these matching algorithms. Once again, either segmenting each frame or using information coming from every frame in order to segment one image (better distinction between blood, intima and plaque) would improve the overall segmentation and the catheter displacement tracking. Both tasks are deeply linked to one another.

Finally, another possibility in coupling one image to the next may arise from the design of catheters, such as the revolutionary micro-motor developed by Lancée et al. [33] at the Thoraxcenter in Rotterdam. Indeed, the two electrical wires connected to the transducer, located at the tip of the catheter are in the field of view. They lie next to the circle representing the transducer and may easily be detected. Thus, they may prove essential in keeping track of the sliding rotation of the catheter within an artery. Nevertheless, these frame-to-frame methods still rely on the assumption that the imaging plane is about orthogonal to the vessel long axis.

Extra information from x-ray imaging

Another source of information is external. The three-dimensional catheter orientation can indeed be computed from two x-ray projections, coming from a biplane system for example [34]. One could also estimate the trajectory of the catheter only from one x-ray projection, by using the dynamic information, but the precision is then questionable.

Present techniques that reconstruct the 3D coronary tree from two x-ray images need to be coupled to the intracoronary ultrasound images. Some authors use bifurcations as landmarks for estimating the amount of rotation of the catheter between two bifurcations [18].

Conclusions

The 3D aspect of intracoronary ultrasound imaging is still being limited by many difficult-to-solve problems. The question to answer is whether three-dimensional intracoronary ultrasound imaging brings relevant and useful information for clinical practice or clinical research, keeping in mind that all 3D information is already present in the acquired 2D images. In fact, 3D ICUS offers a fixed three-dimensional visualisation of the longitudinal aspect of the artery and its atherosclerotic lesion; therefore, a qualitative insight of the plaque is brought to light, along with a quantitative measure (length). Longitudinal details, such as plaque rupture or dissection, directly benefit from this three-dimensional display. On one hand, 3D ICUS could theoretically help our understanding of therapeutic remodelling of the plaque. But in order to be robust and trustworthy, three-dimensional reconstruction must solve many complex limitations. On the other hand, the information present in the 2D images, combined with the knowledge of the catheter displacement, i.e., live temporal images, already permit to work correctly and without limitation.

References

1. Rosenfield K, Losordo DW, Ramaswamy K *et al*. Three-dimensional reconstruction of human coronary and peripheral arteries from images recorded during two-dimensional intravascular ultrasound examination. Circulation 1991;84:1938-56.
2. Rosenfield K, Kaufman J, Pieczek AM *et al*. Human coronary and peripheral arteries. On-line three-dimensional reconstruction from two-dimensional intravascular US scans. Work in progress. Radiology 1992;184:823-32.
3. Coy KM, Park JC, Fishbein MC *et al*. In vitro validation of three-dimensional intravascular ultrasound for the evaluation of arterial injury after balloon angioplasty. J Am Coll Cardiol 1992;20:692-700.
4. Mintz GS, Pichard AD, Satler LF, Popma JJ, Kent KM, Leon MB. Three-dimensional intravascular ultrasonography: reconstructions of endovascular stents in vitro and in vivo. J Clin Ultrasound 1993;21:609-15.
5. Roelandt JRTC, DiMario C, Pandian NG *et al*. Three-dimensional reconstruction of intracoronary ultrasound images. Rationale, approaches,

problems, and directions. Circulation 1994;90:1044-55.

6. Finet G, Maurincomme E, Tabib A et al. Artifacts in intravascular ultrasound imaging: analyses and implications. Ultrasound Med Biol 1993;19:533-47.

7. Lockwood GR, Ryan LK, Gotlieb AI et al. In vitro high resolution intravascular imaging in muscular and elastic arteries. J Am Coll Cardiol 1992;20:153-60.

8. Siegel RJ, Chae JS, Maurer G, Berlin M, Fishbein MC. Histopathologic correlation of the three-layered intravascular ultrasound appearance of normal adult human muscular arteries. Am Heart J 1993;126:872-8.

9. Finet G, Maurincomme E, Douek P, Tabib A, Amiel M, Beaune J. Three-layer appearance of the arterial wall in intravascular ultrasound imaging: artifact or reality ? Implications for accurate measurements in quantitative intravascular ultrasound. Echocardiography 1994;11:343-63.

10. Kitney RI, Moura L, Straughan K. 3-D visualization of arterial structures using ultrasound and voxel modelling. Int J Card Imaging 1989;4:135-43.

11. Kitney RI, Burrell CJ, Straughan K, Moura L, Rothman MT. 3-D modelling techniques of arterial structures and blood flow. Int Congress Sev 1990;916:23-32.

12. Siegel RJ, Ariani M, Fishbein MC, Chae JS, Bowers J, Forrester JS. Intravascular imaging: angioscopy, ultrasound and the development of three dimensional ultrasound reconstruction. Int Congres Sev 1990;916:87-94.

13. Maurincomme E, Magnin I, Finet G, Goutte R. Methodology for three-dimensional reconstruction of intravascular ultrasound images. Proc SPIE 1992;1651:26-34.

14. Chandrasekaran K, D'Adamo AJ, Sehgal CM. Three-dimensional reconstruction of intravascular ultrasound images. In: Tobis JM, Yock PG, editors. Intravascular ultrasound imaging. New York: Churchill Livingstone, 1992:141-7.

15. Klein HM, Günther RW, Verlande M et al. 3D-surface reconstruction of intravascular ultrasound images using personal computer hardware and a motorized catheter control. Cardiovasc Intervent Radiol 1992;15:97-101.

16. Van Egmond FC, Li W, Gussenhoven EJ, Lancée CT. Catheter displacement sensing device: a new tool for standardization of examinations and three-dimensional image reconstruction. Thoraxcentre J 1994;6:9-12.

17. Rothman MT. 3-Dimensional reconstruction of intravascular ultrasound data. In: Reiber JHC, Serruys PW, editors. Progress in quantitative coronary arteriography. Dordrecht: Kluwer Academic Publishers, 1994:405-16.

18. Lengyel J, Greenberg DP, Yeung A, Alderman E, Popp R. Three-dimensional reconstruction and volume rendering of intravascular ultrasound slices imaged on a curved arterial path. Lecture Notes Comput Sci 1995;905:399-405.

19. Bloch I, Pellot C, Sureda F, Herment A. 3D reconstruction of blood vessels by multi-modality data fusion using fuzzy and markovian modelling. Lecture Notes Comput Sci 1995;905:392-8.

20. Evans JL, Ng KH, Vonesh MJ et al. Arterial imaging with a new forward-viewing intravascular ultrasound catheter, I. Initial studies. Circulation 1994;89:712-7.

21. Ng KH, Evans JL, Vonesh MJ et al. Arterial imaging with a new forward-viewing intravascular ultrasound catheter, II. Three-dimensional reconstruction and display of data. Circulation 1994;89:718-23.

22. Hausmann D, Sudhir K, Mullen WL et al. Contrast-enhanced intravascular ultrasound: validation of a new technique for delineation of the vessel wall

boundary. J Am Coll Cardiol 1994;23:981-7.

23. Li W, Gussenhoven EJ, Zhong Y *et al*. Temporal averaging for quantification of lumen dimensions in intravascular ultrasound images. Ultrasound Med Biol 1994;20:117-22.

24. Wenguang L, Gussenhoven WJ, Zhong Y *et al*. Validation of quantitative analysis of intravascular ultrasound images. Int J Card Imaging 1991;6:247-53.

25. Maurincomme E, Friboulet D, Finet G, Magnin IE, Reiber JHC. ADDER: a snake-based segmentation approach for intravascular ultrasound images. In: Fung KK, Ginige A, editors. Conference Proceedings DICTA-93: Digital image computing: techniques and applications. Sydney: Australian Pattern Recognition Society, 1993:422-9.

26. Bosch JG, Reiber JHC, van Burken G, Savalle L, Maurincomme E, Helbing WA. Automated contour detection and acoustic quantification. Eur Heart J 1995;16(Suppl.J):35-41.

27. Li W, Bosch JG, Zhong Y *et al*. Image segmentation and 3D reconstruction of intravascular ultrasound images. In: Wei Y, Gu B, editors. Acoustical imaging. New York: Plenum, 1993:489-96.

28. Kluytmans M, Bouma CJ, ter Haar Romeny BM, Pasterkamp G, Viergever MA. Analysis and 3D display of 30 MHz intravascular ultrasound images. Lecture Notes Comput Sci 1995;905:406-12.

29. Reddy KG, Suneja R, Nair RN, Dhawale P, Hodgson JM. Measurement by intracoronary ultrasound of in vivo arterial distensibility within atherosclerotic lesions. Am J Cardiol 1993;72:1232-7.

30. Rasheed Q, Hodgson JM. Application of intracoronary ultrasonography in the study of coronary artery pathophysiology. J Clin Ultrasound 1993;21:569-78.

31. Feigenbaum H. Echocardiography. 4th ed. Philadelphia: Lea & Febiger, fourth ed., 1986.

32. Maurincomme E, Finet G, Reiber JHC, Savalle L, Magnin I. Quantitative intravascular ultrasound imaging: evaluation of an automatic approach [abstract]. J Am Coll Cardiol 1995;(25e Special Issue):354A.

33. Lancée CT, Bom N, van Egmond FC, Honkoop J, Roelandt JRTC. A micromotor system for intraluminal ultrasound scanning. Thoraxcentre J 1993;5:8-12.

34. Sureda F, Bloch I, Pellot C, Herment A. Reconstruction 3D de vaisseaux sanguins par fusion de donn\'ees \'a partir d'images angiographiques et echographiques. Traitement du Signal 1994;11:525-40.

21. New developments in intracoronary ultrasound

CARLO DI MARIO, PETER J. FITZGERALD & ANTONIO COLOMBO

Introduction

In the last five years, intracoronary ultrasound (ICUS) has progressed from a research tool used only in vitro or in straight large peripheral or coronary arteries by a handful of dedicated investigators [1-8] to a routine diagnostic technique of daily application for guidance of coronary interventions. Miniaturization of transducers, improvement in image quality and increased knowledge of the clinical usefulness of the results of the intracoronary examination in various clinical settings were the pivotal factors of this development. Despite this rapid progress, further technical development is certainly needed to facilitate the integration of ICUS into the various interventional procedures as well as the image interpretation and quantitative assessment. Many fields of development should be considered, from improvement in image quality to forward-looking ultrasound to the combination with interventional devices.

In this manuscript, the interest will be focused on three aspects that we consider the "hot spots" of the future technical development, the miniaturization of the transducer to the diameter of a regular angioplasty guidewire, three-dimensional reconstruction of tomographic ICUS images and the characterization of plaque components with backscatter analysis.

Intracoronary imaging wire

Rationale of the use of an imaging wire

Miniaturization of the transducers has been the primary goal of the technical development in intracoronary ultrasound. The diameter of the first prototypes used for intracardiac imaging was 9 French (1973) [9] and only in the late '80ies 5 French catheters were developed, allowing the first intracoronary examinations in proximal straight coronary arteries. In 1993 the first ultrasound catheters smaller than 1 mm in diameter became available, allowing the assessment of severe stenosis before interventions and of small tortuous distal vessels. In 1995, using these catheters a successful ultrasound examination was obtained in our center in 96% of the intracoronary ultrasound procedures performed for guidance of stent implantation (452 vessels examined). Still, the use of a catheter for this examination has clear disadvantages since a separate insertion of the ultrasound catheter is required before and after each treatment with balloons or other interventional devices. Furthermore, the ultrasound guidance is missing when you need it most, for direct on-line monitoring of the effects of treatment on lumen and plaque. A possible alternative is the combination of therapeutic and imaging capabilities on the same catheter. Balloon catheters mounting 64 crystals in a ring

257

J.H.C. Reiber and E.E. van der Wall (eds.), Cardiovascular Imaging, 257-275.
© *1996 Kluwer Academic Publishers.*

proximal to the balloon are available [10] and combined ultrasound-atherectomy catheters are undergoing advanced clinical testing [11]. The use of these catheters, however, assumes that the selection of the type and size of interventional device to be used is already done, based on angiography, thus limiting the usefulness of these devices. Furthermore, the ultrasound image can be obtained only in one location along the catheter, not always coincident with the area of interest. These limitations have prompted the development of very miniaturized ultrasound transducers, with a diameter comparable to the diameter of regular angioplasty guide wires.

Technical description

The imaging wire tested in our center is, basically, a modification of the driving cable used in the mechanical 2.9 French ultrasound catheters of Cvis/Scimed (Micro View). It consists of metallic interwoven wires forming a flexible cable which is attached to a motor unit and rotated at 1,800 rpm. At the distal end of the cable, a 30 MHz piezoelectric crystal is mounted and connected by electrical cables to the central unit (Insight III, ClearView software, Cvis/Scimed, USA). Although the imaging wire has the diameter of a normal guide wire (0.018 in) and is fairly flexible, its mechanical characteristics are still different from the characteristics of an angioplasty guide wire. The absence of a floppy steerable distal end precludes its use as a rail to insert other devices inside the coronary arteries while, on the contrary, its insertion must be performed through a protective sheath which can be, however, any catheter compatible with 0.018 in guide wires.

Preliminary clinical applications at the Columbus Clinic

The imaging wire was tested in 17 lesions in 14 patients, all undergoing stent implantation because of severe coronary artery disease. The arteries treated were the left anterior descending coronary artery (8 lesions, 47%), the left circumflex (3 lesions, 18%) and the right coronary artery (6 lesions, 35%). The lesion location was in the proximal or mid arterial segment in 12 cases (71%) and in the distal artery in 5 cases (29%). Two protocols of stent implantation and ICUS examination examination were used. In the first 9 patients (11 lesions) a Palmaz-Schatz 14 mm stent (Johnson & Johnson, Warren, NJ) was deployed with a 0.018 in wire compatible over-the-wire catheter (K18, Medtronic, USA). After careful removal of the air inside the balloon by repeatedly applying negative pressure, the stent was hand-crimped and positioned at the stenosis site using a regular angioplasty guide wire. The stent was deployed by inflating the balloon at a pressure of 6-8 atm for 30 seconds and the balloon was deflated and left in place. Afterwards, the guide wire was withdrawn and the imaging wire advanced under fluoroscopy up to the mid-segment of the balloon so that the ultrasonic crystal was positioned within the stent during the subsequent balloon expansion. After positioning, the motor unit was activated but no images could be obtained with the balloon deflated because of persistency of air around the crystal. During inflation, the ICUS image appeared at a pressure of 2 to 4 atm. Occasionally, further application of negative pressure or small changes in the position of the transducer were required. Typically, the image showed a homogeneous black circular area within the balloon, with an echo-dense line representing the balloon membrane (Figure 1) [12]. At low pressure, small spaces filled with highly echogenic blood between balloon and vessel wall were observed and interpreted as sluggish flow around the balloon during inflation. The vessel wall was also visible around the balloon, with bright echodense spots representing the stent struts. "Ghost" images of the stent struts and of the balloon membrane were frequently observed. At balloon pressures of 4 atm and 10 atm, measurements of the area within the stent were obtained [13]. Occasionally, images could be obtained at higher pressures, but in most cases entrapment of the imaging wire occurred at pressures higher than 10 atm because of impingment of the wire lumen, resulting in malrotation artifacts and, eventually, wire rupture (3 cases, 21%). After 30 seconds of inflation at 10 atm, the balloon was deflated and imaging was repeated at the minimal balloon pressure at which an interpretable circumferential image was present. Stent lumen cross-sectional areas and major and minor diameter measurements obtained at 4 and 10 atm are reported in Table 1 and compared with the measurements obtained after deflation (residual pressure of 1-2 atm). The imaging wire was then removed and the regular guide wire inserted, allowing withdrawal of the balloon and insertion of a conventional 2.9 F or 3.2 F ICUS catheter. Since the exact position imaged by the wire was not known, the average of 10 cross-sections in the mid portion of the balloon at 1 mm intervals was used for comparison (Table 1).

Complete Balloon Expansion Assessed with a 0.018 in. Imaging Wire

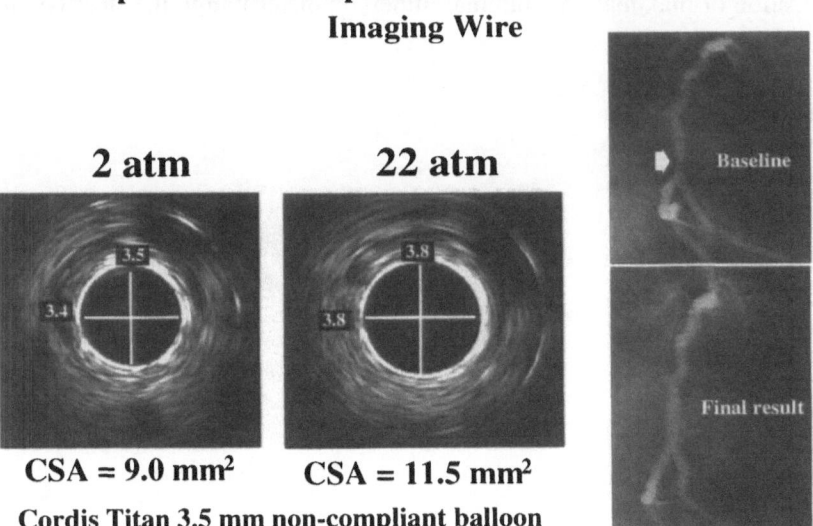

2 atm

22 atm

CSA = 9.0 mm²   CSA = 11.5 mm²

Cordis Titan 3.5 mm non-compliant balloon

Figure 1. Left panels: Cross-sectional images within a Palmaz-Schatz stent during inflation at 2 and 22 atm with a high pressure noncompliant balloon. Right panels: angiograms of the right coronary artery before (upper) and after (lower) stent implantation.

Table 1. Area measurements during balloon inflation within the stent with an imaging wire (n = 8 lesions).

| | IMAGING | WIRE | | 2.9F ICUS |
| | | | After | |
	4 atm	10 atm	deflation	Catheter
Lumen Area mm²	4.4±1.6	6.9±4.0	6.7±2.5	6.4±2.0
Minor Diameter mm	2.3±0.4	2.8±1.1	2.9±0.5	2.8±0.4
Major diameter mm	2.4±0.6	3.1±0.9	2.9±0.5	2.9±0.5

In the last 6 lesions (3 patients), a different type of balloon was used (Titan, Cordis Corporation, Miami, FL), characterized by a very low compliance and high resistance to pressure. In these last cases, the stent was deployed with a second low compliant, 1/2 mm smaller balloon at an average pressure of 14 to 16 atm. In these last cases the imaging wire was advanced after positioning of the Titan balloon within the stent and the measurements were taken at maximal pressure (20-24 atm) and after deflation (at 4 atm). An 18% reduction in stent area from maximal pressure to 4 atm was observed, with a trend to the equalization of maximal and minimal lumen diameter within the stent (Figure 2).

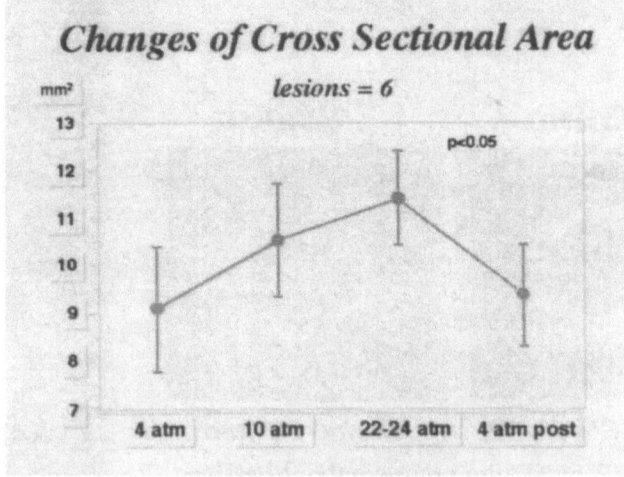

Figure 2. Diagram showing the changes in cross-sectional area within the stent at different balloon pressure in 5 patients assessed with the imaging wire within a Cordis Titan balloon. Note the significant reduction in cross-sectional area after balloon deflation (18% decrease in lumen area in comparison with the area during inflation at 22 atm).

An additional case, shown in Figure 3A, was not included in the analysis summarized in Figure 2, since malrotation artefacts developed at 18 atm, followed by rupture of the rotating cable. The incomplete expansion of the balloon in one of the two positions within the stent assessed with the imaging wire is evident and was confirmed by a subsequent ultrasound examination with a conventional catheter (Figure 3B).

Discussion

These preliminary observations confirm the feasibility of an ICUS examination with a miniaturized imaging wire, compatible with currently available interventional devices. The most important advantage of such a system is that imaging becomes available for guidance during the interventional phase of the procedure, allowing ultrasound directed plaque removal with directional atherectomy and monitoring of the optimal position and expansion of the balloon during balloon angioplasty or stent deployment. Since the first application still requires changes in the design of the atherectomy catheter (0.018 in compatibility, ultrasound window), our attention was focused on this second application, feasible also with the presently available prototypes.

It is common observation after plain balloon angioplasty that the lumen diameter after dilatation is smaller than the nominal balloon diameter. This phenomenon was attributed to wall recoil but it is due, in most cases, to incomplete balloon expansion. Measurement of balloon diameter with quantitative angiography has shown that there are large differences between nominal size of the balloon at a given pressure and true balloon size measured during inflation of stenotic arterial segments [14]. If a stent is present at the site of dilatation, the scaffolding properties and radial force of the stent would limit or prevent wall recoil and prolapse of large dissection flaps inside the vessel lumen but will have little influence in the optimal expansion of the balloon.

Intracoronary ultrasound has shown that incomplete stent expansion/apposition to the vessel wall is present in most cases when balloon dilatation at conventional pressure (up to 8-12 atm) is performed [15,16]. The rationale of the policy of high pressure balloon inflation is the attempt of overcoming the unpredictable mechanical resistance of the vessel wall to stretching, allowing a regular expansion of the balloon [17]. An appropriate monitoring of the balloon expansion would avoid the unnecessary application of high pressure to all lesions, a strategy which potentially increases the wall damage and the consequent hyperplastic response. Considering the frequent eccentricity of the stenotic plaque and of its calcific deposition, it is obvious that only a tomographic technique such as ultrasound can accurately measure the complete and symmetrical balloon expansion. Further modifications of the imaging wire are required to facilitate its use during interventions, including an improved mechanical resistance of the rotating cable, a higher sensitivity of the ultrasound transducer, and the presence of a flexible steerable distal end. Other modifications are probably required for the balloons catheter used in combination with these wires, including an indeformable wire lumen, resistent to high pressure, the use of a special material in the distal segment, allowing imaging through the balloon shaft, and a longer catheter tip at the end of the balloon.

Incomplete Balloon Expansion Detected
with a 0.018 inch Imaging Wire

Distal stent   ## Mid stent

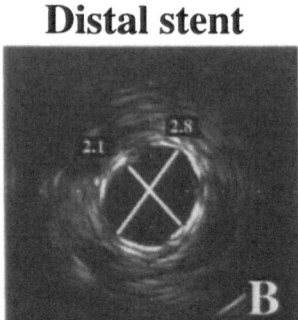
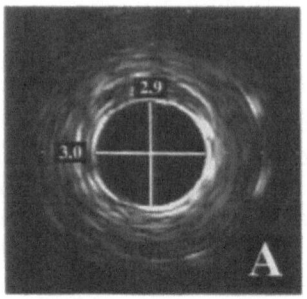

CSA = 6.7 mm²   CSA = 4.9 mm²

Cordis 3.5 mm Titan Balloon 16 atm

a

Incomplete Stent Expansion Detected
with Intracoronary Ultrasound

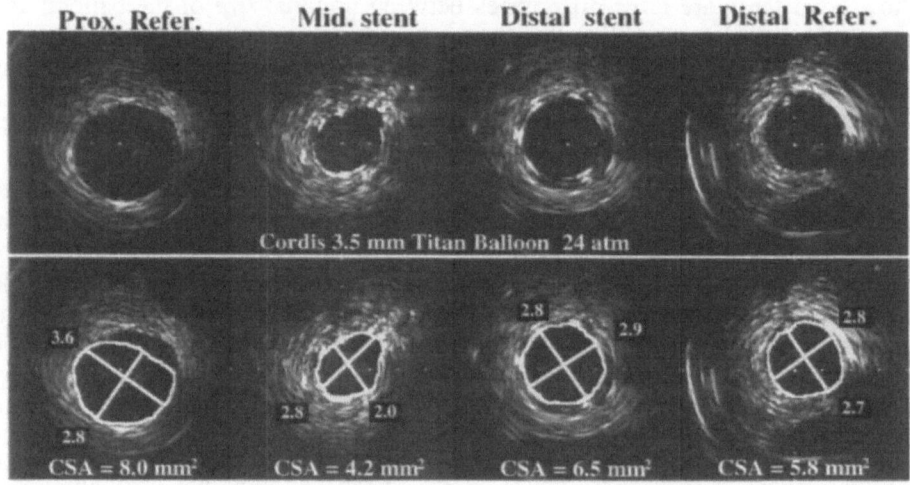

b

Figure 3. (Top set) Left panels: Cross-sectional images within a Palmaz-Schatz stent at two different locations, indicated in the corresponding angiogram of the inflated balloon in two orthogonal projections (right panels). Note that a large reduction in cross-sectional area and asymmetrical stent expansion is observed at site B in comparison with site A, despite the high pressure of inflation. (Bottom set) Multiple cross-sectional images after balloon deflation, confirming the persistence of a segment of severe stent underexpansion.

Conclusions

These encouraging preliminary observations confirm the feasibility of the use of an ultrasound wire for monitoring of balloon expansion during stent implantation. After high pressure inflation, a moderate reduction of the stent lumen was observed during deflation, compatible with the recoil predicted for the stainless-steel mesh stent used. Further improvements of the imaging wire can allow its application to: a) examine the lesion before intervention to select type, size and length of the device to be used; b) guide accurate positioning of the device at the stenosis site and orientation of the cutter to obtain a complete selective plaque removal with directional atherectomy; c) monitoring the expansion of the balloon during inflation over its entire length; d) assess the adequacy of the final result and the need of further interventions.

Three-dimensional reconstruction

Three-dimensional (3-D) reconstruction of ICUS images has the potential to assess the spatial relationship of the structures imaged by ICUS in different tomographic cross-sections and avoid the need of the simultaneous fluoroscopic assessment of the position of the ultrasound probe for orientation [18,19].

Technique

Three-dimensional reconstruction requires acquisition of the basic ultrasonic images and segmentation of the digitized images, two steps which greatly influence the final result.

A prerequisite for reliable longitudinal measurements after 3D-reconstruction is the use of a motorized pullback, allowing the acquisition of successive cross-sections at a known distance.

Two methods can be used:

Continuous pullback at a constant speed: the images are acquired in the form of "slices" during a slow pullback at a constant speed, permitting axial measurements during the image acquisition since the length of the reconstructed segment is defined by the time interval between two cross-sections times the pullback speed. In practice, a pullback speed between 1 and 0.5 mm/sec is used. Typically, a pullback time of 30 to 60 seconds is required to examine a 3 cm long vessel, generally sufficient to include the coronary stenosis and the adjacent reference segments.

ECG-gated motorized pullback and/or image acquisition: Systolic-diastolic movement of the imaging catheter and cyclic changes of the vessel dimensions are major limitations for accurate 3D-reconstruction and quantitative measurements of lumen and vessel wall. An ECG-gated three-dimensional reconstruction can be obtained by using a stepping motor and a dedicated acquisition station [20].

A more simple alternative solution is the ECG-triggered acquisition of images obtained in the same phase of the cardiac cycle during continuous pullback. To maintain a sufficient longitudinal resolution, however, a very slow continuous pullback must be used (0.1-0.25 mm/sec).

Image segmentation

The subsequent essential step after image acquisition and digitization is the image segmentation which distinguishes between blood pool and structures of the vessel wall in all the digitized ultrasound images. The backscatter pattern of flowing blood cells shows a speckle texture which varies over time whereas the echo signal of the vessel wall shows a more fixed pattern. Most blood speckle identification algorithms are based on this principle (Figure 4).

Quantitative 3D Reconstruction of ICUS

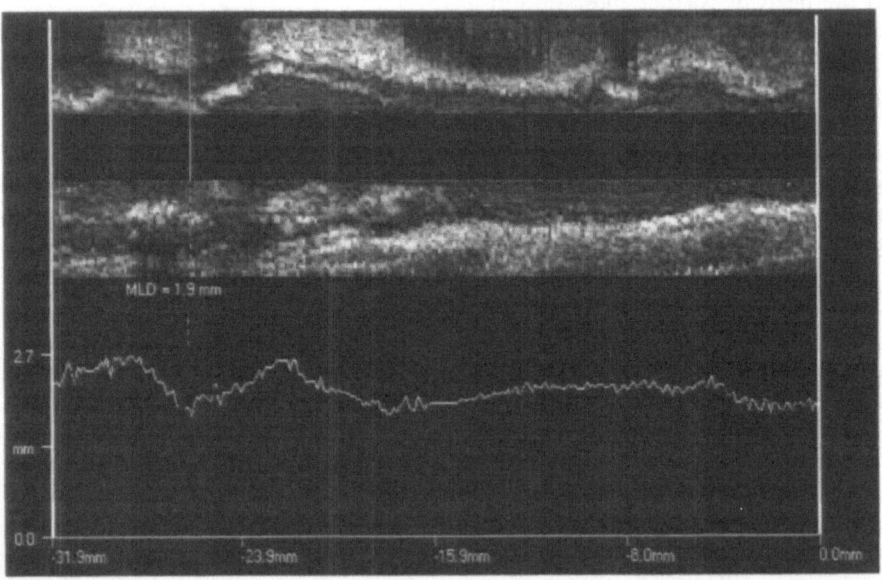

Figure 4. Longitudinal view of the proximal left anterior descending coronary artery after slow pass of a 2.15 mm Rotablator burr. The reconstructed image, obtained after acquisition and segmentation of multiple tomographic ICUS images obtained during a motorized pull-back at 0.5 mm/sec, shows the presence of a large calcific plaque with residual calcification in the proximal vessel, an intermediate normal segment and a new mild stenosis at 5 cm from the coronary ostium. Note that the reconstruction process, including the automatic recognition of the blood pool, encoded in red, and display of the diameter (yellow line) and area (green line) measurements, was completed in 90 seconds after the end of the ICUS examination (EchoLong, Indec, Capitula, CA). (For colour plate of figure 4 see page 560)

An alternative segmentation approach is the contour detection based on the application of a minimum-cost algorithm. In the system developed at the Thoraxcenter, two perpendicular longitudinal views are reconstructed from the series of cross-sectional images [21,22]. A minimum cost algorithm is applied for automated detection of the intimal leading edge and of the external contour of the vessel. Operator interaction is allowed to indicate in the longitudinal images one or more points to be used as fixed constraints for the contour detection process. Four individual edge points, derived from the contours of the longitudinal images, are used as constraints guiding the final contour detection in all the individual cross-sectional images. The cross-sectional image with the minimal luminal cross-sectional area is automatically defined. Lumen area, total vessel area and plaque area are measured for each frame and the corresponding mean diameters are calculated. A high reproducibility of the volumetric measurements of plaque and lumen was observed with mean signed differences between -0.6 and 0.4 % and standard deviations not exceeding ± 2.6 % [23].

Clinical applications

The measurement of plaque volume allows a direct assessment of the changes induced by pharmacological or dietary therapy aiming at regression of atherosclerosis [24-25] and by interventional procedures. Using these algorithms of image segmentation, accurate measurements, were obtained by Hausmann et al. [26] in normal rabbit aortas. On-line 3-D reconstruction offers practical advantages in comparison with a conventional ultrasound examination. The on-line longitudinal view of the stenotic segment before dilatation provides immediate information on the length of the stenosis and on the diameter of the lumen and total vessel in the reference segment. Based on this information, the length and diameter of balloon / device to be used can be more easily selected. The comparison between different cross-sections (i.e. reference and stenosis) can be performed by simply moving a cursor and does not require repeated insertions of the ultrasound probe or a time-consuming review of the video-recordings.

The effects and mechanisms of interventions and of restenosis can be studied using a rigorous comparison of corresponding cross-sections, provided that the pullback maneuver has been started from the same anatomic landmark (i.e. origin of a sidebranch). The depth and length of calcification, an important determinant of results and complications of coronary interventions [27-28], and the spatial geometry of dissections can be better determined [29-33]. Recent reports have also shown that three-dimensional reconstruction facilitates the orientation of the cutter in relation to sidebranches and the detection of deep cuts or spiral cuts from rotation of the atherectomy catheter during plaque removal [34]. The criteria used for guidance of stent implantation can more easily and reliably be applied to a 3-D reconstructed image, displaying the entire stented segment and the adjacent reference segments (Figure 5). The Thoraxcenter group reported that the automatic lumen measurements after on-line three-dimensional reconstruction reduced the time of analysis in comparison with the conventional review of the video taped ICUS examination and manual measurement of the tighest area within the stent and of the proximal and distal reference segments, decreased the interobserver variability of the measurements and more frequently detected stent underexpansion leading to further interventions [35-36].

3-D Reconstruction after Coronary Stenting

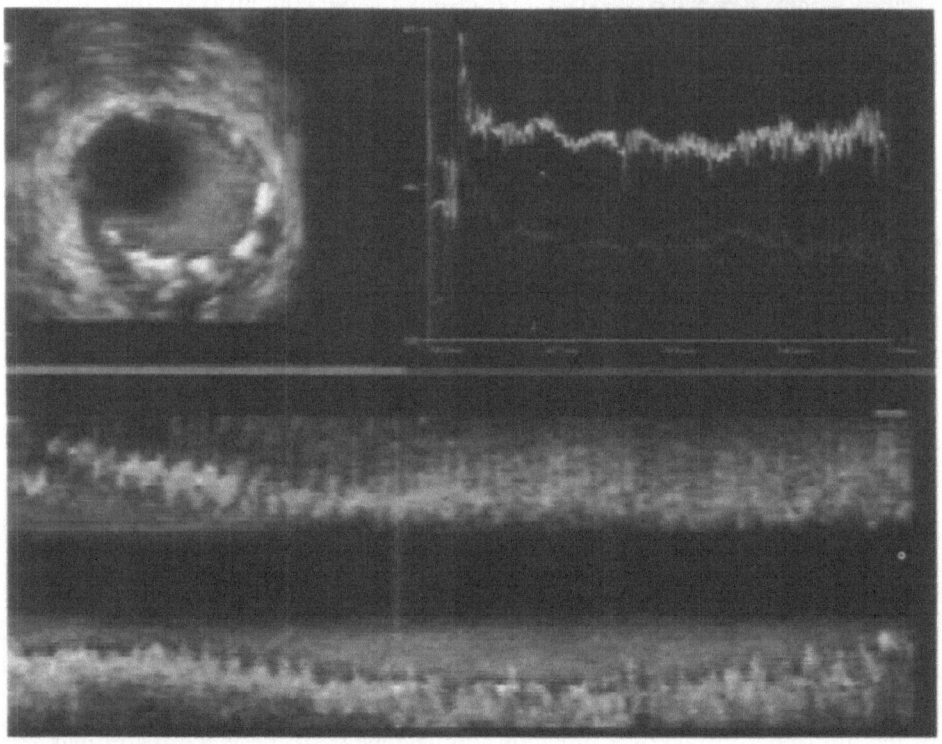

Figure 5. Longitudinal view of the proximal left anterior descending coronary artery after implantation of 3 NIR stenst. Note the perfect matching of the diameter of the proximal reference segment and of the stented segment.
(For colour plate of figure 5 see page 561)

Limitations

The first critical factor conditioning the results of three-dimensional reconstruction is the quality of the acquired echographic cross-sections. An insufficient delineation of the intimal border or the absence or incomplete circumferential detection of the plaque-adventitia interface preclude automated quantitative measurements of lumen and plaque volumes. Calcium shadowing or intraluminal flaps oriented tangentially to the ultrasound beam may also obscure the underlying wall [37]. Curvatures of the vessel also induce a predictable distortion of the 3-D image which is reconstruced along a straight line through the center of successive cross-sections. Expansion or compression of plaques may result in over- or underestimation of the volumes measured from the reconstructed image.

A simultaneous digitized biplane fluoroscopic tracking of the radio-opaque transducer and catheter tip has the potential to overcome this limitation, but is practically applicable only for research purposes [38].

The systolic expansion of the coronary vessel and the movement of the catheter inside the vessel during the cardiac cycle generate a characteristic saw-fish appearance of the vessel, more evident in arteries with large motility such as mid right coronary arteries and bypass grafts. As discussed before, electrocardiographic gating of the image acquisition can eliminate these artefacts, but require at present a significant increase in the time of examination and of the complexity of the instrumentation.

Conclusion

The availability of on-line 3-D reconstruction allows its application to facilitate interpretation and clinical application of intracoronary ultrasound for guidance and immediate assessment of coronary interventions. High quality cross-sectional images are mandatory for the application of algorithms for blood subtraction and quantitative measurement of lumen and plaque volumes.

Tissue characterization by intravascular imaging

Tissue characterization involves the study of the interaction between biologic tissue and various electrical and magnetic signal forms. The goal is to find a method that would obtain 'histologic' information without a biopsy. The composition of plaque in a coronary vessel is thought to have a major impact on its natural history. Spontaneous rupture of a fibrofatty plaque and subsequent thrombosis appear to be the principal substrates for myocardial infarction. Plaque that undergoes disruption tends to be eccentric with a high concentration of extracellular lipid at the base of the plaque. In addition, the composition of plaque also has a critical influence on the response to intervention. For example, thrombus within a target lesion is a negative prognostic factor for acute and, some studies suggest, long-term outcome.

Ultrasound-based strategies

The development of catheter-based ultrasound over the past five years has provided the first opportunity to directly assess tissue composition within a diseased vessel wall in the clinical setting. Initial studies have concentrated on the significance of localized calcium deposits within plaque, since calcium is readily identified by current generation catheters and is found very commonly in target lesions by ultrasound (60-70% of treated segments) [27]. Other studies have demonstrated that even small calcium deposits have a major impact on the response of lesions to both balloon angioplasty and atherectomy [28,39].

While a number of centers are pursuing detection of calcium deposits using intravascular ultrasound, relatively little work is being done in attempting to investigate other aspects of plaque composition. Unfortunately, this reflects a significant limitation in current imaging technology: it is generally not possible, based on images alone, to accurately distinguish different types of noncalcific plaque. Even the differentiation of thrombus and soft plaque is problematic using current intravascular ultrasound equipment.

The impulse response of a 30 MHz transducer has a 1/2 power axial resolution of approximately 80 microns. Thus, tissue with infrastructure containing acoustically reactive components separated by at least 80 microns can be resolved by analysis of the radiofrequency (RF) backscatter signal as long as the signal is sufficiently digitized. To optimize tissue detail, the RF backscatter samples from plaque need to be digitized at a sample frequency of greater than 10 times the center frequency (300 MHz) and transferred directly to computer disc. Figure 6 illustrates an RF sample region from eccentric plaque. The backscatter from the medial layer of muscular arteries reflects less signal power than adjacent plaque and adventitial layers because of the lack of collagen and elastin components. These characteristic signal features of the medial layer aid in the boundary selection of the RF signal, corresponding to plaque for subsequent backscatter analysis.

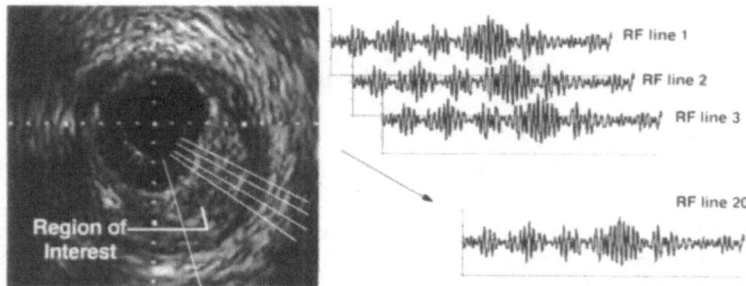

Figure 6. Example of radio-frequency (RF) data sets being acquired from a region-of-interest within an eccentric accumulation of plaque.

Intrinsic characteristics of the backscattered ultrasound signals, including the amplitude distribution, frequency response, and power spectrum of the signal, convey specific information about tissue types. These signal parameters can thus be used to perform "tissue characterization" of coronary plaque [40-41]. Preliminary studies from our laboratory have shown that computer-based analysis of the unprocessed RF backscatter from the vessel wall can clearly differentiate the histologic layers of the normal vessel wall, a key to understanding the effect of atherosclerosis on the images. The cellular infrastructure of noncalcific plaque and thrombus are significantly different. Soft plaque is made up of an amorphous collection of lipid substances, fibrosis, cholesterol clefts, and a variable amount of collagen and elastin. Thrombus, on the other hand, consists of a fairly organized layering of fibrous strands packed with a dense collection of red blood cells. Although these subtleties cannot be appreciated by their gray-scale appearance on the ultrasound image, preliminary results suggest a significant difference in the shape of the probability distribution function (PDF) of the RF backscattered signal from these two tissue types [42]. Figure 7 demonstrates the region in plaque for spatial RF sampling from both fibrofatty plaque and thrombus. Initial results from RF analysis of both thrombus and fibrofatty plaque show that differentiation is possible based on first-order moments of the probability distribution function (PDF); these data are summarized in Figure 7 (lower right). Although these early results are encouraging, additional work is needed in this area.

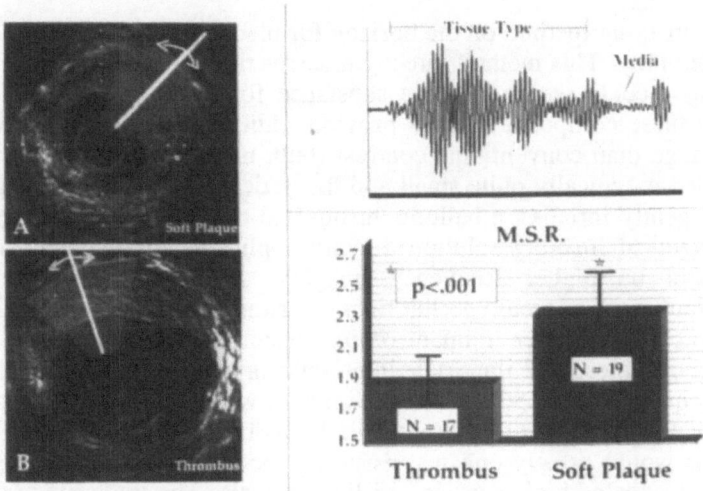

Figure 7. Example of RF regions-of-interest in soft plaque and thrombus. On gray-scale appearance alone, differentiation between these plaque types is rarely possible. Analysis of statistical fluctuation of RF data in each tissue type does allow discrimination based on the MSR (mean to standard deviation ratio).

A plaque can be broadly categorized into two groups. Plaque such as fibrous (de-novo) or intimal hyperplasia (restenosis) can be modeled as homogeneous architecture whereas fibrofatty plaque can be modeled as being inhomogeneous. Each of these plaque types will theoretically scatter ultrasound uniquely. Wave mechanics applied to this model predict that the statistical fluctuation of the RF backscatter, as reflected in the morphology of PDF, will be different for homogeneous and inhomogeneous tissue samples. The presence of fibrotic debris or increase in collagen strands in plaque may be detected by spatial power measurements. Another useful indicator of incoherent specular reflectors (such as cholesterol clefts, calcium deposits, and hyalinization) may be a frequency approach. Computing the power spectral density and autocorrelation functions from the isolated backscattered signal not only recognizes the presence of these specular interfaces, but spatially locates them. The use of a 30 MHz transducer, with the axial resolution on the order of these atheroma components, as well as a wide bandwidth transducer provides a signal from which frequency analysis can take place without significant aliasing artifact.

Up to this point, tissue characterization efforts have been primarily focused on excised cadaveric specimens and in atherosclerotic animal models. In the clinical situation, directional atherectomy may represent a plausible format to correlate tissue specimens with signal features in-vivo. Several groups are testing basic algorithms in human coronary arteries by obtaining RF signals within a region of interest pre-intervention, and then excising this region by directional atherectomy. This should ultimately provide a registry of signal characteristics and histology to test the robust nature of discrimination algorithms, as well as the development of new techniques specifically aimed at plaque typing in human coronary vessels.

One future imaging method on the horizon for plaque typing is a technique called elastography [43]. This method directly assesses tissue elasticity (shear modulus) by tracking speckle within a tissue substance following a displacement force. Essentially these composite images provide additional tissue detail, with larger dynamic range than conventional contrast (bulk modulus) imaging formats. The force applied is typically quite small and theoretically could be applied to plaque in-vivo by gently inflating a balloon during real-time ultrasound imaging.

Another practical imaging solution directly applicable for better characterizing tissue would be higher frequency imaging. Scanning tissue with shorter wavelength ultrasound would permit finer discrimination of spatial detail [44]. As the demand for catheter miniaturization becomes more intense, a shorter wavelength becomes more important in preserving near-field image quality. Using a center frequency of 40-50 MHz, for example, would allow small fatty deposits or zones of fibrous tissue to be separated by as little 3-4 times the size of a red blood. This would greatly enhance tissue distinction based on the images alone without sophisticated higher-order, off-line analysis. The trade-off in the in-vivo situation is a drastic increase in blood backscatter and decreased penetration. One possible format is to have a catheter with two crystals: one of 30 MHz for guidance up to the plaque in question, and a 50 MHz transducer for a more detailed look from an "up close" vantage point. Elevating the higher frequency crystal in close approximation to the plaque would allow a 1-2 mm scan into the tissue, providing additional detail of the contents beneath the tissue surface.

Non-ultrasound strategies

Other non-ultrasound based imaging technologies capable of tissue characterization include Magnetic Resonance Imaging MRI (intravascular and extravascular) and a new modality called OCT (optical coherent tomography). The resolution and reconstruction time have both improved, making MRI a plausible imaging modality for deciphering coronary vessel wall pathology. Figure 8 shows an external MRI scan of a proximal Left Anterior Descending specimen. Note the clear delineation of the vessel wall layers and the perivascular structure. Although most external applications will be limited to the more proximal coronary anatomy, this technique provides the opportunity to accurately distinguish plaque types- including the vulnerable fibrofatty substance from mainly fibrous tissue [45,46]. Additionally, RF coil technology is maturing such that "MRI on a stick" may be possible in the very near future. This would obviously provide one of the most accurate tools for tissue characterization.

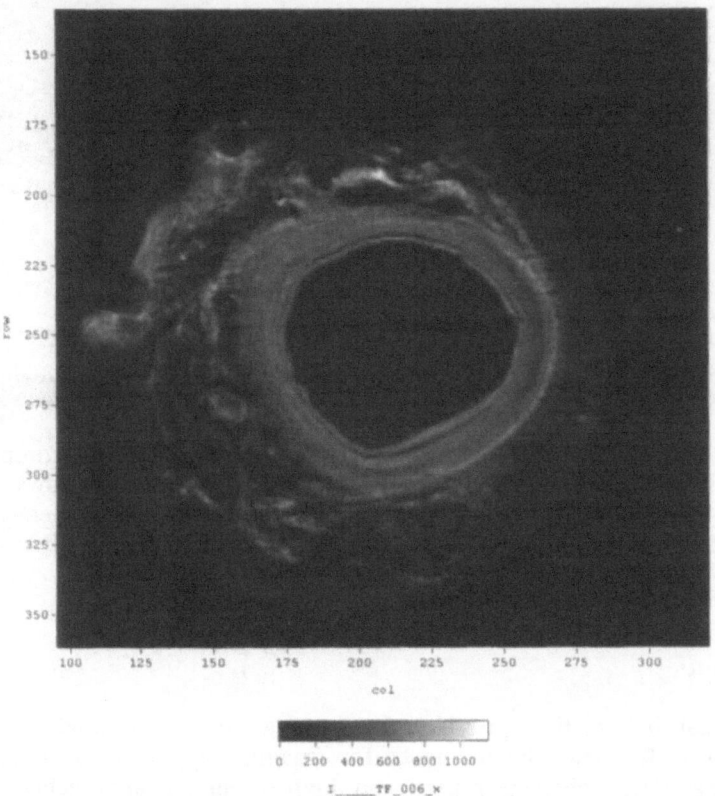

Figure 8. External MRI scan of a proximal left anterior descending (LAD) coronary artery. Various spin echo and gradient echo techniques may permit a high sensitivity for plaque type discrimination.

Although the application of OCT to tomographic vessel imaging is new, the concept itself has been fairly well established [47]. Developed at the Fujimoto Laboratory at MIT, OCT uses coherent infrared light to generate images with significantly improved resolution (4-20 microns) and dynamic range (~ 100 dB), compared to commercially available ultrasound systems. The reflectance patterns received can be transmitted via fiber optic technology, making possible a catheter-based strategy. Early in-vitro work has not only shown this technique possible but has demonstrated precise discrimination of tissue types within the vessel wall [48]. Figure 9 shows correlation between the OCT reflectance pattern from a vessel wall and the corresponding histology in a cadaveric specimen. Further work will determine its usefulness in a blood filled in-vivo environment.

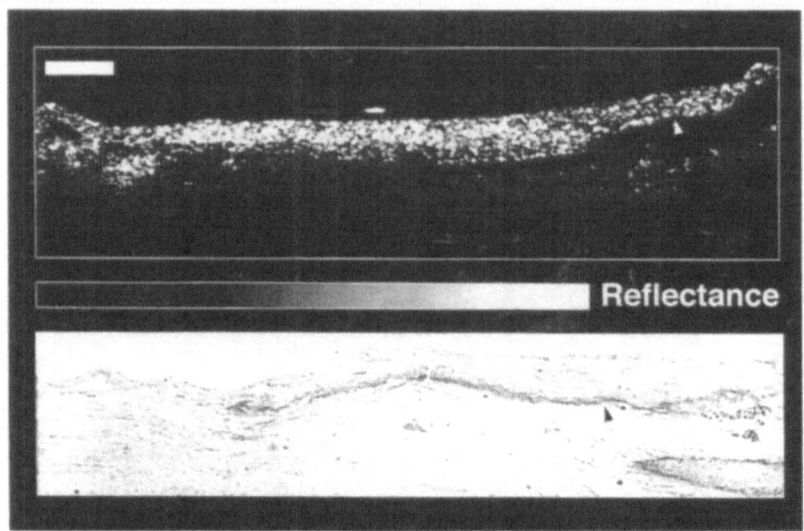

Figure 9. Optical coherence tomographic (OCT) image of a human coronary artery and corresponding histology. The reflectance pattern not only shows a striking difference at tissue transitions zones (arrow) but also tissue type is clearly noted by intensity differences. Courtesy of Dr. Neal Weissman (Georgetown University), and Dr. Mark Brezinski (Massachusetts General Hospital).
(For colour plate of figure 9 see page 562)

Conclusion

The clinical information provided by intravascular ultrasound imaging has stimulated many new developments for imaging applications. In particular, intraluminal tissue characterization and high-frequency approaches are being rapidly explored to better represent various endovascular histologic patterns. Advanced processing of the backscattered ultrasound signal may permit an in-vivo bioassay of plaque and contribute to the understanding of plaque progression, regression, and response to various forms of therapy. Additional non-ultrasound technologies such as MRI and OCT with resolutions approaching the cellular level, hold tremendous promise for catheter-based plaque and tissue characterization.

References

1. Gussenhoven EJ, Essed CE, Lancee CT *et al.* Arterial wall characteristics determined by intravascular ultrasound imaging: an in vitro study. J Am Coll Cardiol 1989;14:947-52.

2. Nishimura RA, Edwards WD, Warner CA *et al*. Intravascular ultrasound imaging: in vitro validation and pathologic correlation. J Am Coll Cardiol 1990;16:145-54.
3. Nissen SE, Gurley JC, Grines CL *et al*. Intravascular ultrasound assessment of lumen size and wall morphology in normal subjects and patients with coronary artery disease. Circulation 1991;84:1087-99.
4. Tobis JM, Mallery J, Mahon D *et al*. Intravascular ultrasound imaging of human coronary arteries in vivo. Analysis of tissue characterization with comparison to in vitro histological specimens. Circulation 1991;83:913-26.
5. Fitzgerald PJ, St. Goar FG, Connolly AJ *et al*. Intravascular ultrasound imaging of coronary arteries. Is three layers the norm? Circulation 1992;86:154-8.
6. Pandian NG, Kreis A, Weintraub A *et al*. Real-time intravascular ultrasound imaging in humans. Am J Cardiol 1990;65:1392-6.
7. Potkin BN, Bartorelli AL, Gessert KM *et al*. Coronary artery imaging with high-frequency ultrasound. Circulation 1990;81:1575-85.
8. Yock PG, Linker Dt. Intravascular ultrasound. Looking below the surface of vascular disease. Circulation 1990;81:1715-8.
9. Bom N, Lancée CT, van Egmond FC. An ultrasonic intracardiac scanner. Ultrasonics 1972;10:71-6.
10. Mudra H, Klauss V, Blasini R *et al*. Ultrasound guidance of Palmaz Schatz intracoronary stenting with a combined intravascular ultrasound balloon catheter. Circulation 1994;90:1252-61.
11. Fitzgerald PJ, Belef M, Connolly Aj, Yock P. Design and initial testing of an ultrasound-guided directional atherectomy device. Am Heart J 1995;129:593-8.
12. Tobis J, Hall P, Maiello L *et al*. Clinical feasibility of an 0.018 intravascular ultrasound imaging device [abstract]. Circulation 1995;92(Suppl.I):I-400.
13. Hall P, Maiello L, Colombo A *et al*. In vivo evidence that Palmaz-Schatz stents do not recoil immediately following deployment [abstract]. Circulation 1995;92(Suppl.I):I-327.
14. Hermans WR, Rensing BJ, Strauss BH, Serruys PW. Methodological problems related to the quantitative assessment of stretch, elastic recoil, and balloon-artery ratio. Cathet Cardiovasc Diagn 1992;25:174-85.
15. Nakamura S, Colombo A, Gaglione A. Intracoronary ultrasound observations during stent implantation. Circulation 1994;89:2026-34.
16. Goldberg SL, Colombo A, Nakamura S, Almagor Y, Maiello L, Tobis JM. Benefit of intracoronary ultrasound in the deployment of Palmaz-Schatz stents. J Am Coll Cardiol 1994;24:996-1003.
17. Colombo A, Hall P, Nakamura S *et al*. Intracoronary stenting without anticoagulation accomplished with intravascular ultrasound guidance. Circulation 1995;91:1676-88.
18. Roelandt JRTC, Di Mario C, Pandian NG *et al*. Three-dimensional reconstruction of intracoronary ultrasound images. Rationale, approaches, problems, and directions. Circulation 1994;90:1044-55.
19. Di Mario C, von Birgelen C, Prati F *et al*. Three dimensional reconstruction of cross-sectional intracoronary ultrasound. Br Heart J 1995;73(Suppl.2):26-32.
20. Bruining N, von Birgelen C, Di Mario C *et al*. Dynamic three-dimensional reconstruction of ICUS images based on an ECG-Gated pull-back device. Comput Cardiol 1995;633-9.
21. Li W, Bosch JG, Zhong Y *et al*. Image segmentation and 3D reconstruction of intravascular ultrasound images. Accoustic imaging 1993;20:489-96.

22. Li W, von Birgelen C, Di Mario C *et al*. Semi-automatic contour detection for volumetric quantification of intracoronary ultrasound. Comput Cardiol 1994;227-80.

23. Von Birgelen C, Di Mario C, Li W *et al*. Volumetric quantification in intracoronary ultrasound: validation of a new automatic contour detection method with integrated user interaction. Am Heart J. In press.

24. Gupta M, Connolly AJ, Zhu BQ *et al*. Quantitative analysis of progression of atherosclerosis by intravascular ultrasound: validation in a rabbit model [abstract]. Circulation 1992;86(Suppl.I):I-518.

25. Galli FC, Sudhir K, Kao AK, Fitzgerald PJ, Yock PG. Direct measurement of plaque volume by three-dimensional ultrasound: potential and pitfalls [abstract]. J Am Coll Cardiol 1992;19(SupplA):115A.

26. Hausman D, Friedrich G, Sudhir K *et al*. 3D intravascular ultrasound imaging with automated border detection using 2.9 F catheters [abstract]. J Am Coll Cardiol 1994;23(Special Issue):174A.

27. Mintz GS, Popma JJ, Pichard AD *et al*. Patterns of calcification in coronary artery disease. A statistical analysis of intravascular ultrasound and coronary angiography in 1155 lesions. Circulation 1995;91:1959-65.

28. Fitzgerald PJ, Ports TA, Yock PG. Contribution of localized calcium deposits to dissection after angioplasty. An observational study using intravascular ultrasound. Circulation 1992;86:64-70.

29. Rosenfield K, Losordo DW, Ramaswamy K *et al*. Three-dimensional reconstruction of human coronary and peripheral arteries from images recorded during two-dimensional intravascular ultrasound examination. Circulation 1991;84:1938-56.

30. Rosenfield K, Kaufman J, Pieczek A, Langevin RE Jr, Razvi S, Isner JM. Real-time three-dimensional reconstruction of intravascular ultrasound images of iliac arteries. Am J Cardiol 1992;70:412-5.

31. Coy KM, Park JC, Fishbein MC *et al*. In vitro validation of three-dimensional intravascular ultrasound for the evaluation of arterial injury after balloon angioplasty. J Am Coll Cardiol 1992;20:692-700.

32. Cavaye DM, White RA, Lerman RD *et al*. Usefulness of intravascular ultrasound imaging for detecting experimentally induced aortic dissection in dogs and for determining the effectiveness of endoluminal stenting. Am J Cardiol 1992;69:705-7.

33. Schryver TE, Popma JJ, Kent KM, Leon MB, Eldridge S, Mintz GS. Use of intracoronary ultrasound to identify the true coronary lumen in chronic coronary dissection treated with intracoronary stenting. Am J Cardiol 1992;69:1107-8.

34. Smucker ML, Kil D, Sarnat WS, Wefald FC, Howard PF. Is 3-dimensional reconstruction a gimmick or a useful clinical tool? Experience in coronary atherectomy [abstract]. J Am Coll Cardiol 1992;19(Suppl.A):115A.

35. Prati F, Di Mario C, von Birgelen C *et al*. Usefulness of on-line 3D reconstruction for stent implantation [abstract]. J Am Coll Cardiol 1995;25(Special Issue):9A-10A.

36. Prati F, Di Mario C, von Birgelen C *et al*. On-line automated lumen volume measurement with 3D intracoronary ultrasound during coronary interventions [abstract]. J Am Coll Cardiol 1995;25(Special Issue):345A.

37. Di Mario C, Madrestma S, Linker D *et al*. The angle of incidence of the ultrasonic beam: a critical factor for the image quality in intravascular ultrasound. Am Heart J 1993;125:442-8.

38. Slager CJ, Laban M, von Birgelen C *et al*. ANGUS: a new approach to three-dimensional reconstruction of geometry and orientation of coronary lumen and plaque by combined use of coronary angiography and IVUS [abstract]. J Am Coll Cardiol 1995;25(Special Issue):144A.

39. DeFranco AC, Nissen SE, Tuzcu EM *et al*. Ultrasound plaque morphology predicts major dissections following stand-alone and adjunctive balloon angioplasty [abstract]. Circulation 1994;90(4 pt 2):I-59.

40. Wickline SA, Barzilai B; Thomas LJ *et al*. Quantification of intimal and medial thickness of human coronary arteries by acoustic microscopy. Coron Artery Dis 1990;1:333-40.

41. Barzilai B, Saffitz JE, Miller JG, Sobel BE. Quantitative ultrasonic characterization of the nature of atherosclerotic plaques in human aorta. Circ Res 1987;60:459-63.

42. Fitzgerald PJ, Connolly AJ, Watkins RD, Hargrave VK, Yock PG. Distinction between soft plaque and thrombus by intravascular tissue characterization [abstract]. J Am Coll Cardiol 1991;17(Suppl.A):11A.

43. Skovoroda AR, Ernelianov SY, Lubinski MA *et al*. Theoretical analysis and verification of ultrasound displacement and strain imaging. IEEE Trans Ultrason Ferroelectr Freq Contr 1994;41:302-11.

44. Lockwood GR, Ryan LK, Gotlieb AI *et al*. In vitro high resolution intravascular imaging in muscular and elastic arteries. J Am Coll Cardiol 1992;20:153-60.

45. Hofman MBM, Paschal CB, Haacke M, van Rossum AC, Sprenger M. MRI of coronary arteries: 2D breath-hold versus 3D respiratory gated acquisition. J Comp Assist Tomogr 1995;19:56-62.

46. Pennell DJ, Keegan J, Firmin DN, Gatehouse PD, Underwood SR, Longmore DB. Magnetic resonance imaging of coronary arteries: technique and preliminary results. Br Heart J 1993;70:315-26.

47. Huang D, Swanson EA, Lin CP *et al*. Optical coherence tomography. Science 1991;254:1178-81.

48. Brezinski ME, Tearney GJ, Bouma BE *et al*. Imaging of coronary artery microstructure (in-vitro) with optical coherence tomography. Am J Cardiol 1996;77:92-3.

22. Practical integration of intravascular ultrasound imaging into the cardiac catheterization laboratory

GARY S. MINTZ, AUGUSTO D. PICHARD, KENNETH M. KENT, JEFFREY J. POPMA, LOWELL F. SATLER, CAROL L. WALSH, PAUL R. MACKELL & MARTIN B. LEON

Summary

By carefully analyzing the catheterization laboratory environment, it is possible to establish a program that facilitates clinical IVUS imaging without adding significant (i.e., more than 5 minutes) to the interventional procedure. This has resulted in the exponential growth of the program. It is currently being used to guide approximately 75% of the interventional procedures we perform. The other limitations to the routine use of IVUS (procedural cost and physician education) will require different solutions.

Introduction

Coronary angiography has been the gold standard for assessing coronary artery disease and for guiding coronary interventions. However, the limitations of coronary angiography are becoming more understood.

Intravascular ultrasound (IVUS) provides transmural images of coronary arteries in vivo. The normal coronary arterial wall, the major components of the atherosclerotic plaque, and the serial changes that occur with the atherosclerotic disease process and as a result transcatheter therapy can be studied in humans in a manner previously not possible. Studies have indicated that IVUS imaging of target lesions before and after catheter-based treatment consistently demonstrates more target lesion calcium, less eccentricity, more extensive reference segment atherosclerosis, larger reference vessel dimensions, smaller final lumen dimensions, inadequate stent expansion, significant residual plaque burden, incomplete stent expansion, and greater degrees of tissue trauma than is evident by angiography. Thus, by providing information that is not available from routine coronary angiography or even from on-line quantitative coronary angiography, IVUS has the potential to influence clinical revascularization treatment strategies. The major limitations to the routine use of IVUS are procedural cost, physician education, equipment complexity, and the difficulties in integrating an ultrasound-based imaging modality into the busy cardiac catheterization laboratory environment. IVUS will be used routinely only if it is quick to set up, easy to perform, does not slow down the flow of the clinical interventional cases in the laboratory, and does cannot interfere with patient care. Each catheterization laboratory is different, and each presents special problems. Even tasks performed by different health care professionals (nurses vs technologists vs cardiology fellows) vary from laboratory to laboratory. The busier the laboratory, the more important are the issues of practical integration and procedural streamlining. At

J.H.C. Reiber and E.E. van der Wall (eds.), Cardiovascular Imaging, 277-282.
© *1996 Kluwer Academic Publishers.*

the Washington Hospital Center, integration of intravascular ultrasound imaging has been successful. The purpose of this review is to describe how this was accomplished.

A cath lab, not an echo lab

The first decision was to create a Clinical IVUS Imaging Program within the administrative structure of the Cardiac Catheterization Laboratory (the busiest interventional program in the United States), not within the administrative structure of the Non-invasive Imaging Laboratory. The temperament of the two environments is very different. For example, interventional procedures cannot be put "on hold" until the equipment is transported from the echocardiography laboratory. The individuals involved in IVUS imaging must have an understanding of interventional procedures.

Director

The second decision was to appoint a Director who is responsible for all aspects of the Clinical IVUS Imaging Program. These include designation and training of technologists, equipment selection, education of physicians, procedural standardization, protocols, etc. The Director also serves as a resource to interpret difficult studies.

Technologists

Even in a busy laboratory with constant IVUS use, it is difficult to have all laboratory personnel trained. Many practical aspects of IVUS imaging are foreign to traditional cath lab practices. These include ordering, handling, and storing of video tapes (especially remembering to advance to the end of the previous study before recording the next one), recording studies, maintaining a log book, maintaining and trouble shooting ultrasound equipment, and stocking ancillary supplies. The individual responsible for IVUS imaging during a particular interventional procedure should not be responsible for patient care or the technical aspects of the interventional procedure itself. Thus, the third decision was to designate specific IVUS technologists.

There are two dedicated IVUS technologists at the Washington Hospital Center. In effect, this represented a new type of position even though, in practice, the IVUS technologists were selected from the general pool of cardiac catheterization laboratory technologists. The first individual that was selected also had extensive experience as an echocardiography technologist. As such, she was the ideal individual to pioneer this new position because she understood ultrasound images in general and interventional procedures in particular. The IVUS technologists are responsible for all practical aspects of IVUS imaging. In particular, their duties include: (1) equipment and catheter set-up; (2) proper recording and documentation of the IVUS imaging runs; (3) interpretation of the IVUS images;

(4) report generation; (5) keeping a procedure log; and (6) equipment maintenance and inventory. By having designated technologists, not only is the flow of the interventional procedure uninterrupted; but just as importantly, the imaging runs are optimized (equipment settings are properly selected) and the correctness of the annotated procedural information is assured. With time, technologists can be trained to interpret the images accurately, to provide the iterative feedback necessary for IVUS-based decision making, and to answer the questions posed by the primary operators. If in doubt (or if the interpretation of the technologist conflicts with that of the operator), the Director is available for assistance.

Catheters and hardware

Different manufacturers produce catheters and hardware that may or may not be interchangeable and that may or may not be appropriate for any given setting. For example, (bigger) catheters with larger transducer apertures will produce superior images and be ideal for diagnostic or post-intervention studies, but their profile may limit use prior to intervention. Short monorail catheters may not perform well in tortuous vessels. Common distal lumen designs (that alternatively house the transducer or the guidewire, but not both) require that the angioplasty guidewire be pulled back before imaging. Catheters designed for coronary use may not be suitable for peripheral applications. Nevertheless, catheter selection is often a matter of personal preference. It is important for all operators to become familiar with the different catheters available and to treat them with the same respect as interventional devices.

{For example, SCIMED manufacturers two types of IVUS catheters originally designed by CVIS: a 3.2F short monorail and a 2.9F long monorail/common distal lumen design. As short monorail catheters go, the 3.2F catheter is well designed. Compared to most short monorail catheters, it tracks well, even through tortuousities; and it crosses most tight lesions. It loses some of its facility in imaging extremely distal lesions (particularly with tortuous, angulated, or extensively diseased proximal vessels) and in crossing tight, calcific stenoses just after a tight bend. However, it has the advantage of being "quick" and less fussy compared to the 2.9F design; importantly, the wire does not have to be pulled back. The 3.2F short monorail catheter should not be used to image coiled stents that don't have an axial spine (the Gianturco-Roubin II stent has an axial spine); the short monorail may trap one of the coils and deform the stent. The 3.2F catheter should also not be used to image the Palmaz-Schatz stent if the guidewire has entered the stent through one of the stent "diamonds". The tip is low-profile enough that the it will go through one of the "diamonds"; however, in withdrawing it from the stent, there is a risk of shearing off the tip. The 2.9F common lumen catheter is the imaging catheter of choice for imaging coiled stents lacking an axial spine, both because of its size and distal design characteristics. If the guidewire path through a Palmaz-Schatz stent is uncertain, then the 2.9F catheter adds a margin of safety to the procedure. The 2.9F catheter is the only design that eliminates the guidewire artifact. It cannot be used with the Transluminal Extraction Catheter wire (the 0.21" ball at the tip of the

TEC wire cannot be withdrawn back in the common lumen).}

Defective catheters (poor images, loss of imaging, excessive NURD, etc.) should be returned to the manufacturer. They are too expensive to be simply discarded. If the catheters are to be reused, they should not be gas sterilized; this effects the quality of the imaging. Instead, soak the catheters in disinfectant solution. Catheters will perform for various lengths of time before failing. Occasionally, catheters have been reported to perform well for hours.

Guiding catheters must be selected according to the imaging catheter being used. In general, all 8F guiding catheters will accommodate all IVUS catheter designs. Some large lumen 7F guiding catheters can be used. However, it is inadvisable to force a catheter with a rotating transducer into a small guiding catheter. This often has the effect of introducing excessive nonuniform rotational distortion (NURD). Some synthetic aperture electronic array IVUS catheters (but no current mechanical devices) will work with some 6F guiding catheters.

The purchase of IVUS equipment, like the purchase of any medical equipment, is typically the responsibility of the program Director. Differences among manufacturers are real, and all choices represent some amount of compromise. Although the diagnostic accuracy is similar, the characteristics of the images vary significantly among the systems. Individuals not familiar with ultrasound imaging technology often find it difficult to switch from one image presentation to another. It is important for the IVUS technologists to become familiar with all of the equipment present in the laboratory.

We have found it useful to "wire" the angiographic suites so that the IVUS images are displayed on the angiographic monitors. The angiographic monitors offer superior resolution, are convenient and readily visible to the operator, and the IVUS machine can then be placed in a position away from the patient table and out of the way of the nurses providing patient care.

We have also fully integrated the IVUS hardware into one of the angiographic suites. The IVUS computer is stored under the patient table and is otherwise "invisible". There is no separate IVUS monitor; the IVUS images are displayed only on one of the angiographic "road map" monitors. The IVUS keyboard and VCR are situated in the angiographic control room. All cables are hidden.

Procedural standardization

In a busy laboratory with multiple operators, it is important to standardize image acquisition so that image analysis can also be standardized. The last major decision was to agree on and enforce a uniform image acquisiton protocol. At the Washington Hospital Center, IVUS imaging is performed the same way in every case. We have found that the use of a motorized transducer pullback device aids (in fact, enforces) procedure standardization. (It also provides useful length measurements.) The catheter is placed in the distal vessel approximately 10 mm beyond the target lesion, the pullback device is activated, imaging is performed (and images are recorded) only during transducer pullback, and transducer pullback is continued until the aortoostial junction is visualized. The catheter is then immediately removed, and the intervention continues. One run usually is sufficient, although additional runs can (and are) made if there is any question about the quality of the image (e.g., inadequate flushing, excessive rotational distortion) or about the pathology present. Measurements are made off-line, not when the catheter is in the vessel; this saves procedure time and minimizes patient ischemia. Not only is the lesion carefully interrogated, but equal attention is paid to the vessel distal and proximal to the lesion. Standardization of image acquisition facilitates off-line image review and analysis; there is no question whether the transducer is being advanced or pulled back. Standardization of image acquisition also facilitates comparison of serial (pre- and post-intervention or post-intervention and follow-up) studies; for example, it is possible to display various imaging runs side-by-side to compare the differences. We prefer a pullback speed of 0.5 mm/sec because we have found (by trial and error) that this is rate at which the trained eye can best assimilate the visual information. However, with very focal stenoses, especially ostial stenoses, we prefer a pullback speed of 0.25 mm/sec. (Conversely, we never use a speed of 1 mm/sec for fear of missing important information.) At a pullback speed of 0.5 mm/sec, an average imaging run takes 90 seconds (4.5 cm of artery); and the average study (three runs: pre-intervention, at some time during the procedure, and post-intervention) takes less than 5 minutes.

We have also found this standardization is especially helpful in coordinating and analyzing IVUS tapes as part of multicenter studies.

Procedure information (including voice annotation) is the responsibility of the IVUS technologist. Even if the microphone is recording verbal commentary, it is very helpful if on-line procedural information is annotated onto the ultrasound system's video screen. Remember, if the image is frozen during replay, there is no sound; and background noise can garble the voice annotation. The temporal relationship of each IVUS imaging run to the sequence of steps during the interventional procedure should be available to anyone viewing the tape. The ideal on screen labeling should contain three elements: (1) the timing of IVUS imaging (e.g., pre-intervention, post PTCA#1, etc.); (2) the procedure being performed (PTCA, DCA, stent, etc.); and (3) the target lesion (vessel and location, e.g., ostial). All IVUS instruments have internal clocks, and the time is automatically recorded onto the videotape. It is helpful to note the "time" that corresponds to the center of the lesion. In the absence of systematic pre-intervention imaging, voice annotation or recording the "time" corresponding to the lesion may be the only way to identify the target lesion on subsequent review. After some procedures (e.g., directional coronary atherectomy with a good result), it is often difficult to identify the target lesion without this information.

Housekeeping issues

Good quality videotapes are essential. It is recommended that virgin (never-used) broadcast quality S-VHS tapes be used. There is a quality difference, and the cost difference is minimal.

Once a tape is finished, remove the tab that allows video images to be recorded. In this way, the tape cannot be accidentally reused.

Videotapes should be stored in a secure place. Although they are not expensive, tapes become irresistible targets for petty thieves because they can be used in home or studio videocassette recorders. Unfortunately, once they contain patient information, videotapes become irreplaceable. If you are worried, copies of each tape can be made by hooking two VCR's together; both VCR's should be medical grade S-VHS units with S-Video turned on. If there is voice annotation information, then the audio circuit must be linked as well. The first generation copy loses some image quality, but is usually acceptable. The second generation copy (copy of a copy) loses too much image information to be useful. It is a good idea to store the originals and copies in separate locations.

Videotape storage can become unwieldy if each patient has his own tape. In general, 20 studies can be recorded on each 2 hour tape. Individual tapes (for each patient) should be reserved for multicenter studies in which the videotape must be sent away to a core laboratory.

A log book should be created. Each video tape should have a unique number. Each tape's studies should be recorded in sequence in the log book. A simple alphabetized data base can also be created to identify individual patient studies for retrieval purposes.

Reports should be generated. The requirements of each institution vary. These reports can also form the nucleus of a data base of patients studied. In some countries, clinical reports cannot be used for research. The clinical reports should become a permanent part of the patient's medical record.

Cath lab environment-related problems

Many cath labs have excessive ambient electrical or radiofrequency noise. Any piece of equipment in the lab can produce electrical "interference". Offenders may include some monitoring equipment, intraaortic balloon pumps, etc. Eliminating these problems requires troubleshooting and working with both the IVUS and non-IVUS equipment vendors.

The Doppler wire causes two types of interference. One is electrical, but the other is ultrasound interference (cross-talk between the two signals). Ultrasonic cross-talk is present whenever two sources of ultrasonic signals are used simultaneously.

In some hospitals the paging system generates a radiofrequency signal that momentarily "blanks out" the ultrasound image. Inexpensive, custom filters will solve this problem.

23. Intravascular ultrasound for evaluation of coronary arteries

GÜNTER GÖRGE, JUNBO GE, MICHAEL HAUDE, VIJAY SHAH, ALLEN JEREMIAS, HELGE SIMON & RAIMUND ERBEL

Summary

Intravascular ultrasound (IVUS) has emerged from a research tool to an intrinsic part of modern invasive cardiology. The main reason is the capability to obtain "in-vivo" histology. For the first time it is possible to base decisions not only on lumenograms but also on vessel wall assessment. The capabilities of IVUS can be divided into its: (a) diagnostic, and (b) intervention associated potentials. Diagnostic strength of IVUS is the ability to monitor compensatory coronary artery enlargement as a response to arteriosclerosis, to assess intermediate lesions, to reveal occult left main stem disease, and angiographycally "silent" arteriosclerosis. The intervention associated potentials of IVUS are the ability to allow optimal device selection, i.e. rotablators in calcified lesions or atherectomy devices in large plaque burden. The effects of PTCA on vessel wall morphology can be studied in great detail and the effect on luminal gain can be assessed almost on-line. Several groups showed, that the residual plaque area even after angiographically successful PTCA lies still in the range of 60%. A significant reduction of this number may influence long-term outcome after PTCA. Minimal luminal areas and residual plaque area after PTCA seem to be an indicator of restenosis, while the presence or absence of dissections seem to be less predictive. Intravascular monitoring of stent expansion led to high-pressure stent deployment with significant increase in post-procedural luminal diameters and finally the ability to withhold anticoagulation in patients with optimal stent deployment. In the future, integrated devices, like balloons on IVUS catheters, steerable catheters, integrated flow and pressure transducers, tissue characterization, and 0.018" IVUS guide-wires will further enhance the usefulness of IVUS.

Introduction

The composition of coronary atheroma and the lumen narrowing are the main factors for the prognosis of patients with diseases of the coronary circulation [1-4]. Unfortunately, only the latter, lumen narrowing, can be determined by angiography [5]. As a silhouette method, angiography does not allow visualization of the plaque and vessel wall composition itself (Figure 1). This limitation makes the results of angiography inferior for the prediction of coronary events, the amount of vessel remodelling, and the effect of various interventional devices [4]. These shortcomings paved the way for the meanwhile wide use and broad acceptance of intravascular ultrasound (IVUS) in clinical cardiology [6-8]. IVUS is a new invasive technique providing tomographic images of coronary

283

J.H.C. Reiber and E.E. van der Wall (eds.), Cardiovascular Imaging, 283-300.
© 1996 *Kluwer Academic Publishers.*

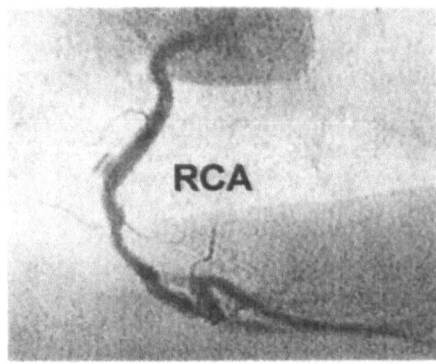 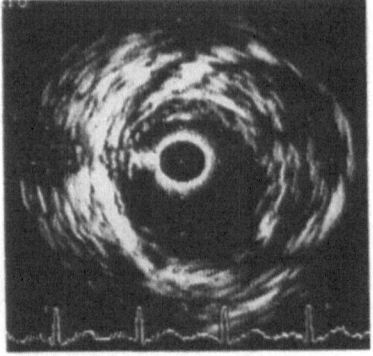

Luminal dimensions   **Cross-sectional images**
"Road-map"   **Luminal and vessel dimensions**
Native calcium   **Wall composition and motion**

Figure 1. Comparison of intravascular ultrasound (IVUS) and angiography. Angiography is a "road map" method, while IVUS allows for tomographic imaging of the lumen and vessel wall.

arteries and other vessels, like aorta or pulmonary arteries [9,10] (Figure 2). Either mechanical or electronical scanners connected to different echo-consoles are currently in use, with diameters of 2.9 -3.5 French for coronary arteries and up to 10 French for peripheral vessels and frequencies from 10 - 30 MHz [11]. For studies in the coronary circulation, the scanners are usually traced over 0.014 - 0.016" guide-wires. The images offer an axial resolution of about 150 - 200 μm and a radial resolution of about 200-400 μm in vivo, which is less than the calculated or measured values in vitro.

IVUS has been used with great success in a variety of indications. The following sections outline the possibilities and promises of IVUS in the understanding of the coronary anatomy in healthy and the coronary pathology in diseased hearts, as well as after heart transplantation (HTX). The second part will summarize the results of IVUS in conjunction with coronary interventions.

IVUS in normal coronary arteries

Most results of IVUS imaging confirm knowledge already published by pathologists two and more decades ago. However, IVUS allows now to study these findings in patients and normal individuals.

VUS has the capability to distinguish between muscular (i.e. coronary arteries, external iliac and femoral arteries) and elastic arteries like the aorta and the pulmonary arteries. IVUS is capable to discover intimal thickening, if it exceeds 150 - 200 μm. The intimal thickening increases with age, with average values of 60 μm from 1 - 5 years, 220 μm at 30 and 250 μm at 40 years, which leads to a typical three-layer appearance of the coronary arteries [12-15]. The value of

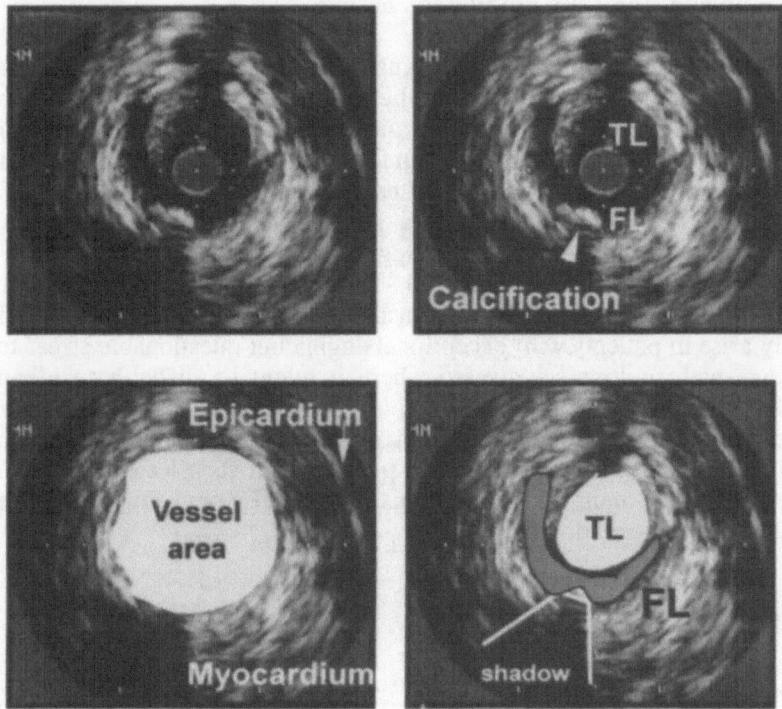

Figure 2. IVUS allows the assessment of complex coronary artery anatomy, like in a patient with circular coronary artery dissection (TL=true lumen, FL = False lumen). Luminal, vessel and adjacent structures are outlined.

intimal thickening should not exceed 300 μm but those values might be higher at bifurcations. This process of intimal thickening seems to be different from the development of atherosclerosis [3]. The image generation of echo images depends on changes in acoustic impedance. Not surprisingly, the lumen-intima border and the media - external elastica lamina can be imaged in great detail, while the external elastica lamina-adventitia border almost never can be distinguished. The same finding is true for the internal elastica lamina. Despite this limitation, IVUS is at present the only method to determine the plaque area and the true percent area stenoses in vivo. IVUS allows the determination of the vessel and lumen size in vivo. In healthy persons, the left coronary system tapers from origin along their length, but the right coronary artery remains constant in diameter until the crux cordis. In patients with beginning of coronary artery disease, IVUS will become positive as early as Stary lesions type 3. Additionally, the compensatory enlargement of coronary arteries during the process of plaque growth, the Glagov principle, could be confirmed by IVUS studies [16,17].

IVUS in angiographically ambiguous lesions

IVUS has the competence to clarify angiographically ambiguous lesions [18]. Ambiguous lesion are often located at the ostium, at bifurcations or the origin of larger side branches. Furthermore, angiographically visualization might be impaired by contrast over- or underflow, by vessel overlapping, or foreshortening. Mintz et al. [19] and Lee et al. [20] reported about a change in approximately 20% of patients with a pre-interventional IVUS study. In our institution, ambiguous lesions are a regular indication to perform IVUS, but lesions with a diameter reduction of 50 - 70% on angiography are often difficult to assess in their functional significance, even after IVUS. These difficulties typically arise in patients with exceptional angina but questionable stress tests, or in patients with multivessel disease where it might be difficult to identify the functional "culprit" lesion. In unclear IVUS results, the estimation of flow reserve after vasodilatation or measurements of the transstenotic pressure gradient is often helpful for decision making in patients with such lesions [21]. The aim for the near future must be the combination of IVUS and Doppler or pressure transducers in a single device.

IVUS in left main disease

Patients with left main (LMCA) disease have a higher incidence of coronary syndromes and an inferior prognosis. Unfortunately, the origin of the left coronary circulation is often difficult to visualize by angiography alone, due to contrast overflow, positioning of the catheter distal to a very proximal lesion or poor image quality by overprojection with the vertebra column. Therefore, various groups investigated the usefulness of IVUS in left mainstem disease [13,22-24]. All showed a higher sensitivity of IVUS to detect left main disease in comparison to angiography, with positive findings in up to 45% of patients studied. Additionally, the coronary artery remodelling with compensatory enlargement as published by Glagov could be verified in vivo by IVUS studies. The discovery of angiographically "occult" left main stem disease may change the therapeutic approach from invasive cardiology to surgical intervention in selected patients [25] (Figure 3).

IVUS in muscle bridging

Patients with muscle bridging present often with exertional angina, do not profit from therapy with nitroglycerin, and present with varying anatomical signs during coronary angiography. Myocardial bridging is described in angiography in 0.5 to 2.5 % of unselected patients. In comparison to pathologic studies, the incidence of muscle bridges is usually underestimated by angiography. While some patients show the typical picture of systolic compression, many are misdiagnosed as having a "normal" coronary angiogram or "spasm". Especially without a pharmacologic challenge like the injection of nitroglycerin or catecholamines. Ge et al. showed the outstanding ability of IVUS for diagnosis

Plaque Rupture Left Main

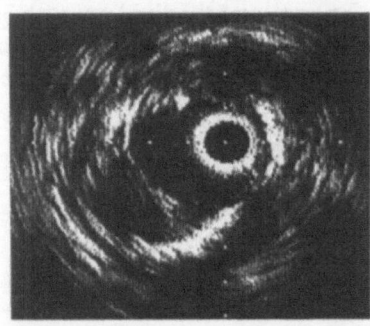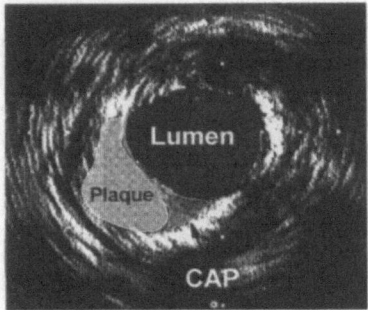

Figure 3. Plaque rupture in the left main in a patient with unstable angina. Ruptured lipid cap and remodelling of the left main with large total vessel area.
(For colour plate of figure 3 see page 563)

of muscle bridging [26,27]. A typical "milking" pattern can be found in these patients in the IVUS image. By a computer assisted automated contour detection, pulsatile variation during cardiac cycle of the normal segment and bridge segment can be quantified. It could be shown that the pulsatile variation of the normal segment is $9\pm7\%$, while the shape change in the bridge segment is $40\pm25\%$. Moreover, the maximal lumen of the bridge segment is seen in mid-diastole rather than in end-systole. Additionally, IVUS revealed the presence of plaque formation at the beginning of the muscle bridge in 45% of all patients with muscle bridging. Further studies will focus on the monitoring of pharmacologic interventions in patients with muscle bridging.

Coronary aneurysm and plaque rupture

Coronary aneurysm is defined as a local coronary artery enlargement with a diameter 1.5 to 2 times larger than that of the adjacent proximal reference segment. The understanding of this syndrome is important because serious complications such as rupture, thrombosis or distal embolization with myocardial infarction occur frequently. As pointed out above, the reference segment is often not normal. Coronary angiography is not able to differentiate true aneurysms and pseudo-aneurysms as the arterial wall is not visualized. We observed in 15% of our patients with angiographically defined aneurysms plaque ruptures.
Pathologic studies have shown that plaque disruption may lead to thrombus formation and can contribute to acute coronary syndromes such as unstable angina, myocardial infarction, and sudden death [2,3]. Analysis of coronary arteries in patients who died of ischemic heart disease showed a morphology consistent with previously healed fissures with various stages of thrombosis and thrombus organization, suggesting that most fissurings probably reseal and incorporate thrombus at the same time but do not produce clinical symptoms.

With the use of IVUS, this process can be demonstrated in vivo [28-31]. Even plaque at an assumed high risk for rupture can be detected with a large lipid core and a thin fibrous cap. We found that plaques are going to rupture (plaque at risk) when the fibrous cap is thinner than 0.5 mm and the lipid core/plaque ratio greater than 20%. However, the capabilities of IVUS to measure very thin "caps" are limited and IVUS is likely to overestimate the true thickness (Figure 4).

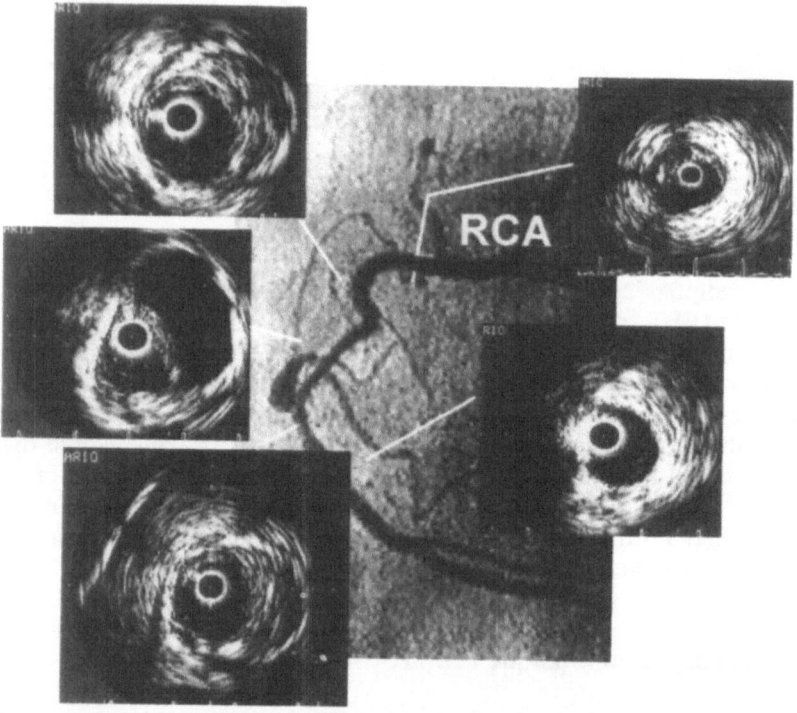

Figure 4. Complex coronary anatomy in a patient with ruptured plaque in his mid right coronary artery and unstable angina. The proximal and distal parts of the RCA show also eccentric plaque (proximal) and focal calcification (distal RCA).

IVUS after in transplanted hearts

Transplant vasculopathy is the main limiting factor of patients after the initially successful procedure. IVUS is the new standard in the evaluation of transplanted hearts. IVUS seems to be safe in patients with transplanted hearts [32,33]. Pinto et al. did not find an accelerated progression of transplant vasculopathy in coronary arteries studied by IVUS [34].

Coronary "Syndrome X"

Since the introduction of diagnostic coronary angiography, patients with chest pain but with normal coronary angiograms were considered as syndrome X. In a group of 44 patients with chest pain and normal coronary angiograms, we found plaque formation in 48% of the patients [35]. Most of the plaques (87%) were eccentric and only 16% calcified. Based on the detection of plaque formation by IVUS and reduction of coronary flow reserve by intracoronary Doppler, Erbel et al. divided these patients into four groups. Just 36% of all patients studied had no evidence of atherosclerosis and a normal coronary flow reserve. Consequently, only patients without plaque formation and reduced coronary flow reserve can be considered as coronary "Syndrome X" patients [34]. Additionally, IVUS provides morphological evidence of early signs of atherosclerosis in a large part of the patients which were previously considered as pure "Syndrome X" patients. It explains the reason why angiography cannot detect the early signs of atherosclerosis and the large discrepancy in results in patients. However, at present it is not clear, if atherosclerotic lesions seen in patients with angina or positive stress tests but normal flow reserve and angiography, can explain the clinical symptoms.

Tissue characterization

Whereas IVUS offers detailed morphology of the atherosclerotic lesions, it is sometimes difficult to differentiate the tissue characteristics e.g. thrombus from soft plaque. Frimerman et al. recently demonstrated that IVUS can differentiate thrombi with different composition [36]. They concluded that platelet-rich thrombi are echolucent, and the main echogenic structures of thrombi originates from red blood cells. Lee et al. indicates that thrombus presents a fine, homogeneous speckled pattern or a smooth pedunculated appearance, whereas plaque is an intrinsic component of the arterial wall and a more heterogeneous reflector of echo signals [37]. We noticed that fresh thrombus is characterized by a mobile appearance during IVUS imaging.

Three-dimensional reconstruction

IVUS provides information of the vessel wall in cross section. In order to better understand the spatial orientation of the plaques and to quantify the plaque volumes, it is essential to reconstruct the IVUS images in three dimensions [38-40]. Although the basic principle for three-dimensional reconstruction is known and studies were done over the last several years, yet some of the technical problems remain unsolved. This is mainly related to pulsation of the artery, catheter rotation and spatial orientation [41]. In fact, the present socalled three-dimensional reconstruction is not truly three-dimensional for the entire coronary artery studied but only for very short segments. Just recently, the first report on a true three-dimensional reconstruction with advanced registration of biplane coronary angiography has been published [42]. In the future, regression-progression studies will depend on the high reproducibilty of IVUS measurements [43]. Additional impact on three-dimensional reconstruction can be expected by the development of steerable and forward-looking IVUS catheters [44,45].

Evaluation of the development of atherosclerosis

Stary classified the development of atherosclerosis into seven stages for coronary and eight stages for peripheral lesions by pathologic examinations [3]. It is now possible to identify these stages from Stary (II)-III to VIII in patients by IVUS [25,46]. A normal coronary artery presents itself in an IVUS image with a monolayer appearance. Because the resolution of the IVUS catheter used today is approximately 150-200 μm, IVUS is not able to differentiate Stary I and early Stary II lesions from normal coronary arteries. Stary III lesions are portrayed in IVUS image with eccentric focal intimal thickening or three-layer appearance. Stary IV lesions (atheroma) can clearly be identified and Stary V lesions (fibroatheroma) are presented with a lipid core. Patients with Stary VI plaques may present with acute clinical syndromes such as unstable angina, acute myocardial infarction [47]. Therefore, the diagnosis of this stage is important as timely treatment may improve prognosis. Stary VII and VIII are going to stabilize, but are the final stages of the atherosclerosis.

IVUS in acute myocardial infarction

IVUS in acute myocardial infarction is useful as a diagnostic and therapeutic device, leading to recanalization by its "dottering" effect. Bocksch et al. reported of patients with pre-PTCA IVUS in acute myocardial infarction [48]. The studies were safe, and IVUS was able to characterize the geometry of the target lesion and to allow the detection of calcium in many patients. Nevertheless, the differentiation of thrombus from plaque was not possible in most cases, and only indirect markers like "foot-prints" of the IVUS catheter in the thrombus allowed to differentiate between both. The therapeutic approach was not changed by IVUS.

While Bocksch et al. reported mainly on patients with acute occlusions, IVUS in myocardial infarction may also identify patients with plaque rupture. In this patient population, the underlying lesion may be overlooked by angiography alone and the patient may be misdiagnozed of having "normal" coronary arteries [30,31].

IVUS and coronary interventions

The success of therapeutic interventions is mainly determined by the acute gain in free lumen, avoidance of acute complications, and the prevention of restenosis [49-51]. Acute complications are mainly related to the development of flow-limiting coronary artery dissections with or without thrombus formation. The two most important questions to be answered by IVUS in coronary interventions therefore are:

(1): can pre-interventional IVUS predict the outcome of the intervention; and
(2): can post-interventional IVUS optimize the result?
One principal problem is, that pre-interventional IVUS is only possible, if the lesion can be crossed before the intervention. Despite the small IVUS probes available today, pre-interventional IVUS often occludes the target lesion and may cause ischemic complications, although Alfonso et al. showed even a beneficial effect of pre-PTCA IVUS on minimal luminal diameter, increasing from 0.84 to 1.16 mm in patients with pre-PTCA IVUS studies using 4.8 French catheters [52].
The additional information from IVUS concerning lesion geometry and composition led to a different interventional strategy in 20% of cases, as reported by Mintz et al. The same group reported in 1,155 lesions on the presence and distribution of calcium, where IVUS was superior to angiography in revealing the presence, length, and arch of calcification [53]. The arch of calcification is predictive for the occurrence of dissections after PTCA. Rotablation instead of PTCA or atherectomy might be superior in patients with heavy calcification discovered during pre-interventional IVUS [54]. However, until present no study showed a superior outcome in patients with a pre-interventional IVUS compared to bare angiographic assessment. This is not a shortcoming of IVUS, but rather reflects the need for prospective studies addressing this question.
IVUS can reveal the vessel wall changes after PTCA (Figure 5). Several groups focused their interest on IVUS after PTCA to better understand the mechanisms

Proximal LAD

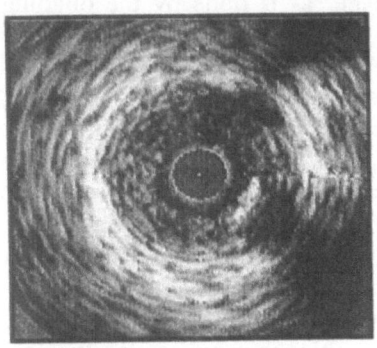
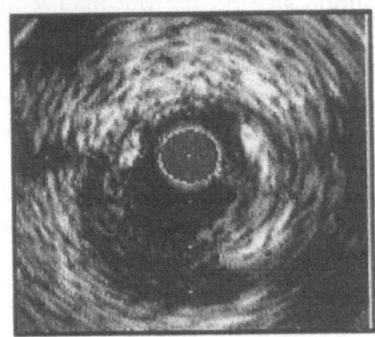

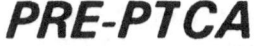

PRE-PTCA   **POST-PTCA**

Figure 5. IVUS before and after PTCA in an LAD lesion. Deep dissection with flap. Patient was symptomatic and a stent was implanted.

of the procedure and to find predictors of restenosis [55-60]. The findings in post-PTCA IVUS studies led to various classifications of the effect of balloon angioplasty on the vessel wall. The most detailed classification has been published by Gerber et al. It could be shown, that most lesions are eccentric in nature, and that tears and dissections are the main mechanisms leading to luminal enlargement, while stretching of the diseased free wall or plaque compression is found less frequently after PTCA (Figure 6).

The implication of the post-interventional morphologic description alone seems to be limited and interest focuses at present on the definition of residual stenosis by IVUS after angiographycally "optimal" PTCA [61,62]. Because of the limitations of angiography to reveal changes of the coronary artery wall, IVUS is at present the only method to measure exactly the residual area stenoses in vivo. Different groups showed an average residual stenosis of approximately 60% after PTCA [57,63-65].

The PICTURE trial (Post Intra-Coronary Treatment Ultrasound Restenosis Evaluation) is the first larger trial to be completed looking at ultrasound markers for restenosis. The results were discouraging, because in about 200 patients no correlation was found between various morphologic and dimensional parameters and the outcome of the patients [58]. On the contrary, the GUIDE II trial showed a significant predictive value of residual plaque burden and luminal cross-sectional area to predict restenosis [61]. Similar results were published by Mintz et al. who found a >50% restenosis rate in patients with a >70% area stenosis after PTCA [62]. In our group, the minimal residual stenosis assessed by IVUS, circular dissections after PTCA seen by IVUS, and the residual plaque area were IVUS-related markers for the development of restenosis [64].

Therefore, the future in PTCA seems to be an IVUS-guided approach, identifying patients with a "false-optimal" angiographic results. Modifications of PTCA to provide a larger increase in gained lumen are limited to higher balloon inflation pressures and larger balloons. However, a ratio of the reference segment to the expected balloon diameter of >1.1 leads to a higher complication rate without a clear benefit in long-term outcome [50]. An interesting approach is to select the balloon size on the pre-interventional IVUS image, as is done by the ongoing CLOUT trial by Hodgson et al. [66].

Patients with large residual stenosis after PTCA are a prime target for further "IVUS-guided" patient management, which could include the use of larger balloons, perfusion balloons, directional atherectomy (DCA) or coronary artery stents [67]. The mechanisms of action of perfusion balloons are incompletely understood, and preliminary IVUS data indicate that the main mechanism is the increase in lumen area and not the attachment of the dissection membrane [68]. Theoretically, IVUS has the potential to identify stenoses ideally treated by DCA (large plaque burden, "soft" plaque, no superficial calcium). IVUS analysis pre- and post-DCA showed that DCA does not depend on the presence of an eccentric lesion. In fact, DCA is most effective in large plaques, no matter whether eccentric or concentric in nature. In both types of lesions, IVUS imaging after the initial DCA cuts may be helpful to guide further and deeper cuts. But this more aggressive approach requires multiple exchanging of the equipment (IVUS versus DCA device) and prolongs the catheter laboratory time. To give a more precise answer to the usefulness of IVUS in DCA procedures, various ongoing trials

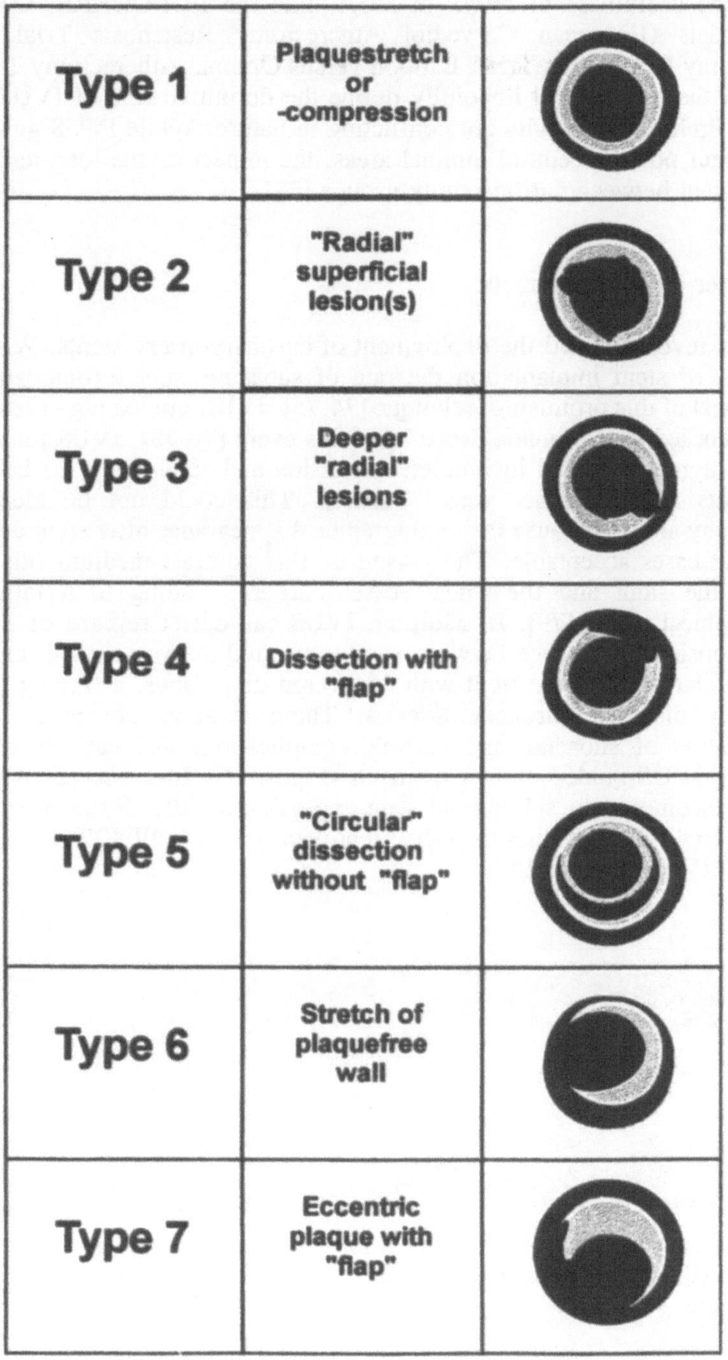

Figure 6. Seven types of vessel wall morphology can be found after PTCA. Types 1-4 occur in concentric, types 6 and 7 in eccentric lesions, while circular dissections can be found in either eccentric or concentric lesions.

address the usefulness of IVUS in DCA, like the EUROCARE, OARS, and BOAT trials (European Carvediol Atherectomy Restenosis Trial, Optimal Atherectomy Restensosis Trial, Balloon versus Optimal Atherectomy Trial). The results of these trails will hopefully define the definitive role of IVUS in DCA [69-72]. Preliminary results are conflicting in nature. While IVUS-guided DCA led to larger post-procedural luminal areas, the impact on the long-term success was different between various study groups [73].

IVUS after stent deployment

IVUS has revolutionized the deployment of coronary artery stents. While in the beginning of stent implantation the rate of subacute stent thrombosis was the achilles heal of this promising technique [74,75], IVUS-guided high pressure stent deployment led to a dramatic decrease of this event [76-78]. IVUS imaging after stent deployment showed incomplete expansion and echo free gaps between the stent struts and the inner vessel borders. This could not be identified by angiography alone, because the angiographical appearance after stent deployment is in most cases acceptable. The reason is, that contrast medium fills the gaps between the stent and the inner vessel borders, leading to a false-positive angiographical result [79]. In addition, IVUS can detect regions of incomplete stent expansion, free space between stent struts and the vessel wall, and regions proximal and distal to the stent with uncovered dissections, a finding often seen in heavily diseased coronary arteries. These findings are most likely the determinators of subacute and chronic complications and can be avoided by complete, IVUS-guided stent expansion (Figure 7). In a recent study, IVUS revealed incomplete or suboptimal stent expansion in 80% of the cases and even after the application of high pressure stent deployment, still 40% of patients had abnormal IVUS findings [80].

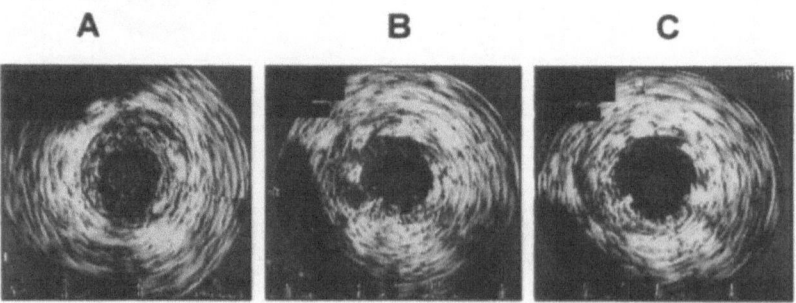

Figure 7. Stent implantation after PTCA for a restenotic lesion (A). Incomplete stent expansion (B) with additional, high pressure inflations leading to a further increasse in lumen area (C).

IVUS guided, high-pressure stent deployment led to a dramatic increase in mean minimal luminal area, with an increase from 4.58 mm² to 8.5 mm² seen in a population of 52 patients with high or low pressure stent deployment [81]. Based on this knowledge, beneficial results with high-pressure stent deployment alone but without IVUS have been reported [82]. Nevertheless, IVUS will most likely have its place in the future in all complicated stent deployments (long lesions, diffuse disease, very proximal or side-branch implantation) and during follow-up studies to reveal the amount of intimal hyperplasia within the stent.

Conclusion

IVUS has emerged from a research tool to a work-horse device in many laboratories. The fascination to image the vessel wall and complex vessel wall morphologies before and after coronary interventions has broadened the understanding of coronary artery pathology. IVUS helps to withhold interventions in a minority of patients with ambiguous lesions, and allows quantitative estimation of left mainstem involvement. It is at present the gold standard for evaluation of patients after heart transplantation. The main advantage of IVUS is to allow for rapid estimation of the effects of PTCA or DCA, in terms of quantification of luminal diameters and residual area stenosis, which can be determined exactly by IVUS only. The results of larger prospective studies currently underway addressing the effects of IVUS on device selection or the predictability of long-term results will give the answer to the cost-benefit ratio of peri-interventional intravascular ultrasound.

Acknowledgement

The continuous help of the catheterization laboratory staff for preparation of the IVUS studies is gratefully acknowledged.

References

1. Falk E. Plaque rupture with severe pre-existing stenosis precipitating coronary thrombosis. Characteristics of coronary atherosclerotic plaques underlying fatal occlusive thrombi. Br Heart J 1983;50:127-34.
2. Falk E, Shah PK, Fuster V. Coronary plaque disruption. Circulation 1995;92:657-71.
3. Stary HC, Chandler B, Dinsmore RE *et al.* A definition of advanced types of atherosclerotic lesions and a histological classification of atherosclerosis. A report from the Committee on Vascular Lesions of the Council on Arteriosclerosis, American Heart Association. Circulation 1995;92:1355-74.
4. Waller BF, Pinkerton CA, Slack JD. Intravascular ultrasound: a histological study of vessels during life. The new 'gold standard' for vascular imaging. Circulation 1992;85:2305-10.
5. Sones FM, Shirey EK. Cine coronary angiography. Mod Concepts Cardiovasc Dis 1962;31:735-8.
6. Hodgson JM, Graham SP, Savakus AD *et al.* Clinical percutaneous imaging of coronary anatomy using an over-the-wire ultrasound catheter system. Int J Card Imaging 1989;4:187-93.

7. Tobis JM, Yock PG, editors. Intravascular ultrasound imaging. New York, Churchill Livingston, 1992.

8. Yock PG, Linker DT, Angelsen BA. Two-dimensional intravascular ultrasound: technical development and initial clinical experience. J Am Soc Echocardiogr 1989;2:296-304.

9. Görge G, Erbel R, Gerber T *et al.* Intravasalar Ultraschall bei Patienten mit Verdacht aug Aortendissektion: Vergleich zur transesophagealen Echokardiographie. Z Kardiol 1992;81:37-43.

10. Görge G, Erbel R, Schuster S, Ge J, Meyer J. Intravascular ultrasound in diagnosis of acute pulmonary embolism [letter]. Lancet 1991;337:623-4.

11. Bom N, Lancee CT, van Egmond FC. An ultrasonic intracardiac scanner. Ultrasonics 1972;10:72-6.

12. Di Mario C, The SH, Madretsma S *et al.* Detection and characterization of vascular lesions by intravascular ultrasound: an in vitro study correlated with histology. J Am Soc Echocardiogr 1992;5:135-46.

13. Ge J, Erbel R, Gerber T *et al.* Intravascular ultrasound imaging of angiographically normal coronary arteries: a prospective study in vivo. Br Heart J 1994;71:572-8.

14. Hausmann D, Lundkvist AJ, Friedrich G, Sudhir K, Fitzgerald PJ, Yock PG. Lumen and plaque shape in atherosclerotic coronary arteries assessed by in vivo intracoronary ultrasound. Am J Cardiol 1994;74:857-63.

15. Nissen SE, Gurley JC, Grines CL *et al.* Intravascular ultrasound assessment of lumen size and wall morphology in normal subjects and patients with coronary artery disease. Circulation 1991;84:1087-99.

16. Ge J, Erbel R, Zamorano J *et al.* Coronary artery remodeling in atherosclerotic disease: An intravascular ultrasonic study in vivo. Coron Artery Dis 1993;4:981-6.

17. Glagov S, Weisenberg E, Zarins CK, Stankunavicius R, Kolettis GJ. Compensatory emlargement of human arherosclerotic coronary arteries. N Engl J Med 1987;316:1371-5.

18. Fortin DF, Spero LA, Cusma JT *et al.* Pitfalls in the determination of absolute dimensions uesing angiographic catheters as calibration devices in quantitative coornary angiography. Am J Cardiol 1991;68:1176-82.

19. Mintz GS, Pichard AD, Kovach JA *et al.* Impact of preintervention intravascular ultrasound imaging on transcatheter treatment strategies in coronary artery disease. Am J Cardiol 1994;73:423-30.

20. Lee DY, Eigler N, Luo H *et al.* Effect of intracoronary ultrasound imaging on clinical decision making. Am Heart J 1995;129:1084-93.

21. Di Mario C, de Feyter PJ, Slager CJ, de Jaegere P, Roelandt JR, Serruys PW. Intracoronary blood flow velocity and transstenotic pressure gradient using sensor-tip pressure and Doppler guidewires: a new technology for the assessment of stenosis severity in the catheterization laboratory. Cathet Cardiovasc Diagn 1993;28:311-9.

22. Davies SW, Winterton SJ, Rothman MT. Intravascular ultrasound to assess left main stem coronary artery lesion. Br Heart J 1992;68:524-6.

23. Gerber TC, Erbel R, Görge G, Ge J, Rupprecht HJ, Meyer J. Extent of atherosclerosis and remodeling of the left main coronary artery determined by intravascular ultrasound. Am J Cardiol 1994;73:666-71.

24. Hermiller JB, Buller CE, Tenaglia AN *et al.* Unrecognized left main coronary artery disease in patients undergoing interventional procedures. Am J Cardiol

1993;71:173-6.
25. Erbel R, Ge J, Görge G *et al*. Intravaskuläre Sonographie bei koronarer Herzkrankheit. Neue Aspekte zur Pathogenese. Dtsch Med Wochenschr 1995;120:847-54.
26. Erbel R, Rupprecht H, Ge J, Gerber T, Görge G, Meyer J. Coronary artery shape and flow changes induced by myocardial bridging. Echocardiography 1993;10:71-7.
27. Ge J, Erbel R, Rupprecht HJ *et al*. Comparison of intravascular ultrasound and angiography in the assessment of myocardial bridging. Circulation 1994;89:1725-32.
28. Erbel R, Ge J, Schümann D *et al*. Differentiation of coronary syndroms with intracoronary ultrasound. In: Roelandt JRTC, Gussenhoven EJ, Bom N, editors. Intravascular ultrasound. Dordrecht: Kluwer Academic Publishers, 1993:33-44.
29. Kearney P, Erbel R. Imaging in the catheterization laboratory. Curr Opin Cardiol 1993;8:988-99.
30. Kearney P, Erbel R, Ge J *et al*. Assessment of spontaneous coronary artery dissection by intravascular ultrasound in a patient with unstable angina. Cathet Cardiovasc Diagn 1994;32:58-61.
31. Zamorano J, Erbel R, Ge J *et al*. Spontaneous plaque rupture visualized by intravascular ultrasound. Eur Heart J 1994;15:131-3.
32. Kerber S, Rahmel A, Karbenn U *et al*. Allograft vasculopathy in the early phase of orthotopic heart transplantation: angiography, intravascular ultrasound and functional in vivo findings. Z Kardiol 1994;83:215-24.
33. St.-Goar FG, Pinto FJ, Alderman EL *et al*. Intracoronary ultrasound in cardiac transplant recipients. In vivo evidence of "angiographically silent" intimal thickening. Circulation 1992;85:979-87.
34. Pinto FJ, St.-Goar FG, Gao SZ *et al*. Immediate and one-year safety of intracoronary ultrasonic imaging. Evaluation with serial quantitative angiography. Circulation 1993;88:1709-14.
35. Erbel R, Ge J, Rupprecht HJ, Görge G, Gerber T. Intravascular ultrasound and Doppler in angiographically normal coronary arteries [abstract]. Circulation 1992;86(Suppl.I):I-122.
36. Frimerman A, Miller HI, Hallman M, Laniado S, Keren G. Intravascular ultrasound characterization of thrombi of different composition. Am J Cardiol 1994;73:1053-7.
37. Lee DY, Eigler N, Fishbein MC, Bhambi B, Maurer G, Siegel RJ. Identification of intracoronary thrombus and demonstration of thrombectomy by intravascular ultrasound imaging. Am J Cardiol 1994;73:522-3.
38. Cavaye DM, White RA, Kopchok GE, Mueller MP, Maselly MJ, Tabbara MR. Three-dimensional intravascular ultrasound imaging of normal and diseased canine and human arteries. J Vasc Surg 1992;16:509-17.
39. Mintz GS, Pichard AD, Satler LF, Popma JJ, Kent KM, Leon MB. Three-dimensional intravascular ultrasonography: reconstruction of endovascular stents in vitro and in vivo. J Clin Ultrasound 1993;21:609-15.
40. Rosenfield K, Losordo DW, Ramaswamy K *et al*. Three-dimensional reconstruction of human coronary and peripheral arteries from images recorded during two-dimensional intravascular ultrasound examination. Circulation 1991;84:1938-56.
41. Roelandt JR, di-Mario C, Pandian NG *et al*. Three-dimensional reconstruction of intracoronary ultrasound images. Rationale, approaches, problems, and

directions. Circulation 1994;90:1044-55.

42. Evans JL, Ng K-H, Wiet SG *et al*. Accurate three-dimensional reconstruction of intravascular data. Spatially correct three-dimensional reconstructions. Circulation 1996;93:567-76.

43. Von Birgelen C, di Mario C, Li W *et al*. Volumetric quantification by intracoronary ultrasound. In: de Feyter PJ, di Mario C, Serruys PW, editors. Quantitative coronary imaging. Delft: Barjesteh, Meeuwes & Co, 1995:211-23.

44. Görge G, Ge J, Haude M, Baumgart D, Buck T, Erbel R. Initial experience with a steerable intravascular ultrasound catheter in the aorta and pulmonary artery. Am J Card Imagaging 1995;9:180-4.

45. Ng KH, Evans JL, Vonesh MJ *et al*. Arterial imaging with a new forward-viewing intravascular ultrasound catheter, II. Three-dimensional reconstruction and display of data. Circulation 1994;89:718-23.

46. Hausmann D, Mugge A, Daniel WG. Die Form atherosklerotischer Koronarplaques: Pathoanatomische Konzepte und neue Einblicke mittels intravaskularen Ultraschalls. Z Kardiol 1994;83:717-26.

47. Ge J, Erbel R, Gorge G *et al*. Intravascular ultrasound imaging of arterial wall architecture. Echocardiography 1992;9:475-83.

48. Bocksch WG, Schartl M, Beckmann SH, Dreysse S, Paeprer H. Intravascular ultrasound imaging in patients with acute myocardial infarction: comparison with chronic stable angina pectoris. Coron Artery Dis 1994;5:727-35.

49. De Feyter PJ, van den Brand M, Jaarman G, van Domburg R, Serruys PW, Suryapranata H. Acute coronary artery occlusion during and after percutaneous transluminal coronary angioplasty. Frequency, prediction, clinical course, management, and follow-up. Circulation 1991;83:927-36.

50. Roubin GS, Douglas JS Jr, King SB III *et al*. Influence of balloon size on initial success, acute complications, and restenosis after percutaneous transluminal coronary angioplasty. A prospective randomized study. Circulation 1988;78:557-65.

51. Zijlstra F, den Boer A, Reiber JHC, Van-Es GA, Lubsen J, Serruys PW. Assessment of immediate and long-term functional results of percutaneous transluminal coronary angioplasty. Circulation 1988;78:15-24.

52. Alfonso F, Macaya C, Goicolea J *et al*. Angiographic changes induced by intracoronary ultrasound imaging before and after coronary angioplasty. Am Heart J 1993;125:877-80.

53. Mintz GS, Popma JJ, Pichard AD *et al*. Patterns of calcification in coronary artery disease. A statistical analysis of intravascular ultrasound and coronary angiography in 1155 lesions. Circulation 1995;91:1959-65.

54. Matar FA, Mintz GS, Pinnow E *et al*. Multivariate predictors of intravascular ultrasound end points after directional coronary atherectomy. J Am Coll Cardiol 1995;25:318-24.

55. Gerber TC, Erbel R, Görge G, Ge J, Rupprecht HJ, Meyer J. Classification of morphologic effects of percutaneous transluminal coronary angioplasty assessed by intravascular ultrasound. Am J Cardiol 1992;70:1546-54.

56. Görge G, Erbel R, Gerber TC, Ge J, Trauth B, Meyer J. Morphologic findings by intravascular ultrasound and clinical outcome after PTCA [abstract]. Circulation 1992;84(Suppl.I):I-518

57. Honye J, Mahon DJ, Jain A *et al*. Morphological effects of coronary balloon angioplasty in vivo assessed by intravascular ultrasound imaging. Circulation 1992;85:1012-25.

58. Peters RJG. Prediction of the risk of angiographic restenosis by intracoronary ultrasound imaging after coronary balloon angioplasty [abstract]. J Am Coll Cardiol 1995;25(Special Issue):35A-36A.

59. Tenaglia AN, Buller CE, Kisslo KB, Phillips HR, Stack RS, Davidson CJ. Intracoronary ultrasound predictors of adverse outcomes after coronary artery interventions. J Am Coll Cardiol 1992;20:1385-90.

60. Tenaglia AN, Buller CE, Kisslo KB, Stack RS, Davidson CJ. Mechanisms of balloon angioplasty and directional coronary atherectomy as assessed by intracoronary ultrasound. J Am Coll Cardiol 1992;20:685-91.

61. The GUIDE Trial investigators. IVUS-determined predictors of restenosis in PTCA and DCA: an interim report from the GUIDE trail, phase II [abstract]. Circulation 1994;90(4 pt 2):I-23.

62. Mintz G, Chang YC, Popma JJ *et al*. The final percent cross-sectional narrowing (residual plaque burden) is the strongest intravascular ultrasound predictor of angiographic restenosis [abstract]. J Am Coll Cardiol 1995;25 (Special Issue):35A.

63. Gerber TC, Erbel R, Görge G, Ge J, Rupprecht H-J, Meyer J. Classification of morphologic effects of percutaneous transluminal coronary angioplasty assessed by intravascular ultrasound. Am J Cardiol 1992;70:1546-54.

64. Görge G, Liu F, Ge J, Haude M, Baumgart D, Caspari G. Intravascular ultrasound variables predict restenosis after PTCA [abstract]. Circulation 1995;92(Suppl.I):I-148.

65. Jain SP, Jain A, Collins TJ, Ramee SR, White CJ. Predictors of restenosis: A morphometric and quantitative evaluation by intravascular ultrasound. Am Heart J 1994;128:664-73.

66. Hodgson JMcB, Stone GW, Linnemeier TJ, Sheehan HM, St. Goar FG, Berry JL. Oversized balloons defined by intracoronary ultrasound results in dramatic improvements in angioplasty results: initial ultrasound analysis of the CLOUT pilot study [abstract]. Eur Heart J 1995;16(Abstract Suppl):427.

67. Serruys PW, de-Jaegere P, Kiemeneij F *et al*. A comparison of balloon-expandable-stent implantation with balloon angioplasty in patients with coronary artery disease. Benestent Study Group. N Engl J Med 1994;331:489-95.

68. Görge G, Erbel R, Haude M *et al*. Continous coronary perfusion balloon catheters in coronary dissections after percutaneous transluminal coronary angioplasty. Acute clinical results and 6-months follow-up. Eur Heart J 1994;15:908-14.

69. Aretz HT, Gregory KW, Martinelli MA *et al*. Ultrasound guidance of laser atherectomy. Int J Card Imaging 1991;6:231-7.

70. Fitzgerald PJ, Yock PG. Mechanisms and outcomes of angioplasty and atherectomy assessed by intravascular ultrasound imaging. J Clin Ultrasound 1993;21:579-88.

71. Mintz GS, Pichard AD, Popma JJ, Kent KM, Satler LF, Leon MB. Preliminary experience with adjunct directional coronary atherectomy after high-speed rotational atherectomy in the treatment of calcific coronary artery disease. Am J Cardiol 1993;71:799-804.

72. Suneja R, Nair RN, Reddy KG, Rasheed Q, Sheehan HM, Hodgson JM. Mechanisms of angiographically successful directional coronary atherectomy: evaluation by intracoronary ultrasound and comparison with transluminal coronary angioplasty. Am Heart J 1993;126:507-14.

73. Nakamura S, Mahon DJ, Leung CY *et al*. Intracoronary ultrasound imaging

before and after directional coronary atherectomy: in vitro and clinical observations. Am Heart J 1995;129:841-51.

74. Haude M, Erbel R, Straub U, Dietz U, Meyer J. Short and long term results after intracoronary stenting in human coronary arteries: monocentre experience with the balloon-expandable Palmaz-Schatz stent. Br Heart J 1991;66:337-45.

75. Sigwart U, Puel J, Mirkovitch V, Joffre F, Kappenberger L. Intravascular stents to prevent occlusion and restenosis after transluminal angioplasty. N Engl J Med 1987;316:701-6.

76. Colombo A, Goldberg SL, Almagor Y, Maiello L, Finci L. A novel strategy for stent deployment in the treatment of acute or threatened closure complicating balloon coronary angioplasty. Use of short or standard (or both) single or multiple Palmaz-Schatz stents. J Am Coll Cardiol 1993;22:1887-91.

77. Mudra H, Klauss V, Blasini R *et al*. Ultrasound guidance of Palmaz-Schatz intracoronary stenting with a combined intravascular ultrasound balloon catheter. Circulation 1994;90:1252-61.

78. Nakamura S, Colombo A, Gaglione A *et al*. Intracoronary ultrasound observations during stent implantation. Circulation 1994;89:2026-34.

79. Blasini R, Schühlen H, Mudra H *et al*. Angiographic overestimation of lumen size after coronary stent placement: Impact of high pressure dilatation [abstract]. Circulation 1995;92(Suppl.I):I-223.

80. Serruys PW, Di Mario C. Who was the thrombogenic: the stent or the doctor? Circulation 1995;91:1676-88.

81. Görge G, Haude M, Ge J *et al*. Intravascular ultrasound after low and high inflation pressure coronary artery stent implantation. J Am Coll Cardiol 1995;26:725-30.

82. Morice MC, Breton C, Bunouf P *et al*. Coronary stenting without anticoagulation, without intravascular ultrasound. Results of the french registry [abstract]. Circulation 1995;92(Suppl.I):I-796.

24. To which extent can the coronary artery tree be imaged and quantified with the current MR technology?

ALBERT C. VAN ROSSUM & JOHANNES C. POST

*** Adapted with permission from Herz 1996;21:97-105. Coronary imaging using MRI, by AC van Rossum, JC Post, CA Visser.***

Summary

Without use of ionizing radiation and injection of contrast material magnetic resonance (MR) imaging can be applied to generate signal from flowing blood and create tomographic images of the blood stream in coronary arteries, which resemble conventional contrast enhanced x-ray angiograms. The tortuosity, small diameter and motion of the coronary arteries provided technically demanding problems, which had to be solved before MR coronary angiography became realistic. Faster pulse sequences, dedicated radiofrequency receiver coils, cardiac and respiratory gating techniques were introduced and are still in the process of constant development to improve the quality of the images.

To date, most clinical experience has been obtained using two-dimensional (2D) approaches, necessitating repetitive breath-holds to encompass the coronary artery tree. A substantial part of the proximal and middle parts of the coronary arteries can be visualized, which has proven to be accurate in identifying anomalous coronary anatomy and patency of proximal coronary artery bypass grafts. With respect to detection of coronary artery disease, studies in limited numbers of patients indicate that the sensitivity for detection of stenoses > 50% of luminal diameter narrowing is high in left main disease, moderate in LAD and RCA disease, and low in LCX disease.

Another approach is a single acquisition respiratory gated three-dimensional (3D) technique which is less operator and patient dependent, requires less imaging time for an entire coronary protocol and is more comfortable for the patient than the 2D breath-hold approach. Initial experience demonstrates the capability to identify the major epicardial coronary vessels to at least a similar extent as with the 2D technique. But here too, further development is required to demonstrate coronary stenoses.

It can be envisaged that, although currently not apt to replace conventional coronary angiography, MR coronary angiography will become of use in the evaluation of specific, well defined clinical issues in coronary artery disease.

Introduction

Since its introduction in the clinical field during the last decade, MR imaging has proven to be of value in the diagnosis of a variety of cardiovascular diseases.

J.H.C. Reiber and E.E. van der Wall (eds.), Cardiovascular Imaging, 301-314.
© 1996 *Kluwer Academic Publishers.*

General advantages of this non-invasive technique include that the images are obtained without exposure to x-rays, with free choice of the orientation of tomographic imaging planes, and with a wide field of view. Thus, the information of the cardiovascular anatomy is basically three-dimensional and is shown in clear relation to surrounding structures.

Of importance to angiographic applications of MR is that blood flow can be manipulated to generate a MR signal. This signal can be used to create images of the blood stream in coronary arteries resembling conventional contrast enhanced x-ray angiography, without the necessity to inject contrast material. The MR blood signal can also be used to measure flow velocity and volume flow within the vessel. The capability of obtaining angiographic as well as functional information noninvasively, without contrast injection, is a very powerful combination which is likely to make MR imaging an important tool in the assessment of coronary artery disease.

Considerations in MR imaging of coronary arteries

Early studies which made use of conventional spin-echo and gradient-echo techniques reported that proximal parts of coronary arteries could be visualized occasionally [1-3]. However, for more consistent imaging of coronary arteries several technically demanding improvements with regard to hardware and pulse sequence design had to be made.

Spatial resolution and MR signal

The small calibre and tortuosity of the coronary vessels requires a high spatial resolution, preferably of less than 1 mm^3 per volume element (voxel). Although this goal, which technically is a function of the performance of the magnetic field gradients, is not yet achieved with the routine scan techniques, it has come within reach of the current state-of-the-art generation of MR scanners. Going to such high resolution images will decrease the signal within the voxel and the signal-to-noise ratio, which can be partially retrieved by using high field MR scanners (generally 1.5 to 2.0 Tesla) and locally applied radiofrequency receiver coils. Another problem which had to be addressed was the high signal generated by fat that surrounds the epicardial coronary arteries and hampers their identification. The introduction of fat suppression techniques by use of selective fat saturation radiofrequency pulses, greatly enhanced the contrast between intraluminal blood and surrounding epicardial fat.

Cardiac and respiratory motion

The quality of the MR images, which are usually acquired during several seconds or minutes, is negatively influenced by motion. The coronary vessels are subdue to the intrinsic motion from the cardiac cycle and to the displacement within the chest that results from respiration. Without adaptation of the imaging pulse sequences to these sources of motion, images of the heart and coronary vessels would suffer from severe artifacts and blurring.

The solution to deal with cardiac motion is to synchronize MR data acquisition with the ECG. Motion can be minimized when the acquisition window is set to middiastole, which is a period of relative diastasis.

Artifacts resulting from respiratory motion can be suppressed by acquiring data during breath-holding, thereby limiting the time available for imaging [4,5]. Alternatively, one can also synchronize the data acquisition with the respiratory cycle. This may be achieved by using a belt with sensors to monitor the thoraco-abdominal expansion [6]. More recently techniques have been introduced that rapidly image the cranio-caudal displacement of the diaphragm prior to the regular imaging radiofrequency pulse, thus allowing to reconstruct data obtained during a certain 'window' (generally the expiration phase) of the respiratory cycle [7,8]. These respiratory navigator techniques will allow the patient to breath freely without setting limitations to the available imaging time.

Fast MR imaging techniques

Whatever specific technique is used to image the coronary arteries, it is very clear that these techniques have to be fast in order to reduce the motion-associated problems. Rapid progress in this area is being made and several methods have been reported, although with only very limited clinical experience. The most widely used method is a fast segmented k-space gradient-echo technique applied during breath-holding [4,9-12]. Other techniques include interleaved spiral k-space imaging [5], subtraction techniques [13] and 3D data acquisition [8,14].

Two-dimensional MR coronary angiography

Technique

The presently most employed 2D MR angiographic technique was first described by Edelman et al. [4] and clinically applied by Manning et al. [9]. It consists of a fast flow-compensated gradient-echo sequence, using incremental flip angles, k-space segmentation and fat suppression. Using typical imaging parameters, such a technique will allow to obtain a single 2D image within 16 or 18 heart beats. The data are acquired within a time frame of 90-100 ms per heart beat, during middiastole to minimize the influence of cardiac motion. Respiratory motion is reduced by imaging within a breath-hold, usually during end-expiration. The latter is the most effective in obtaining a reproducible position of the heart, required to avoid misregistration between contiguous parallel slices. Patients may be positioned prone on a standard spine RF receiver coil, which is somewhat uncomfortable but has the advantage of a close proximity of the heart to the surface coil, restriction of the chest movements, and in our experience a decrease in the incidence of claustrophobia. However, newly developed coils using phased-array technology may favor a supine position. Typically, the in-plane resolution is 1.5-1.8 x 1 mm^2, with a slice thickness of 4 mm. Multiple series of oblique parallel slices are required to cover the tortuous course of each of the major proximal coronary arteries, which are then displayed in oscillating cine-loops for diagnostic evaluation. By overlapping the parallel slices (e.g. by 1 or 2 mm) misregistration is reduced. Recently we described a standardized protocol, derived from multiple three-dimensional data sets, to image the proximal coronary arteries with an optimal efficacy [15]. In that study a standard transverse imaging plane and a left-anterior-oblique equivalent plane proved to be valuable, whereas the right-anterior-oblique plane was of no use. Total examination time would require 45-60 minutes.

Advantages of the 2D breath-hold technique are the good image quality and the rapid on-screen availability of the images. Disadvantages include the need of repetitive breath-holds - which is strenuous for the patient and a source of misregistration -, the on-site requirement of operators with knowledge of the (pathological) coronary anatomy, the dependence on the skill and experience of the investigator, and the necessity of a regular heart rate.

Coronary artery length and diameter

Several studies using the 2D approach demonstrated that nearly all of the proximal segments of the major epicardial coronary arteries could be visualized (Figure 1) [9-11,16]. Most exceptions occurred for the left circumflex coronary artery (LCX), visualized in 76% [9], 77% [10], and 76% [11] respectively. This is mainly due to the posterior localization of the LCX, which is the coronary artery most distant from the RF receiver coil applied on the chest wall. The use

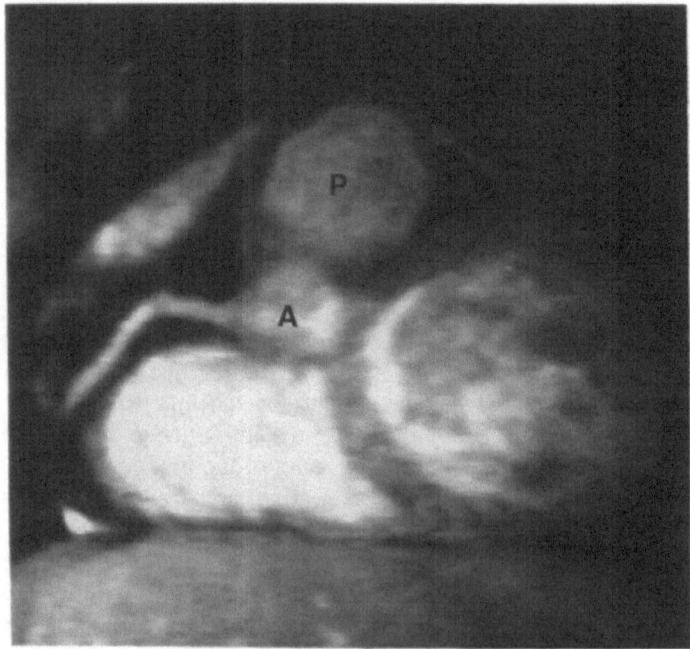

Figure 1. MR angiographic image of the right coronary artery obtained with a 2D breath-hold technique. Oblique coronal plane comparable to left anterior oblique view of x-ray angiography. A = aorta; P = pulmonary artery.

of newer multiple circularly polarized surface coils wrapped around the chest and coupled in an array may become beneficial in this respect [17]. Furthermore side branches of the right coronary artery (RCA), left anterior descending artery (LAD) and LCX were identified in 65%, 53% and 6% respectively [16]. Figures 2 and 3 show the mean lengths and diameters of the proximal coronary arteries as assessed by MR imaging in different centers.

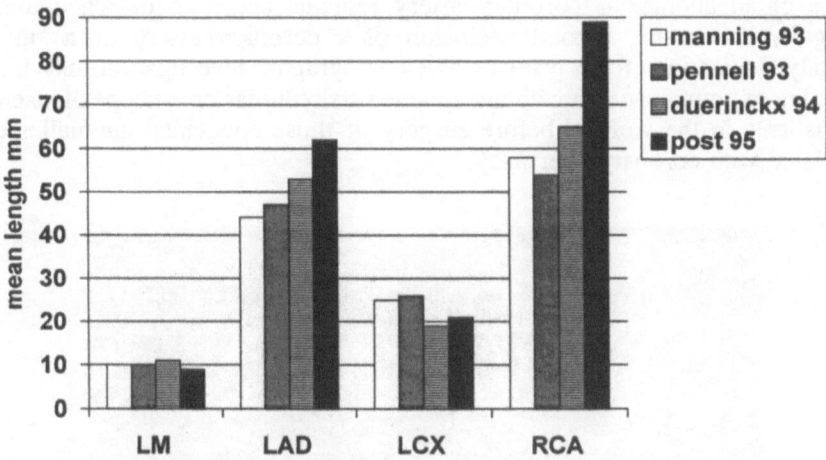

Figure 2. Mean lengths of coronary arteries as visualized with 2D breath-hold MR angiography in four studies [9-10,21].

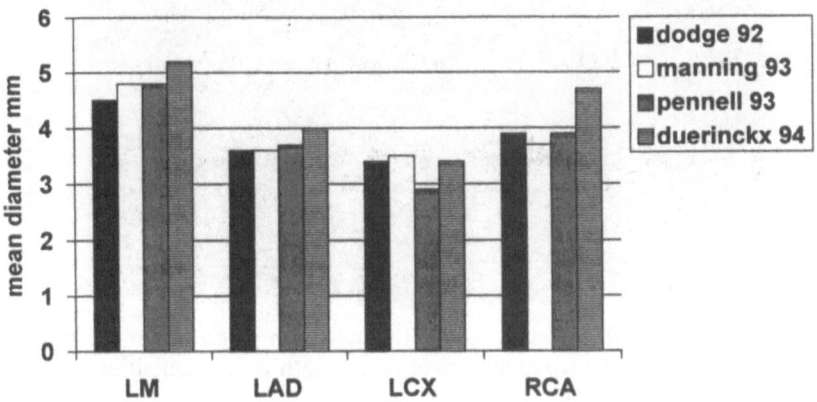

Figure 3. Mean diameters of proximal coronary arteries obtained with 2D breath-hold MR angiography in three studies [9-11] and compared to x-ray angiographic reference values reported by Dodge et al. [18].

Coronary artery anomalies

Two recent studies demonstrated the high accuracy of 2D MR angiography for

delineating the proximal course of anomalous coronary arteries [12,19]. MR
angiography proved especially useful when differentiation had to be made
between a prognostic 'low risk' retro-aortic, septal or anterior free wall course
and a 'high risk' interarterial course (Figure 4). The noninvasive MR assessment
was less ambiguous and had a higher interobserver agreement than the invasive
x-ray angiographic approach. Therefore, MR angiography may be clinically
indicated secondary to conventional contrast angiography when the proximal
course of an anomalous coronary artery remains uncertain or when there is
ambiguity concerning a total occlusion of a coronary artery or a 'missed'
anomaly. Indications for a primary MR angiographic investigation may include
screening of young patients with unexplained arrhythmias or syncope on exercise,
and patients in the workup before surgery of those congenital anomalies often
associated with coronary aberrancy.

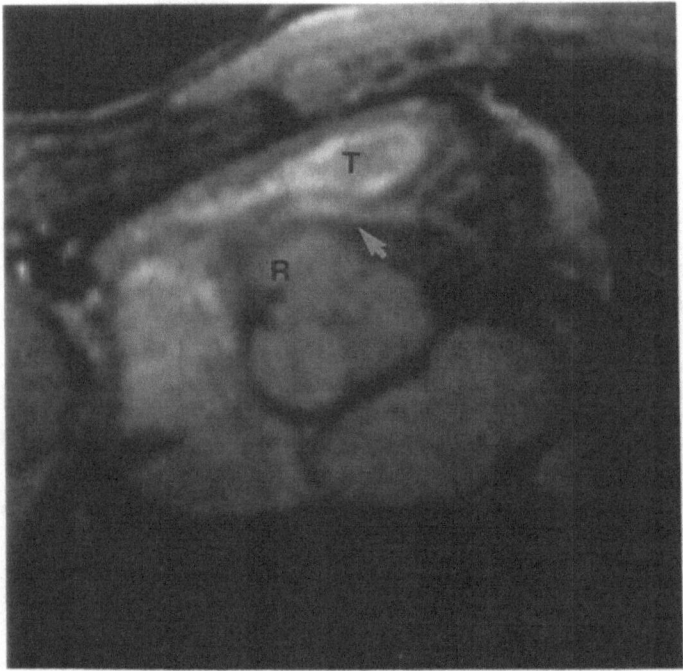

Figure 4. Anomalous left coronary artery (arrow) with origin from the right aortic
sinus (R) and interarterial proximal course (2D breath-hold acquisition). T = right
ventricular outflow tract.

Coronary artery stenoses

Because the spatial resolution and image quality of currently available human
studies is insufficient to reliably determine a coronary artery diameter narrowing,
assessment of coronary artery stenoses is based on detection of the attenuation or
complete loss of the normally bright intravascular blood signal [10,11,20,21].

This signal void is caused by turbulent flow in or distal to the stenosis (Figures 5 and 6). Thus, the detection of hemodynamically severe stenoses is based on aphysiological phenomenon rather than on a direct determination of the luminal narrowing. From this, one might expect that not only stenosis severity, but also other factors such as stenosis morphology, bending and branching, and collateral supply may be important determinants of flow disturbance and signal voids. MR angiographic signal voids therefore, do not necessarily have to correspond with stenoses based on luminal diameter narrowing as assessed by conventional contrast angiography. Table 1 is an overview of sensitivities and specificities reported in three comparative studies concerning the detection of x-ray angiographic stenosis >50% in the four major epicardial coronary arteries [10,20,21].

The variability of the results can be partially explained by bias from differing patient selection criteria, but it also reflects the present lack of robustness of the MR coronary angiography technique and of its data analysis. Pitfalls leading to false negative results include misinterpretation of pericardium or veins and collateral blood supply, whereas misregistration between overlapping slices due to inconsistent breath-holding and noisy images may lead to false positive results. In its present state 2D MR coronary angiography can not yet be considered a reasonable alternative to conventional angiography for imaging of coronary artery stenoses.

Nonetheless, subcategories of patients with coronary artery disease may already benefit from MR coronary angiography. Hundley et al. [22] recently described the use of cine MR angiography in combination with presaturating pulses to determine the patency and direction of flow in the infarct related artery. Also, in patients with coronary artery bypass vein grafts, patency of proximal graft segments can be predicted with a high accuracy using conventional MR techniques (Table 2) [23-29]. Coronary artery bypass stenoses, however, are difficult to predict and it is likely that results in these patients will further improve using the newer 2D MR angiography techniques.

Three-dimensional MR coronary angiography

Techniques

As in 2D imaging, 3D data are acquired during middiastole by means of ECG gating. Imaging of the 3D data set requires more time than imaging of a single 2D image, and therefore breath-holding is not feasible. In an early study respiratory motion artifacts were reduced by averaging multiple data acquisitions [14]. A further refinement was obtained by using respiratory navigator echoes of the position of the diaphragm, followed by reconstruction of the end-expiratory acquired data [8]. Thus, within 10-13 minutes, a volume-slab is imaged of e.g. 30 x 30 x 6.4 cm^3 with a spatial resolution of 1 x 2 x 2 mm^3. The slab is positioned to encompass the aortic root and the proximal coronary arteries. Using multiplanar reformatting software, contiguous thin sections can be reconstructed on a 3D workstation in any desired orientation to optimally display the coronary arteries (Figure 7). To visualize distal parts of the coronary arteries one or two

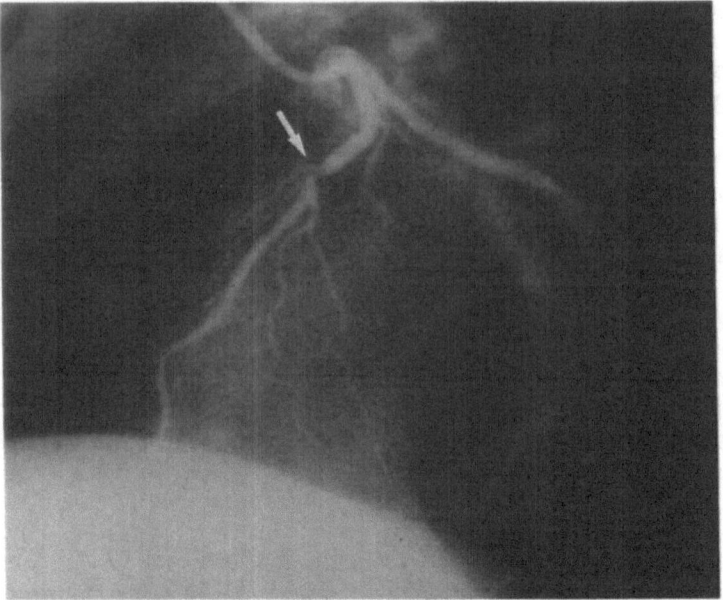

a

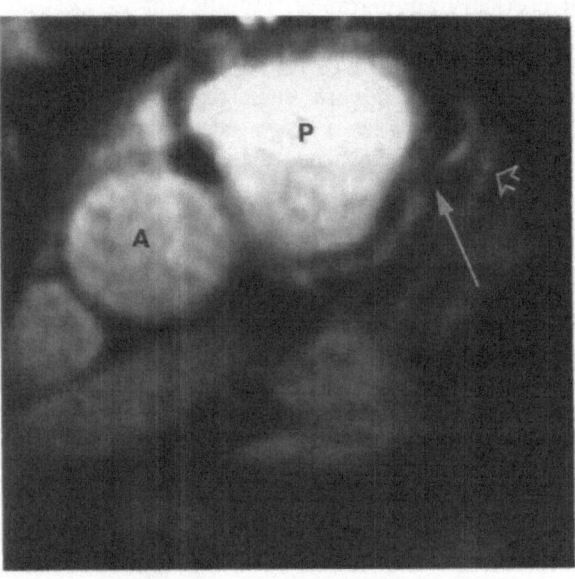

b

Figure 5. A) Left anterior oblique projection by x-ray coronary angiography of a significant LAD stenosis (arrow). B) Transverse image obtained by 2D breath-hold MR coronary angiography demonstrating a signal void at the site of the LAD stenosis (arrow). The great cardiac vein (open arrow) is visualized parallel and left lateral from the LAD. A = aorta; P = pulmonary artery.

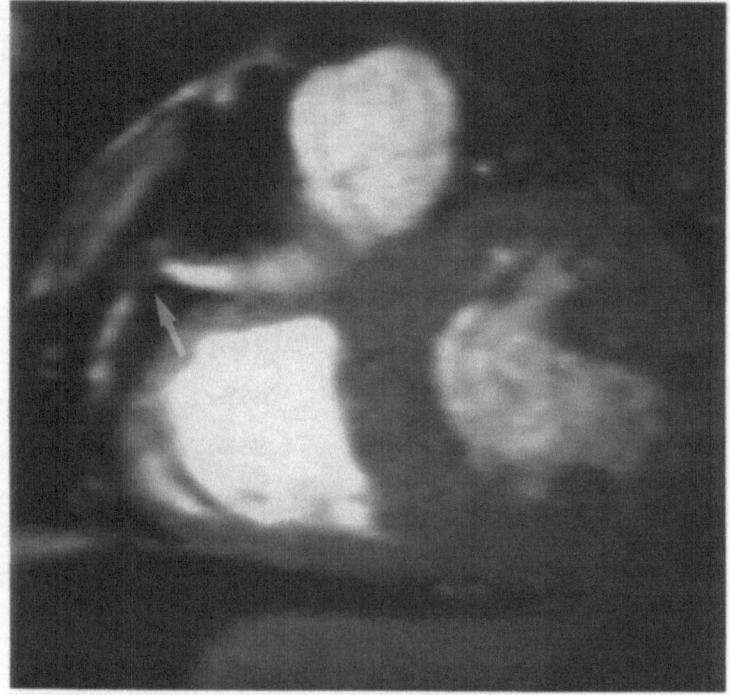

Figure 6. Signal void due to stenosis (arrow) in the proximal right coronary artery (2D breath-hold acquisition).

Table 1. Sensitivity (sens) and specificity (spec) of 2D MR angiography in detection of coronary artery stenoses >50%.

Reference	LM		LAD		LCX		RCA	
	sens	spec	sens	spec	sens	spec	sens	spec
Manning [20]	100%	100%	87%	92%	71%	90%	100%	78%
Duerinckx [10]	50%	84%	73%	37%	0%	82%	62%	56%
Post [21]	100%	93%	53%	73%	0%	96%	71%	82%

LM = left main; LAD = left anterior descending coronary artery; LCX = left circumflex coronary artery; RCA = right coronary artery

Table 2. Detection of bypass graft patency using conventional 2D MRI.

Reference	technique	no. of grafts	sensitivity	specificity	accuracy
White et al. [23]	SE-MRI	65	91%	72%	86%
Rubinstein et al. [24]	SE-MRI	44	92%	85%	89%
Jenkins et al. [25]	SE-MRI	60	90%	90%	90%
Frija et al. [26]	SE-MRI	52	98%	78%	94%
White et al. [27]	cine-MRI	28	93%	86%	89%
Aurigemma et al. [28]	cine-MRI	45	88%	100%	91%
Galjee et al. [29]	SE-MRI	98	98%	85%	96%
	cine-MRI		98%	88%	96%
	combined		98%	76%	94%

SE-MRI = spin-echo magnetic resonance imaging; cine-MRI = gradient-echo
magnetic resonance imaging

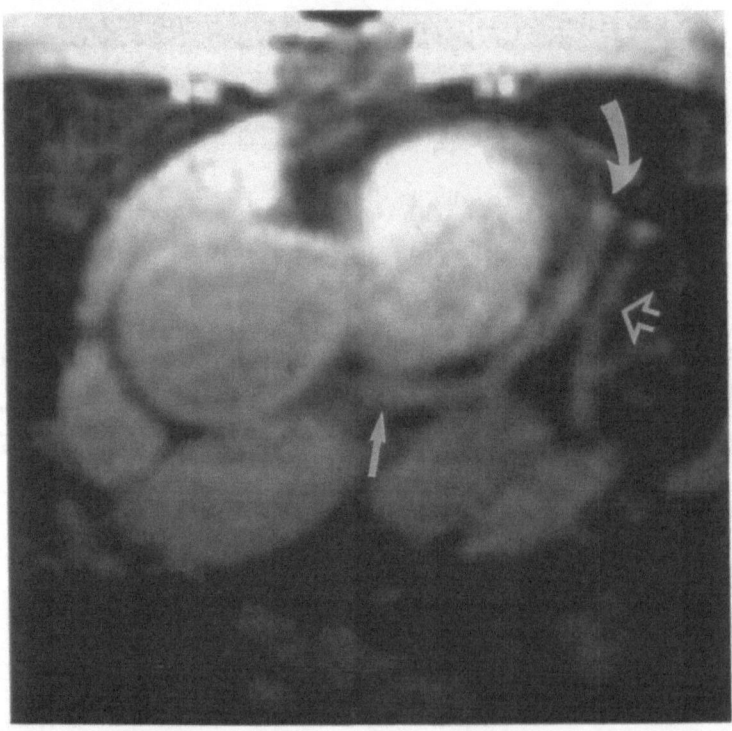

Figure 7. Imaging plane reformatted from 3D MR data set shows normal left
coronary artery artery. Straight arrow = left main coronary artery; curved arrow =
LAD; open arrow = great cardiac vein.

additional slabs must be acquired. Postprocessing techniques which make use of 3D surface rendering may yield a 'holographic' representation of the coronary arteries (Figure 8) [30].

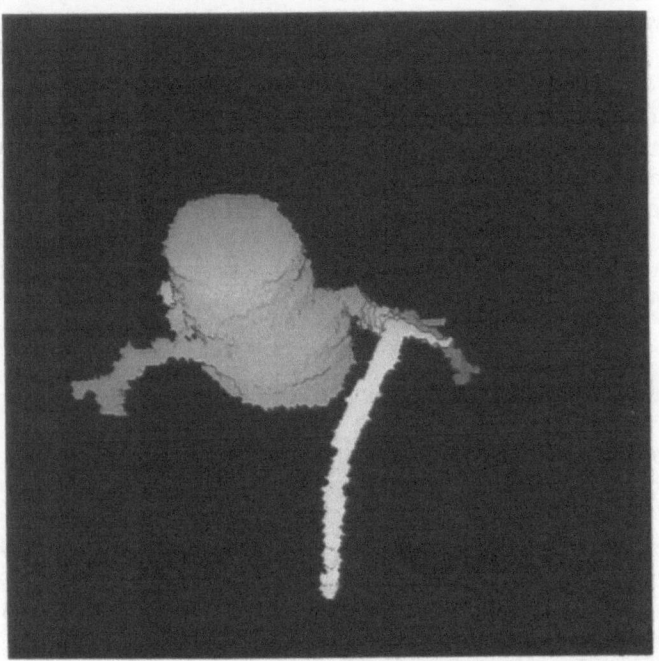

Figure 8. Cranially angulated left anterior oblique view of a 3D surface rendered reconstruction of the aortic root and the major proximal epicardial coronary arteries [30]. The bright artery with anterior course is the LAD.

Clinical results

So far, clinical data regarding the use of 3D coronary angiography are scarce. We performed a study [30] in 20 patients suspected of having coronary artery disease, in which a comparison was made with conventional contrast angiography using the same 3D technique as described by Hofman [8]. Of the 80 major coronary arteries 96% were positively identified, with an average length of the RCA, LM, LAD and LCX of 58 ± 13 mm, 9 ± 5 mm, 59 ± 16 mm and 24 ± 10 mm, respectively. In this study only 1 slab was imaged, thereby restricting the visualization of longer vessel segments. The sensitivity for detecting 21 stenoses with > 50% luminal diameter narrowing was only 38% with a specificity of 95%. Several factors may have contributed to this result: 1) in 3D imaging a progressive saturation of blood signal leads to decreasing contrast between blood and surrounding tissue; 2) the use of a short echo-time (TE), one of the imaging parameters, is likely to make the pulse sequence less sensitive to blood flow turbulence and hence to the detection of stenoses; and 3) in spite of cardiac and respiratory gating techniques, residual motion may have occurred due to patient movement, imperfect respiratory gating, and a large acquisition window in the cardiac cycle. In a comparative study between 2D breath-hold and 3D respiratory gated MR coronary angiography by Hofman et al. [8], this seemed to be confirmed. The 3D images were of lesser quality and coronary arteries showed more blurring of vessel edges.

In spite of these provisional shortcomings, imaging of the complicated 3D structure of the coronary vessel tree within a single 3D data acquisition is a very appealing concept. As compared to 2D MR coronary angiography, a major advantage is that imaging can easily be performed by persons without specific knowledge of the coronary anatomy. The latter is required only afterwards, when data are analyzed at the 3D workstation. Also, 3D MR angiography is more comfortable for the patient because repetitive breath-holds are not required, it is less subdue to misregistrations artifacts, thinner sections may be obtained, and total imaging time is shorter than in a full 2D MR angiographic protocol.

Prospects of MR coronary artery imaging

Clinical applications of MR coronary angiography already include imaging of anomalous coronary arteries and coronary artery bypass grafts. Concerning the detection of coronary artery stenoses, it is clear that the MR technology requires further development in terms of hardware, pulse sequence design, and postprocessing of the data. Breath-hold techniques limit the time available to increase spatial and temporal resolution, but the newer respiratory gating techniques will help to overcome this restriction. Improved surface coil design can further increase the signal to noise ratio, and contrast can be augmented with magnetization transfer techniques [14,17]. MR contrast agents may be needed which, as opposed to the currently available interstitial agents, remain in the bloodpool. At present, this type of contrast agent is still investigational and not yet available for clinical application. By postprocessing the MR data, a projectional display can be obtained, facilitating the evaluation of the tortuous coronary anatomy [31]. These are only a few of the refinements that will help to improve MR coronary angiography in the very near future.

Although imaging of the entire coronary vessel tree with sufficient spatial resolution to assess stenoses is presently not attainable, applications focused on specific clinical questions are within reach. Noninvasive determination of the infarct artery patency [22] is an example of this. Evaluation of restenosis after PTCA, when the localization of the stenosis is already known, might be another possibility. The feasibility of noninvasively adding flow information to the angiographic findings is unique to MR imaging [32-34].

Finally, imaging of coronary arteries should be looked upon as only one of the aspects in the evaluation of coronary artery disease. Other aspects are the assessment of myocardial function, perfusion and metabolism, which can all be addressed by MR and may ultimately lead to an integrated MR imaging approach.

References

1. Paulin S, von Schulthess GK, Fossel E, Krayenbuehl HP. MR imaging of the aortic root and proximal coronary arteries. AJR Am J Roentgenol 1987;148:665-70.
2. Alfidi RJ, Masaryk TJ, Haacke EM *et al*. MR angiography of peripheral, carotid, and coronary arteries. AJR Am J Roentgenol 1987;149:1097-109.
3. Cho ZH, Mun CW, Friedenberg RM. NMR angiography of coronary vessels with 2-D planar image scanning. Magn Reson Med 1991;20:134-43.
4. Edelman RR, Manning WJ, Burstein D, Paulin S. Coronary arteries: breath-hold MR angiography. Radiology 1991;181:641-3.
5. Meyer CH, Hu BS, Nishimura DG, Macovski A. Fast spiral coronary artery imaging. Magn Reson Med 1992;28:202-13.
6. Ehman RL, McNamara MT, Pallack M, Hricak H, Higgins CB. Magnetic resonance imaging with respiratory gating: techniques and advantages. AJR Am J Roentgenol 1984;143:1175-82.
7. Ehman RL, Felmlea JP. Adaptive technique for high definition MR imaging of moving structures. Radiology 1989;173:255-63.
8. Hofman MBM, Paschal CB, Li D, Haacke EM, van Rossum AC, Sprenger M. MRI of coronary arteries: 2D breath-hold vs 3D respiratory-gated acquisition. J Comput Assist Tomogr 1995;19:56-62.
9. Manning WJ, Li W, Boyle NG, Edelman RR. Fat-suppressed breath-hold magnetic resonance coronary angiography. Circulation 1993;87:94-104.
10. Duerinckx AJ, Urman MK. Two-dimensional coronary MR angiography: analysis of initial clinical results. Radiology 1994;193:731-8.
11. Pennell DJ, Keegan J, Firmin DN, Gatehouse PD, Underwood SR, Longmore DB. Magnetic resonance imaging of coronary arteries: technique and preliminary results. Br Heart J 1993;70:315-26.
12. Post JC, van Rossum AC, Bronzwaer JGF *et al*. Magnetic resonance angiography of anomalous coronary arteries: a new gold standard for delineating the proximal course? Circulation 1995;92:3163-71.
13. Wang SJ, Hu BS, Macovski A, Nishimura DG. Coronary angiography using fast selective inversion recovery. Magn Reson Med 1991;18:417-23.
14. Li D, Paschal CB, Haacke EM, Adler LP. Coronary arteries: three-dimensional MR imaging with fat saturation and magnetization transfer contrast. Radiology 1993;187:401-6.
15. Post JC, van Rossum AC, Hofman MBM, Valk J, Visser CA. Protocol for two-dimensional magnetic resonance coronary angiography studied in three-dimensional magnetic resonance data sets. Am Heart J 1995;130:167-73.
16. Van Rossum AC, Post JC, Hofman MBM, Valk J, Visser CA. Current limitations of two-dimensional breath-hold magnetic resonance coronary angiography [abstract]. J Am Coll Cardiol 1995;25 Special Issue:134A.
17. Fayad ZA, Connick TJ, Axel L. An improved quadrature or phased-array coil for MR cardiac imaging. Magn Reson Med 1995;34:186-93.
18. Dodge JT Jr, Brown BG, Bolson EL, Dodge HT. Lumen diameter of normal human coronary arteries. Influence of age, sex, anatomic variation, and left ventricular hypertrophy and dilation. Circulation 1992;86:232-46.
19. McConnell MV, Ganz P, Selwyn AP, Li W, Edelman RR, Manning WJ. Identification of anomalous coronary arteries and their anatomic course by magnetic resonance coronary angiography. Circulation 1995;92:3158-62.

20. Manning WJ, Li W, Edelman RR. A preliminary report comparing magnetic resonance coronary angiography with conventional angiography. N Engl J Med 1993;328:828-32.

21. Post JC, van Rossum AC, Hofman MBM, Valk J, Visser CA. Clinical utility of two-dimensional breath-hold MR angiography in coronary artery disease. Proc Soc Magn Reson 1995:1394.

22. Hundley WG, Clarke GD, Landau C et al. Noninvasive determination of infarct artery patency by cine magnetic resonance angiography. Circulation 1995;91:1347-53.

23. White RD, Caputo GR, Mark AS, Modin GW, Higgins CB. Coronary artery bypass graft patency: noninvasive evaluation with MR imaging. Radiology 1987;164:681-6.

24. Rubinstein RI, Askenase AD, Thickman D, Feldman MS, Agarwal JB, Helfant RH. Magnetic resonance imaging to evaluate patency of aortocoronary bypass grafts. Circulation 1987;76:786-91.

25. Jenkins JPR, Love HG, Foster CJ, Isherwood I, Rowlands DJ. Detection of coronary artery bypass graft patency as assessed by magnetic resonance imaging. Br J Radiol 1988;61:2-4.

26. Frija G, Schouman-Claeys E, Lacombe P, Bismuth V, Ollivier J-P. A study of coronary artery bypass graft patency using MR imaging. J Comput Assist Tomogr 1989;13:226-32.

27. White RD, Pflugfelder PW, Lipton MJ, Higgins CB. Coronary artery bypass grafts: evaluation of patency with cine MR imaging. AJR Am J Roentgenol 1988;150:1271-4.

28. Aurigemma GP, Reichek N, Axel L, Schiebler M, Harris C, Kressel HY. Noninvasive determination of coronary artery bypass graft patency by cine magnetic resonance imaging. Circulation 1989;80:1595-602.

29. Galjee MA, van Rossum AC, Doesburg T, van Eenige MJ, Visser CA. Value of magnetic resonance imaging in assessing patency and function of coronary artery bypass grafts: an angiographically controlled study. Circulation 1996;93:660-6.

30. Post JC, van Rossum AC, Hofman MBM, Valk J, Visser CA. Three-dimensional respiratory gated MR angiography of coronary arteries: comparison with conventional coronary angiography. AJR Am J Roentgenol. In press.

31. Edelman RR, Manning WJ, Pearlman J, Li W. Human coronary arteries: projection angiograms reconstructed from breath-hold two-dimensional MR images. Radiology 1993;187:719-22.

32. Edelman RR, Manning WJ, Gervino E, Li W. Flow velocity quantification in human coronary arteries with fast, breath-hold MR angiography. J Magn Reson Imaging 1993;3:699-703.

33. Keegan J, Firmin D, Gatehouse P, Longmore D. The application of breath hold phase velocity mapping techniques to the measurement of coronary artery blood flow velocity: phantom data and initial in vivo results. Magn Reson Med 1994;31:526-36.

34. Hofman MBM, van Rossum AC, Sprenger M, Westerhof N. Assessment of flow in the right human coronary artery by magnetic resonance phase contrast velocity measurements: effects of cardiac and respiratory motion. Magn Reson Med. In press.

25. Flow measurements in coronary arteries using MRI

MICHEL A. GALJEE

Summary

A noninvasive approach to visualize the coronary arteries would be a very desirable asset in clinical cardiology. Over the past few years, magnetic resonance angiography has rapidly evolved to become a feasible modality for imaging of the coronary arteries. However, the technical demands for imaging the coronary arteries are considerable, particularly with respect to cardiac and respiratory motion, and the small size and tortuosity of the vessels. To date, magnetic resonance angiography is only capable of visualizing the proximal course of the coronary arteries. To become a clinical reality, magnetic resonance coronary angiography has to undergo several substantial developments. The necessary advances to be made are: 1) improved breath-hold reproducibility with faster imaging techniques (spiral imaging); 2) sophisticated respiratory gating and triggering techniques by navigator-echo real-time imaging; 3) higher spatial resolution using phased-array body surface coils; and 4) accurate flow-velocity measurements by echo-planar time-of-flight imaging. When these conditions are fulfilled, it is expected that magnetic resonance angiography will further mature into a clinically applicable method for reliable noninvasive imaging of coronary artery morphology and function.

Introduction

Until now, the gold standard for the evaluation of coronary artery disease is x-ray contrast angiography. With this technique we can assess the coronary anatomy, degree of patency and the therapeutical options. However, it has limited capability for determining the functional significance of a stenosis. Repeat studies, to evaluate treatment strategies, cannot be undertaken lightly due to its character and the radiation exposure.

True assessment of coronary artery function requires quantification of coronary blood flow. By using Doppler flow-wire technique in addition to the standard x-ray contrast angiography, the velocity and stenotic velocity gradients within the coronary vessel can be assessed. The velocity data are influenced by limitations of guidewire positioning and the influence of the guidewire on stenotic velocity gradients. Therefore, the flow reserve as assessed by the current Doppler flow-wire technique, is a relative measure of flow. Noninvasive methods as stress thallium imaging, PET and stress-echocardiography are indirect methods for the assessment of coronary flow.

Phase contrast velocity magnetic resonance imaging (MRI) offers the potential for noninvasive measurement of absolute coronary artery flow [1]. This technique can be combined with other MRI options as MR coronary angiography and cine MRI to assess cardiac function. The presently available clinical methods for direct

J.H.C. Reiber and E.E. van der Wall (eds.), Cardiovascular Imaging, 315-327.
© 1996 *Kluwer Academic Publishers.*

detection of differences in myocardial perfusion such as thallium-201 scintigraphy, positron emission tomography, technetium-99m sestamibi imaging, contrast echocardiography and videodensitometry all have certain drawbacks.

MR techniques for flow imaging

Blood flow can be studied in two ways by standard MR imaging techniques. Firstly, routinely used MR spin-echo and gradient-echo imaging has the unique feature of yielding qualitative flow information without the need of administrating contrast agents. Flowing blood can appear bright or dark, depending on the velocity, velocity profile and pulse sequence. The signal emitted by the flowing protons depends on the "magnetization history" of the spins. These time-of-flight effects have no linear relation with the signal amplitude, which complicates its application for flow quantification.

The MR imaging method which is capable of assessing flow quantitatively is called MR phase velocity mapping. This technique is used for blood flow quantification in coronary arteries.

Quantification of flow can be obtained when the phase-shifts are measured, induced by the motion of spinning protons along an imaging gradient. The phase-shifts are proportional to the velocity of the moving spins. An image can then be constructed in which the signal intensity is proportional to the phase of moving spins relative to stationary spins. These images provide pixel-by-pixel information of velocity on a grey scale. The grey scale is made such that zero velocity has medium grey intensity, whereas increasing flow in one direction become gradually darker, and in the opposite direction gradually brighter. The component of flow can be measured perpendicular to the image (along the phase-encoding direction), or within the image (along the frequency-encoding direction). The strength of the imaging gradient and the time during which the spins are exposed to the gradient prescribe the velocity sensitivity. Therefore, it is important to adjust these parameters for the anticipated flow velocity to prevent spin phase-shifts by more than one-half cycle, or 180°, which cause wraparound or aliasing [2].

An additional extension is the use of "flow compensating" gradients. This compensates for the signal loss that results from phase dispersion due to different velocities within a single voxel. It is beyond the scope of this introduction to go into the details of this modulation [3-5].

As gradient-echo imaging techniques are very sensitive to magnetic field inhomogeneities, a correction has to be made for non velocity-related background phase. This is obtained by subtraction of two sets of phase-images which are acquired in an interleaved scheme: one with flow compensation and the other with the velocity encoding gradient modulation. The subtraction will eliminate the background phase without affecting the velocity encoding phase-shifts [2,4,5].

The temporal resolution depends mainly on the power of the gradient system. The spatial resolution depends on the slice thickness, matrix and field of view that is used. The voxel dimensions which can be obtained by using a (phased array) surface coil are nowadays 0.8x1.6x4 mm. The total imaging time varies depending on the technique used. This can be from a breath-hold up to 17 minutes for a respiratory-gated technique.

Reconstruction of the amplitude data yields a conventional cine-image which serves as an anatomical reference, and the subtracted phase data are used for reconstruction of a velocity map (Figure 1).

After identification of the object of interest on the conventional cine-image, the velocity within a vessel or other structure can now be measured on the velocity map with a region-of-interest function. The velocity can be measured in a single pixel within the vessel or as an average value over an area of multiple pixels. From the assessment of flow at consecutive phases throughout the cardiac cycle one can derive mean volume flow or, by integration of the area under the curve, the volume of flow per cardiac cycle.

MR phase-velocity mapping has the unique advantage of measuring the flow velocity in each voxel of the vascular image. Therefore, MR phase-velocity mapping allows the determination of blood flow profiles irrespective of whether the distribution of velocities is flat or not. This may be important for characterizing cardiovascular abnormalities in which the velocity profiles are not flat and influenced by diameter variations during the cardiac cycle, as is the case in most vessels.

Other techniques such as Doppler ultrasound and catheter-tip velocity transducers can determine velocity in only a single point of a cross-sectional area and therefore can not measure real volumetric flow.

Validation of MR phase velocity mapping technique

The theoretically expected accuracy of phase velocity mapping is confirmed by several phantom and in vivo studies. Phantom studies of a wide range of steady flow and of pulsatile flow showed a great accuracy of the MR pulsatile flow measurements [6-9].

In-vivo validation has been performed by comparisons within the MR technique and with Doppler ultrasound in healthy volunteers. Comparison of quantitative flow rates obtained by MR imaging in the pulmonary artery and the aorta showed an acceptable average difference between the two measurements of 5% [6]. A high correlation between right ventricular stroke volume and volumetric pulmonary stroke volume was demonstrated in investigations with volunteers [10]. We demonstrated a high correlation between stroke volume measured in the ascending aorta and venous return through superior and inferior vena cava per cardiac cycle [5].

In addition, the accuracy of MR flow measurements has been established by comparison of MR flow measurements with Doppler ultrasound in healthy volunteers for left ventricular stroke volume, cardiac output and blood flow in human abdominal aorta [5,11]. Hence, the expected accuracy of phase velocity mapping in large vessels has been confirmed by several phantom and in-vivo studies.

However, the accuracy of the volume flow measurements can be affected when the vessel diameter is small relative to the spatial resolution. This is the case in imaging of the coronary arteries. The relative amount of pixels at the vessel boundary increases as the vessel diameter becomes smaller. This leads to a larger contribution of the partial volume effect at the vessel boundary. An in-vivo

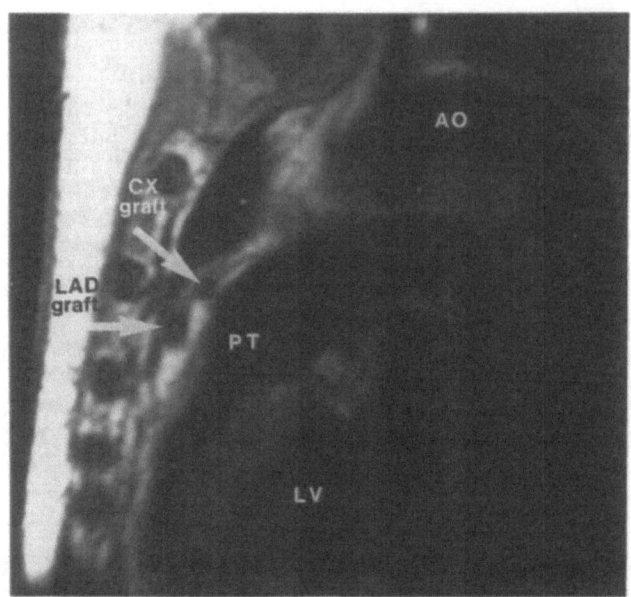

Figure 1A. Spin-echo image perpendicular to a left anterior descending (LAD) and circumflex (CX) graft in a sagital plane at the level of the pulmonary trunk (PT). LV: left ventricle. Ao: aorta.

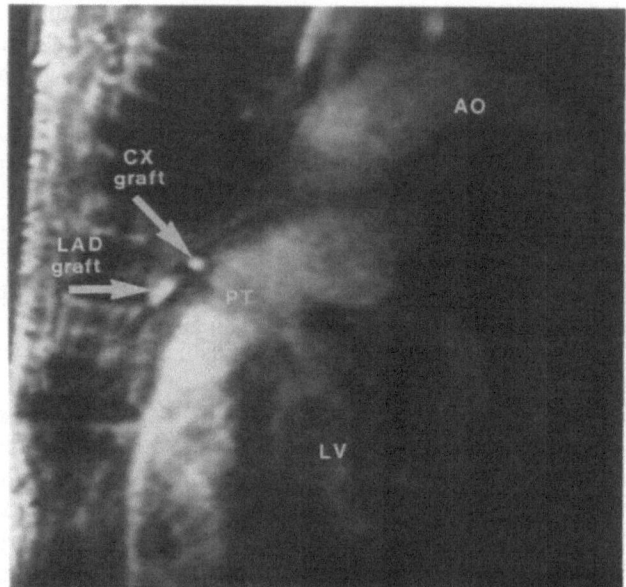

Figure 1B. Anatomic gradient-echo image at the same level as in Figure 1A. Flowing blood has a high signal intensity. The grafts are depicted as bright dots.

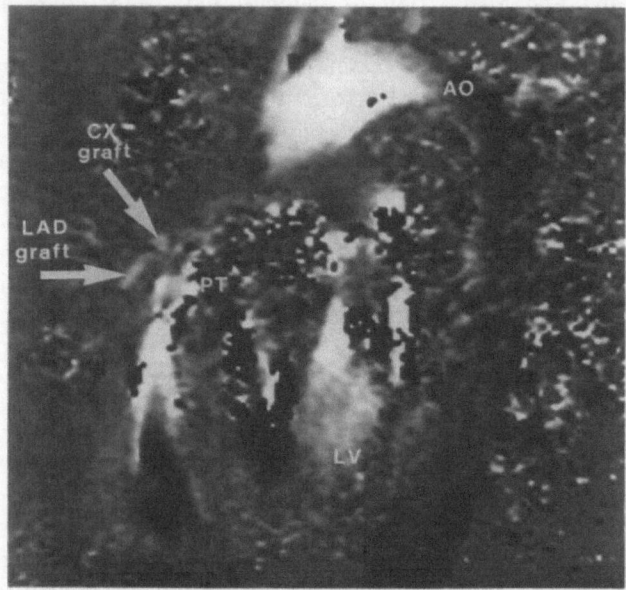

Figure 1C. Corresponding velocity image. On the phase-encoded velocity images flow in the grafts is depicted in shades from mid grey to white, proportional to the flow velocity.

validation study of MR phase velocity mapping with limited resolution (1x1 mm², slice thickness of 6 mm) in small vessels (diameter 3 mm) demonstrated a good correlation of MR volume flow measurements compared with ultrasonic transit-time method [12].

Potential errors

In clinical practice some aspects need to be considered to avoid errors or misinterpretation of data [2].

For quantification of blood flow it is essential that the imaging plane is at right angles to the vessel and that the flow sensitivity is encoded perpendicularly to the imaging plane. Otherwise, the flow velocity will be underestimated and the area of the object overestimated. Because there is a cosine relationship between measured flow velocity and true flow velocity, small angles of misalignment will only lead to small errors: a misalignment of 5°, 20° or 30° produces an underestimation of <1%, 6% and 13%, respectively. When the angle between the vessel and the image plane is in between 90⁰ and 120⁰, no major errors will be made for volume flow measurements as the lower measured mean velocity is partially compensated by a greater measured area of the vessel. When calculating volume flow by multiplying area with velocity, the errors made by overestimation of the area and underestimation of velocity will cancel out, as was shown experimentally.

Motion and curvature of the vessels can cause partial volume effects and misregistration. These sources of error, in general, can be avoided by adjusting the technique.

Of greater importance is the limitation to quantify flow when signal loss occurs due to higher orders of motion, such as acceleration and turbulence [13]. These effects can occur in case of vascular stenoses, in the vicinity of cardiac valves and in the great vessels at points of great turbulence. Improvement can be obtained by using pulse sequences with short echo times, combined with thin imaging sections, thereby minimizing the disparity of higher orders of velocity within a voxel and raising the threshold at which signal loss occurs [14]. However, these measurements require the use of powerful gradient supplies which may not be available as a standard.

Studies of flow measurements in coronary arteries

MR imaging has evolved as the main imaging tool of the great vessels and particularly of the aorta. Not only because of its high spatial resolution in any desired plane, but also because of its flexibility and sensitivity to characterize flow phenomena and motion using standard imaging techniques. MR imaging is currently the standard in evaluating congenital anomalies such as coarctation, Marfan´s syndrome, pulmonary atresia, patent ductus arteriosus, malrotations, palliative subacute and chronic aortic dissections, aortic aneurysm. The following section will primarily focus on the aspect of flow measurements.

The aorta is relatively easy to access for phase velocity mapping as it has an uncomplicated geometry and large diameter over a long distance. Measurements of phasic flow in the aorta is a powerful potential of MR phase velocity mapping techniques. By this means quantification of cardiac output, aortic valve stenoses and insufficiency, shunt measurements, regurgitant fractions and aortic distensibility can be performed in a noninvasive manner [5,15].

Visualization of the coronary arteries and determination of the coronary flow are some of the most challenging tasks of MRI. A complete vizualisation of the coronary vessels on conventional spin-echo and gradient-echo images is hindered by their small calibre, tortuosity, proximity to other tissue, cardiac motion and respiratory motion. The proximal part of the vessels can, however, be visualized by conventional techniques. Coronary artery aneurysms, fistulas are often incompletely visualized with routine angiography. MR images improve preoperative assessment of patients with these anomalies [16]. Recently, rapid imaging sequences have been developed which allow the acquisition of images of coronary arteries within a breath-hold [17]. Also, three-dimensional approaches of MR coronary angiography have now been introduced using respiratory gating [18].

In a study to assess the feasibility of conventional magnetic resonance velocity mapping to quantitate coronary flow, 10 patients with an angiographically patent right coronary artery (RCA) and 10 healthy controls underwent ECG gated MRI at 0.6 Tesla with the subject in prone position on a surface coil [19].

First, multislice sagital and transverse SE scout views were performed for identification of the RCA. These scout views were used to obtain magnitude and phase velocity maps perpendicular to the coronary artery throughout the cardiac cycle (flip angle 25°, TE 24 ms, matrix 160x256, FOV 25.6x25.6 cm, slice thickness 5 mm, 4 averages). Cross-sections of the RCA were determined on magnitude images. The component of flow perpencicular to the imaging plane was measured over each cross-section on corresponding velocity maps (Figure 2). From these measurements we calculated volume flow (ml/min).

In all subjects the RCA was identified on subsequent transverse SE tomograms. Adequate flow measurements were obtained in 8 patients and 7 volunteers. In 3 subjects LCA flow was measured in addition. RCA flow was best measured at a transverse plane, 1-2 cm distal from the origo as the LCA flow was best measured at a sagital plane 1 cm distal from the origin. Figure 3 shows an example of a flow pattern. The flow data are shown in Table 1.

Measured flow rates were in the physiologic range, although significant higher flow rates were found in the control group and the LCA.

By fast breath-hold MR velocity mapping techniques for coronary flow measurements, the total scan time is shortened by using k-space segmentation to reduce the number of cardiac phases [19,20]. With k-space segmentation several (e.g. 4) phase encoding steps are applied per cardiac cycle. Therefore the number of cardiac phases to complete the image is reduced four fold. A matrix of 256x96 is completed with $96/4 = 24$ cardiac cycles. When the heart rate is 75 beats/min the scan duration will be 34 seconds. Better delineation of the vessel is obtained by using a pulse sequence which suppresses fat. The signal-to-noise ratio is improved by using a surface coil.

These techniques have also limitations. Firstly, the relatively long time window per velocity image (160 ms). On the images this can result in "blurring" of the coronary vessels, especially during systole when the displacement of the coronary vessels is large. Therefore, flow is only measured at a single time-point in diastole and phasic flow measurements or flow quantification over the cardiac cycle is hardly possible. Secondly, the spatial resolution is relatively low (1.6x1.6mm).

Echo-planar MRI using time-of-flight techniques is very fast. The main limitations are the lower spatial resolution and the lesser accuracy of time-of-flight techniques for quantification of flow [21].

Recently, fast breath-hold techniques with high-performance gradient coils have been developed. These techniques allow phasic flow measurements with high spatial resolution (submillimeter pixel sizes) [12,22,23]. This technique is not ideal. It also has a relative large acquisition time window (126 ms) within the cardiac cycle. Although phasic flow can be measured by this technique, the temporal resolution is only 5 images per cardiac cycle.

The long acquisiton time window within the cardiac cycle is the result of k-space segmentation which is needed to acquire images within one breath-hold. Without k-space segmentation respiratory gating is needed to reduce respiratory motion artefacts. Respiratory gating can be performed by applying a projection spin echo for diaphragm location. As no k-space segmentation is performed the acquistion time window (16 ms) is small. This significantly reduces the sensitivity to cardiac motion. However, the total acquistion time is much longer and may be up to 17

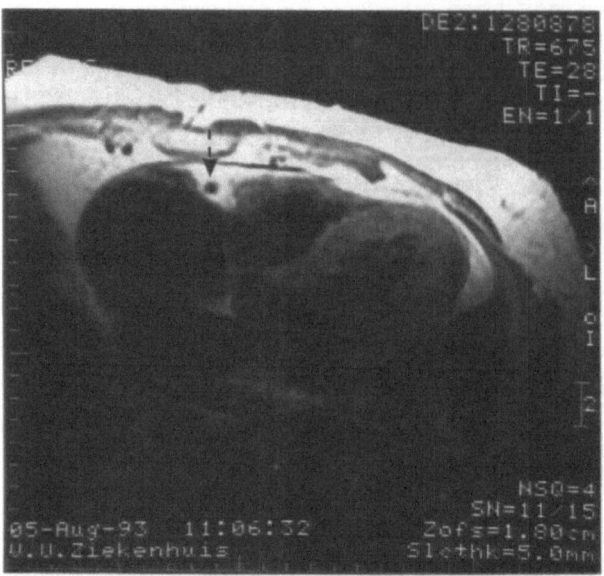

Figure 2A. Spin-echo image perpendicular to the right coronary artery (arrow) in a transverse plane at the level of the right atrial-ventricular grove.

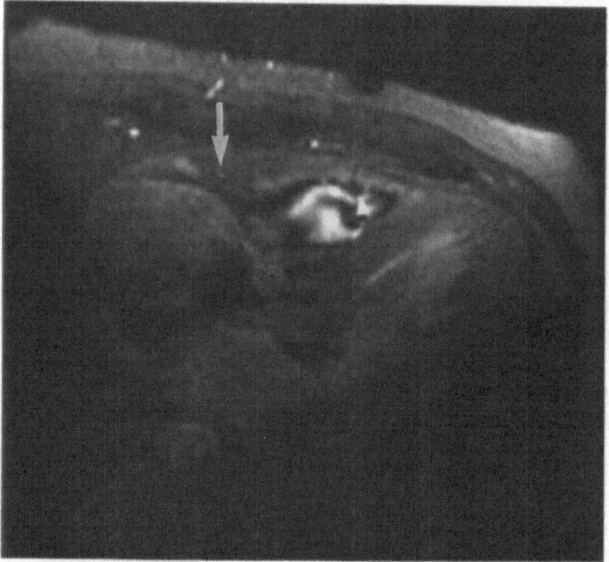

Figure 2B. Anatomic gradient-echo image at the same level as in figure 2A. Flowing blood has a high signal intensity. The right coronary artery is depicted as a bright dot (arrow).

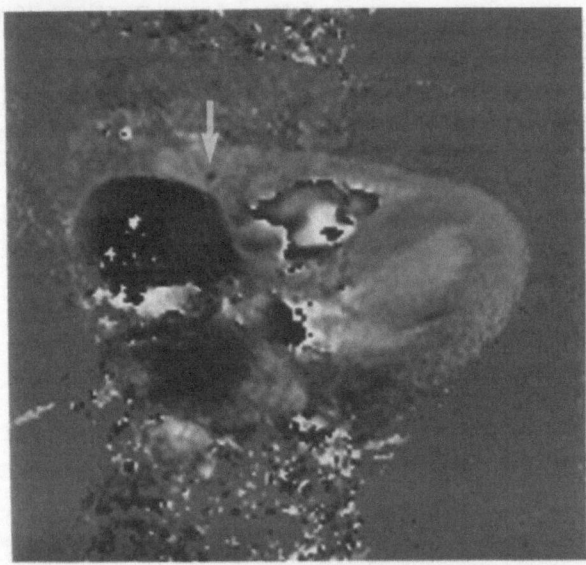

Figure 2C. Corresponding velocity image. On the phase-encoded velocity images flow in the right coronary artery (arrow) is depicted in shades from mid grey to black, proportional to the flow velocity.

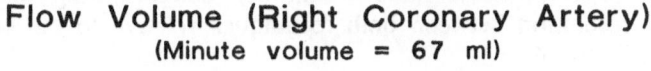

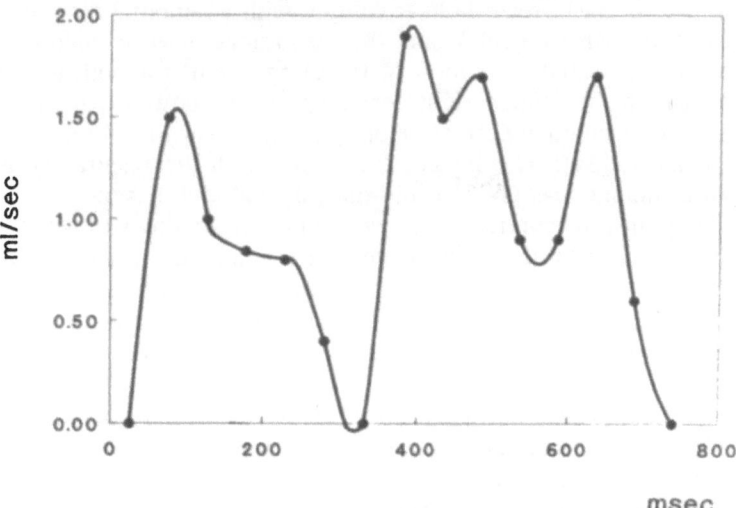

Figure 3. Example of a blood flow pattern acquired from the right coronary artery by MR phase velocity mapping techniques. The blood flow in the right coronary artery is characterized by a biphasic flow pattern, with one peak in systole and a second one in diastole. The volume flow in this case was 67 ml/min.

Table 1. MR phase velocity mapping data of coronary artery flow in patients and healthy controls.

	CORONARY FLOW (ml/min)	
	mean ± SD	range
RCA all (n=15)	50 ± 19	21 - 81
RCA controls (n=7)	62 ± 18	33 - 81
RCA patients (n=8)	40 ± 13*	21 - 57
LCA (n=3)	112 ± 41	68 - 148

* p=0.0173

min.

The time diagram of the pulse sequences of the breath-hold technique and the retrospective respiratory gated technique, demonstrating the differences in temporal resolution between both techniques relative to the cardiac cycle are shown in Figure 4.

Comparison of the fast breath-hold technique with a temporal resolution of 155 ms (5 images per cardiac cycle), and the respiratory gated technique (temporal resolution 16 ms, spatial resolution of 0.8x1.6x4 mm^3 for both techniques) to assess the flow in the human right coronary artery showed that only with the respiratory gated technique correct velocity images over the whole cardiac cycle could be obtained [24]. The image quality for both the respiratory gated and breath-hold technique was good at mid-diastole and end-diastole.

At those time points the contrast of the vessel to surrounding structures was high. When systolic and early diastolic images were compared, a large difference in image quality was found in favor of the respiratory gated technique.

The image obtained during breath-holding demonstrated a strongly blurred image of the vessel, whereas a sharper image is obtained by the respiratory gated technique.

The displacement of the coronary artery is large with respect to the vessel diameter in systole and early-diastole. During mid- to end-diastole the displacement of the vessel was in the range of the spatial resolution of the image, or less. The breath-hold technique showed a strong overestimation of the area of the vessel during the time intervals with large vessel displacement. The time averaged ratio was 1.9. During mid-diastole this ratio was 0.94, not significantly different from unity.

The ratios of the velocity obtained by the breath-hold and respiratory gated technique was 0.82 for the time-averages value, and 0.84 for the mid-diastolic

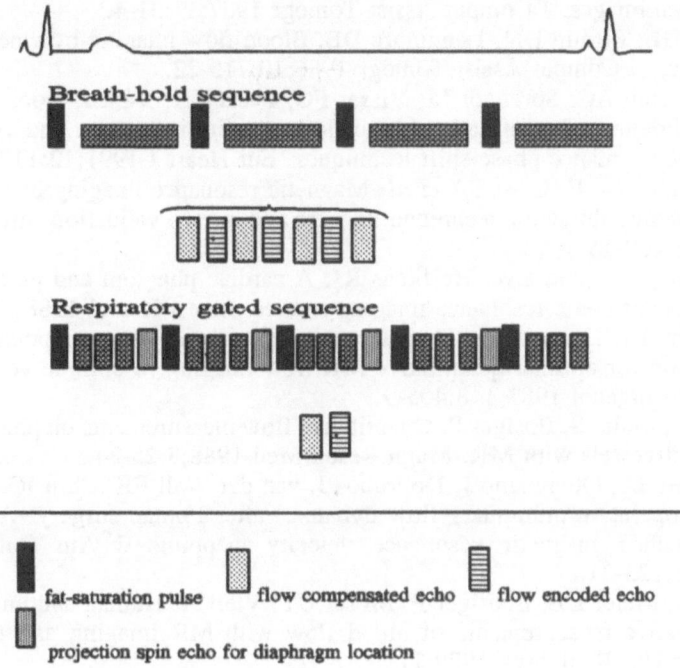

Figure 4. Time diagram of the pulse sequences of the breath-hold techniques and the retrospective respiratory gated techniques.

value (both not significant). The volume flow ratios were 1.6 (p=0.05) and 0.86 (p=0.19), respectively.

Noticeable was the finding that there was no major effect of respiratory gating on the flow measurements as compared to the nonrespiratory gated data. The ratio of the nongated data to the respiratory gated data for the volume flow was 1.15 ± 0.20 (NS). This can mean that respiratory gating will not be neccessary. Probably due to the fact that most of the data will be collected at expiration.

Future developments of hardware should improve spatial and temporal resolution to make MRI a clinical useful tool in the assessment of coronary artery flow. The use of phased-array coils and spiral imaging with phase velocity imaging has the potential to become this useful instrument [25].

References

1   Galjee MA, van Rossum AC, Doesburg T, van Eenige MJ, Visser CA. Value of magnetic resonance imaging in assessing patency and function of coronary artery bypass grafts: an angiographically controlled study. Circulation 1996;93:660-6.

2.   Firmin DN, Nayler GL, Kilner PJ, Longmore DB. The application of phase shifts in NMR for flow measurement. Magn Reson Med 1990;14:230-41.

3.   Axel L, Morton D. MR flow imaging by velocity-compensated/uncompensated

difference images. J Comput Assist Tomogr 1987;11:31-4.

4.   Nayler GL, Firmin DN, Longmore DB. Blood flow imaging by cine magnetic resonance. J Comput Assist Tomogr 1986;10:715-22.
5.   Van Rossum AC, Sprenger M, Visser FC, Peels KH, Valk J, Roos JP. An in vivo validation of quantitative blood flow imaging in arteries and veins using magnetic resonance phase-shift techniques. Eur Heart J 1991;12:117-26.
6.   Evans AJ, Iwai F, Grist TA *et al*. Magnetic resonance imaging of blood flow with a phase subtraction technique. In vitro and in vivo validation. Invest Radiol 1993;28:109-15.
7.   Evans AJ, Hedlund LW, Herfkens RJ. A cardiac phantom and pulsatile flow pump for magnetic resonance imaging studies. Invest Radiol 1988;23:579-83.
8.   Pettigrew RI, Dannels W. Use of standard gradients with compound oblique angulation for optimal quantitative MR flow imaging in oblique vessels. AJR Am J Roentgenol 1987;148:405-9.
9.   Meier D, Maier S, Bosiger P. Quantitative flow measurements on phantoms and on blood vessels with MR. Magn Reson Med 1988;8:25-34.
10. Rebergen SA, Ottenkamp J, Doornbos J, van der Wall EE, Chin JGJ, de Roos A. Postoperative pulmonary flow dynamics after Fontan surgery: Assessment with nuclear magnetic resonance velocity mapping. J Am Coll Cardiol 1993;21:123-31.
11. Maier S, Meier DE, Boesiger P, Moser UT, Vieli A. Human abdominal aorta: Comparative measurements of blood flow with MR imaging and multigated Doppler US. Radiology 1989;171:487-92.
12. Hofman MBM, Visser FC, van Rossum AC, Vink GQM, Sprenger M, Westerhof N. In vivo validation of magnetic resonance blood volume flow measurements with limited spatial resolution in small vessels. Magn Reson Med 1995;33:778-84.
13. Podolak MJ, Hedlund LW, Evans AJ, Herfkens RJ. Evaluation of flow through simulated vascular stenoses with gradient echo magnetic resonance imaging. Invest Radiol 1989;24:184-9.
14. Kilner PJ, Manzara CC, Mohiaddin RH *et al*. Magnetic resonance jet velocity mapping in mitral and aortic valve stenosis. Circulation 1993;87:1239-48.
15. Bogren HG, Klipstein RK, Firmin N *et al*. Quantitation of antegrade and retrograde blood flow in the human aorta by magnetic resonance velocity mapping. Am Heart J 1989;117:1214-22.
16. Post JC, van Rossum AC, Bronzwaer JGF *et al*. Magnetic resonance angiography of anomalous coronary arteries. A new gold standard for delineating the proximal course? Circulation 1995;92:3163-71.
17. Manning WJ, Li W, Edelman RR. A preliminary report comparing magnetic resonance coronary angiography with conventional angiography. N Engl J Med 1993;328:828-32.
18. Pennell DJ, Keegan J, Firmin DN, Gatehouse PD, Underwood SR, Longmore DB. Magnetic resonance imaging of coronary arteries: technique and preliminary results. Br Heart J 1993;70:315-26.
19. Galjee MA, van Rossum AC, Doesburg T, Hofman MBA, Visser CA. Coronary artery flow in humans measured by magnetic resonance phase velocity mapping, Proc Soc Magn Reson Med 1993:552.
20. Edelman RR, Manning WJ, Gervino E, Li W. Flow velocity quantification in human coronary arteries with fast, breath-hold MR angiography. J Magn Reson Imagin 1993;3:699-703.

21. Keegan J, Firmin D, Gatehouse P, Longmore D. The application of breath hold phase velocity mapping techniques to the measurement of coronary artery blood flow velocity: phantom data and initial in vivo results. Magn Reson Med 1994;31:526-35.

22. Poncelet BP, Weisskoff RM, Wedeen VJ, Brady TJ, Kantor H. Time of flight quantification of coronary flow with echo-planar MRI. Magn Reson Med 1993;30:447-57.

23. Clarke GD, Eckels R, Chaney C *et al*. Measurement of absolute epicardial coronary artery flow and flow reserve with breath-hold cine phase-contrast magnetic resonance imaging. Circulation 1995;91:2627-34.

24. Hofman MBM, van Rossum AC, Sprenger M, Westerhof N. Assessment of flow in the right human coronary artery by magnetic resonance phase contrast velocity measurement. Magn Reson Med. In press.

25. Gatehouse PD, Firmin DN, Collins S, Longmore DB. Real time blood flow imaging by spiral scan phase velocity mapping. Magn Reson Med 1994;31:504-12.

26. Current and future applications of magnetic resonance coronary angiography

WARREN J. MANNING

Summary

Despite their small size, tortuosity, and mobility, noninvasive imaging of the proximal and mid-portions of the major coronary arteries is now possible using breath-hold magnetic resonance (MR) techniques. Current technology offers relatively limited spatial resolution and quantitation of coronary artery stenoses is not possible. Clinically, MR coronary angiography has been most useful for the identification of coronary artery anomalies, and MR is likely to become the "gold standard" for the delineation of the course of these vessels. MR has also been shown to allow for characterization of bypass graft patency and infarct artery patency. Further improvements and testing are needed before more widespread clinical applications can be advocated. The use of non-breathhold solutions, stronger gradients, and improved receiver coils are likely to allow for many of the needed improvements in spatial resolution and slice registration, and thereby allow for reliable identification of focal stenoses in the native coronary arteries.

Introduction

Among its many applications to the cardiovascular system, magnetic resonance (MR) has had its greatest clinical impact in the evaluation of suspected thoracic aortic aneurysm and dissection [1]. At most institutions, thoracic MR is now routinely performed for the evaluation of patients presenting with symptoms or signs of aortic dissection. Unlike the 3-4 cm diameter of the aorta, however, the epicardial coronary arteries are only 3-4 mm in diameter, or 1/100th the cross-sectional area of the thoracic aorta. In addition, the epicardial coronary arteries are surrounded by epicardial fat and undergo complex three-dimensional motion during the cardiac cycle and with normal respiration.

Despite initial pessimism, MR coronary angiography (MRCA) is being successfully implemented at many centers around the world, and it is likely that in the future, MRCA will emerge as the dominant indication for a clinical MR examination. "Replacement" of the contrast angiogram is many years away, but current and future indications for clinical MRCA are now being identified.

MR coronary angiography - current applications

Current MRCA techniques

While conventional ECG-gated spin-echo imaging will occasionally depict the

329

J.H.C. Reiber and E.E. van der Wall (eds.), Cardiovascular Imaging, 329-355.
© 1996 *Kluwer Academic Publishers.*

proximal portions of the major coronary arteries [2], reliable depiction of the native coronary arteries awaited the development of 2D segmented k-space gradient-echo sequences, as first reported in humans by Edelman et al. [3]. Typically, a frequency-selective pre-pulse is used to suppress signal from surrounding epicardial fat and breath-holding is used to minimize respiratory artifacts. Multiple phase encoding steps are also acquired during each heart beat [3,4]. Commonly, 128 phase encoding steps (128 x 256 matrix) are acquired during 16 successive heart beats (i.e., 8 phase encoding steps per heart beat). This approach permits each 2D image to be acquired during a single 15-20 second breath-hold. To minimize blurring associated with cardiac motion, the segment or group of phase encoding steps is acquired during a brief interval (100 ms), gated by the electrocardiogram (ECG) to mid-diastole, a period of relative diastasis. Typical imaging parameters include a repetition time of 13 msec, echo time of 7 msec, 3-4 mm slice thickness and a field-of-view of 240 mm (in-plane spatial resolution of approximately 1.9 x 0.9 mm). Thirty or more breath-hold images are often needed to completely define the major coronary artery anatomy. A cine variation of the sequence permits visualization of long segments of the left anterior descending and right coronary arteries [5].

In addition to the 2D approach mentioned above, MRCA has been described using multiple other MR sequences, including 3D techniques [6], subtraction methods with selective tagging/stimulation of blood in the aortic root with subsequent wash-in of "tagged" blood into the native coronaries [7], as well as the more rapid spiral scanning [8] and echo-planar imaging (EPI) [9-11] methods. EPI methods fill k-space with one (single-shot EPI) or several (multi-shot EPI) radiofrequency pulses, offering extremely rapid data acquisition, but more limited spatial resolution and more pronounced flow artifacts. Such a sequence may be ideal as a "localizer" for rapidly defining the location and orientation of the major coronary vessels, with subsequent higher resolution scanning using either segmented 2D or 3D approaches.

MRCA of normal coronary anatomy

Using the breath-hold 2D segmented k-space gradient-echo MRCA approach, the coronary ostia may be identified initially in the transverse plane (Figures 1,2). Further definition of the coronary anatomy can be performed using additional (superior/inferior) transverse images as well as with obliquely oriented images acquired along the major or minor axis of the major coronary arteries (Figure 3). In studies of normal coronary anatomy in young adult volunteers [4,12,13] the left main, left anterior descending, and right coronary arteries have been identified in nearly all patients. The left circumflex coronary artery, however, is more difficult to visualize and has been identified in 74 - 94% of patients [4,5,12-15], a finding likely related to the frequent use of an anteriorly placed surface coil as radiofrequency (RF) receiver, with a relative decrease in signal/noise in the area of the posteriorly directed circumflex coronary artery. In addition to these major vessels, diagonal branches of the left anterior descending coronary artery may be identified in up to 80% of subjects and the great cardiac vein in 88% of subjects [4,12]. The obtuse marginal branches of the left circumflex coronary artery are more difficult to visualize using breath-hold 2D

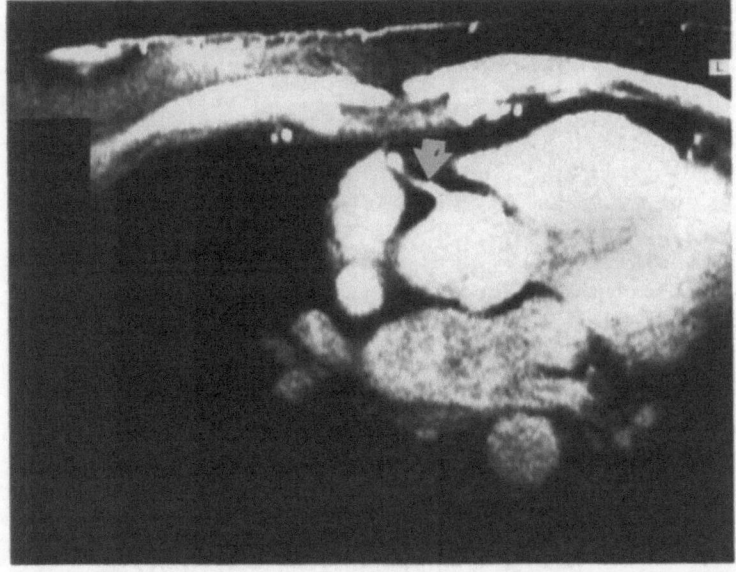

a

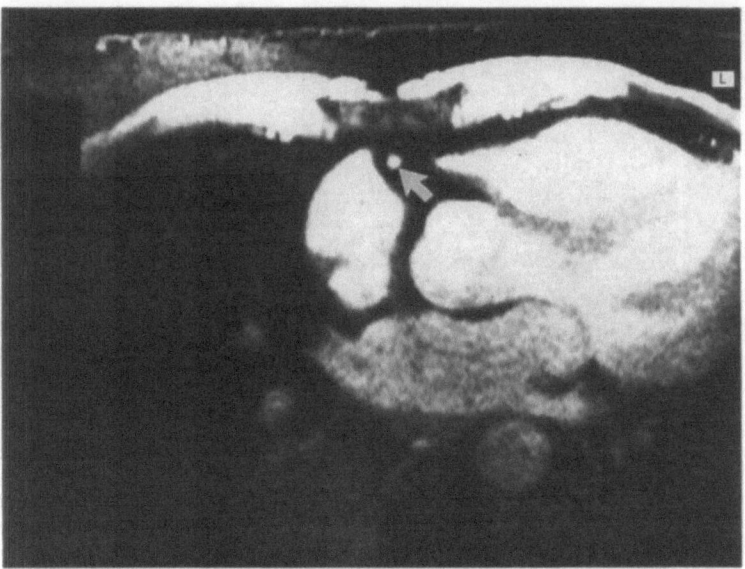

b

Figure 1. Transverse 3 mm thick breath-hold axial MR sections in a healthy volunteer at A) the level of the proximal right coronary artery (RCA) (solid white arrow); B) subsequent transverse section of RCA at a more inferior level (white arrow) identifying the vessel in cross-section. Ao = aortic root. Reprinted with permission of the American Heart Association [4].

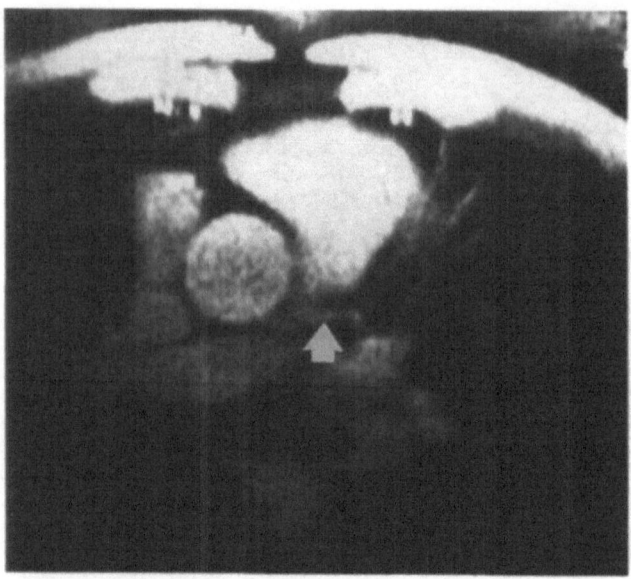

a

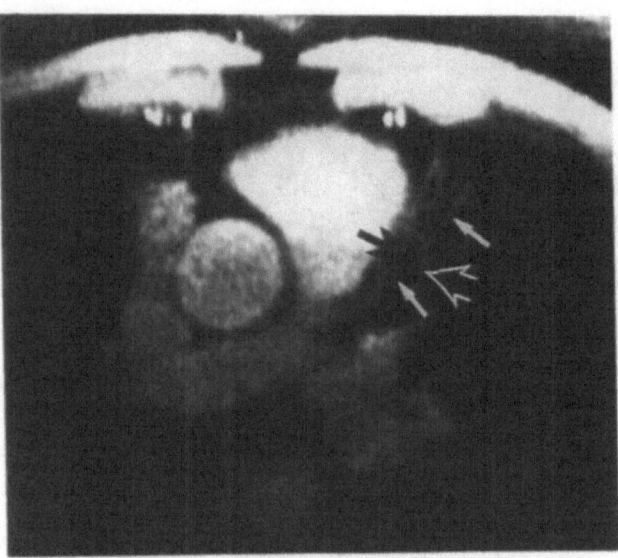

b

Figure 2.(A) Transverse MR section of the left main coronary artery (solid white arrow) continuing on into the B) left anterior descending (LAD) (black arrows) coronary artery. Note the diagonal branches of the LAD (solid white arrows) and the great cardiac vein (open white arrow); Reprinted with permission of the American Heart Association [4].

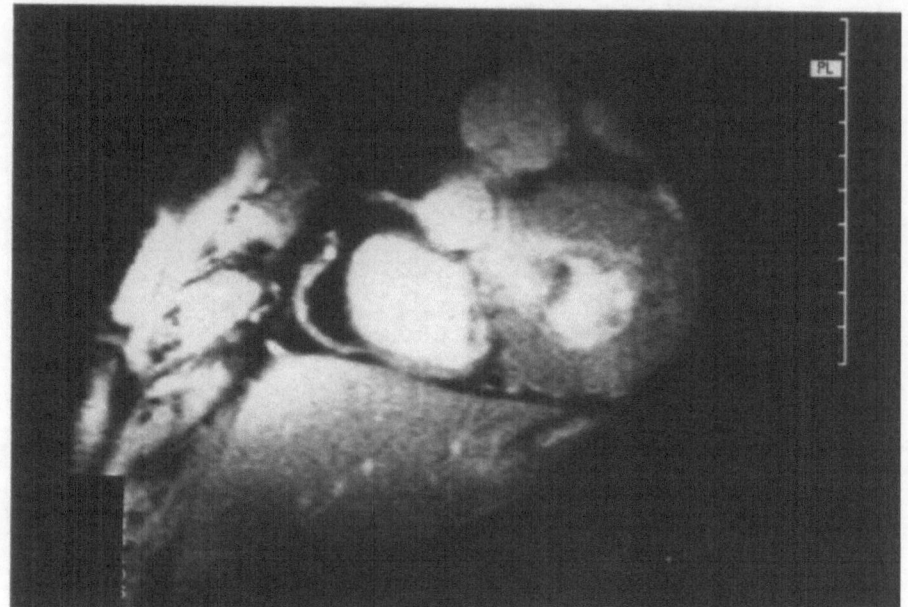

a

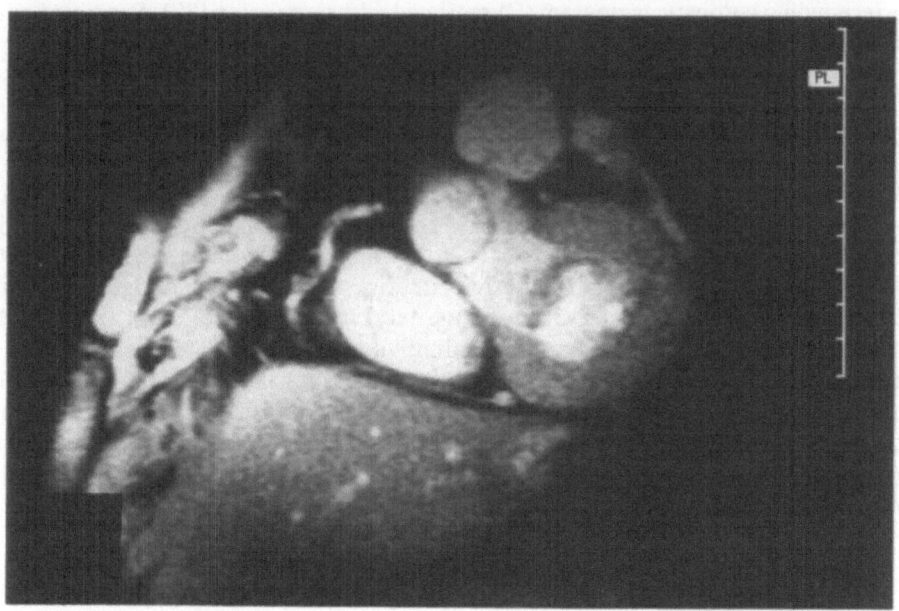

b

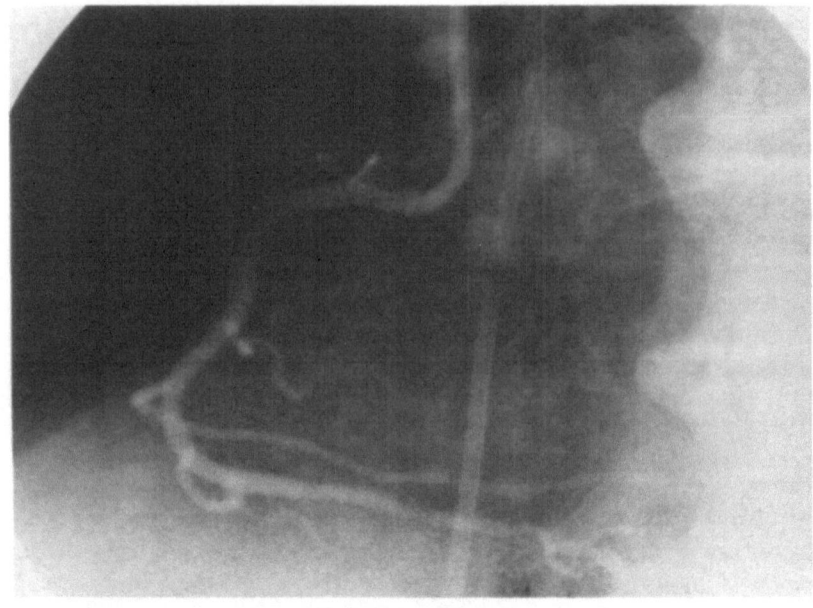

c

Figure 3. (A) (B) Single oblique MRCA along the long axis of the RCA with corresponding coronary angiogram (C) reprinted with permission [32]. Reprinted with permission of the New England Journal of Medicine [46].

approaches, a problem likely related to their oblique orientation, small size, and relative posterior location.

MRCA data on the average vessel diameter and the average length of contiguously observed major coronary artery in normals are summarized in Figure 4. The entire left main coronary artery is generally visualized, along with 5-8 cm contiguous segments of the left anterior descending and right coronary arteries. Only the proximal 2-3 cm of the left circumflex are seen, again likely related to the posterior location and diminutive size of this vessel as it continues in the atrio-ventricular groove. Though in-plane spatial resolution is relatively limited, MR coronary angiographic proximal coronary artery diameter corresponds well to angiographic and autopsy data [4,16] (Figure 5). Fewer data are available using 3D MRCA methods, though the extent of contiguous coronary artery visualization appears comparable [17-19].

Evaluation of anomalous coronary arteries

The ability of MRCA to visualize the proximal and mid portions of the native coronary arteries, and to define their position with respect to other major vessels/chambers, makes MRCA an ideal clinical tool for the identification of anomalous coronary arteries and delineation of their subsequent course. Among adults referred for contrast x-ray coronary angiography, anomalous origins of the epicardial coronary arteries are found in 0.6-1.2% of patients [20,21].

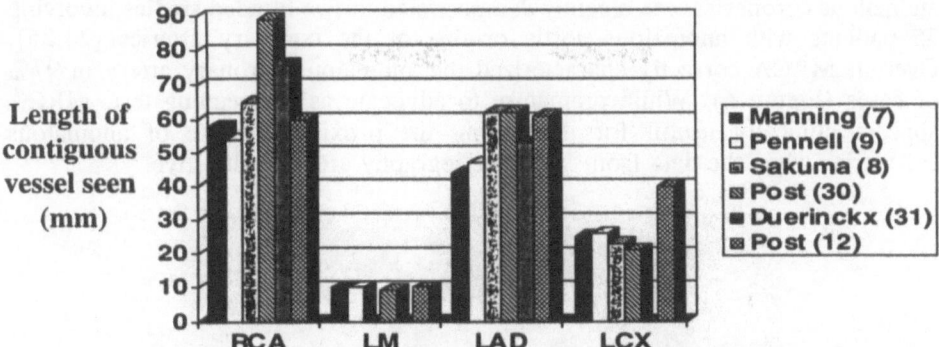

Figure 4. Contiguous length of native coronary artery visualized using 2D segmented k-space and 3D MR coronary angiographic techniques. RCA = right coronary artery; LM = left main; LAD = left anterior descending; LCX = left circumflex coronary artery.

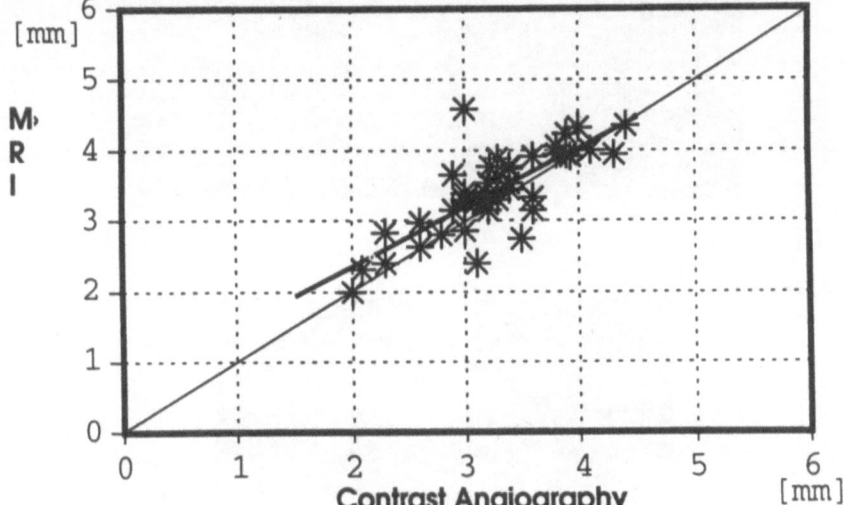

Figure 5. Scatterplot showing comparison of normal proximal vessel diameter as assessed by MR coronary angiography in a subset of patients who also underwent quantitative (digital caliper) contrast angiography. Reprinted with permission [16].

Fortunately, the majority of these anomalies are clinically benign. However, origin of a coronary artery from the contralateral side, with subsequent passage posterior to the pulmonary artery and anterior to the ascending aorta is associated with sudden death [22,23]. Conventional contrast x-ray coronary angiography identifies the presence of an anomalous vessel quite reliably, but the course of these anomalous vessels with respect to the aorta and pulmonary artery may be difficult to discern.

The superior ability of MRCA to delineate the three-dimensional path of anomalous coronaries was recently demonstrated in two blinded studies involving 35 patients with anomalous aortic origins of the coronary arteries [24,25]. Overall, MRCA correctly characterized the anomalous coronary artery in 97% of cases (Figure 6). While premature to advocate as a screening test, MRCA appears clinically useful for delineating the proximal course of anomalous coronaries when the data from x-ray angiography are not definitive.

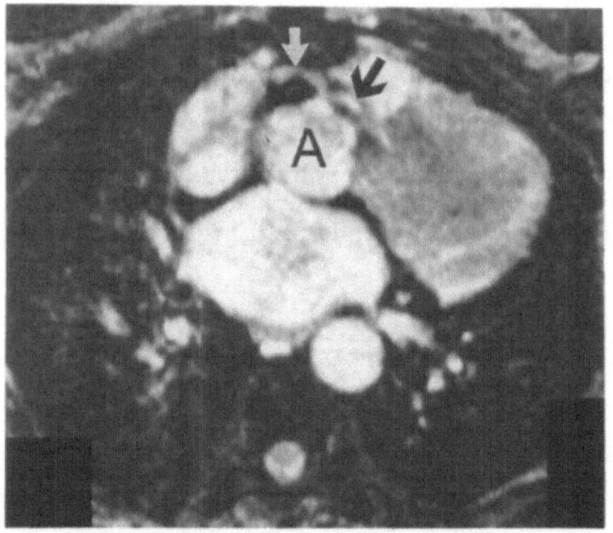

a

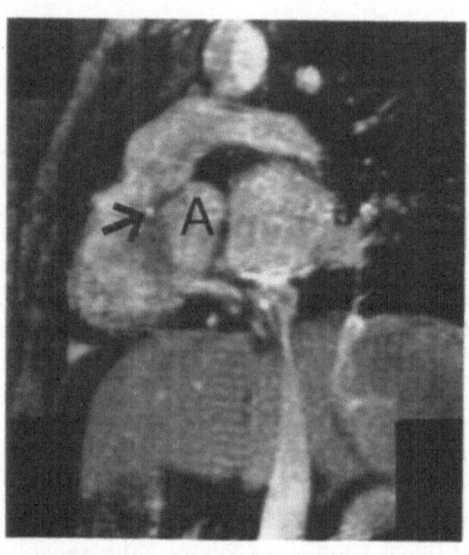

b

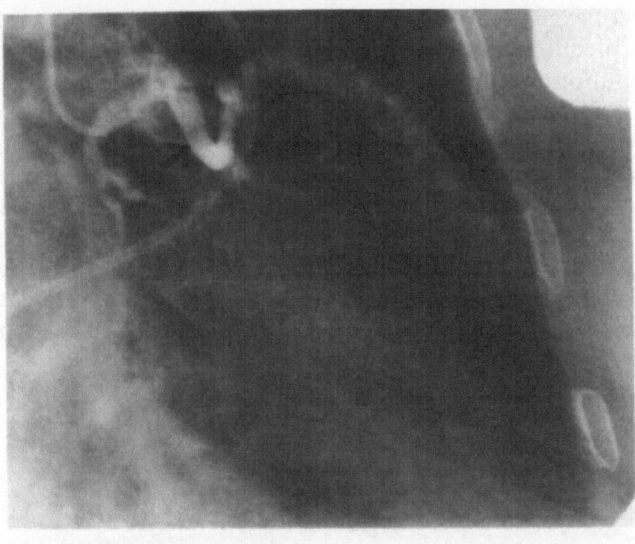

c

Figure 6. A) Transverse MRCA from a 61 year-old woman with an anomalous origin of the left main coronary artery (black arrow) from the right coronary artery (solid white arrow) with subsequent passage anterior to the aorta (A) and posterior to the right ventricular outflow tract. B) Oblique MRCA demonstrating the anomalous left coronary artery (black arrow) anterior to the aorta and posterior to the pulmonary artery. C) Corresponding contrast x-ray angiogram (RAO view) demonstrating the left main coronary artery (black arrow) coursing anterior to the aorta and posterior to the pulmonary artery (note the pulmonary artery catheter). Reprinted with permission of the American Heart Association [24].

Assessment of infarct artery patency

Over the past decade it has been recognized that among patients with myocardial infarction, restoration of antegrade flow in the infarct artery serves to improve both left ventricular function and survival [26-28]. Despite rapid initiation of thrombolytic therapy, 25% of infarct-related arteries will remain occluded [29]. If lack of patency could be quickly recognized, such patients could be referred for rescue angioplasty or other therapies. Contrast x-ray coronary angiography is a reliable method for determining infarct artery patency, but it is invasive and costly. Typically, MRCA methods are not sensitive to the direction of blood flow. Thus, infarct-related arteries with significant stenoses yet antegrade distal flow might appear similar to those with total occlusions and prominent retrograde blood flow in the distal vessel due to collaterals. By combining the previously described breath-hold MRCA methods with a saturation pre-pulse in the proximal portion of the infarct-related artery, blood flow direction distal to the infarct-related lesion can be assessed. Such an approach was recently reported by

Hundley and colleagues [30]. They used a cine version of a segmented k-space gradient-echo breath-hold technique to image the infarct artery both with and without a saturation pre-pulse applied proximal to the point of signal dropout. Signal loss occurs in the distal vessel if it received antegrade flow, while signal in the distal vessel would persists if there is retrograde blood flow to this region (Figures 7,8). Among patients with a prior history of myocardial infarction, these investigators were successful at characterizing antegrade or retrograde blood flow in all 18 vessels studied [30]. Data on a cohort with acute infarction have not been reported, but presumably would be similar. An alternative MR approach might be to directly measure coronary blood flow among patients with acute infarction using phase velocity methods [31-33], but this has not been reported in a clinical series.

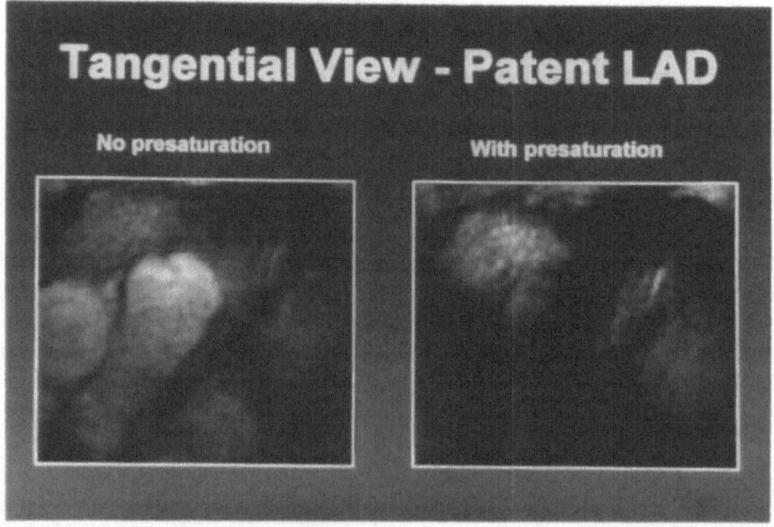

Figure 7. Oblique image of the distal left anterior descending (LAD) without (left) and with (right) presaturation pulses. Loss of signal in the LAD after presaturation (right) is consistent with antegrade blood flow in the LAD. Reprinted with permission of the American Heart Association [30].

Assessment of coronary artery bypass graft patency

Reverse saphenous vein and internal mammary artery bypass grafts have been easier to image using conventional MR imaging techniques due to their larger size (typically 5-10 mm in diameter) and more limited mobility associated with cardiac and respiration motion. Conventional ECG-gated spin-echo [34-36] and gradient-echo [37,38] methods have both been used to assess bypass graft patency for several years. Typically, transverse images are obtained at a level corresponding to that expected for the bypass graft. A graft is then characterized

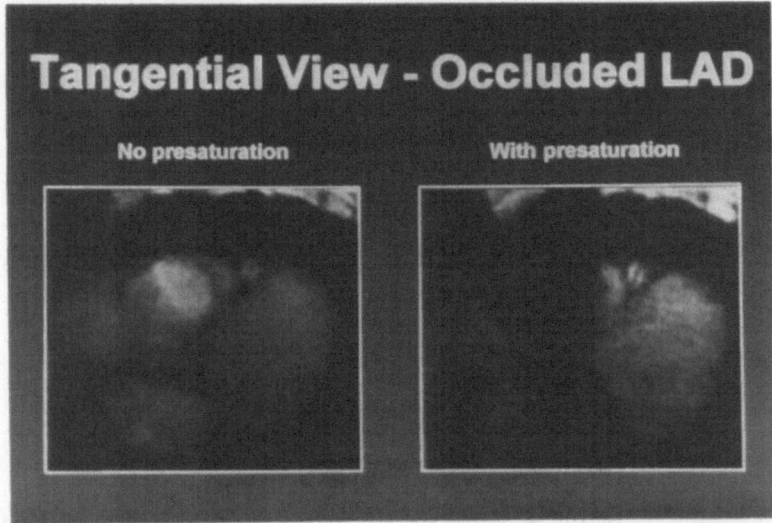

Figure 8. Oblique images of the LAD from another patient without (left) and with (right) presaturation pulses demonstrates persistence of signal in the distal LAD (white arrows) after presaturation, consistent with retrograde filling of this portion of the vessel. Reprinted with permission of the American Heart Association [30].

as "patent" if a signal void (spin echo) or bright signal (gradient echo) (Figure 9) of rapidly moving laminar blood flow is seen in at least two anatomic levels in the expected region of the bypass graft. Data from several clinical studies comparing MR data with contrast x-ray angiography are summarized in Table 1. Combined analysis of spin-echo and gradient-echo data do not appear to improve accuracy [39].

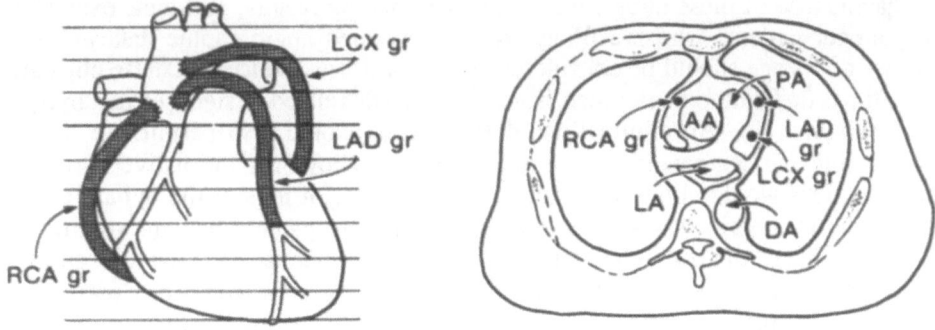

a

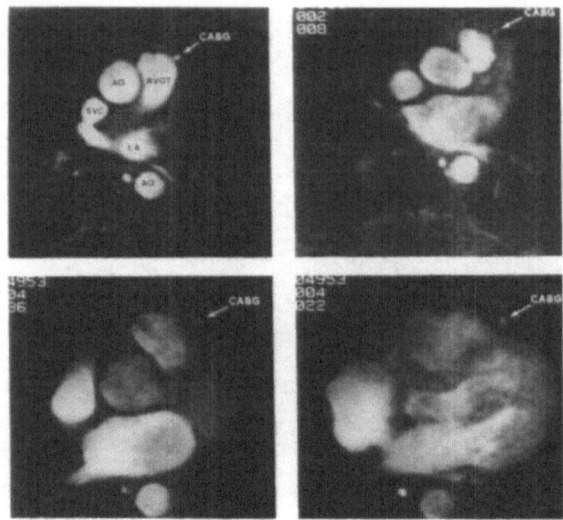

b

Figure 9. A) Typical location of bypass grafts coming off the proximal ascending aorta and anastomosing with the distal native coronaries with location of contiguous transaxial slices. B) The grafts as they might appear in a single transaxial slice (white arrows). AA = ascending aorta; DA = descending thoracic aorta; PA = pulmonary artery; RCA gr = graft to the right coronary artery (RCA); LAD gr = graft to the LAD; LCX gr = graft to the left circumflex coronary artery (LCX). Reprinted with permission of the American Heart Association [35].

Major obstacles to bypass graft imaging are the local signal artifacts associated with metallic hemostatic clips, sternal wires, and graft markers (Figure 10), especially with more sensitive gradient-echo sequences. The use of these metallic clips is especially common among patients with internal mammary artery grafts. The avoidance of these clips would improve imaging results, and their exclusion in younger patients who are likely to need repeated angiographic data as their bypass grafts age should be considered. Image artifacts induced by these clips are sometimes difficult to distinguish from signal voids related to stenoses in a bypass graft (Figure 10). An elimination of these clips would also permit use of the breath-hold 2D segmented approaches described above for the native coronary arteries. This would allow for imaging along the major axis of the bypass grafts and serve to identify saphenous vein grafts that are patent but with significant stenoses. Such stenoses can cause myocardial ischemia, yet for the studies reported to date, a bypass graft with a significant stenosis would be "correctly" classified as patent using conventional spin-echo or gradient-echo imaging [34-38]. Because of the frequent use of metallic intrathoracic clips, few data utilizing segmented gradient-echo approaches for imaging of vein grafts have been reported [40], though extensive portions of saphenous vein grafts are visible in selected patients (Figure 11).

In addition to MR imaging, phase velocity mapping has also been used to measure blood flow in native and grafted internal mammary arteries as well as saphenous vein grafts. The utility of MR phase mapping to assess bypass graft patency has been studied in approximately 135 bypass grafts [41-43]. Typical internal mammary artery bypass graft flow is 80 ml/min. Two studies [42,43] found saphenous vein grafts to be characterized by a biphasic flow pattern, the absence of which was useful for identifying diseased grafts. Another indicator of saphenous vein graft dysfunction is flow < 20 ml/min [42]. Grafts with three touch-down sites have greater volume flows as compared with grafts with a single touch-down site [43].

Table 1. Sensitivity/specificity of MR for characterizing CABGs as patent or occluded.

Author	Technique	#Pts	#Grafts	%SVG	%Patent	Sens	Spec
White [34]	Spin-echo	25	72	88	69	0.86	0.72
Rubinstein [35]	Spin-echo	20	47	100	62*	0.90	0.72
Jenkins [36]	Spin-echo	16†	41	100	63	0.89	0.73
Galjee [39]	Spin-echo	47	98	100	74	0.98**	0.85**
White [37]	Cine gradient-echo	10	28	96	52	0.93	0.86
Aurigemma [38]	Cine gradient-echo	20	45	91	73	0.88	1.00
Galjee [39]	Cine gradient-echo	47	98	100	74	0.98**	0.88**

* graft with 99% diameter stenosis was considered occluded
†# of pts who had comparison angiograms
** data for 7 grafts were inconclusive and excluded from analysis
SVG = reverse saphenous vein bypass graft; Pts = patients; Sens = sensitivity; Spec = specificity

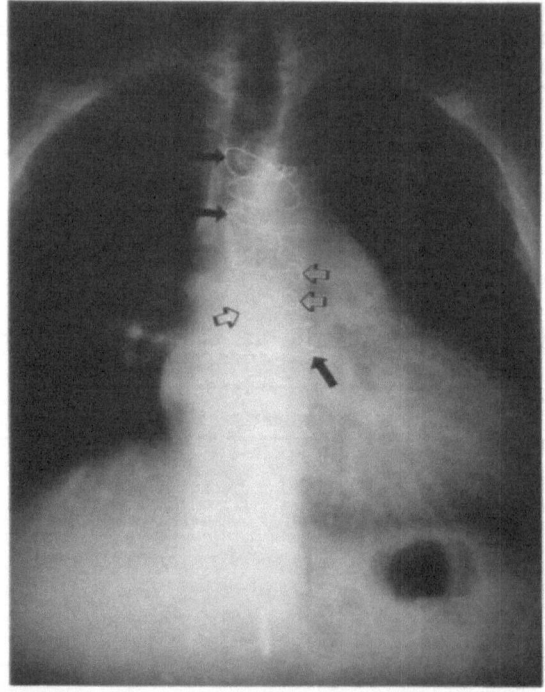

a

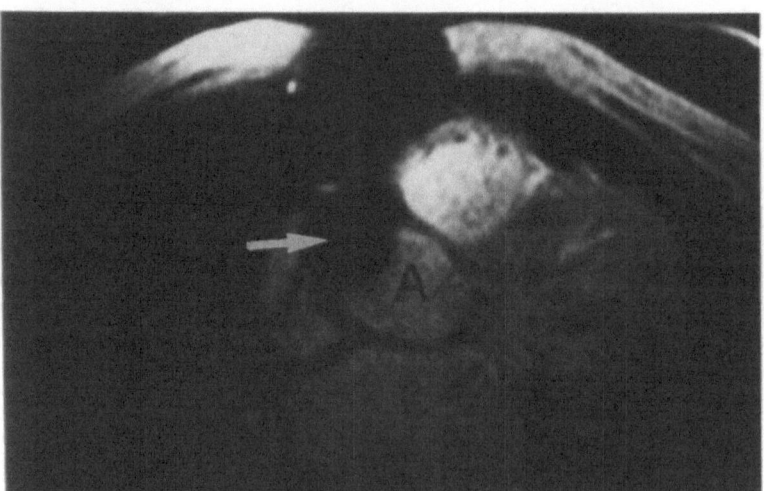

b

Figure 10. A) Posterior-anterior chest x-ray demonstrating sternal wires (solid black arrows) and graft markers (open black arrows). B) Transverse breath-hold MRCA showing signal voids in the sternum as well as area corresponding to the graft markers.

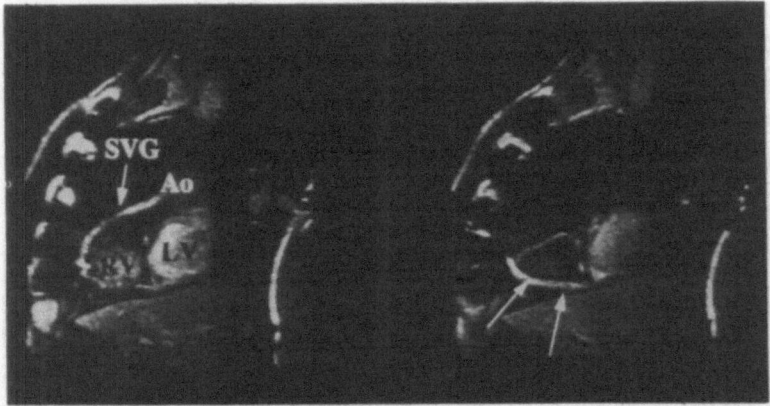

Figure 11. Oblique breath-hold MRCA of a widely patent saphenous vein bypass graft (SVG) (white arrows) extending from the aorta (Ao) to an acute marginal and posterior descending coronary artery.

Identification of coronary artery stenoses

Despite ongoing improvements in both prevention and treatment, coronary artery disease remains the leading cause of morbidity and mortality in the developed world. In the U.S. alone, there are over 1.5 million myocardial infarctions and 490,000 cardiac deaths per year, at an estimated cost of $66 billion [44]. Numerous noninvasive tests for identifying patients with coronary artery disease have been developed, yet at least 20% of diagnostic contrast x-ray coronary angiograms demonstrate no significant stenoses [45]. The ability of MRA to non-invasively assess coronary artery integrity would therefore represent an important advance in patient care.

The small caliber of the native coronary arteries (3-4 mm in diameter) and relatively limited spatial resolution of current breath-hold MRCA methods (1.9 x 0.9 mm; vs 300μ for contrast angiography), makes quantitative MRCA impractical using current approaches. Instead, we and others have used the blood-flow sensitivity of gradient-echo MR to identify focal coronary stenoses. Coronary artery stenoses are characterized by signal "voids" due to turbulent (proton dephasing) or from markedly diminished, or absent blood flow (due to saturation effects) which contrasts with the "bright" signal from rapidly moving, laminar blood flow (due to inflow of unsaturated protons). Therefore, coronary arteries with severe stenoses but significant antegrade blood flow would be expected to have a focal loss of signal, followed by bright signal depicting laminar flow in the more distal lumen, and the extent (length) of the stenosis would be expected to be exaggerated on MRCA due to post-stenosis flow abnormalities. A total occlusion or severe stenosis with poor distal blood flow, on the other hand, would be expected to appear as an abrupt loss of signal (Figure 12). As MRCA spatial resolution is currently relatively limited, quantitative MRCA is not possible.

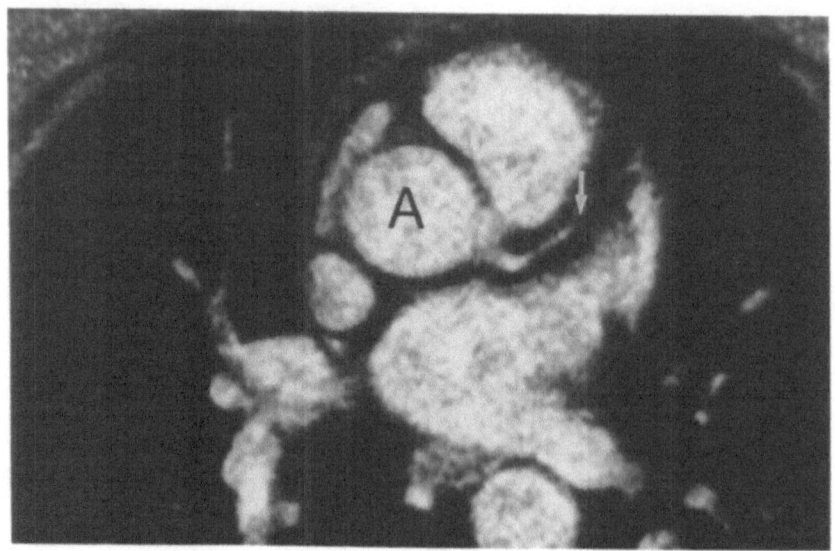

a

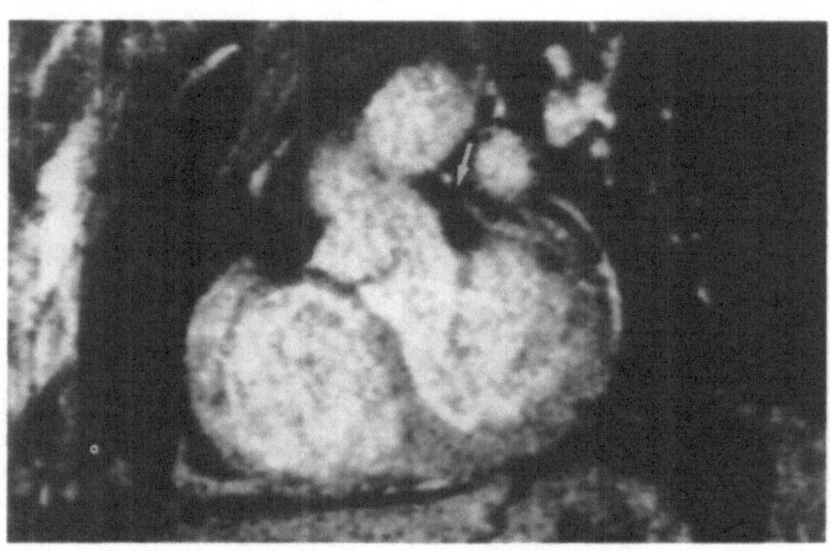

b

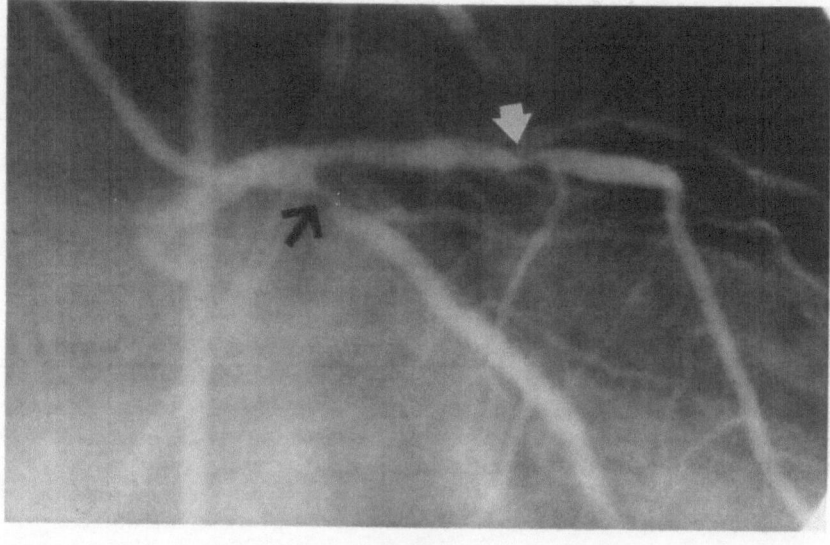

c

Figure 12. A) Transverse MRCA demonstrating a signal void in the proximal-mid LAD (white arrow). B) Oblique MRCA demonstrating a signal void in the proximal left circumflex coronary artery (white arrow). C) Contrast x-ray angiogram demonstrating the stenoses in the proximal-mid LAD(white arrow) and proximal left cirumflex coronary arteries (black arrow).

We have reported on a group of 39 patients referred for elective coronary angiography who also underwent breath-hold MRCA examination either immediately before or after conventional contrast x-ray angiography [46]. Individual major coronary arteries were graded as "normal or having minimal disease" if there were minimal or no luminal irregularities, or as having "substantial disease" if there was marked attenuation of the luminal diameter or a signal void. MRCA images of 98% of the major coronary arteries were adequate for evaluation. In a blinded analysis, overall sensitivity and specificity of the 2D MRA technique for correctly classifying individual vessels as with (50% diameter stenosis on conventional contrast x-ray angiography) or without disease, was 90% and 92%, respectively. The corresponding positive and negative predictive values were 0.85 and 0.95, respectively. Data for individual vessels are shown in Table 2. The sensitivity and specificity of the MRCA technique for correctly classifying individual patients as having or not having significant coronary disease, in this population with an prevalence of coronary disease of 0.74, was 97% and 70%, respectively. Using similar methodology, comparable data have been reported by others [47-49] and appears quite favorable for left main stenoses or proximal right and left anterior descending coronary artery stenoses.

Using a similar approach, Pennell and co-workers [49] graded MRCA data as severe (complete signal loss), moderate (partial signal loss) and mild (wall irregularity only) stenoses and found a significant relationship between angiographic diameter stenoses based on these classifications. Preliminary data

Table 2. Sensitivity, specificity, positive/negative predictive value of MRCA

	# (%) with disease	sensitivity (%)	specificity (%)	PV (+)	PV (−)
LM	2 (5%)	100	100	1.00	1.00
LAD	23 (64%)	87	92	0.95	0.80
LCX	7 (20%)	71	90	0.63	0.93
RCA	20 (53%)	100	78	0.83	1.00
Patient	29 (74%)	97	70	0.90	0.88

Abbreviations as in Table 1.
PV (+) = predictive value positive; PV (−) = predictive value negative
Modified from [46] and printed with permission

from Rogers and co-workers [50], however, suggest computer-assisted measurement of the coronary signal intensity does not correlate with severity of stenoses. A recent study using flow phantoms by Oshinski et al. [51] suggests that the magnitude of the turbulent fluctuation velocity, and not merely the presence of turbulence or the Reynolds number, was the parameter that determined the extent of signal loss in the area of stenosis.
In contrast, Duerinckx and Urman [14], as well as Post and colleagues [12]), have had more limited success utilizing 2D segmented MRA for identification of coronary stenoses. This may be related to their use of longer acquisition times [14], a shorter echo time [12], poor patient cooperation with breath-holding, or irregular cardiac rhythms, all of which will contribute to image degradation. 3D MRCA also appears to be far more limited in the ability to detect stenoses using non-breath-hold or breath-hold techniques [12], though the use of 3D MRCA in combination with navigator gating shows great promise (Figure 13).

MR coronary angiography - future directions

Considerable work needs to be done before MRCA can be advocated for the routine clinical evaluation of patients with multiple risk factors or suspected coronary artery disease. For now MRCA has relatively limited clinical applications - primarily evaluation of anomalous coronary arteries, determination of infarct artery patency, and potentially the identification or patent saphenous vein grafts and exclusion of left main coronary artery disease. Before MRCA can be advocated for the detection of native epicardial disease of the major branch vessels, improvements in spatial resolution and respiratory motion suppression are needed.

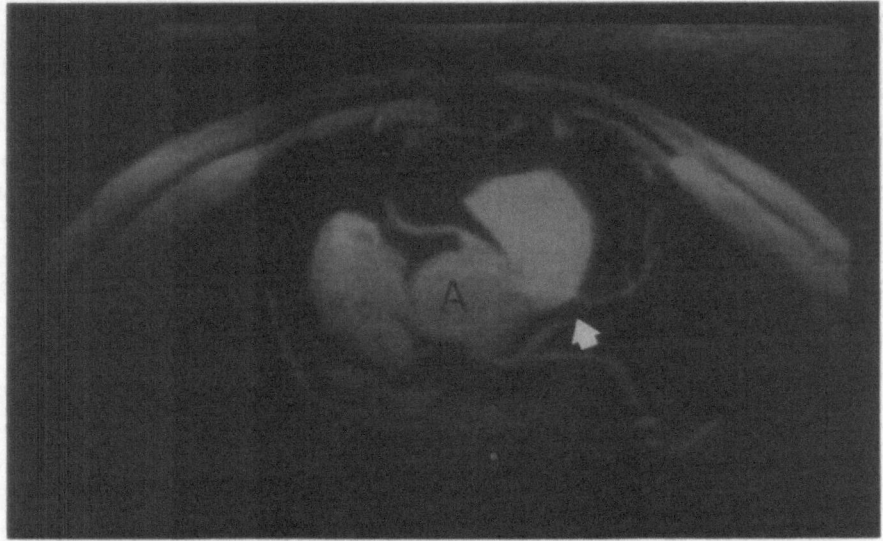

Figure 13. Maximum intensity projection showing the coronary arteries of a patient with a 50% proximal left anterior descending coronary artery stenosis (arrow). The original images were collected using a 3D acquisition sequence with retrospective respiratory gating. The left ventricle was removed by post-processing before projection to avoid overlapping with the coronary arteries. Reprinted with permission (Haacke EM, Li D, Kaushikkar S, Cardiac MR imaging: Principles and techniques. Topics Magn Reson Imaging 1995; 7: 200-217).

Respiratory suppression methods

Suppression of respiratory motion artifacts is essential for MRCA. The current use of breath-holds to minimize respiratory artifacts has many limitations, including registration errors related to breath-hold variability, variable image quality due to the need for significant patient cooperation and experienced operator involvement, and relatively limited spatial resolution due to time constraints.

Alternatives to standard breath-holding that reduce breath-hold variability include multiple 1-s breath-holds [43] and respiratory feedback monitoring systems [52-54]. It is likely that these methods will also have limited clinical utility as they also require significant patient cooperation and operator instruction. Respiratory gating to an external (bellows) sensor monitoring chest/abdominal wall expansion has been proposed as a method for respiratory motion suppression during free breathing [55]. This technique assumes that chest/abdominal wall motion correlates closely with respiratory motion of the heart. While time efficient, preliminary data from our laboratory [56] and Oshinski et al. [57] suggest that simple bellows gating results in inferior image quality as compared to breath-holding.

A more eloquent approach involves the use of MR navigator echos to directly track the respiratory motion of the heart or diaphragm during free breathing

(Figure 14) and appears to offer a more optimal solution for respiratory motion suppression [58]. End-expiratory gating may be performed retrospectively [59] or prospectively [60]. Such an approach requires minimal patient and operator involvement. Most importantly, given the linear relationship between diaphragmatic, cardiac, and coronary position [61] navigator position can also be used for prospective adaptive correction of the image slice position to improve image quality and time efficiency [62]. In our experience, navigator gating significantly reduces registration error (thus requiring fewer slices to complete imaging of the coronary imaging) with similar image quality [56]. The use of navigator gating also improves image quality for 3D coronary MRCA [63] (Figure 13).

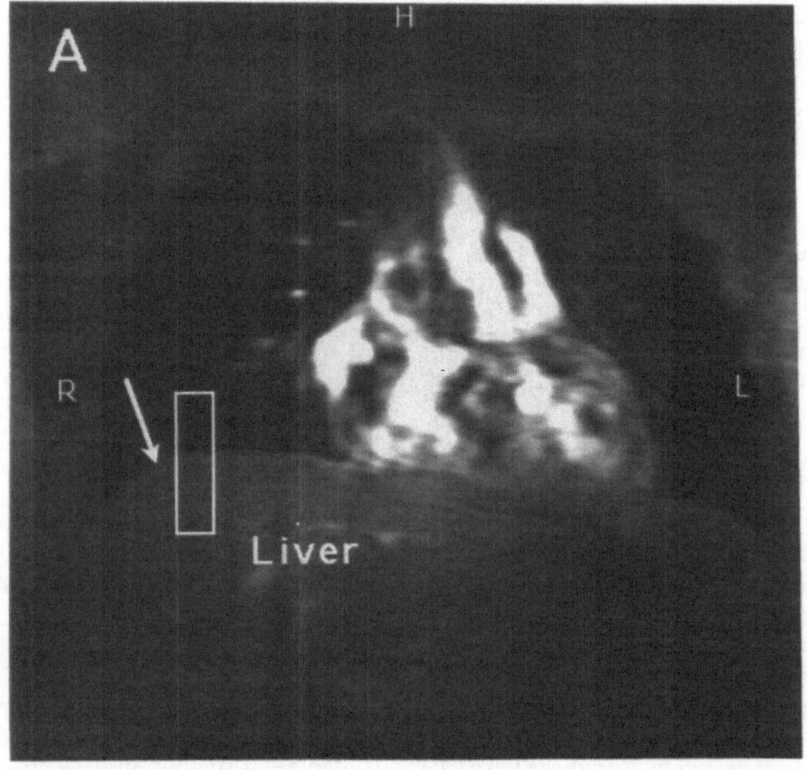

a

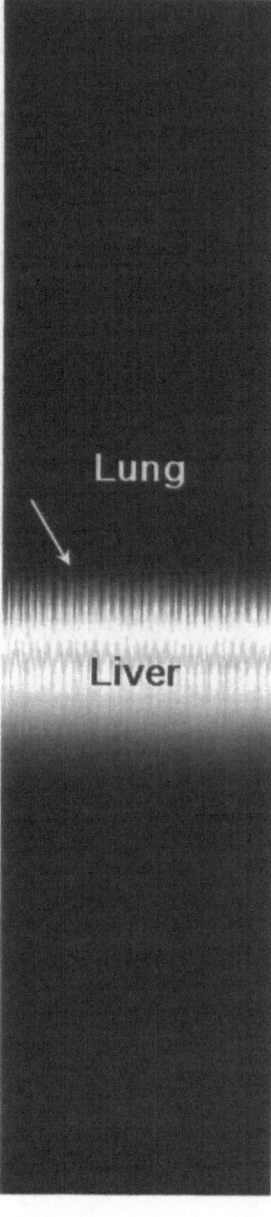

b

Figure 14. A) Turbo field echo coronal scout depicting the location of a vertical navigator (white rectangle) through the dome of the right hemidiaphragm (white arrow). B) Navigator echoes through the right hemidiaphragm are shown as a vertical one-dimensional line image with the lung appearing dark and the diaphragm and liver appearing bright. The rise and fall of the diaphragm with normal respiration is visible. Approximately 1 minute of data are depicted in this figure.

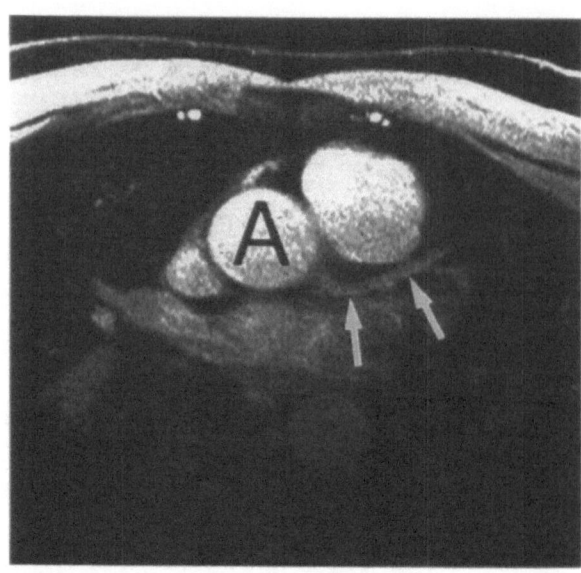

Figure 15. High-resolution transverse MRCA acquired using navigator gating depicting the left main and LAD (arrows). Spatial resolution is 950 μ x 475 μ.

Advances in MR hardware

Much of current MR hardware has been optimized for brain and body imaging. Only recently have manufacturer's begun developing cardiac specific hardware. One important advance is the development of phased-array surface coils specifically adapted for the size and location of the heart [64,65]. Initial experience has shown improved signal/noise compared to surface and body coils, with the greatest benefit is likely to be for visualization of posterior cardiac structures, such as the left circumflex coronary artery.

Stronger and faster gradients are also being developed, which can enhance signal/noise and allow for more rapid imaging [66], including EPI techniques [11]. High-field systems (3T) have also been installed at several centers. They offer the potential for improved signal/noise, but also require significant adaptation of other equipment to function at high field [67]. Specific advantages for such high field systems for coronary imaging remain to be determined.

High-resolution coronary MRA

While MRCA will likely not supplant diagnostic x-ray coronary angiography for several years to come, the field is advancing very quickly. The recent advances discussed above -navigator gating, cardiac RF coils, improved gradients - will likely be combined to allow rapid, high-resolution 2D or 3D MRCA [68] (Figures 13,15). In-plane resolution of 500 μ or less will begin to approach that of x-ray angiography (300 μ). This approach will allow for a quantitative or semi-quantitative assessment of coronary stenosis, which clinicians need for guiding therapeutic decisions. In addition, improved visualization and evaluation of the smaller, but clinically relevant major diagonal and obtuse marginal arteries will likely be obtained.

Conclusion

Over the past five years, tremendous strides have been made in the development of MRCA, but considerable hurdles remain before its routine clinical use can be advocated. Using breath-hold 2D approaches, extensive portions of the native coronary arteries can now be seen in the vast majority of subjects. While it is premature to advocate MRCA for the identification of native coronary artery stenoses, recent improvements in software and hardware suggest that clinical MRCA made soon find a role in the evaluation of specific patient subgroups, such as patients presenting with a dilated cardiomyopathy or those requiring surgery for primary valvular heart disease. Standardization of methodology, large multicenter trials, and outcomes research will need to be performed, but the future of MRCA looks very promising.

Acknowledgments

Supported in part by grants from the National Institute of Health (RO1 HL48538), Bethesda, MD, and the Edward J. Mallinkrodt, Jr. Foundation, Saint Louis, MO.

References

1. Nienaber CA, von Kodolitsch Y, Nicolas V *et al*. The diagnosis of thoracic aortic dissection by noninvasive imaging procedures. N Engl J Med 1993;328:1-9.
2. Paulin S, von Schulthess GK, Fossel E, Krayenbuehl HP. MR imaging of the aortic root and proximal coronary arteries. AJR Am J Roentgenol 1987;148:665-70.
3. Edelman RR, Manning WJ, Burstein D, Paulin S. Coronary arteries: breath-hold MR angiography. Radiology 1991;181:641-3.
4. Manning WJ, Li W, Boyle NG, Edelman RR. Fat-suppressed breath-hold magnetic resonance coronary angiography. Circulation 1993;87:94-104.
5. Sakuma H, Caputo GR, Steffens JC *et al*. Breath-hold MR cine angiography of coronary arteries in healthy volunteers: value of multiangle oblique imaging planes. AJR Am J Roentgenol 1994;163:533-7.
6. Wang Y, Grist TM, Korosec FR *et al*. Respiratory blur in 3D coronary MR imaging. Magn Reson Med 1995;33:541-8.
7. Wang SJ, Hu BS, Macovski A, Nishimura DG. Coronary angiography using fast selective inversion recovery. Magn Reson Med 1991;18:417-23.
8. Meyer CH, Hu BS, Nishimura DG, Macovski A. Fast spiral coronary artery imaging. Magn Reson Med 1992;28:202-13.
9. BÜrnert P, Jensen D. Coronary artery imaging at 0.5T using segmented echo

planar imaging. Magn Reson Med 1995;34:779-85.

10. Edelman RR. Cardiac angiography [abstract]. Proc Soc Magn Reson 1994:104.

11. Wielopolski PA, Manning WJ, Edelman RR. Breath-hold volumetric imaging of the heart using magnetization prepared 3D segmented echo planar imaging. J Magn Reson Imaging 1995;5:403-9.

12. Post JC, van Rossum AC, Hofman MBM *et al*. Current limitations of two-dimensional breath-hold MR angiography in coronary artery disease [abstract]. Proc Soc Magn Reson 1994:508.

13. Pennell DJ, Keegan J, Firmin DN, Gatehouse PD, Underwood SR, Longmore DS. Magnetic resonance imaging of coronary arteries: Technique and preliminary results. Br Heart J 1993;70:315-26.

14. Duerinckx AJ, Urman MK. Two-dimensional coronary MR angiography: analysis of initial clinical results. Radiology 1994;193:731-8.

15. Post JC, van Rossum AC, Hofman MBM *et al*. Clinical utility of two-dimensional breath-hold MR angiography in coronary artery disease [abstract]. Proc Soc Magn Reson 1995:1394.

16. Scheidegger MB, Vassalli G, Hess OM, Boesiger P. Validation of coronary artery MR angiography: comparison of measured vessel diameters with quantitative contrast angiography [abstract]. Proc Soc Magn Reson 1994:497.

17. Li D, Paschal CB, Haacke EM, Adler LP. Coronary arteries: Three-dimensional MR imaging with fat saturation and magnetization transfer contrast. Radiology 1993;187:401-6.

18. Post JC, van Rossum AC, Hofman MBM, Valk J, Visser CA. Respiratory-gated three-dimensional MR angiography of coronary arteries and comparison with x-ray contrast angiography [abstract]. Proc Soc Magn Reson 1994:509.

19. Dogherty L, Schnall MD, Holland GA, Greenman BL, Axel L. Fast 3D imaging of coronary arteries using Gd-DTPA enhancement [abstract]. Proc Soc Magn Reson 1995:1397.

20. Engel HJ, Torres C, Page HL Jr. Major variations in anatomical origin of the coronary arteries: angiographic observations in 4,250 patients without associated congenital heart disease. Cathet Cardiovasc Diagn 1975;1:157-69.

21. Kimbiris D, Iskandrian AS, Segal BL, Bemis CE. Anomalous aortic origin of coronary arteries. Circulation 1978;58:606-15.

22. Cheitlin MD, De Castro DM, McAllister HA. Sudden death as a complication of anomalous left coronary origin from the anterior sinus of Valsalva. A not-so-minor congenital anomaly. Circulation 1974;50:780-7.

23. Levin DC, Fellows KE, Abrams HL. Hemodynamically significant primary anomalies of the coronary arteries: Angiographic aspects. Circulation 1978;58:25-34.

24. McConnell MV, Ganz P, Selwyn AP, Li W, Edelman RR, Manning WJ. Identification of anomalous coronary arteries and their anatomic course by magnetic resonance coronary angiography. Circulation 1995;92:3158-62.

25. Post JC, van Rossum AC, Bronzwaer JGF *et al*. Magnetic resonance angiography of anomalous coronary arteries. A new gold standard for delineating the proximal course? Circulation 1995;92:3163-71.

26. Cigarro RG, Lange RA, Hillis LD. Prognosis after acute myocardial infarction in patients with an without residual antegrade coronary blood flow. Am J Cardiol 1989;64:155-60.

27. Holmes DR Jr, Califf RM, Topol EJ. Lessons we have learned from the GUSTO trial. Global Utilization of Streptokinase and Tissue Plasminogen

Activator for Occluded Arteries. J Am Coll Cardiol 1995;25(7 Suppl.):10S-17S.

28. Lamas G, Flaker F, Mitchell G *et al* for the SAVE investigators. Effect of captopril therapy on post MI outcome in patients with and without a patent infarct-related artery [abstract]. J Am Coll Cardiol 1993;21(2 Suppl.A):44A.

29. Topol EJ, Califf RM, George BS *et al*. A randomized trial of immediate versus delayed elective angioplasty after intravenous tissue plasminogen activator in acute myocardial infarction. N Engl J Med 1987;317:581-8.

30. Hundley WG, Clarke GD, Landau C *et al*. Noninvasive determination of infarct artery patency by cine magnetic resonance angiography. Circulation 1995;91:1347-53.

31. Edelman RR, Manning WJ, Gervino E, Li W. Flow velocity quantification in human coronary arteries using fast, breath-hold MR angiography. J Magn Reson Imaging 1993;3:699-703.

32. Keegan J, Firmin D, Gatehouse P, Longmore D. The application of breathhold phase velocity mapping techniques to the measurement of coronary artery blood flow velocity: Phantom data and initial in vivo results. Magn Reson Med 1994;31:526-36.

33. Poncelet BP, Weisskoff RM, Wedeen VJ, Brady TJ, Kantor H. Time of flight quantification of coronary flow with echo-planar MRI. Magn Reson Med 1993;30:447-57.

34. White RD, Caputo GR, Mark AS, Modin GW, Higgins CB. Coronary artery bypass graft patency: noninvasive evaluation with MR imaging. Radiology 1987;164:681-6.

35. Rubinstein RI, Askenase AD, Thickman D, Feldman MS, Agarwal JB, Helfant RH. Magnetic resonance imaging to evaluate patency of aortocoronary bypass grafts. Circulation 1987;76:786-91.

36. Jenkins JPR, Love HG, Foster CJ, Isherwood I, Rowlands DJ. Detection of coronary artery bypass graft patency as assessed by magnetic resonance imaging. Br J Radiol 1988;61:2-4.

37. White RD, Pflugfelder PW, Lipton MJ, Higgins CB. Coronary artery bypass grafts: evaluation of patency with cine MR imaging. AJR Am J Roentgenol 1988;150:1271-4.

38. Aurigemma GP, Reichek N, Axel L, Schiebler M, Harris C, Kressel HY. Noninvasive determination of coronary artery bypass graft patency by cine magnetic resonance imaging. Circulation 1989;80:1595-602.

39. Galjee MA, van Rossum AC, Doesburg T, van Eenige MJ, Visser CA. Value of magnetic resonance imaging in assessing patency and function of coronary artery bypass grafts: an angiographically controlled study. Circulation 1996;93:660-6.

40. Pennell DJ, Keegan J, Firmin DN *et al*. Magnetic resonance coronary angiography: Early experience in coronary artery disease and visualization of vein grafts [abstract]. Proc Soc Magn Reson Med 1993:219.

41. Debatin JF, Strong JA, Sostman HD *et al*. MR characterization of blood flow in native and grafted internal mammary arteries. J Magn Reson Imaging 1993;3:443-50.

42. Hoogendoorn LI, Pattynama PM, Buis B, van der Geest RJ, van der Wall EE, de Roos A. Noninvasive evaluation of aortocoronary bypass grafts with magnetic resonance flow mapping. Am J Cardiol 1995;75:845-8.

43. Doyle M, Scheidegger MB, de Graaf RG, Vermeulen J, Pohost GM. Coronary artery imaging in multiple 1-sec breath holds. Magn Reson Imaging

1993;11:3-6.

44. Heart and stroke facts: 1996 statistical supplement. Dallas: American Heart Association, 1996:9,22,23.

45. Kaski JC, Elliott PM. Angina pectoris and normal coronary arteriograms: clinical presentation and hemodynamic characteristics. Am J Cardiol 1995;76:35D-42D.

46. Manning WJ, Li W, Edelman RR. A preliminary report comparing magnetic resonance coronary angiography with conventional angiography. N Engl J Med 1993;328:828-32.

47. Nitatori T, Hachiya J, Korenaga T et al. Clinical application of coronary MR angiography: studies on shortening of time for examinatino [abstract]. Proc Society Magn Reson, 1995:1390.

48. Post JC, van Rossum AC, Hofman MBM et al. Clinical utility of two-dimensional breath-hold MR angiography in coronary artery disease [abstract]. Proc Society Magn Reson, 1995:1394.

49. Pennell DJ, Bogren HG, Keegan J et al. Detection, localisation and assessment of coronary artery stenosis by magnetic resonance imaging [abstract]. Proc Soc Magn Reson 1994:369.

50. Rogers WJ, Kramer CM, Simonetti OP, Reichek N. Quantification of human coronary stenoses by magnetic resonance angiography [abstract]. Proc Soc Magn Reson 1994:370.

51. Oshinski JN, Ku DN, Pettigrew RI. Turbulent fluctuation velocity: the most significant determinant of signal loss in stenotic vessels. Magn Reson Med 1995;33:193-9.

52. Liu YL, Riederer SJ, Rossman PJ, Grimm RC, Debbins JP, Ehman RL. A monitoring, feedback, and triggering system for reproducible breath-hold MR imaging. Magn Reson Med 1993; 30:507-11.

53. Wang Y, Christy PS, Korosec FR et al. Coronary MRI with a respiratory feedback monitor: the 2D imaging case. Magn Reson Med 1995;33:116-21.

54. Wang Y, Grimm RC, Rossman PJ, Debbins JP, Riederer SJ, Ehman RL. 3D coronary MR angiography in multiple breath-holds using a respiratory feedback monitor. Magn Reson Med 1995;34:11-6.

55. Ehman RL, McNamara MT, Pallack M, Hricak H, Higgins CB. Magnetic resonance imaging with respiratory gating: techniques and advantages. AJR Am J Roentgenol 1984;143:1175-82.

56. Khasgiwala VC, McConnell MV, Savord BJ et al. Comparison of respiratory gating techniques and navigator locations for magnetic resonance coronary angiography [abstract]. Circulation. In press.

57. Oshinski JN, Hofland L, Mukundan S Jr, Dixon WT, Parks WJ, Pettigrew RI. Respiratory gated coronary magnetic resonance angiography compares favorably with breath-hold imaging [abstract]. Proc Soc Magn Reson 1995:22.

58. Ehman RL, Felmlee JP. Adaptive technique for high-definition MR imaging of moving structures. Radiology 1989; 173:255-63.

59. Hofman MBM, Paschal CB, Li D, Haacke EM, van Rossum AC, Sprenger M. MRI of coronary arteries: 2D breathhold vs 3D respiratory-gated acquisition. J Comput Assist Tomogr 1995;19:56-62.

60. Sachs TS, Meyer CH, Hu BS, Kuhli J, Nishimura DG, Macovski A. Real-time motion detection in spiral MRI using navigators. Magn Reson Med 1994;32:639-45.

61. Wang Y, Riederer SJ, Ehman RL. Respiratory motion of the heart: kinematics

and the implications for the spatial resolution in coronary imaging. Magn Reson Med 1995;33:713-9.

62. McConnell MV, Khasgiwala VC, Savord BJ *et al.* Prospective navigator correction of slice position during magnetic resonance coronary angiography [abstract]. Circulation. In press.

63. Wang Y, Rossman PJ, Grimm RC, Riederer SJ, Ehman RL. Navigator-echo-based real-time respiratory gating and triggering for reduction of respiration effects in three-dimensional coronary MR angiography. Radiology 1996;198:55-60.

64. Constantinides CD, Westgate CR, O'Dell WG, Zerhouni EA, McVeigh ER. A phased array coil for human cardiac imaging. Magn Reson Med 1995;34:92-8.

65. Fayad ZA, Connick TJ, Axel L. An improved quadrature or phased-array coil for MR cardiac imaging. Magn Reson Med 1995;34:186-93.

66. Reeder SB, McVeigh ER. The effect of high performance gradients on fast gradient echo imaging. Magn Reson Med 1994;32:612-21.

67. Jaffer FA, Duewell S, Chesnick AS, Wen H, Balaban RS. Cardiac imaging at 4.0 Tesla using a local volume coil [abstract]. Proc Soc Magn Reson 1994;1511.

68. Li D, Dhawale PJ, Kaushikkar S, Haacke EM. High resolution magnetic resonance imaging of coronary arteries [abstract]. Circulation 1995;92(Suppl.I):I-224.

27. Advantages and limitations of coronary MR angiography

ANDRÉ J. DUERINCKX

Summary

The principles underlying coronary MR angiographic pulse sequences are reviewed, including basic coronary anatomy, motion and flow physiology. Coronary MR angiographic techniques can be subdivided in breath-hold (single or repeated breath-hold) and non-breath-hold techniques. Most of the clinical experience so far has been with a single breath-hold technique, and was limited to cooperative patients. The recent introduction of navigator pulses for real-time respiratory gating or triggering allows non-breath-hold or repeated breath-hold 3-D coronary MR angiography, and will allow a more widespread use of this technique. Although the role of coronary MR angiography in screening for coronary artery lesions has not yet been established, coronary MR angiography has been very successful in the detection of coronary artery variants, and the imaging of coronary stents and bypass grafts. These new MRI techniques can be adapted to quantitate velocity in native coronary arteries.

Introduction

Coronary arteries are small tortuous vessels subjected to significant physiological motion, both cardiac and respiratory, which present a tremendous challenge to conventional magnetic resonance imaging (MRI) and magnetic resonance angiography (MRA) techniques. With the development of a new group of ultrafast MR imaging pulse sequences "reliable" magnetic resonance angiography (MRA) of the coronary arteries has gradually become possible during the last five years [1-8]. The term "reliable" means simply that images of good reproducible quality can routinely be obtained in the majority of patients [9-12]. The potential diagnostic value or clinical utility of these coronary MR images is still unproven [13]. We will first review the history of the development of coronary MRA.

Conventional cardiac triggered MRI has provided reliable, clinically useful and diagnostic images of cardiac structures and large vessels within the thorax for many years [14]. Imaging of coronary bypass grafts with these techniques has also been possible partially because these vessels are subjected to less respiratory motion than native coronary vessels. With conventional cardiac MRI it has been possible to visualize coronary bypass grafts, evaluate bypass graft patency [15,16] and quantitate flow in bypass grafts [17]. Although small portions of the native coronary artery tree are also occasionally seen on traditional cardiac triggered spin-echo (SE) and gradient-recalled-echo (GRE) images [18], the new coronary MR angiographic techniques allow much more reliable and consistent visualization of the proximal coronary tree [9-12].

Conventional MRA techniques depict and characterize blood vessels and blood

357

J.H.C. Reiber and E.E. van der Wall (eds.), Cardiovascular Imaging, 357-365.
© *1996 Kluwer Academic Publishers.*

flow and are relatively well established in clinical practice [19,20]. MR angiographic techniques traditionally rely on either time of flight (TOF) or a phase contrast (PC) approaches. When it comes to imaging small tortuous vessels in the chest or abdomen, none of these traditional MRA techniques have been able to perform consistently or adequately [21-24].

Recent advances in MR pulse sequence design have resulted in a significant reduction of both respiratory motion artifacts (by eliminating, correcting or compensating for respiratory motion) and pulsatile flow artifacts (by always using cardiac triggering and mid-diastolic acquisitions), while maintaining a reasonable short image acquisition time (by segmenting the data acquisition in k-space) [25,26]. Coronary MR angiography does significantly differ from conventional MRA in that it incorporates mechanisms to compensate for both cardiac and respiratory motion. Most of the new coronary MR angiography techniques can also be applied to image vessels elsewhere in the body.

The physiology of blood flow in coronary arteries is very different from the physiology of blood flow in large vessels such as the carotid arteries and the abdominal aorta. In the coronary arteries flow velocities are lower than in other large vessels; there is less or no turbulent flow and there is potential for collateral blood flow. Normal coronary arteries and veins appear as high signal linear structures on coronary MR angiograms. Distal to a total occlusion vessels with no collateral flow have decreased signal intensity or background (fat-suppressed) signal intensity .

Clinical applications

Significant clinical applications of coronary MRA have been defined and include: determining the patency of and direction of flow in native coronary arteries [13,27-29]; evaluation of coronary bypass grafts and native vessels after coronary stent placement [30-33]; evaluation of coronary variants, both congenital [34-37] and acquired; and the follow-up of the status of a-priori known coronary lesions, such as after treatment with angioplasty [38]. Another obvious application for coronary MR angiography would be the screening and evaluation of patients with ischemic heart disease and atherosclerotic coronary disease.

It was originally hoped that coronary MR angiography could become a noninvasive screening tool for detection of coronary artery lesions. Unfortunately, after three years of pre-clinical trials of coronary MRA, no technique has yet emerged which can provide a sensitivity and specificity for coronary lesion detection which compares to traditional contrast coronary angiography [13,27,29,38-42]. All published coronary MRA studies used the 2-D ECG-triggered k-space segmented breath-hold GRE technique. Initial clinical testing of this 2-D coronary MRA technique at Beth-Israel Hospital in Boston in a group of 39 selected patients demonstrated the capability to detect coronary occlusion and stenosis [27]. MRI coronary angiography had a 90% sensitivity and a 92% specificity, as compared with conventional angiography, for correctly identifying individual vessels with $\geq$ 50 % angiographic stenoses. Subsequent attempts by other investigators to reproduce these results based on blinded studies have not been as successful. The sensitivity for detection of significant ($\geq$ 50%) lesions in these subsequent studies has been varied: 36 % based on an initial study by Post et al. [42] of 14 patients with 14 significant lesions; 33% to 75 % based on a follow-up study by Post et al. [29] of 35 patients with 35 stenoses; 63% average sensitivity (range: 0% to 75%) based on a study by Duerinckx et al. [13] of 20 patients with 27 proximal lesions; 65% based on an initial study by Pennell et al. [38] of 17 patients with 23 lesions; 88% based on a follow-up study by Pennell et al. [39] using a non-blinded analysis of 31 patients with 41 lesions; 83% to 100% in a study by Nitatori et al. [43] in 50 patients; 56% in a study by Mohiaddin, Bogren et al. [41] in 16 heart transplant patients with 9 lesions. These results for 2-D techniques are summarized in Figure 1. The very first clinical results with a non-breathhold 3-D coronary MRA technique were disappointing, with a 0% sensitivity for significant lesion detection [44]. However several other promising 3-D coronary MRA techniques will soon undergo pre-clinical trials [45]. It is still premature to judge the ultimate capability of these newer coronary MRA techniques in screening for significant coronary lesions.

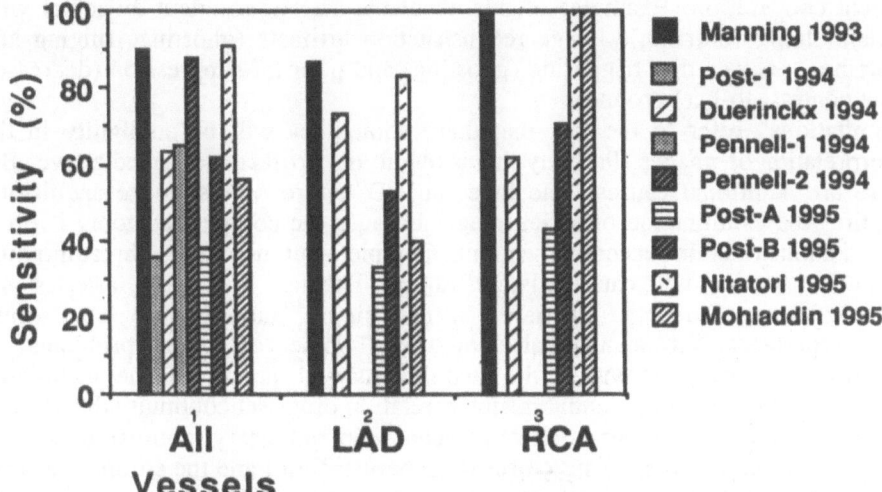

Figure 1. Plot of the sensitivities for detection of hemodynamically significant ($\geq$ 50%) coronary lesion as published in clinical studies: 1) All vessels; 2) LAD only; and 3) RCA only . The legend on the left lists the studies in the same sequence as the bars along the horizontal axis (from left to right). For two studies (Post et al., 1995 and Nitatori et al., 1995) the average of the sensitivities for detection of $\geq$ 50% lesions in the LAD and RCA was taken as the overall sensitivity. (*From* Duerinckx AJ. Coronary MR angiography. Magnetic Resonance Imaging Clinics of North America, May 1996; with permission)

Limitations

Limitations and artifacts of two-dimensional coronary MR angiography have been described in detail by Duerinckx et al. [46,47]. The most important limitation of today's coronary MR angiography is still the great variation in the appearance of significant (> 50%) coronary lesions and the large number of image artifacts which can be misinterpreted as representing lesions. It can be very tempting to interpret an artifactual change in the signal intensity of flow in a vessel as representing a lesion, especially if the artifact just happens to be located in the vicinity of the real lesion. Such erroneous overinterpretation of artifacts as lesions will increase the sensitivity for lesion detection, as will be explained and illustrated in the next section. Unfortunately if done consistently, it would also significantly reduce the specificity of the technique, thus ultimately reducing its clinical impact.

In the study by Duerinckx et al. [46] problems were divided into two areas: data acquisition problems (artifacts) and image interpretation problems (limitations).

"Artifacts" refer to the consequences of data acquisition problems that preclude the gathering of good quality images at the desired anatomic locations. These items can cause image degradation, poor image quality, and diminish the number of high-quality images available for the clinical study. In some cases, these can be overcome during the examination by readjustment of the systems or better patient cooperation. Examples of this problems are: intermittent difficulty with breathholding (blurring), image reconstruction artifacts (ghosting, ringing and blurring), poor cardiac triggering (ghosting) and poor fat-suppression (decreased flow contrast-to-background).

"Limitations" refer to the fact that there sometimes will be ambiguity in the interpretation of images. Partially this is due to the artifacts described above. But there are additional causes. The inherent 2-D nature of the image acquisition requires the examination of serial images because the complex anatomy is often only demonstrated in successive sections. Complete but inconsistent breathholding or patient motion will cause misregistration. The fact that veins, arteries and pericardial sac contents all have similar signal intensity can also cause misinterpretation of anatomical structures. Some of these problems of interpretation are inherent in the two-dimensional nature of the technique. Examples of these are: potential misinterpretation of vessel continuity due to slice misregistration, misidentification of adjacent vein and artery, confusion between a superimposed anatomical structures (e.g. pericardium) and the coronary artery, confusion between a vessel and the upper pericardial recess area, and susceptibility artifacts caused by sternal wires, surgical clips or coronary stents. Duerinckx et al. quantitated the frequency of occurrence of these problems (see Table 1) and recommended possible methods to overcome artifacts and deal with limitations.

Developing coronary MR angiography technology is part of a greater effort to speed up and improve the quality of cardiac and thoracic MR imaging [25]. The new breathhold MR techniques provide better spatial resolution and tissue characterization than color Doppler echocardiography. When compared to conventional cardiac MRI, breathhold MRI allows more interactive and faster selection of imaging planes to study the anatomy of and the flow patterns within the cardiac chambers. Breathhold MRI techniques have also helped to improve MR studies of myocardial perfusion and cardiac function (wall motion studies and myocardial tagging).

Table 1. Frequency of artifacts and limitations with 2-D breathhold coronary MR angiography (based on a study in 27 subjects by Duerinckx et al. [46].

Artifacts	Description	Frequency (%)
	1. Intermittent difficulty with breathholding	40 %
	2. Ghosting	22 %
	3. Ringing	19 %
	4. Blurring	22 %
	5. Poor fat-suppression	19 %
Limitations		
	1. Misregistration due to inconsistent breath-holding	37 %
	2. Difficulty distinguishing arteries from veins	37 %
	3. Overlapping structures	26 %
	4. Poor visualization of the left main artery	59 %

(From Duerinckx AJ. Coronary MR angiography. Magnetic Resonance Imaging Clinics of North America, May 1996; with permission)

3-D techniques with navigator-echo feedback

More recently "non-breathhold" and "repeated breathhold" 3-D coronary MRA pulse sequences have been developed, which although they do not offer the same advantages of speed and interactive imaging, have several significant advantages [45,48,49]. These techniques use respiratory gating and/or respiratory triggering to eliminate respiratory motion. Most importantly, they provide higher spatial resolution, continuous and consistent coverage of the coronary arteries, and the capability for postprocessing (multiplanar reconstruction). Also, they can be used with elderly and very young pediatric patients who can not cooperate with breathholding requirements. The search for the ultimate coronary MR angiography technique is part of an effort to provide a "one stop imaging shop" for the cardiac patient in general and specifically for the patient with ischemic heart disease. When perfected, these new cardiac triggered MRI techniques will provide anatomical information, flow quantification, functional information and myocardial viability information all during a single MRI/MRA examination, and equivalent to the information gained today from multiple traditional cardiac examinations.

Alternatives

Today's alternatives to noninvasive coronary MR angiography include: traditional contrast based coronary angiography (invasive, using x-rays and iodinated contrast); transthoracic echocardiography and transesophageal echocardiography (TEE) (semi-invasive, requiring intubation) [50,51]; and electron-beam computed tomography (EBCT) (noninvasive, but requiring x-rays and iodinated contrast) [52]. The advantage of coronary MR angiography over all of these techniques is its noninvasive nature and the fact that it does not require the use of iodinated contrast agents or intubation of the patient. Coronary MRA routinely provides visualization of a much larger portion of the proximal coronary tree than TEE [53]. Early three-dimensional (3-D) coronary angiography using MRI or EBCT look very similar [52,54].

Conclusions

The fact that early commercial implementations of coronary MR angiography pulse sequences have now become available has dramatically increased interest in their use. The techniques developed for coronary MR angiography will affect the way MR angiography of the thorax and abdomen will be done in the future. This chapter has reviewed the established and most likely to succeed coronary MR angiographic techniques. While coronary MR angiography may be relatively easy to perform for a cardiac trained clinician, it still represents a challenge to the general radiologist and MR technologist. The coronary MR angiographic techniques are in continual flux and will continue to evolve. We hope to motivate clinicians to use these and similar techniques to image other vessels such as the thoracic arch, arch vessels, pulmonary arteries and renal arteries.

References:

1.   Atkinson DJ, Edelman RR. Cineangiography of the heart in a single breath hold with a segmented turboFLASH sequence. Radiology 1991;178:357-60.
2.   Edelman RR, Manning WJ, Burstein D, Paulin S. Coronary arteries: breath-hold MR angiography. Radiology 1991;181:641-3.
3.   Wang SJ, Hu BS, Macovski A, Nishimura DG. Coronary angiography using fast selective inversion recovery. Magn Reson Med 1991;18:417-23.
4.   Meyer CH, Hu BS, Nishimura DG, Macovski A. Fast spiral coronary artery imaging. Magn Reson Med 1992;28:202-13.
5.   Manning WJ, Li W, Boyle NG, Edelman RR. Fat-suppressed breath-hold magnetic resonance coronary angiography. Circulation 1993;87:94-104.
6.   Paschal CB, Haacke EM, Adler LP. Three-dimensional MR Imaging of the coronary arteries: preliminary clinical experience. J Magn Reson Imaging 1993;3:491-500.
7.   Wielopolski PA, Manning WJ, Edelman RR. Single breath-hold volumetric imaging of the heart using magnetization-prepared 3-dimensional segmented echo planar imaging. J Magn Reson Imaging 1995;5:403-9.
8.   Wang Y, Christy PS, Korosec FR *et al*. Coronary MRI with a respiratory feedback monitor: the 2D imaging case. Magn Reson Med 1995;33:116-21.
9.   Manning WJ, Edelman RR. Magnetic resonance coronary angiography. Magn Reson Q 1993;9:131-51.
10. Pennell DJ, Keegan J, Firmin DN, Gatehouse PD, Underwood SR, Longmore DB. Magnetic resonance imaging of coronary arteries: technique and preliminary results. Br Heart J 1993;70:315-26.

11. Duerinckx AJ. MR Angiography of the coronary arteries [review]. Top Magn Reson Imaging 1995;7:267-85.

12. Bogaert J, Duerinckx AJ, Baert AL. Coronary MR angiography: a review. J Belge Radiol 1994;77:255-61.

13. Duerinckx AJ, Urman MK. Two-dimensional coronary MR angiography: analysis of initial clinical results. Radiology 1994;193:731-8.

14. Duerinckx A, Higgins C, Pettigrew R, editors. MRI of the cardiovascular system. New York: Raven Press, 1994.

15. White R, Caputo GR, Mark AS, Modin GW, Higgins CB. Coronary artery bypass graft patency: noninvasive evaluation with MR imaging. Radiology 1987;164:681-6.

16. Buser PT, Higgins CB. Coronary artery graft disease: diagnosis of graft failure by magnetic resonance imaging. In: Lüscher TF, Turina M, Braunwald E, editors. Coronary artery graft disease: mechanisms and prevention. Berlin: Springer-Verlag, 1994:99-112.

17. Debatin JF, Strong JA, Sostman HD *et al.* MR Characterization of blood flow in native and grafted internal mammary arteries. J Magn Reson Imaging 1993;3:443-50.

18. Paulin S, von Schulthess GK, Fossel E, Krayenbuehl HP. MR Imaging of the aortic root and proximal coronary arteries. AJR Am J Roentgenol 1987;148:665-70.

19. Anderson CM, Edelman RR, Turski PA, editors. Clinical magnetic resonance angiography . New York: Raven Press, 1993.

20. Potchen EJ, Haacke EM, Siebert JE, Gottschalk A. Magnetic resonance angiography: concepts & applications. St. Louis: Mosby, 1993.

21. Debatin JF, Ting RH, Wegmuller H *et al.* Renal artery blood flow: quantification with phase-contrast MR imaging with and without breath holding. Radiology 1994;190:371-8.

22. Atkinson D, Teresi L. Magnetic resonance angiography [review]. Magn Reson Q 1995;10:149-72.

23. Duerinckx AJ, Sinha U, Atkinson DJ, Simonetti OP. MRA in the upper thorax using segmented breathhold 2D-TOF [abstract]. J Magn Reson Imaging 1994;(4 Suppl.):93.

24. Hartnell GG, Finn JP, Zenni M *et al.* MR imaging of the thoracic aorta: comparison of spin-echo, angiographic and breath-hold techniques. Radiology 1994;191:697-704.

25. Pearlman JD, Edelman RR. Ultrafast magnetic resonance imaging. Segmented turboflash, echo-planar, and real-time nuclear magnetic resonance. Radiol Clin North Am 1994;32:593-612.

26. Mezrich R. A perspective on K-space. Radiology 1995;195:297-315.

27. Manning WJ, Li W, Edelman RR. A preliminary report comparing magnetic resonance coronary angiography with conventional angiography. N Engl J Med 1993;328:828-32.

28. Hundley WG, Clarke GD, Landau C *et al.* Noninvasive determination of infarct artery patency by cine magnetic resonance angiography. Circulation 1995;91:1347-53.

29. Post JC, van Rossum AC, Hofman MBM, Valk J, Visser CA. Clinical Utility of Two Dimensional Breathhold MR Angiography in Coronary Artery Disease. [abstract]. In: Book of abstracts of the 3rd Meeting of the Society of Magnetic Resonance (SMR) and the 12th Annual Scientific Meeting of the European

Society for Magnetic Resonance in Medicine and Biology (ESMRMB). Nice, France, August 20-25.: 1995.

30. Duerinckx AJ, Urman MK, Lewis B. Coronary artery bypass graft imaging using MR coronary angiography [abstract]. J Magn Reson Imaging 1994;(4 Suppl.):122.

31. Duerinckx AJ, Atkinson D, Hurwitz R, Mintorovitch J, Whitney W. Coronary MR angiography after coronary stent placement. AJR Am J Roentgenol 1995;165:662-4.

32. Scott NA, Pettigrew RI. Absence of movement of coronary stents after placement in a magnetic resonance imaging field. Am J Cardiol 1994;73:900-1.

33. Duerinckx AJ, Atkinson D, Hurwitz R. Coronary Stent Imaging with Coronary MR Angiography [abstract]. In: Book of abstracts of the 3rd Meeting of the Society of Magnetic Resonance (SMR) and the 12th Annual Scientific Meeting of the European Society for Magnetic Resonance in Medicine and Biology (ESMRMB). Nice, France, August 20-25.:1995.

34. Duerinckx AJ, Bogaert J, Jiang H, Lewis BS. Anomalous origin of the left coronary artery: diagnosis by coronary MR angiography. AJR Am J Roentgenol 1995;164:1095-7.

35. Manning WJ, Li W, Cohen SI, Johnson RG, Edelman RR. Improved definition of anomalous left coronary artery by magnetic resonance corornary angiography. Am Heart J 1995;130:615-7.

36. Post JC, van Rossum AC, Bronzwaer JGF *et al*. Magnetic resonance angiography of anomalous coronary arteries. A new gold standard for delineating the proximal course? Circulation 1995;92:3163-71.

37. McConnell MV, Ganz P, Selwyn AP, Li W, Edelman RR, Manning WJ. Identification of anomalous coronary arteries and their anatomic course by magnetic resonance coronary angiography. Circulation 1995;92:3158-62.

38. Pennell DJ, Bogren HG, Keegan J, Firmin DW, Underwood SR. Coronary artery stenosis: Assessment by magnetic resonance imaging [abstract]. In: Book of Abstracts of the 11th Annual Scientific Meeting of the European Society for Magnetic Resonance in Medicine and Biology. Vienna, Austria, April 20-24.: 1994; 374.

39. Pennell DJ, Bogren HG, Keegan J, Firmin DN, Underwood SR. Detection, localization and assessment of coronary artery stenosis by magnetic resonance imaging [abstract]. In: Printed program of the second meeting of the Society of Magnetic Resonance (SMR). San Francisco, California, August 6-12.: 1994.

40. Rogers WJ, Kramer CM, Simonetti OP, Reichek N. Quantification of human coronary stenoses by magnetic resonance angiography [abstract]. In: Printed program of the second meeting of the Society of Magnetic Resonance (SMR). San Francisco, California, August 6-12.: 1994:370.

41. Mohiaddin RH, Bogren HG, Firmin DN, Keegan J. MR Angiography of the coronary arteries in heart transplants [abstract]. In: Book of Abstracts of VII International Workshop on Magnetic Resonance Angiography. Matsuyama, Japan; Oct 12-14.: 1995.

42. Post JC, vanRossum AC, Hofman MBM, Valk J, Visser CA. Current limitations of two dimensional breathhold MR angiography in coronary artery disease [abstract]. In: Printed program of the second meeting of the Society of Magnetic Resonance (SMR). San Francisco, California, August 7-12.: 1994.

43. Nitatori T, Hachiya J, Korenaga T, Hanaoka H, Yoshino. A. Clinical Application of Coronary MR Angiography. Studies on Shortening of Time for

Examination [abstract] In: Book of abstracts of the 3rd Meeting of the Society of Magnetic Resonance (SMR) and the 12th Annual Scientific Meeting of the European Society for Magnetic Resonance in Medicine and Biology (ESMRMB). Nice, France, August 20-25.: 1995.

44. Post JC, vanRossum AC, Hofman MBM, Valk J, Visser CA. Respiratory-gated three dimensional MR angiography of coronary arteries and comparison with x-ray contrast angiography [abstract]. In: Printed program of the second meeting of the Society of Magnetic Resonance (SMR). San Francisco, California, August 7-12.: 1994.

45. Wang Y, Rossman PJ, Grimm RC, Riederer SJ, Ehman RL. Navigator-echo-based real-time respiratory gating and triggering for reduction of respiration effects in three-dimensional coronary MR angiography. Radiology 1996;198:55-60.

46. Duerinckx AJ, Atkinson DP, Mintorovitch J, Simonetti OP. Two-dimensional coronary MR Angiography: limitations and artifacts. Eur Radiol. In Press.

47. Duerinckx AJ. Coronary MR Angiography [review article]. MRI Clin North Am. In press.

48. Li D, Kaushikkar S, Woodard P, Dhawale P, Haacke EM. Three-dimensional MRI of Coronary Arteries [abstract]. In: Book of Abstracts of VII International Workshop on Magnetic Resonance Angiography. Matsuyama, Japan; Oct 12-14.: 1995.

49. Haacke EM, Li D, Kaushikkar S. Cardiac MR Imaging: principles and techniques. Top Magn Reson Imaging 1995;7:200-17.

50. Iliceto S, Marangelli V, Memmola C, Rizzon P. Transesophageal Doppler echocardiography evaluation of coronary blood flow velocity in baseline conditions and during dipyridamole-induced coronary vasodilation. Circulation 1991;83:61-9.

51. Iliceto S, Memmola C, Marangelli V, Caiato C, Rizzon P. Evaluation of coronary artery anatomy and physiology with the use of transesophageal echocardiography. Coron Artery Dis 1992;3:357-63.

52. Moshage WEL, Achenbach S, Seese B, Bachman K, Kirchgeorg M. Coronary artery stenoses: three-dimensional imaging with electrocardiographicaly triggered, contrast agent-enhanced, electron-beam CT. Radiology 1995;196:707-14.

53. Tardif JC, Vannan MA, Taylor K, Schwartz SL, Pandian NG. Delineation of extended lengths of coronary arteries by multiplane transesophageal echocardiography. J Am Coll Cardiol 1994;24:909-19.

54. Doyle M, Scheidegger MB, DeGraaf RG, Vermeulen J, Pohost GM. Coronary artery imaging in multiple 1-sec breath holds. Magn Reson Imaging 1993;11:3-6.

28. Color quantization in angioscopic images

JAN A. OOMEN, J.C. HANS SCHUURBIERS, KENNETH G. LEHMANN, CEES J. SLAGER & PATRICK W. SERRUYS

Summary

The angioscopic image gives us access to a property heretofore not available by other means: the color of the vessel wall. Colors in video representations of angioscopic images are up until now described by a human observer. Differences in settings of the monitor and the inherent poor ability of the human eye to classify colors objectively results in a very poor intraobserver as well as interobserver reproducibility. A PC-based method is described to measure colors in a video image and to present the results in a novel C-diagram. Results with this method for standard calibrated colors are given. Possible sources of error are discussed and methods to minimize these errors are presented.

Introduction

In recent years it has become possible to obtain intraluminal images of coronary arteries by means of a small and flexible fiber optic viewing system, connected to a standard color video camera [1,2]. This intraluminal application is an extension of the longer existing technique of endoscopy, which also is capable of providing video color images from inner surfaces of the human body. These images are viewed on a video monitor and can be recorded using a commercially available (S)VHS recorder. One characteristic property these systems open for investigation, and which is not available by other means, is the color of the inner surfaces at its normal and diseased parts. However, the ability of the human observer to distinguish between different colors in an objective way is relatively weak. Attempts at description of a color often result in vague terms like yellowish-white or whitish-yellow. This was confirmed by the observer panel of the European Working Group on Coronary Angioscopy [3]. If one wants to make use of color data in multicenter studies or longitudinal clinical trials, however, the use of an objective and reproducible numeric description of color is highly preferred. Our aim is to describe a method of processing video color signals in such a way, that an objective and reproducible measurement of the color of a surface can be established.

Color perception

It has been found that color perception is achieved by the human eye through the color cones in the retina. Three different kind of cones can be found, each with a specific response to light of different wavelengths. One type is mostly responsive to red light, a second type has its maximum response at green wave-

J.H.C. Reiber and E.E. van der Wall (eds.), Cardiovascular Imaging, 367-377.
© 1996 *Kluwer Academic Publishers.*

lengths and the third type is most sensitive to blue, as indicated in Figure 1.

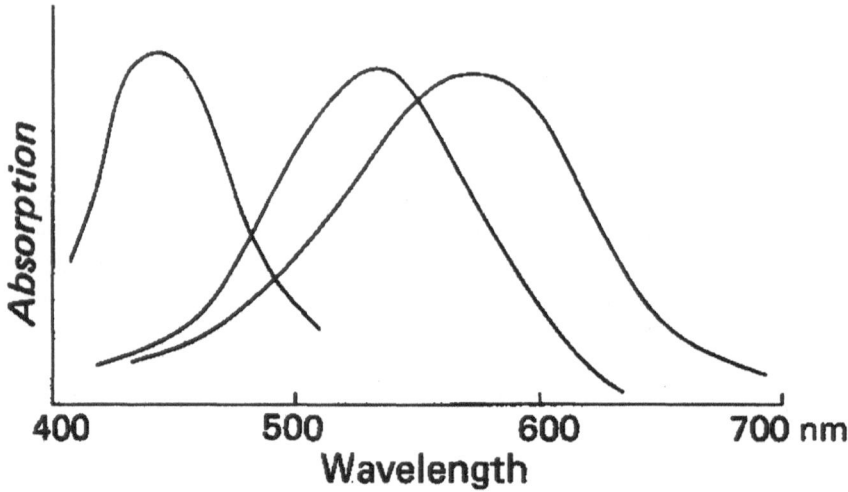

Figure 1. Absorption of light of different wavelengths for the 3 different types of cones in the human.

The perceived color is dictated by the ratio in which neurons receive signals from the red, green and blue sensitive cones. If three monochromatic primary colors could be found, such that each of them would stimulate only one type of cone, all perceivable colors could be presented to the human eye, using the right mixture of these three monochromatic colors. At the same time, this would give us a way of describing each possible color, by specifying the ratio of the monochromatic components.

Unfortunately, as can be seen from Figure 1, stimulating 'green' cones is impossible, without also stimulating the 'red' and/or 'blue' types.

As a result of this it is not possible to reproduce all observable colors by mixing three fixed colors in different ratios. Thus color slides, color printing and video images each are able to reproduce only part of the noticeable color differences as perceived by the human eye.

The CIE1931/D65 diagram in Figure 2 is used to specify the coordinates of all colors that can be perceived by humans. Using this diagram, colors can be specified by giving the x and y coordinates within this diagram. The diagram possesses the 'additive mixing property', i.e. given any three points c_1, c_2 and c_3 in this diagram, all colors within the c_1,c_2,c_3-triangle can be made by mixing the appropriate amounts of light with colors defined by c_1, c_2 and c_3. The area numbered 1 defines the colors achievable by paint and ink and area 2 contains all colors which can be reproduced on color film.[1] The solid line triangle, marked R,G,B at its corners, contains all colors achievable by color TV and video systems. The position of the corners R, G and B of this triangle is defined by international agreement and thus constitutes a suitable standard to be used in the definition of color in video images.

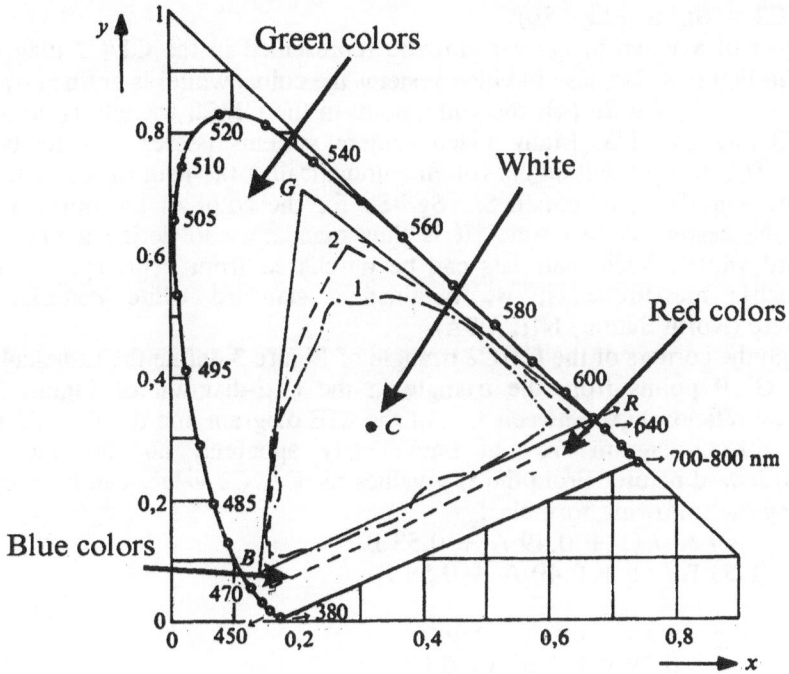

Figure 2. The CIE diagram. The outermost rounded triangle contains all colors discernible by the human eye. The areas 1 and 2 contain the colors reproducible by ink and paint (1) or color film (2). The triangle RGB contains the colors reproducible by video systems.

The C1/C2 diagram

A color video signal can easily be decomposed into the three signal values Sr (red), Sg (green) and Sb (blue). These so-called RGB-signals can be fed to a suitable monitor to display a color picture. Other monitors are fed a composite video signal, meaning that luminosity and color information is coded in one signal. The composite monitors have internal circuitry to derive the Sr, Sg and Sb signals, which are necessary to drive the color tube. So the ratio of Sr, Sg and

---

[1]These areas are not pure triangles, because paint, ink and photographic rendition of colors depend on color subtracting methods instead of color addition processes.

Sb values can be used to define a color at a certain spot in the video picture. We decided to define two numbers C1 and C2, where C1 stands for the ratio of the Sr signal and the total luminosity and C2 the ratio of Sg and the total luminosity. Luminosity is here defined as the sum of the Sr, Sg and Sb signals. Thus in formula form:

$$C1 = Sr/(Sr+Sg+Sb) \text{ and}$$
$$C2 = Sg/(Sr+Sg+Sb)$$

All colors of a video image can now be represented in the C1/C2 diagram as shown in Figure 3. Because in video systems the color 'white' is defined by equal values of Sr, Sg and Sb [4], the white point in the C1/C2 triangle is defined as C1=1/3 and C2=1/3. Many video camera systems posses a white balance feature. This feature will adjust (often automatically) the gain of the red, green and blue amplifiers, to obtain Sr=Sg=Sb for the color of the object present before the camera at that time. It is thus mandatory to define a material as 'standard white'. Such materials can be purchased from firms specializing in colorimetric measurements; we obtained a standard white material from Labsphere (North Sutton, NH, USA).

Although the corners of the C1/C2 triangle of Figure 3 define the same colors as the R, G, B points from the triangle in the CIE-diagram of Figure 2, the numerical relationships between x, y of the CIE diagram and the C1, C2 values of the C1/C2-diagram are not immediately apparent, nor are they of a straightforward nature. From the x, y values the C1, C2 values can be computed [5] using the following formulas:

$$C1 = (1.49 \ A) / (1 + 0.49 \ A + 0.53 \ B) \qquad (1a)$$
$$C2 = (1.53 \ B / (1 + 0.49 \ A + 0.53 \ B) \qquad (1b)$$

where:

$$A = 1.99 \ x - 0.22 \ y - 0.26 \qquad (2a)$$
$$B = - 0.79 \ x + 1.68 \ y - 0.02 \qquad (2b)$$

These linear transformations were derived making use of the fact that the corners of the RGB-triangle in the CIE diagram are defined as:

R: x = 0.67, y = 0.33;
G: x = 0.21, y = 0.71;
B: x = 0.14, y = 0.08

which should correspond to the corners of the C1/C2-diagram, defined by:

R: C1=1, C2=0;
G: C1=0, C2=1;
B: C1=0, C2=0

Furthermore, 'D65 white'[2] in the CIE1931/D65 coordinates is defined to be:

x = 0.3127;   y = 0.3291

---

[2]D65 white has been chosen, because the x, y figures for this white were available for our color standards and the CIE1931 diagram is based on this color, hence the addition: CIE1931/D65.

and, as stated above, TV-white[3] is defined as:
$$C1 = 1/3; \qquad C2 = 1/3.$$

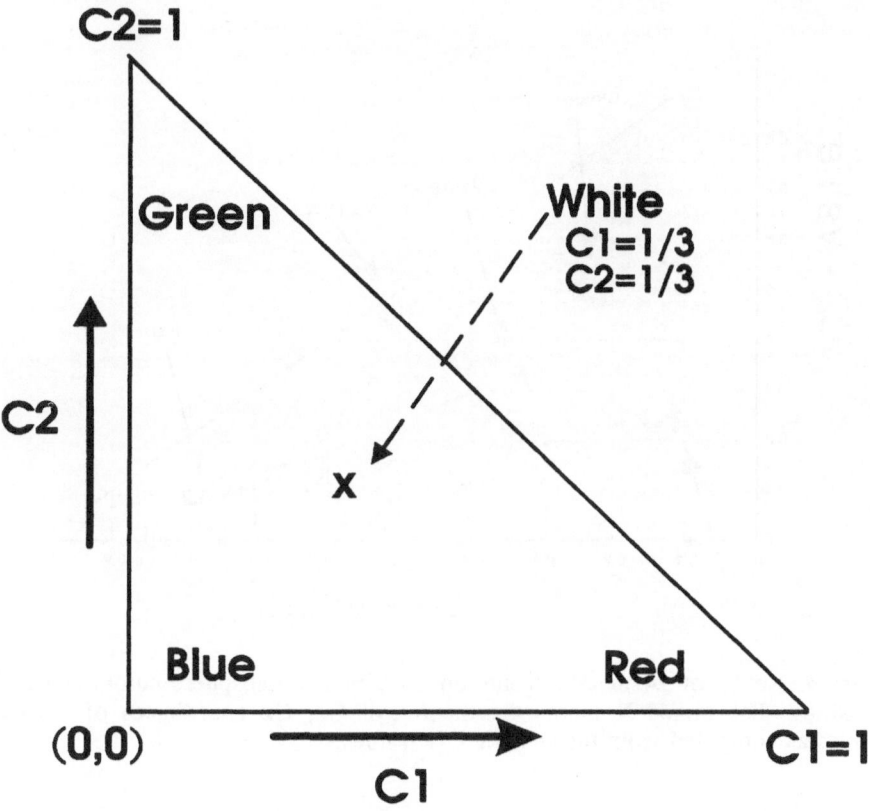

Figure 3. The C1/C2 triangle encompassing all possible colors in a video image.

The above transformations make use of these definitions, to arrive at the correct transformation constants.

We acquired four samples of certified color standards (Labsphere, North Sutton, NH, USA) and made images of these colors, using the model 2075 angioscope camera (Baxter, Irvine, CA, USA), with different levels of illumination by the Baxter Xenon light source through the accompanying light transmitting fibers. These images were measured using the method described below and Figure 4

[3]The actual color of a white signal on the TV or monitor screen varies between countries and manufacturers, probably due to differences in local taste. The European white has a color temperature around 5600° Kelvin, while American sets produce a more bluish white of around 9300° Kelvin.

shows the results plotted in the C1/C2 triangle. In the same triangle the C1/C2 values as computed from the known CIE1931/D65 *x, y* values are shown, showing a close relationship between measured and computed values.

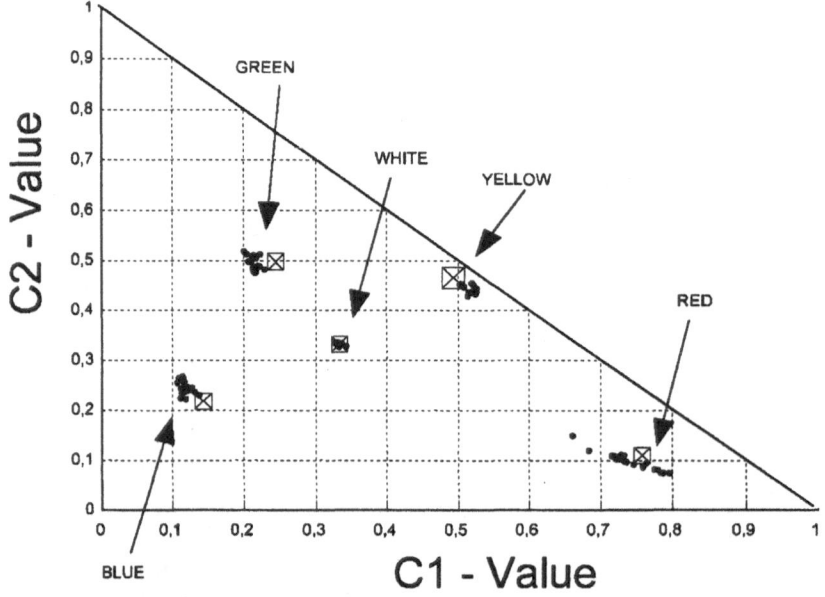

Figure 4. Result of 24 measurements on 5 calibrated Labsphere colors at varying intensities. The boxed X marks the theoretical C1, C2 coordinates of the color samples as computed from the specific CIE values.

Measuring C1 and C2

In order to measure the C1 and C2 components of a certain color in a video image, the image is fed, either directly or after recording on a VCR, to a frame grabber board, mounted in a PC. Such a frame grabber will translate the analog composite video signal into a series of numbers. This process is called: digitization. Out of the range of numbers representing the image it is easy to distill the value of the red (R), green (G) and blue (B) component of any part of the picture. If we call these numerical values Sr, Sg and Sb respectively, then C1 and C2 can be found using the expressions:

$$C1 = Sr/(Sr+Sb+Sc) \qquad \text{and} \qquad C2 = Sg/(Sr+Sg+Sb)$$

A computer program can be written to 'grab' a video image present at its video input connector. With suitable software the numerical data describing the picture now can be processed, resulting in C1 and C2 values for any part of the image one cares to select. However, this method of computing C1 and C2 albeit simple, is not directly useful, because of specific sources of error inherent in the way in which a video picture is processed by the related electronic circuitry.

White balance

An image of a white object should result in C1 and C2 values of 0.33. However this may not always be the case and the aberration has these possible causes:
a. The object is not pure white.
b. The illuminating light is not pure white.
c. The fiber is coloring the light.
d. The video camera is not sufficiently 'white balanced'.
Problems caused by a): an object that is not pure white, can easily be avoided by using a standard white object as a color balance test object. The other problems can be solved by the 'white balance' feature of the software. It operates as follows:
Before each measurement an image is recorded of the standard white test object. Our test objects are blocks of 1x1x1 cm, machined from the commercially available standard white material. Into this cube a little hole is drilled and the test blocks are sterilized. Before an angioscopy is performed, a white image is acquired by inserting the angioscope catheter tip into the hole of the test cube. This ensures an image of a white material, illuminated by the same light used for the diagnostic pictures and processed through the same equipment.
While analyzing the pictures for colorimetric values, the standard white image is used to set a correction factor for Sr and Sg component values, such that the white test image results in the correct C1 and C2 values of 0.33.
This white balance method will thus correct for color aberrations in the light source, the optic fibers, the video recorder and associated electronics, thus assuring reproducible results under different circumstances and with different types of equipment.

Black level offset

The signals Sr, Sg and Sb are numerically represented by values between 0 and 255 ([4]). The relationship between luminance of a white object and the digital value of the Sr, Sg and Sb signals is depicted in Figure 5. This relationship has been measured by varying the light intensity of the Baxter Xenon light source with the aid of its mechanical shutter. In this type of measurement one should avoid changing the supply voltage of the light source, because this will influence the spectral composition of the light. The light intensity reaching the color standards was measured independently with the aid of a photo-diode.
Figure 5 shows the digital values leveling off for high amounts of illumination. This is a result of the workings of the automatic exposure feature, so the real dynamic range of interest lies between the illumination levels of 0 and 1000. The linear approximation of this section of the graph, shown as a dotted line in Figure 5, intersects the y-axis for a negative value of y. We call this value 'the dynamic offset' and this value should be taken into account when calculating color signal

---

[4]This is a consequence of these values being represented by bytes. A byte contains eight bits, resulting in $2^8 = 256$ values.

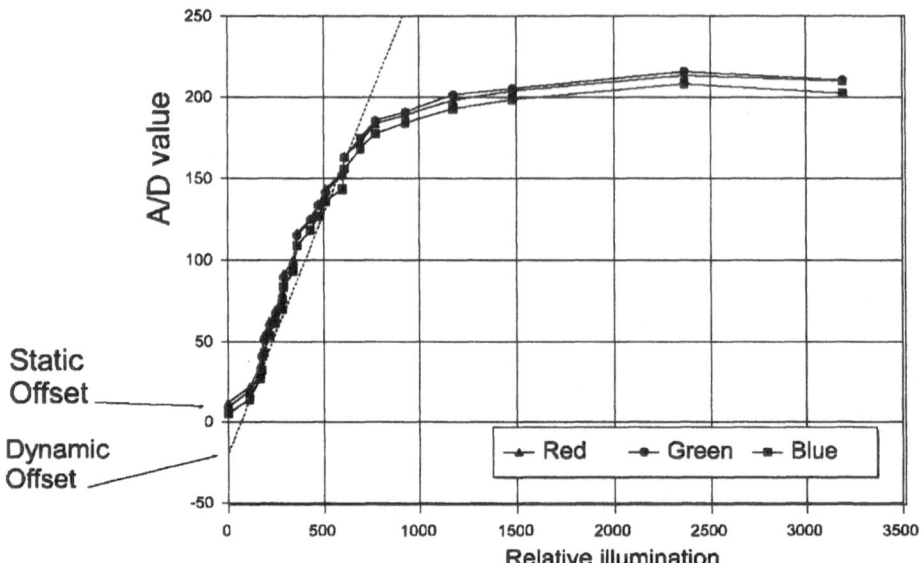

Figure 5. Relation between luminance of a white object and digital value for a Baxter cameras/IRIS frame grabber combination. The dotted line is a linear approximation over the range of interest i.e the range not affected by the automatic exposure.

values. We have introduced three constants Kr, Kg and Kb, representing the dynamic offset for each of the three color values. As shown before, the dynamic offset may be a negative number, resulting in positive correction factors Kr, Kg and Kb. The values of these constants for a specific set up can be measured using the method described below under 'Correction Values'.

Different combinations of camera and frame grabber will give different numbers, and especially replacing one or both of these with a different model or brand might change the optimal corrective value appreciably. Thus each equipment set up should be calibrated to obtain the most suitable K-factors for that specific set up.

With a completely black image the digital value of the three color signals lies around 10. This is to be expected, because frame grabbers do not use the full 0..255 range in order to be able to adopt to small changes in gain and offset of the related electronic circuitry. For the same reason 'full white' never reaches the theoretical maximum of 255 [6].

Gamma correction

With video cameras, the signal level as provided by the light sensitive element is customarily raised to the power $1/\gamma$, where γ is chosen to fall between 1.5 and 2.5. This is done to account for the non-linear characteristic of the light emitting phosphors of the picture tube and is referred to as 'gamma correction'. Because the viewing system: monitor and picture tube, is not part of the measuring system, we separately correct for the gamma through raising the measured and offset corrected digital value to the power γ, where γ has to be set at a value which is specific for the camera/frame grabber system in use.

Correction values

To find the most suitable values for each of the K constants and the value of γ, we measured five standard colors (red, green, blue, yellow and white) for which the x,y values in the CIE1931/D65 diagram were known. Using the formulas (1a), (1b), (2a), (2b) the corresponding C1 and C2 values can be calculated. Different levels of illumination were used on these samples and a spreadsheet (Quattro Pro, Borland, Scotts Valley, Ca, USA) was used to introduce variable K-factors and γ. Using the optimization function provided by Quattro Pro, these values were optimized for the closest correlation between known and measured C1/C2 values of the color standards. For our set up the γ was found to have a value of 1.8, with K-factors of Kr = 4, Kg = 7 and Kb = 10.

Results

The measuring system described above has subsequently been used to quantify the color of different types of intraluminal wall, as seen through an angioscope system. The results are shown in Figure 6. Twenty-four wall sections have been subdivided by a skilled angioscopist into 5 different classes: normal, white plaque, yellow plaque, mural thrombus and protruding thrombus. The average value of C1 and C2 for each of these five classes is depicted in Figure 6. As could be expected, the more reddish lesions gave rise to higher C1 values, but the difference between the color of normal wall and white plaque, although less obvious to the human observer, is readily recognizable in the C1/C2 diagram of Figure 6.

Discussion

Due to the nature of the wide angle lens system of the angioscopy catheter, dimensions in angioscopic images are very hard to quantify, although some efforts to solve this problem have been reported [7]. On the other hand the image gives access to the color of lesions and normal sections of the intraluminal wall. Using a system as described here, these colors can be quantified and using the CIE1931/D65 system, which is internationally agreed upon, a standard calibration and correction procedure is available, so results from several systems can be compared, without the need to restrict the user to a specific type and brand of video imaging system.

However, it should be realized that color is decoded as a phase relationship into the video signal during transmission and recording of this signal and phase errors in this process might effect the color appreciably. The European PAL system has safeguards protecting from the adverse effects of such a phase distortion, the NTSC system used in the USA however lacks this feature.

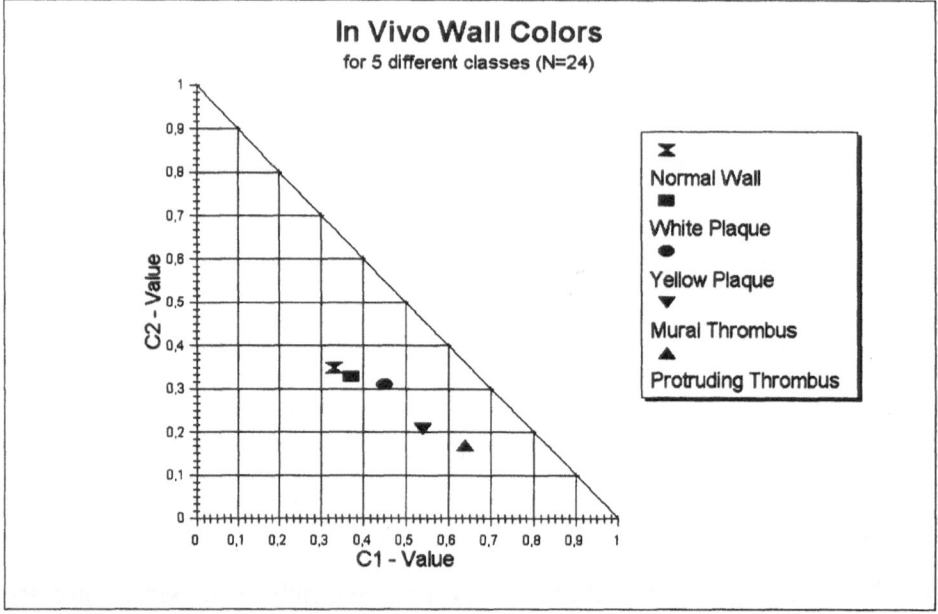

*Figure 6.*Result of measuring specific intraluminal wall categories in normal and diseased vessels.

We have used PAL type equipment during all our experiments and we expect a lower reproducibility using NTSC, especially if the image is recorded on a VCR using that system.

Finally, we would like to stress the point that our system of measurement does not include the video monitor. These monitors have user settings for color intensity, and its position is dependent on user taste. Lowering the color intensity however, will move the colors in the C1/C2 triangle closer to white (C1 = 0.33, C2 = 0.33). NTSC type monitors have an additional setting for 'hue', which influences the color proper. The human observer, judging colors on a monitor, thus has the additional problem of how to adjust the monitor settings in such a way that a standard color rendition is achieved. Our system does not include the monitor in its chain of measurement and the setting of the monitor does not influence the results.

References

1.   Forrester JS, Litvack F, Grundfest W, Hickey A. A perspective of coronary disease seen through the arteries of living man. Circulation 1987;75:505-13.

2. White CJ, Ramee SR, Collius TJ, Mesa JE, Jain A. Percutaneous angioscopy of saphenous vein coronary bypass grafts. J Am Coll Card 1993;21:1181-5.
3. Den Heijer P, Foley DP, Hillege HL *et al*. The "Ermenonville" classification of observations at coronary angioscopy. Evaluation of intra- and inter-observer agreement. European Working Group on Coronary Angioscopy. Eur Heart J 1994;15:815-22.
4. Hunt RW. The reproduction of colour. 3rd ed. Kings Langley: Fountain Press, 1975.
5. Oomen JA, Slager CJ, Lehmann KG, Schuurbiers JC, Serruys PW. Color quantification in angioscopic images. Med Prog Technol 1995;21:39-46.
6. Davidoff F. Digital television coding standards. In: Friedmann JB, editor. Video pictures of the future. Scarsdale: Society of Motion Picture and Television Engineers, 1983.
7. Schuurbiers JC, Slager CJ, Serruys PW. Luminal volume reconstruction from angioscopic video images of casts from human coronary arteries. Am J Cardiol 1994;74:764-8.

29. The use of coronary angioscopy in diagnosis and clinical decision making

PETER den HEIJER

Summary

Although coronary angioscopy, shortly after its introduction in 1991, seemed promising as a clinical decision tool in interventional cardiology, it has until now mainly been used as a device for clinical research. It is somewhat surprising that this imaging modality proved to be in lack of practical applications. Nevertheless, angioscopy can reliably discriminate unstable from stable lesions, and be of value in the management of threatened acute closure after PTCA or stenting. Its sensitivity and specificity in the detection of intracoronary thrombus is unsurpassed. A new class of drugs, the glycoprotein IIb/IIIa inhibitors, is presently making a large impact on interventional cardiology. Coronary angioscopy can potentially play an important role in research as well as clinical use of such drugs, because it is essentially the only reliable tool for intracoronary thrombus detection.

Introduction

Coronary angioscopy in its present form was introduced in interventional cardiology in late 1991. The image quality and the ease of use of the ImageCath™ system were such that angioscopy at that time seemed extremely promising as a tool for clinical decision making in intracoronary interventions. However, the following years have shown that angioscopy certainly has attributed to clinical research, but that its practical role in clinical patient management has remained very limited. In this paper, we will discuss the additional imaging information that angioscopy has given in certain situations, and try to identify a potential new role that this tool can play in decision making.

Angioscopic assessment of lesions in stable and unstable angina

The clinical syndrome of unstable angina pectoris has been associated with platelet aggregation, intracoronary thrombosis, alterations in vasomotor tone, and complicated and ruptured atheromatous plaque [1]. In fact, angioscopy has contributed significantly in recent years to the pathophysiological insights in unstable angina [2,3], identifying a complex lesion morphology and a high incidence of thrombus in the culprit lesions of patients with unstable angina. In order to demonstrate whether culprit lesions in unstable angina could be angioscopically distinguished from stenotic lesions in stable angina by means of the modified Ermenonville classification [4], we have analyzed 33 undisturbed native coronary stenoses in patients with unstable angina pectoris, and compared

379

J.H.C. Reiber and E.E. van der Wall (eds.), Cardiovascular Imaging, 379-388.
© 1996 *Kluwer Academic Publishers.*

these lesions to those of a control group consisting of 19 patients with stable angina. Unstable angina pectoris was defined as the presence of one or more of the following three features: 1) crescendo angina superimposed on a preexisting pattern of relatively stable, exertion-related angina pectoris; 2) angina at rest or with minimal exertion; 3) new onset angina pectoris, which is brought on by minimal exertion. The classification data were compared between the two groups using the Chi-Square test. There were no significant differences between the groups in the grading or shape of the narrowings. Although 13 of 33 (39.4%) of patients with unstable angina proved to have lining red thrombus at angioscopy, versus 4 of 19 (21.1%) of the stable angina group, this difference was not significant with this sample size (Figure 1). There was, however, a significant difference in the incidence of white thrombus: eleven (33.3%) of the unstable angina patients had lining (n=5) or protruding (n=6) white thrombus, which could not be demonstrated in any of the stable angina patients (Figure 2). We found a highly significant difference in the distribution of the atheroma types.

Red thrombus

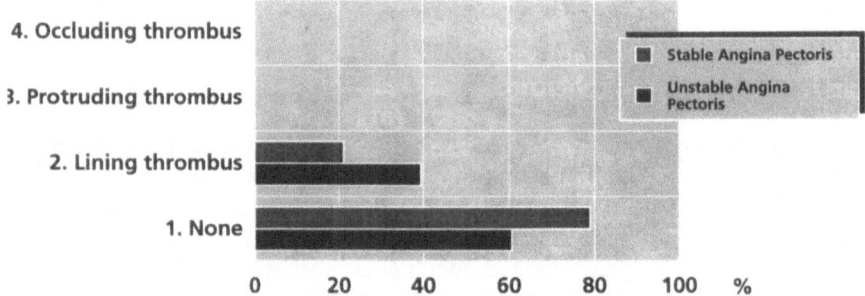

Figure 1. Distribution of angioscopically observed red thrombus in patients with stable and unstable angina.

White thrombus

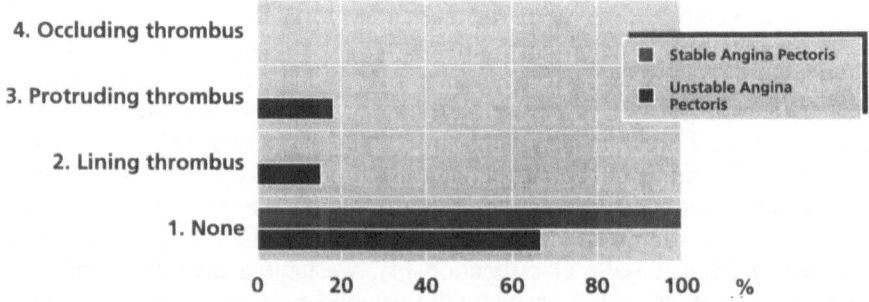

Figure 2. Distribution of white thrombus.

A so-called "complicated lesion" was identified in 25 of 33 (75.8%) patients of the unstable angina group, versus 2 of 19 (10.5%) patients of the stable angina group (Figure 3). The observation of a grade 5 ("complicated") lesion had a sensitivity of 85%, and a specificity of 83% for the clinical syndrome of angina pectoris. It is evident that unstable angina is associated with a specific angioscopic lesion morphology, and that the finding of such a morphology is highly predictive for an unstable lesion. A study to establish if such angioscopically unstable lesions are associated with primary PTCA outcome and post-PTCA events is underway. An alternative to PTCA might, in certain cases, be the stabilization of unstable plaques by cholesterol-lowering "statin"-therapy. Such a strategy can perhaps in the future be controlled by angioscopic and/or ultrasound imaging of the vessel wall.

Atheroma

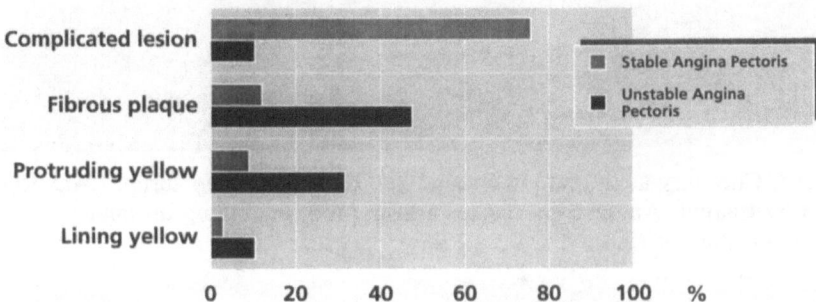

Figure 3. Classification of type of lesion in stable versus unstable angina.

Acute myocardial infarction

Although coronary angioscopy, with its potential for intracoronary thrombus detection, can be used to assess the occluding lesion in acute myocardial infarction, its clinical use for this indication is limited. In fact, red thrombus was found by angioscopy in almost all cases of acute myocardial infarction [5]. Lablanche et al. [6] have demonstrated that red thrombus can even be found up to 60 days after clinically and angiographically successful thrombolysis in a large majority of patients. Of course, such findings generally have no bearing on the therapeutic options available. We have seen one exception in an unusual case of acute myocardial infarction caused by trauma. A 32-year old goalkeeper in amateur football was admitted with an acute anterior infarction after stopping a penalty ball with his sternum. Angiography showed abrupt closure of the Left Anterior Descending artery. Angioscopy was performed in order to prove the presence of occlusive red thrombus, excluding such causes as intramural or extravascular compression (Figure 4). Vessel patency was restored by direct PTCA, and follow-up angioscopy confirmed absence of thrombus 10 days after intravenous heparin treatment (Figure 5).

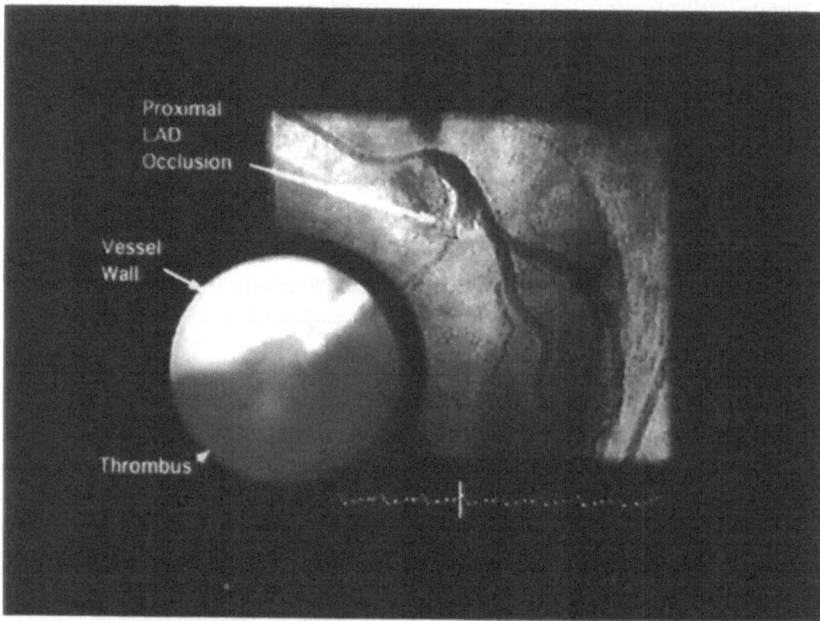

Figure 4. Coronary angiogram in Cranial LAO view showing abrupt LAD occlusion caused by trauma. Angioscopy reveals a large, red, occluding thrombus.
(For colour plate of figure 4 see page 564)

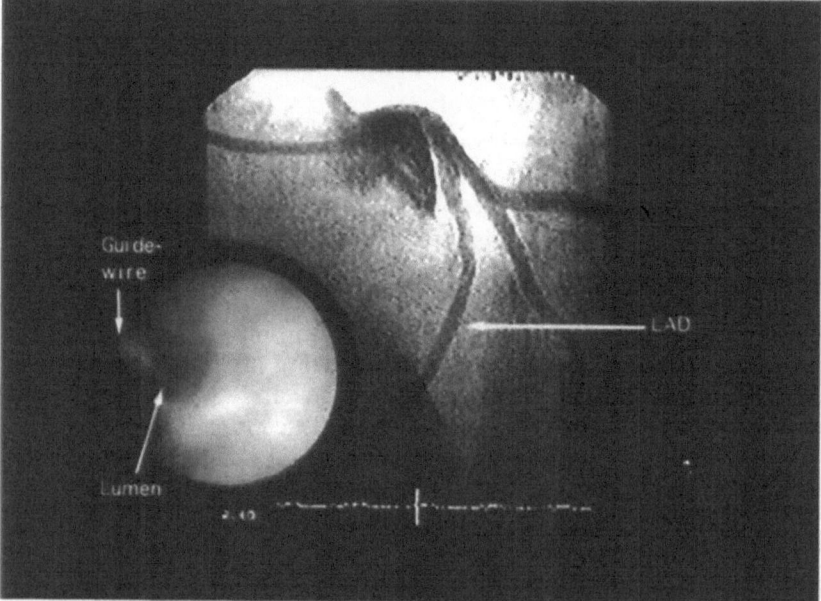

Figure 5. The same patient, 10 days following PTCA and intravenous heparin treatment. The patency of the LAD is fully restored. Angioscopy shows brown/yellow discoloration, probably remnants from balloon dilatation, but absence of thrombus.
(For colour plate of figure 5 see page 564)

Threatened or acute closure after PTCA

Only two years ago, this particular situation seemed to be the one in which angioscopy was most promising as a tool which could actually guide the interventional procedure [7]. Acute closure at the site of dilatation of course is a major potential hazard during or immediately after balloon angioplasty [8]. It occurs in 2-12% of patients undergoing PTCA, and is usually caused by major intimal dissection, intracoronary thrombosis, or a combination of both. Untreated, it can lead to death, acute myocardial infarction, or emergency coronary bypass surgery. In recent years, coronary stents have successfully been employed to counteract impending or complete acute coronary occlusions during PTCA. Prolonged inflation with autoperfusion balloons can be used as an alternative bail-out strategy [9,10]. Fischman and Herrman and co-workers have demonstrated that intracoronary thrombus, angiographically detected prior to stent deployment, increases the risk of subacute stent closure because of the inherent thrombogenicity of stents [9,11]. Angiography, compared to angioscopy, grossly underestimates the presence of intracoronary thrombus. It is therefore logical to assume that bail-out strategies, and in particular the choice between stent implantation and a more conservative therapy, can be improved by angioscopic examination of the occluded or threatened angioplasty segment. In such a setting, angioscopy can be used to determine whether the obstruction is caused by thrombus, dissection, or both. If a large thrombus load is encountered, the operator should, if possible, avoid stent implantation, and try to restore patency by means of prolonged balloon inflation and/or thrombolytic therapy. We have attempted angioscopic imaging of threatened or frank occlusion in 18 patients. Successful angioscopy was possible in 17 of these patients. Acute occlusion was present in 5 patients, and impending occlusion or subtotal occlusion in 12 patients. Angioscopy confirmed large intimal dissection and absence of thrombus in 9 of these patients. Palmaz-Schatz™ coronary stents (Johnson & Johnson Interventional Systems Corp., Warren, NJ, USA) were implanted in 7 of these 9 patients. Two of these patients with obstructing dissections and absence of thrombus had unfavorable anatomies for stent placement, and were successfully treated with autoperfusion balloon inflations during 20 minutes. Obstructing thrombus, without evidence of dissection, was encountered in 2 of the 17 patients. These 2 patients were treated with infusion of streptokinase through the irrigation lumen of the angioscopy. The remaining 6 patients proved to have dissection as well as thrombus at angioscopy. They were treated with autoperfusion balloon inflation and adjunctive intracoronary thrombolytic therapy (150000 - 400000 units of Streptokinase). A 100% procedural success, with fully restored TIMI 3 patency, was reached in these 17 angioscopy guided bail-out procedures. One patient had a subacute stent reclosure after 5 days, while the other 16 patients remained free from further events until discharge from the hospital. Thus, the overall clinical success rate in this group was 94%. The results of the angioscopy guided bail-out suggest that angioscopy can play a role in the selection of treatment strategies for acute or threatened closure during PTCA, and that it potentially can contribute to improve the outcome of such cases. However, it has to be recognized that acute and in-hospital results of bail-out stenting have improved substantially during the last years, to the point where one must assume that stents now stay open even in the presence of (angiographically undetected) thrombus.

Coronary stenting

Angioscopy can be used to assess the correct deployment, adequate expansion, and possible presence of thrombotic material following stent implantation [12]. We have studied 5 patients with freshly implanted stents. Three of these stents were delivered in vein grafts, the other two in native coronary arteries. Imaging was successful in all 5 patients. At angioscopy, all stents were found to be well expanded, although small intima flaps (grade 2 dissection) were seen to protrude through the gaps between the stent wires in 3 patients. One patient, who had received a Strecker™ (Boston Scientific, Watertown, MA, USA) in a vein graft, even had a grade 3, large, dissection visible within the stent, although the angiographic result was satisfactory. Even more disturbing was the finding of lining red thrombus within the stented area of the vein graft in 2 patients, and a protruding red thrombus in one patient with a Palmaz-Schatz stent in a vein graft. These patients received additional intracoronary infusion of thrombolytic agents. Follow-up was uneventful in all patients. Whereas intravascular ultrasound imaging is superior in assessing the optimal expansion of a stent [13], angioscopy is useful to check for remaining thrombotic or intimal material that may remain undetected at angiography [12,14].

Angioscopy can also be useful when adverse results are encountered during follow-up after stent implantation, again by providing the ability to discern thrombus from other intraluminal filling defects. Resar and Brinker have described a case where renarrowing inside a coronary stent, 6 weeks after its delivery, proved to consist of intimal hyperplasia, although thrombus was suspected angiographically [15]. Similarly, Strumpf et al. [14] have reported 2 cases in which thrombolytic therapy was avoided because stent restenosis proved to exist of tissue instead of thrombus. We have used angioscopy to determine the cause of subacute stent closure in 3 patients. Although subacute stent occlusion has been attributed in the literature exclusively to thrombosis [9,16], we discovered that the occlusion was caused by dissection rather than thrombus in 2 of these patients [17]. The third patient with subacute stent occlusion appeared to have an occluding mixed red and white thrombus within his stent, and was treated with PTCA and intracoronary thrombolytic therapy.

Restenosis

The response of the coronary vascular wall to balloon dilatation and other angioplasty modalities is still the subject of numerous studies. Luminal renarrowing, occurring in 25-45% of the dilated lesions, remains the "Achilles heel" of balloon angioplasty [18,19]. Restenosis is the result of a complex process involving platelets, growth factors, endothelial cells, smooth muscle cells, mechanical injury, wall shear stress, and probably other unknown factors. Although many questions concerning the pathophysiological mechanisms of restenosis still are unanswered, it is generally accepted that secondary hyperplasia of the intima is the major mechanism. Endothelial injury may play an important role in the development of intimal hyperplasia leading to re-narrowing of the lumen within the first months after PTCA [20-22]. Neither mechanical interventions, such as laser angioplasty or atherectomy, nor drug therapy, have so far contributed much to reduce this intima hyperplasia [23-29]. It has now been proven that intracoronary stents reduce restenosis, but the mechanism is probably one of achieving a larger initial lumen rather than preventing intima hyperplasia [30,31]. On the assumption that angioscopy could demonstrate a possible relationship of the magnitude and amount of arterial wall damage and thrombus caused by PTCA to restenosis, we have undertaken a pilot study, in which we documented the angioscopic changes that occur during the first hour after PTCA [32]. Recently, Bauters and Lablanche and co-workers published their angioscopic restenosis study, in which they confirmed a high angiographic restenosis rate in lesions that contained thrombus at the time of PTCA [33]. The next important question of course is, whether this restenosis rate can be influenced by effective management of intracoronary thrombus. This leads us to a promising new class of drugs: the glycoprotein IIb/IIIa inhibitors.

Glycoprotein IIb/IIIa inhibitors

The first available drug of this new class was produced in 1985 [34]. It is a mouse monoclonal antibody, known as c7E3 Fab, against the glycoprotein IIb/IIIa receptor on the surface of the platelet. Its effectiveness was first demonstrated on a large scale in the EPIC study, in which 2099 patients in 56 centers received a bolus and an infusion of placebo or c7E3 Fab prior to scheduled coronary angioplasty or atherectomy in high risk PTCA (refractory angina pectoris, evolving acute myocardial infarction, or complex coronary morphology). Treatment with c7E3 Fab bolus plus infusion resulted in a 35 percent reduction in primary events, death, nonfatal myocardial infarction, unplanned revascularization, or intervention (12.8 vs 8.3 percent, p = 0.008) [35]. Treatment before or after PTCA with c7E3 Fab is getting widespread acceptance in interventional cardiology, and remarkable cases of rapid solution of thrombus related coronary problems are now being reported. In addition, these glycoprotein IIb/IIIa inhibitors may have an effect on late restenosis. We are presently conducting a pilot trial to study the effect of c7E3 Fab on the angiographic presentation of intracoronary thrombus. A possible role of angioscopy not only is the further investigation of IIb/IIIa inhibition, but may also, as a clinical decision tool, may be one of identifying patients who benefit most from these powerful new drugs.

Discussion

It appears that the clinical utility of coronary angioscopy is related directly to its ability to visualize unstable lesions and especially to its high sensitivity for demonstrating intracoronary thrombus. There is no doubt about the superiority of angioscopy in this respect. In a comparative, retrospective study, we have found that 48% of angioscopically observed thrombi remained undetected at angiography [36]. Comparable results were published by Uretsky et al. [37]. Nevertheless, at the current time angioscopy still has to be regarded mainly as a very useful research tool, rather than a method that has a large impact on decision making in interventional cardiology. To become an indispensable tool in the interventional cathlab, it should have a specific clinical applicability. Research using angioscopy should be aimed at the stabilization of atheromatous plaque by lipid lowering agents, and the effects on intracoronary thrombus of glycoprotein IIb/IIIa inhibitors. These are the areas where angioscopy may find its place in diagnosis and clinical decision making.

References

1. Ambrose JA, Winters SL, Stern A *et al.* Angiographic morphology and the pathogenesis of unstable angina pectoris. J Am Coll Cardiol 1985;5:609-16.
2. De Feyter PJ, Ozaki Y, Baptista J *et al.* Ischemia-related lesion characteristics in patients with stable or unstable angina. A study with intracoronary angioscopy and ultrasound. Circulation 1995;92:1408-13.
3. Mizuno K, Satomura K, Miyamoto A *et al.* Angioscopic evaluation of coronary-artery thrombi in acute coronary syndromes. N Engl J Med 1992;326:287-91.
4. Den Heijer P, Foley DP Hillege HL, *et al.* The "Ermenonville" classification of observations at coronary angioscopy - evaluation of intra- and inter observer agreement. European Working Group on Coronary Angioscopy. Eur Heart J 1994;15:815-22.
5. Knopf WD, Cates CU, Doby B, Langlois K. Coronary angioscopy influences intervention in patients with unstable angina and recent myocardial infarction [abstract]. Circulation 1992;86(Suppl.I):I-651.
6. Lablanche JM, Hamon M, McFadden EP, Bauters C, Quandalle P, Bertrand ME. Angiographically silent thrombus frequently persists after thrombolytic therapy for acute myocardial infarction: a prospective angioscopic study [abstract]. Circulation 1993;88(4 pt 2):I-595.
7. White CJ, Ramee SR, Collins TJ. Percutaneous coronary angioscopy: a tool in clinical decision-making. Choices Cardiol 1994;8:53-6.
8. Lincoff AM, Popma JJ, Ellis SG, Hacker JA, Topol EJ. Abrupt vessel closure complicating coronary angioplasty: clinical, angiographic and therapeutic profile. J Am Coll Cardiol 1992;19:926-35.
9. Herrmann HC, Buchbinder M, Clemen MW *et al.* Emergent use of balloon-expandable coronary artery stenting for failed percutaneous transluminal coronary angioplasty. Circulation 1992;86:812-9.
10. De Muinck ED, den Heijer P, van Dijk RB *et al.* Autoperfusion balloon versus stent for acute or threatened closure during percutaneous transluminal coronary angioplasty. Am J Cardiol 1994;74:1002-5.
11. Fischman DL, Savage MP, Leon MB *et al.* Angiographic predictors of subacute thrombosis following coronary artery stenting [abstract]. Circulation 1991;84(Suppl.II):II-588.
12. Teirstein PS, Schatz RA, Wong SC, Rocha-Singh K. Coronary stenting with

angioscopic guidance. Am J Cardiol 1995;75:344-7.

13. Nakamura S, Colombo A, Gaglione A *et al*. Intracoronary ultrasound observations during stent implantation. Circulation 1994;89:2026-34.

14. Strumpf RK, Heuser RR, Eagan JT Jr. Angioscopy: a valuable tool in the deployment and evaluation of intracoronary stents. Am Heart J 1993;126:1204-10.

15. Resar JR, Brinker J. Early coronary artery stent restenosis: utility of percutaneous coronary angioscopy. Cathet Cardiovasc Diagn 1992;27:276-9.

16. Schatz RA, Baim DS, Leon M *et al*. Clinical experience with the Palmaz-Schatz coronary stent. Initial results of a multicenter study. Circulation 1991;83:148-61.

17. Den Heijer P, van Dijk RB, Twisk S, Lie KI. Early stent occlusion is not always caused by thrombosis. Cathet Cardiovasc Diagn 1993;29:136-40.

18. Ryan TJ, Faxon DP, Gunnar RM *et al*. Guidelines for percutaneous transluminal coronary angioplasty. A report of the American College of Cardiology/American Heart Association Task Force on Assessment of Diagnostic and Therapeutic Cardiovascular Procedures (Subcommittee on Percutaneous Transluminal Coronary Angioplasty). Circulation 1988;78:486-502.

19. Foley DP, Hermans WM, Rensing BJ, De Feyter PJ, Serruys PW. Restenosis after percutaneous transluminal coronary angioplasty. Herz 1992;17:1-17.

20. Ferns GA, Stewart-Lee LA, Anggard EE. Arterial response to mechanical injury: balloon catheter de-endothelialization. Atherosclerosis 1992;92:89-104.

21. Harrison DG. Endothelial modulation of vascular tone: relevance to coronary angioplasty and restenosis. J Am Coll Cardiol 1991;17(6 Suppl.B):71B-76B.

22. Liu MW, Roubin GS, King SB 3rd. Restenosis after coronary angioplasty: Potential biologic determinants and role of intimal hyperplasia. Circulation 1989;79:1374-87.

23. Kuntz RE, Safian RD, Levine MJ, Reis GJ, Diver DJ, Baim DS. Novel approach to the analysis of restenosis after the use of three new coronary devices. J Am Coll Cardiol 1992;19:1493-9.

24. Umans VA, Beatt KJ, Rensing B, Hermans WR, De Feyter PJ, Serruys PW. Comparative quantitative angiographic analysis of directional coronary atherectomy and balloon coronary angioplasty. Am J Cardiol 1991;68:1556-63.

25. White CW, Chaitman B, Knudtson ML, Chisholm RJ. Antiplatelet agents are effective in reducing the acute ischemic complications of angioplasty but do not prevent restenosis: Results from the ticlopidine trial. Coron Artery Dis 1991;2:757-67.

26. Serruys PW, Rutsch W, Heyndrickx GR *et al*. Prevention of restenosis after percutaneous transluminal coronary angioplasty with thromboxane A2-receptor blockade. A randomized, double-blind, placebo-controlled trial. Coronary Artery Restenosis Prevention on Repeated Thromboxane-Antagonism Study (CARPORT). Circulation 1991;84:1568-80.

27. Bairati I, Roy L, Meyer F. Double-blind, randomized, controlled trial of fish oil supplements in prevention of recurrence of stenosis after coronary angioplasty. Circulation 1992;85:950-6.

28. Kaul U, Sanghvi S, Bahl VK, Dev V, Wasir HS. Fish oil supplements for prevention of restenosis after coronary angioplasty. Int J Cardiol 1992;35:87-93.

29. Margolis JR, Mehta S. Excimer laser coronary angioplasty. Am J Cardiol 1992;69:3F-11F.

30. Serruys PW, De Jaegere P, Kiemeneij F *et al.* A comparison of balloon-expandable-stent implantation with balloon angioplasty in patients with coronary artery disease. Benestent Study Group. N Engl J Med 1994;331:489-95.

31. Fischman DL, Leon MB, Baim DS *et al.* A randomized comparison of coronary-stent placement and balloon angioplasty in the treatment of coronary artery disease. Stent Restenosis Study Investigators. N Engl J Med 1994;331:496-501.

32. Den Heijer P, van Dijk RB, Hillege HL, Pentinga ML, Serruys PW, Lie KI. Serial angioscopic and angiographic observations during the first hour after successful coronary angioplasty: a preamble to a multicenter trial addressing angioscopic markers for restenosis. Am Heart J 1994;128:656-63.

33. Bauters C, Lablanche JM, McFadden EP, Hamon M, Bertrand ME. Relation of coronary angioscopic findings at coronary angioplasty to angiographic restenosis. Circulation 1995;92:2473-9.

34. Coller BS. A new murine monoclonal antibody reports an activation dependent change in the conformation and/or microenvironment of the platelet glycoprotein IIb/IIIa complex. J Clin Invest 1985;76:101-8.

35. Use of a monoclonal antibody directed against the platelet glycoprotein IIb/IIIa receptor in high-risk coronary angioplasty. The EPIC Investigators. N Engl J Med 1994;330:956-61.

36. Den Heijer P, Foley DP, Escaned J *et al.* Angioscopic versus angiographic detection of intimal dissection and intracoronary thrombus. J Am Coll Cardiol 1994;24:649-54.

37. Uretsky BF, Denys BG, Counihan PC, Ragosta M. Angioscopic evaluation of incompletely obstructing coronary intraluminal filling defects: comparison to angiography. Cathet Cardiovasc Diagn 1994;33:323-9.

30. Current status and future expectations of the flow velocity guidewire

RICHARD G. BACH

Summary

Coronary angiography incompletely delineates the physiologic consequences of many epicardial stenoses and is unable to diagnose microvascular abnormalities. Intracoronary flow velocity measurements with the Doppler guidewire contribute physiologic data regarding the hemodynamic significance of coronary stenoses and the functional capacity of the coronary microvasculature. Flow velocity analysis can provide objective criteria for refining the selection of cases for revascularization, and prospective clinical data have confirmed the safety of deferring intervention on lesions with normal physiologic assessment. Translesional and distal coronary flow velocity dynamics during procedures also yield immediate information regarding the physiologic adequacy of intervention. The preliminary results of the DEBATE study indicate that impaired post-PTCA coronary flow reserve (CFR) predicts subsequent clinical events, and data comparing flow velocity indices pre- and post-stenting suggest physiologically inadequate results of PTCA may be improved by additional intervention. Flow velocity assessment may also have utility in profiling the adequacy of infarct artery reperfusion following acute myocardial infarction. Evidence has been accumulated to support an expanding use of Doppler flow velocity analysis as a clinically relevant and cost-effective technique for improving both diagnostic and therapeutic decisions in interventional cardiology.

Introduction: clinical application of flow velocity assessment

In the evaluation of coronary artery disease, coronary arteriography provides essential information regarding the anatomic presence, location and extent of coronary obstructions, but only indirectly images plaque geometry, may be subject to interobserver variability in interpretation, and incompletely delineates the physiologic consequences of many stenoses [1]. Myocardial perfusion inadequacy related to microvascular disease or functional supply-demand imbalance is inaccessible to angiographic diagnosis. Uncertainty regarding lesional functional significance is especially problematic among stenoses with intermediate severity or complex morphology, characteristics which also typically describe most lesions resulting from coronary angioplasty.

Given the limitations of angiography, adjunctive techniques have been developed to improve diagnostic accuracy. Some of these techniques, such as computer-assisted quantitative analysis (QCA) or intravascular ultrasound (IVUS), enhance the ability to define lesion geometry. Others, such as Doppler flow velocity assessment and intracoronary pressure measurement, explore the physiology of coronary blood flow and the functional consequences of coronary

389

J.H.C. Reiber and E.E. van der Wall (eds.), Cardiovascular Imaging, 389-402.
© 1996 *Kluwer Academic Publishers.*

obstructive disease. While providing a detailed and highly refined geometric description of an individual lesion, both QCA and IVUS remain limited to morphologic data: physiologic consequences must be extrapolated from assumptions based on physical principles which may be difficult to generalize to individual patients. Intracoronary flow interrogation using Doppler velocimetry and intracoronary pressure measurement are two relatively new and complementary techniques which directly assess coronary physiology and hemodynamics. With its miniaturized size and validated ability to quantitate flow velocity instantaneously in real time [2], the 0.014-in or 0.018-in Doppler-tipped angioplasty guidewire (Flowire, Cardiometrics, Inc) can provide data useful in certain clinical situations which are common to the invasive cardiologist. Doppler velocimetry by the flow velocity guidewire allows quantitation of blood flow velocity and of the phasic components of flow velocity both in proximal and post-stenotic distal coronary arteries, and has emerged as a practical and clinically useful tool for providing physiologic assessment of the adequacy of coronary blood flow and of coronary artery lesion significance. Use of intracoronary flow velocity for diagnostic functional assessment can refine the selection of cases for revascularization. Translesional and distal coronary flow velocity dynamics during procedures, furthermore, provide immediate data regarding the physiologic adequacy of intervention.

Chest pain with normal coronary arteries

Angiographically normal or nonobstructed coronary arteries are encountered in a substantial minority of patients with chest pain syndromes undergoing cardiac catheterization. Some of these patients have noninvasive testing data suggesting impaired myocardial perfusion or ischemia. These patients often represent a diagnostic and therapeutic dilemma. When epicardial coronary vasospasm has been excluded, clinicians often infer coronary microvascular disease and/or myocardial supply-demand imbalance. "Syndrome X" has been a term widely used to describe this clinical scenario. In patients with chest pain syndromes but angiographically nonobstructed epicardial coronary arteries, flow velocity analysis in conjunction with pharmacologic vasodilatation can investigate the functional integrity of the coronary microvasculature. Coronary flow reserve (CFR), the ratio of maximal hyperemic flow velocity to basal flow velocity, has been shown to be a sensitive indicator of the functional capacity of the coronary resistive microvessels to accommodate increased blood flow. Previous studies have demonstrated an impairment of CFR in a proportion of patients with syndrome X, implying microvascular disease [3], although this remains controversial. Since the flow velocity guidewire can be inserted into the coronary artery via standard diagnostic angiographic catheters, Doppler velocimetry in conjunction with stimulation of maximal hyperemia by intracoronary adenosine (12 to 18 μg bolus) provides a convenient method whereby CFR can be routinely assessed in such patients. In our laboratory, the mean CFR in over 400 arteries in 196 patients with chest pain syndromes and angiographically normal coronary arteries was 2.7 $\pm$ 0.6 [4]. While it must be remembered that CFR can be influenced by changes in resting blood flow and factors such as myocardial hypertrophy and heart rate, the documentation of a "normal" CFR in such patients may enhance confidence that impaired coronary perfusion is not the etiology of chest pain and redirect the evaluation towards a non-cardiac etiology of symptoms.

Physiologic assessment of coronary stenosis severity

The Doppler guide wire has provided the first method by which *post-stenotic* coronary blood flow can be practically and directly measured in the catheterization laboratory. In patients with coronary stenoses which fall into an angiographically indeterminate or intermediate range of severity ($\sim$40-70%), interrogation of blood flow velocity distal to a stenosis can demonstrate the degree of consequent flow impairment to the relevant myocardial bed. This provides data which differentiates hemodynamically significant from insignificant stenoses, and refines the selection of lesions for revascularization.

Regarding clinical application of this technology, certain statements can be made: (1) intracoronary flow velocity measurements using the flow velocity guidewire are valid, safe and reproducible; (2) due to the branching nature of the coronary tree, flow velocity and CFR measurements made proximal to a coronary stenosis do not reliably predict flow velocity in the relevant post-stenotic artery [5-7]; (3) resting absolute flow velocity values alone cannot discriminate lesion significance [5]; (4) direct measurements of distal flow velocity have correlated poorly with lesional flow indices predicted from QCA [5,8]; (5) directly measured post-stenotic CFR correlates very well with non-invasive stress imaging results for determining impairment of regional perfusion [6,9].

In the assessment of intermediate coronary stenoses, three parameters have been determined to have relevance for predicting lesional hemodynamic significance: (1) an impairment of maximal hyperemic flow expressed in the post-stenotic CFR, (2) an impairment of resting flow velocity across the stenosis, expressed in the translesional proximal-to-distal (P/D) flow velocity ratio, and (3) an impairment of the normal phasic pattern of flow velocity expressed in the post-stenotic diastolic-to-systolic velocity ratio (DSVR).

P/D Doppler velocity ratio

The presence of an abnormal P/D ratio in the post-stenotic artery provides relatively specific evidence of severe epicardial obstruction. In patients with predominantly left coronary lesions studied in our laboratory, a P/D ratio of > 1.7 predicted a translesional gradient of > 30 mmHg with 95% accuracy (Figure 1) [5]. Importantly, among angiographically intermediate stenoses this parameter continued to show excellent correlation with translesional gradients (r = 0.8, p < 0.001), while QCA (ACA program) percent diameter stenosis showed a poor correlation (r = 0.2, p = NS).

Diastolic-to-systolic velocity ratio

Due to the interaction of aortic driving pressure and intramyocardial compressive pressure, normal flow velocity spectra in the left coronary and left ventricular

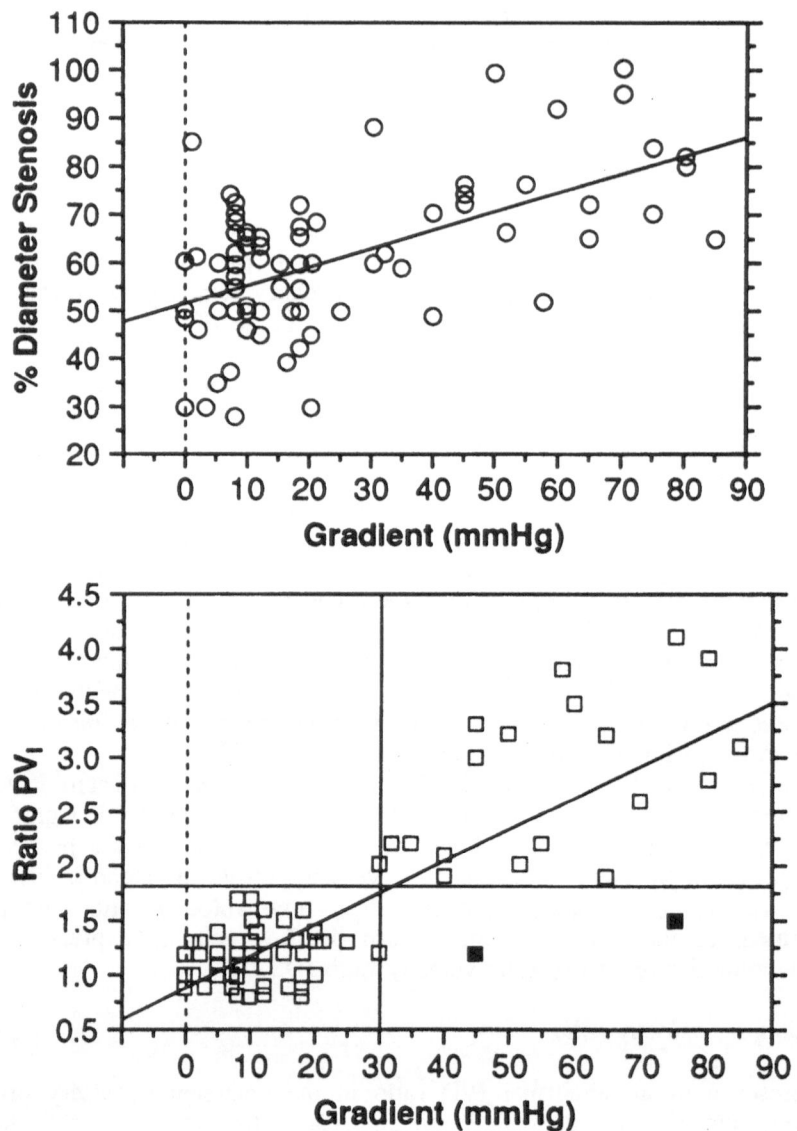

Figure 1. Linear regression analyses depicting relationships between translesional hemodynamics and percent diameter stenosis by quantitative coronary angiography (top panel) and the ratio of proximal-to-distal peak velocity integral obtained using the Doppler wire (lower panel). Note the weak correlation (r=0.2,p=NS) between percent diameter stenosis and translesional gradient for intermediate (40-70%) stenoses, while proximal-to-distal velocity ratio of > 1.7 correlated highly (90%) with translesional gradients of > 30 mmHg. (Reproduced with permission from Donohue TJ, Kern MJ, Aguirre FV, Bach RG, Wolford T, Bell CA, Segal J. Assessing the hemodynamic significance of coronary artery stenoses: analysis of translesional pressure-flow velocity relations in patients. J Am Coll Cardiol 1993;22:449-58.)

branches of the right coronary show a diastolic-predominant waveform, resulting in a normal DSVR of > 1.5. In animal models, as an epicardial stenosis increases in severity to the point at which autoregulation is exhausted, viscous pressure losses across the stenosis become dominant and the distal phasic flow pattern becomes altered [10,11]. Using Doppler flow wires during coronary angioplasty in a total of 67 patients, Segal et al. [12] and Ofili et al. [13] demonstrated a reduction in DSVR distal to significant stenoses prior to intervention. In >50% of angiographically severe lesions studied, post-stenotic phasic predominance was reversed and systolic velocity higher than diastolic velocity. In response to successful PTCA, there was a return of the normal phasic pattern to distal flow velocity and therefore normalization of the distal DSVR.

Post-stenotic coronary flow reserve

As might be expected due to the compensatory effects of coronary autoregulation on basal blood flow, absolute resting flow velocity measurements in either the proximal or distal artery are poorly predictive of lesional significance. As a ratio normalizing maximal hyperemic flow to basal flow, the CFR has been shown in animal models to correlate with the severity of coronary stenoses [14]. However, due to the effect of pre-stenotic branches with low resistance, CFR measured proximal to a stenosis can differ substantially from CFR measured distally, obviating the ability to reliably assess a stenosis by proximal flow velocity measurements [5-7,9]. For the assessment of lesion functional significance, therefore, the post-stenotic CFR has emerged as the most clinically important of the Doppler velocity parameters. A case example illustrating intermediate lesion assessment using the flow velocity guidewire is shown in Figure 2.

In a recent comparison of pharmacologic stress ^{99m}Tc-sestamibi tomographic perfusion imaging with quantitative coronary angiography and coronary flow velocities in 33 patients with intermediately severe coronary artery disease [6], among all variables tested the strongest correlation (89%) was found between an abnormal post-stenotic coronary flow reserve ($\leq$ 2.0) and the presence of reversible perfusion defects in the target perfusion zone. Similar results were reported by Joye et al. [9] comparing flow velocity with stress tomographic thallium-201 imaging in 30 patients with intermediate stenoses. In that study, the sensitivity, specificity, and overall predictive accuracy of post-stenotic coronary flow reserve for stress imaging results were 94%, 95% and 94%, respectively. These and other studies now establishing an excellent correlation between invasive and non-invasive physiologic testing suggest that, while recognizing certain limits, the data provided by lesion assessment in the catheterization laboratory using the flow velocity guidewire can serve as a reliable indicator of the functional significance of coronary stenoses.

There are limitations in the use of Doppler flow velocity parameters for lesion assessment. CFR can be potentially affected by factors other than lesion severity, such as heart rate, blood pressure, left ventricular hypertrophy, previous infarction, and anemia. Coronary flow velocity can be affected by all lesions within a vessel, and serial stenoses may complicate the interpretation of velocity measurements across any one site. While an accurately measured abnormal P/D ratio alone may have high specificity for very significant stenoses (> 30 mmHg

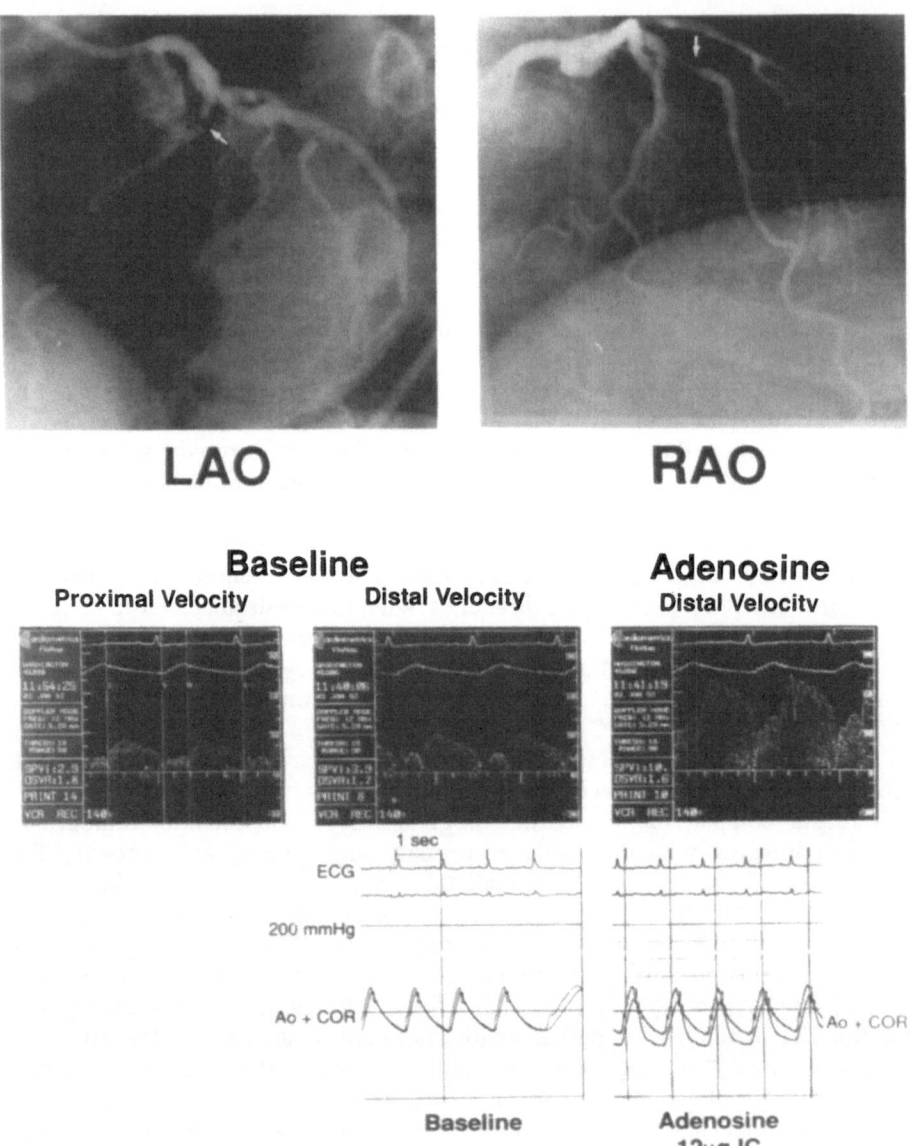

Figure 2. Translesional flow velocity assessment of intermediate stenosis in a 59-year old man with chest pain and equivocal radionuclide stress test, demonstrating absence of hemodynamic significance. Upper panel shows cineangiographic frames of an eccentric stenosis in the proximal left anterior descending artery; left anterior oblique (LAO) view shows > 80% diameter stenosis. In the right anterior oblique (RAO) view, the diameter stenosis was < 50%. Lower panel shows flow velocity guidewire and translesional gradient (tracking catheter) measurements. Proximal average peak velocity was 22 cm/sec, distal post-stenotic velocity was 26 cm/sec, with a normal phasic pattern and diastolic/systolic velocity ratio (1.8). Hyperemia induced a 2.5-fold increase in post-stenotic flow velocity. These findings corresponded to a translesional

pressure gradient of 0 mmHg at rest and 10 mmHg at peak hyperemia. Ao=aorta; COR=coronary pressure; flow velocity scale=0-140 cm/sec. (Reproduced with permission from Donohue TJ, Kern MJ, Aguirre FV, Bach RG, Wolford T, Bell CA, Segal J. Assessing the hemodynamic significance of coronary artery stenoses: analysis of translesional pressure-flow velocity relationships in patients. J Am Coll Cardiol 1993;22:449-58.)

resting gradient), this parameter can remain insensitive to functionally significant lesions with lower resting gradients. Vasoconstriction or angiographically inapparent luminal narrowing can accelerate resting flow velocity at a particular site, affecting comparisons with other sites. Accurate velocities proximal to the zone of acceleration may also be difficult to obtain for very proximal coronary lesions. The degree of proximal arterial branching also has a strong influence on the ability of P/D ratios to discriminate lesions, as non-branching conduits must maintain equivalent proximal and distal flow by the continuity equation. In a study limited to right coronary arteries, Heller et al. [7] reported the P/D ratio was not helpful in functional lesion assessment in the proximal and mid vessel, potentially a result of the lack of significant branching typical for this portion of the right coronary artery. In addition, the diastolic-to-systolic velocity ratio of flow velocity in the proximal to mid right coronary artery is typically less than 1.5, likely due to the lower systolic resistance in the right heart. This may limit the use of distal diastolic-to-systolic velocity ratio in discriminating lesion significance in those segments.

Comparison of flow-derived and pressure-derived indices of lesion significance

Translesional pressure gradients measured using miniaturized, high fidelity transducers have also been proposed as an alternative method for assessing the hemodynamic significance of intermediate lesions. DeBruyne et al. [15,16] and Pijls et al. [17] have developed the concept of myocardial fractional flow reserve (FFR_{myo}). FFR_{myo} is calculated from the ratio of post-stenotic coronary pressure to aortic pressure at maximal hyperemia corrected for the mean central venous pressure (assumed at 5 mmHg). In comparisons of translesional pressure-derived indices with stress testing and positron emission tomography, an FFR_{myo} below 0.7 correlated well with evidence of abnormal myocardial perfusion [15,16]. In an attempt to correlate flow velocity indices of lesional physiology with pressure-derived measurements, Tron and colleagues [18] directly compared post-stenotic CFR with FFR_{myo} determined using a flow velocity guidewire and 2.7F fluid-filled tracking catheter, respectively, with the results of stress perfusion imaging in 70 arteries with stenoses in 62 patients. (Of note, the tracking catheter is larger in cross sectional area than the 0.018-in pressure guidewire used in other studies.) Mean angiographic diameter stenosis was 56 ± 15% (range 14% to 94%). While there was a correlation between post-stenotic CFR and FFR_{myo} ($r = 0.45$, $p < 0.0001$), the strongest predictor of stress myocardial imaging results was the post-stenotic CFR (Figure 3). As shown in Table 1, a FFR_{myo} of ≤ 0.69 had positive and negative predictive values for stress perfusion results (reversible defect) of 71% and 63%, respectively, while

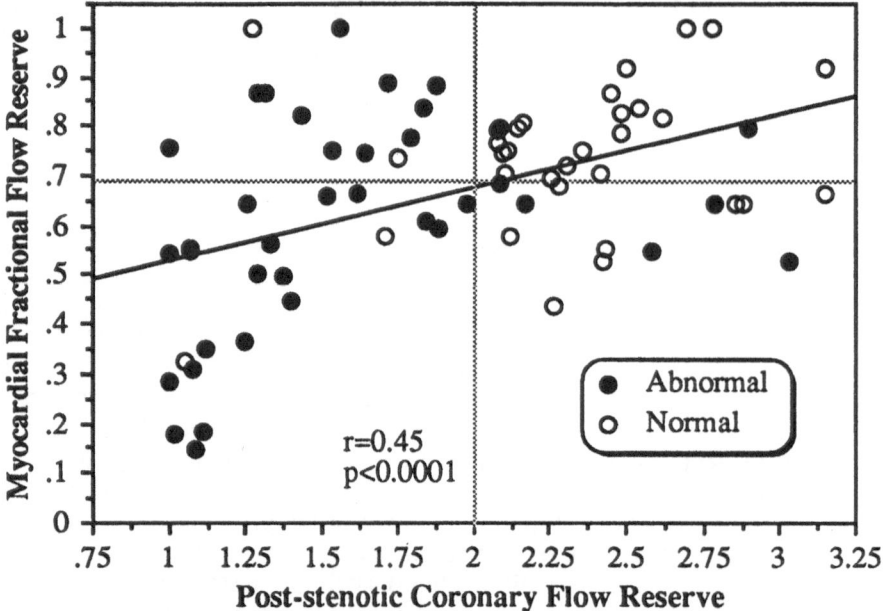

Figure 3. Correlation of post-stenotic CFR and FFR_myo. *Solid circles,* patients with abnormal stress myocardial perfusion imaging results; *open circles,* patients with normal stress myocardial perfusion imaging results; *dashed lines,* best cutoff points for prediction of stress myocardial perfusion imaging results (2.0 for post-stenotic CFR and 0.69 for FFR_myo). (Reproduced with permission from Tron C, Donohue TJ, Bach RG, Aguirre FV, Caracciolo EA, Wolford TL, Miller DD, Kern MJ. Comparison of pressure-derived fractional flow reserve with post-stenotic coronary flow reserve for prediction of stress myocardial perfusion imaging results. Am Heart J 1995;130:723-33.)

Table 1. Prediction of myocardial imaging results by flow velocity-, pressure-, and QCA-derived indices.

	Sensitivity	Specificity	Positive Predictive Value	Negative Predictive Value	Accuracy
Distal coronary flow reserve ≤2	82	87	89	80	84
FFR_myo ≤0.69	66	69	71	63	67
Diameter stenosis >56%	63	62	67	59	60
Minimal lumen diameter ≤1.2 mm	54	56	59	51	55

Reproduced with permission from Tron et al. Comparison of pressure-derived fractional flow reserve with poststenotic coronary flow velocity reserve for prediction of stress myocardial perfusion imaging results. Am Heart J 1995;130:723-33.

a post-stenotic CFR ≤ 2.0 had positive and negative predictive values of 89% and 80%, respectively. These data highlight the strong correlation between post-stenotic CFR and stress myocardial perfusion imaging.

These results further suggest that flow velocity analysis and translesional pressure measurements may provide complementary information in assessing impaired hyperemic responses related to epicardial obstruction and microvascular abnormalities. To overcome limitations related to the interpretation of CFR, Mancini et al. [19] provided data in an animal model which proposed the instantaneous hyperemic diastolic flow versus pressure slope index as an alternative and potentially more sensitive indicator of stenosis severity which was independent of heart rate, contractility, aortic pressure and preload. Di Mario et al. [20] applied this concept to the evaluation of coronary stenoses in patients using separate high-fidelity pressure and Doppler-tipped guidewires, with high sensitivity and specificity in discriminating stenoses, and with the potential advantage of independence from changes in basal velocity and hemodynamic conditions. The practical application of these and other similar techniques to clinical use will depend on confirmation of these results in larger studies and ultimately on technical advancements allowing incorporation of both Doppler flow velocity and high-fidelity pressure sensors on a single angioplasty guidewire.

Practical utility of lesion assessment: clinical outcomes

The practical clinical applicability of Doppler flow velocity measurement has been documented both in the diagnostic setting and during intervention. Our experience has suggested that a proportion of coronary stenoses suspected to be functionally significant by angiography will be found non-flow limiting by direct assessment, and therefore, regional myocardial perfusion is unlikely to be improved by angioplasty or bypass grafting. In a study involving 100 lesions in 88 patients undergoing translesional flow and hemodynamic assessment who were followed over a mean of 9 months, angioplasty was deferred safely in patients with normal translesional flow velocity-pressure parameters [21].

Conversely, using flow wire assessment, we have not infrequently encountered lesions which appear angiographically moderate but which are flow limiting [22], and even lesions of equal angiographic severity in different arteries of the same patient which differ markedly in hemodynamic significance [23].

Physiologic angioplasty endpoint guidance

While employed as an angioplasty guidewire, a distally placed flow velocity guidewire can theoretically provide immediate data regarding the functional adequacy of luminal expansion by intervention, and thereby guide the potential need for additional intervention. Use of the flow wire for continuous distal flow velocity monitoring during the immediate post-intervention period has allowed identification of patterns of the coronary flow velocity trend which are unstable and associated with impending occlusion or inadequate results. These include cyclic flow variations, steadily declining average peak velocity, and abrupt cessation of flow [24,25]. Interestingly, similar to animal models where cyclic flow variations have been found due to intermittent platelet aggregation and dissolution, Anderson et al. [26] have shown that cyclic flow variations detected by the flow wire in patients following PTCA can be abolished by a chimeric monoclonal antibody agent, c7E3 Fab, which blocks platelet aggregability.

In the post-intervention setting, angiography may be limited in accurately representing the luminal encroachment by residual plaque or dissection. Studies employing post-interventional IVUS and angioscopy have highlighted the lack of sensitivity of the angiogram in depicting significant dissection or inadequate results. The DEBATE trial explored the hypothesis that persistently impaired distal flow velocity and CFR after PTCA could predict clinical events or restenosis during 6 month follow-up. The findings of this important prospective multicenter trial have been presented in preliminary form [27]. Approximately 300 patients with single-vessel disease and no previous Q-wave myocardial infarction undergoing PTCA were studied. PTCA success was guided angiographically. Before and 15 minutes after angiographically successful PTCA, baseline and hyperemic flow velocity measurements were obtained proximal and distal to the lesion. Only 4 patients had cyclic flow variabilities detected in the immediate post-PTCA period by distal flow velocity monitoring, but of those 3/4 developed abrupt closure. Among patients with successful PTCA but recurrence of symptoms or positive exercise test within 1 month, the immediate post-PTCA distal CFR was significantly lower than among patients who remained asymptomatic. The post-PTCA minimal luminal diameter by QCA did not discriminate these groups. Compared to patients with higher CFR, patients with a post-PTCA distal CFR of ≤ 2.5 had a more than twofold increase in the relative risk of clinical recurrence by 6 months. These results suggest that immediate post-PTCA distal flow velocity and CFR measurements have value in predicting subsequent clinical events.

Future expectations of the Flowire for interventional decisions

Given the correlation between reduced CFR in the immediate post-PTCA period and subsequent clinical ischemic events despite equivalent angiographic results in DEBATE, it follows that clinical failure within 6 months may be related to angiographic PTCA pseudo-success. In order to explore this hypothesis, sequential coronary flow velocity and IVUS measurements were obtained before and after balloon dilatation followed by stenting using Palmaz-Schatz coronary stents in 10 patients in our laboratory [28]. In this series, balloon dilatation was performed with PTCA balloons selected for 1:1 balloon:artery size-matching, and an effort was made to achieve an angiographically "acceptable" PTCA result prior to flow and IVUS assessment and stenting. Results are shown in Table 2. The IVUS lesional cross-sectional area increased from 5.4 ± 1.4 mm^2 after balloon to 7.7 ± 3.0 mm^2 (p < 0.01) after stent, associated with an improvement in mean CFR from 1.5 ± 0.3 after PTCA to 2.4 ± 0.7. These results suggest that the failure to normalize CFR in many patients after PTCA may be due to persistent but angiographically unrecognized inadequate luminal expansion. Nevertheless, as highlighted by the results of DEBATE, a majority of patients are in fact adequately treated by PTCA alone, and coronary stents carry their own added risks and costs. Therefore, physiologic guidance of coronary angioplasty

Table 2. Flow velocity and intravascular ultrasound measurements after PTCA and after stenting.

	Angio Diameter (%)	Angio MLD (mm)	IVUS area (mm^2)	Rest APV (cm/sec)	CFR
Base	70±12	0.98±0.35	-----	17.0±6.9	1.47±0.34
Post-PTCA	41±13	2.1±0.6	5.4±1.4	17.1±4.7	1.54±0.26
Post-stent	11±4*	3.0±0.49*	7.7±3.0*	20.3±8.5	2.4±0.7*

*p<0.01 vs PTCA
Reproduced with permission of Kern et al. Impact of residual lumen narrowing on coronary flow after angioplasty and stent: intravascular ultrasound, Doppler and imaging data in support of physiologically-guided coronary angioplasty [abstract]. Circulation 1995;92:I-263.

by distal Doppler guide wire flow velocity assessment may allow appropriate discrimination of lesions where PTCA results are adequate versus those with unresolved and unappreciated residual stenosis where additional intervention (for example, stenting) may be indicated in an effort to improve clinical outcome. This hypothesis awaits testing in prospective clinical trials.

Infarct artery flow in acute MI

The assessment of coronary flow velocity as a quantitative means for determining the adequacy of reperfusion in patients following thrombolysis or intervention for acute myocardial infarction represents another active topic of current investigation. In patients with acute myocardial infarction, prognosis has been correlated with the degree of restoration of infarct-related artery blood flow based on the angiographic rate of contrast opacification. According to the Thrombolysis in Myocardial Infarction Study Group (TIMI) semi-quantitative grading scale, patients with complete or TIMI grade 3 flow in the infarct artery have improved regional and global left ventricular function and reduced morbidity and mortality compared with patients with TIMI flow grade of ≤ 2 [29]. In preliminary data from Aguirre et al. [30] acquired by use of flow velocity guidewires in 29 patients undergoing angioplasty in the setting of acute myocardial infarction, angiographic flow grade and directly measured intracoronary flow velocity were compared. Arteries with TIMI grades 0, 1, and 2 filling consistently had very low flow velocities and there were no significant differences in the post-stenotic flow velocity values among these groups. There was, however, a difference in flow velocity detected between arteries with TIMI grade ≤ 2 versus those with TIMI grade 3 opacification . In arteries with TIMI grade ≤ 2 filling, the flow velocity was significantly lower on average than in arteries with TIMI grade 3 filling (distal average peak velocity = 12.5 ± 7.6 vs 21.2 ± 12.4 cm/sec, respectively, p<0.008). Importantly, arteries with TIMI grade 3 opacification showed a wide range of flow velocities, with some overlap with the low flow values of the TIMI grade ≤ 2 group. Thus, differences in semi-quantitative TIMI perfusion grades with clinical relevance (≤ 2 vs 3) were distinguished by differences in coronary flow velocity.

By examining the potential correlation between directly measured flow velocities in the infarct-related artery obtained acutely and subsequent clinical outcomes, clinically useful physiologic and prognostic information may be derived from a quantitative analysis of coronary blood flow during myocardial infarction, and in the future, analysis of coronary physiology during acute infarction may supersede the qualitative information of angiography.

Issues of cost efficiency

Given the ongoing trend toward managed care and capitated costs in the United States, questions have arisen regarding the cost effectiveness of various diagnostic and therapeutic procedures. As alluded to by Miller et al. [6], charges for stress perfusion imaging may be comparable to those for cardiac catheterization including flow wire lesion assessment. In a trial reported by Joye et al. [31] designed to compare the cost of stenosis flow velocity assessment using the Flowire with post-angiographic thallium imaging, 53 patients with intermediate coronary lesions (40-70%) were prospectively randomized to undergo distal CFR measurement or stress thallium perfusion scintigraphy. Preliminary results suggest that use of the flow velocity guidewire for decision making shortens average length of hospital stay by approximately two days and reduces hospital direct costs substantially compared with post-angiographic thallium imaging.

Conclusion

Translesional flow velocity measurements are easily incorporated into invasive diagnostic or therapeutic cardiac procedures. This technology has been validated as a cost-effective method for diagnosing the hemodynamic significance of intermediate coronary lesions and for providing clinically relevant physiologic endpoint data after PTCA. It has also opened new doors to research on coronary physiology, and allowed previously impossible direct investigations into distal coronary blood flow in response to various pharmacologic factors, distal coronary blood flow in the setting of acute myocardial infarction, collateral blood flow, and blood flow in bypass conduits. Since coronary blood flow and myocardial perfusion are central to cardiac pathophysiology, in the future, such research will likely translate into additional clinically important applications of flow velocity measurement.

References

1.   Zir LM, Miller SW, Dinsmore RE, Gilbert JP, Harthorne JW. Interobserver variability in coronary angiography. Circulation 1976;53:627-32.
2.   Doucette JW, Corl PD, Payne HM *et al*. Validation of a doppler guide wire for

intravascular measurement of coronary artery flow velocity. Circulation 1992;85:1899-911.

3. Chauhan A, Mullins PA, Petch MC, Schofield PM. Is coronary flow reserve in response to papaverine really normal in syndrome X? Circulation 1994;89:1998-2004.

4. Kern MJ, Aguirre FV, Bach RG *et al*. Variations in coronary vasodilatory reserve by artery, sex, status post transplantation and remote coronary disease [abstract]. Circulation 1994;90(4 pt 2):I-154.

5. Donohue TJ, Kern MJ, Aguirre FV *et al*. Assessing the hemodynamic significance of coronary artery stenoses: analysis of translesional pressure-flow velocity relationships in patients. J Am Coll Cardiol 1993;22:449-58.

6. Miller DD, Donohue TJ, Younis LT *et al*. Correlation of pharmacological ^{99m}Tc-sestamibi myocardial perfusion imaging with poststenotic coronary flow reserve in patients with angiographically intermediate coronary artery stenoses. Circulation 1994;89:2150-60.

7. Heller LI, Silver KH, Villegas BJ, Balcom SJ, Weiner BH. Blood flow velocity in the right coronary artery: assessment before and after angioplasty. J Am Coll Cardiol 1994;24:1012-7.

8. Tron C, Kern MJ, Donohue TJ *et al*. Comparison of quantitative angiographically derived and measured translesion pressure and flow velocity in coronary artery disease. Am J Cardiol 1995;75:111-7.

9. Joye JD, Schulman DS, Lasorda D, Farah T, Donohue BC, Reichek N. Intracoronary Doppler guide wire versus stress single-photon emission computed tomographic thallium-201 imaging in assessment of intermediate coronary stenoses. J Am Coll Cardiol 1994;24:940-7.

10. Manor D, Shofti R, Sideman S, Beyar R. Quantitative sorting of normal and abnormal coronary flow wave form shapes. IEEE Trans Biomed Eng 1994;41:846-53.

11. Kajiya F, Tsujioka K, Ogasawara Y *et al*. Analysis of flow characteristics in poststenotic regions of the human coronary artery during bypass graft surgery. Circulation 1987;76:1092-100.

12. Segal J, Kern MJ, Scott NA *et al*. Alterations of phasic coronary artery flow velocity in humans during percutaneous coronary angioplasty. J Am Coll Cardiol 1992;20:276-86.

13. Ofili EO, Kern MJ, Labovitz AJ *et al*. Analysis of coronary blood flow velocity dynamics in angiographically normal and stenosed arteries before and after endolumen enlargement by angioplasty. J Am Coll Cardiol 1993;21:308-16.

14. Gould KL, Lipscomb K, Hamilton GW. Physiologic basis for assessing critical coronary stenosis. Instantaneous flow response and regional distribution during coronary hyperemia as measures of coronary flow reserve. Am J Cardiol 1974;33:87-94.

15. De Bruyne B, Baudhuin T, Melin JA *et al*. Coronary flow reserve calculated from pressure measurements in humans. Validation with positron emission tomography. Circulation 1994;89:1013-22.

16. De Bruyne B, Bartunek J, Sys SU, Heyndrickx GR. Relation between myocardial fractional flow reserve calculated from coronary pressure measurements and exercise-induced myocardial ischemia. Circulation 1995;92:39-46.

17. Pijls NHJ, van Gelder B, van der Voort P *et al*. Fractional flow reserve. A useful index to evaluate the influence of an epicardial coronary stenosis on

myocardial blood flow. Circulation 1995;92:3183-93.

18. Tron C, Donohue TJ, Bach RG et al. Comparison of pressure-derived fractional flow reserve with poststenotic coronary flow velocity reserve for prediction of stress myocardial perfusion imaging results. Am Heart J 1995;130:723-33.

19. Mancini GBJ, McGillem MJ, DeBoe SF, Gallagher KP. The diastolic hyperemic flow versus pressure relation. A new index of coronary stenosis severity and flow reserve. Circulation 1989;80:941-50.

20. Di Mario C, Krams R, Gil R, Serruys PW. Slope of the instantaneous hyperemic diastolic coronary flow velocity-pressure relation. A new index for assessment of the physiologic significance of coronary stenosis in humans. Circulation 1994;90:1215-24.

21. Kern MJ, Donohue TJ, Aguirre FV et al. Clinical outcome of deferring angioplasty in patients with normal translesional pressure-flow velocity measurements. J Am Coll Cardiol 1995;25:178-87.

22. Kern MJ, Donohue TJ, Aguirre FV et al. Assessment of angiographically intermediate coronary artery stenosis using the doppler flowire. Am J Cardiol 1993;71:26D-33D.

23. Kern MJ, Flynn MS, Caracciolo EA, Bach RG, Donohue TJ, Aguirre FV. Use of translesional coronary flow velocity for interventional decisions in a patient with multiple intermediately severe coronary stenoses. Cathet Cardiovasc Diagn 1993;29:148-53.

24. Anderson HV, Kirkeeide RL, Stuart Y, Smalling RW, Heibig J, Willerson, JT. Coronary artery flow monitoring following coronary interventions. Am J Cardiol 1993;71:62D-69D.

25. Kern MJ, Aguirre FV, Donohue TJ et al. Continuous coronary flow velocity monitoring during coronary interventions: velocity trend patterns associated with adverse events. Am Heart J 1994;128:426-34.

26. Anderson HV, Kirkeeide RL, Krishnaswami A et al. Cyclic flow variations after coronary angioplasty in humans: clinical and angiographic characteristics and elimination with 7E3 monoclonal antiplatelet antibody. J Am Coll Cardiol 1994;23:1031-7.

27. DEBATE Study Group. Are flow velocity measurements after PTCA predictive of recurrence of angina or of a positive exercise test early after balloon angioplasty? [abstract] Circulation 1995;92(Suppl.I):I-264.

28. Kern MJ, Aguirre FV, Donohue TJ et al. Impact of residual lumen narrowing on coronary flow after angioplasty and stent: intravascular ultrasound Doppler and imaging data in support of physiologically-guided coronary angioplasty [abstract]. Circulation 1995;92(Suppl.I):I-263.

29. Anderson JL, Karagounis LA, Becker LC, Sorensen SG, Menlove RL. TIMI perfusion grade 3 but not grade 2 results in improved outcome after thrombolysis for myocardial infarction. Ventriculographic, enzymatic, and electrocardiographic evidence from the TEAM-3 study. Circulation 1993;87:1829-39.

30. Aguirre FV, Donohue TJ, Bach RG et al. Coronary flow velocity of infarct-related arteries: physiologic differences between complete (TIMI III) and incomplete (TIMI O,I,II) angiographic coronary perfusion [abstract]. J Am Coll Cardiol 1995;25(Special Issue):401A.

31. Joye JD, Cates CU, Farah T et al. Cost analysis of intracoronary Doppler determination of lesion significance: preliminary results of the PEACH Study [abstract]. J Invasive Cardiol 1995;7:22A.

31. Coronary pressure measurements and myocardial
fractional flow reserve for clinical decision making
in the catheterization laboratory

NICO H.J. PIJLS & BERNARD DE BRUYNE

Myocardial fractional flow reserve is a lesion-specific index to assess the
influence of an epicardial coronary stenosis on myocardial perfusion.
It is defined as:

$$FFR_{myo} = \frac{\text{maximum attainable flow in the presence of a stenosis}}{\text{normal maximum flow}}$$

FFR_{myo} represents that very fraction of normal maximum flow that has been
maintained in spite of the presence of the stenosis. FFR_{myo} can be easily determined by high-fidelity intracoronary pressure measurements (Figure 1).

Unique features of myocardial fractional flow reserve are:
* FFRmyo can be easily obtained by pressure recordings at maximum coronary
  vasodilation by the equation:

$$FFRmyo = P_d/P_a$$

where P_d is mean hyperemic distal (transstenotic) coronary pressure and P_a is
mean aortic pressure.

* **FFR_{myo} can be obtained both at diagnostic catheterization and at PTCA.**

* FFR_{myo} is independent of changes in systemic blood pressure, heart rate, or
  contractility.

* FFR_{myo} includes collateral flow.

* FFR_{myo} is applicable in multivessel disease.

* FFR_{myo} has an unequivocal normal value of 1.0 for every patient, and every
  coronary artery.

* $FFR_{myo} < 0.75$ or ≥ 0.75 distinguishes lesions which are functionally
  significant or not. The accuracy for that purpose is almost 100%.

The concept of fractional flow is further clarified in the Figures 1 to 6.

J.H.C. Reiber and E.E. van der Wall (eds.), Cardiovascular Imaging, 403-410.
© 1996 *Kluwer Academic Publishers.*

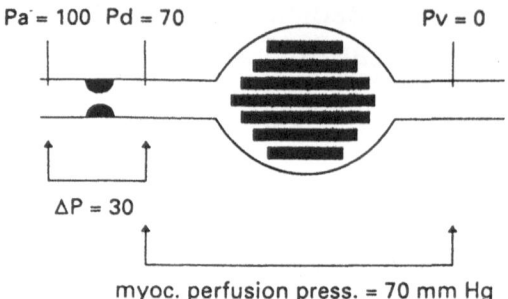

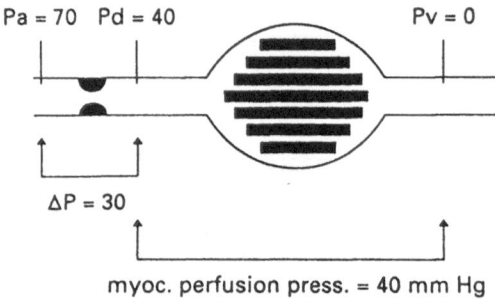

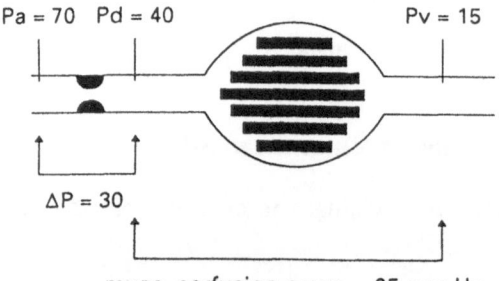

Figure 1. Suppose that the patient in the upper part of the figure is studied at maximum coronary vasodilation, when flow is proportional to driving pressure. Looking at this figure, it is intuitively clear that hyperemic myocardial flow is determined by $(P_d - P_v)/(P_a - P_v)$ which is called myocardial fractional flow reserve (FFR$_{myo}$), and represents that fraction of maximum flow which has still been preserved despite the stenosis. If P_v is not elevated, as will be the case most often, FFR$_{myo}$ equals hyperemic distal to proximal pressure. The figure also illustrates why Δ P alone cannot be used as a reliable index of stenosis severity: in all three examples in this figure transstenotic pressure gradient at maximum vasodilation (corresponding with minimal resistance) equals 30 mmHg. However, the driving pressure over the myocardium (which determines myocardial perfusion at maximum vasodilation) largely varies from 25 to 70 mmHg.

Separate calculation of coronary and collateral blood flow at PTCA

If the concept of Fractional Flow Reserve is applied during PTCA, where also coronary wedge pressure can be measured, it is even possible to calculate the separate contribution of coronary arterial ànd collateral blood flow to maximum myocardial flow. The 3 equations to do so, are tabulated in Table 1. Remember however, that from a patient's point of view, myocardial fractional flow reserve is the most important index.

Table 1. Pressure-flow equations.

1. Myocardial Fractional Flow Reserve (FFR$_{myo}$):

$$\text{FFR}_{myo} = \frac{P_d - P_v}{P_a - P_v} \approx \frac{P_d}{P_a}$$ [If central venous pressure is not elevated (i.e $\cong 0$)]

2. Coronary Fractional Flow Reserve (FFR$_{cor}$):

$$\text{FFR}_{cor} = \frac{P_d - P_w}{P_a - P_w}$$

3. Fractional Collateral Flow (Q$_c$ / Q^N):

$$Q_c / Q^N = (\text{FFR}_{myo} - \text{FFR}_{cor})$$

Abbreviations: P_a = mean arterial pressure at maximum hyperemia; P_d mean distal coronary pressure at maximum hyperemia; P_w = mean distal coronary pressure at coronary artery occlusion, (wedge pressure); P_v = mean central venous pressure at maximum hyperemia; Q^N = normal maximum myocardial blood flow; Q_c = collateral blood flow. From Pijls NHJ, De Bruyne B et al., Circulation 1993;87:1354-67.

A detailed example how to apply these 3 equations at PTCA, is given in Figure 7 and Table 2.

Table 2. Matrix describing FFR$_{myo}$, FFR$_{cor}$, and fractional collateral blood flow before and after PTCA and at balloon occlusion in the patient of Figure 7.

	Before PTCA	At Occlusion	After PTCA
FFR$_{myo}$	0.50	0.18	0.97
FFR$_{cor}$	0.39	0.00	0.96
Q$_c$/Q^N	0.11	0.18	0.01

Q_c/Q^N indicates fractional collateral blood flow. The values in such a matrix are independent of loading conditions.

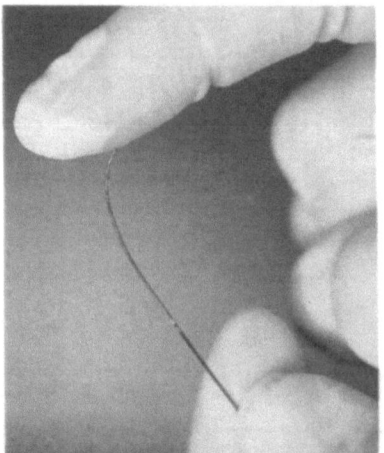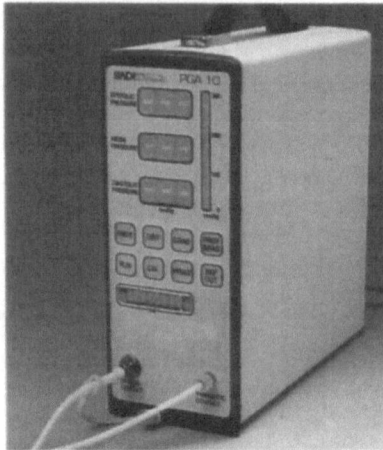

Figure 2. High fidelity 0.014 fiberoptic pressure monitoring guide wire and corresponding interface. The pressure sensor is located at the transition of the 3 cm long radiopaque floppy tip and the radiolucent part of the wire.

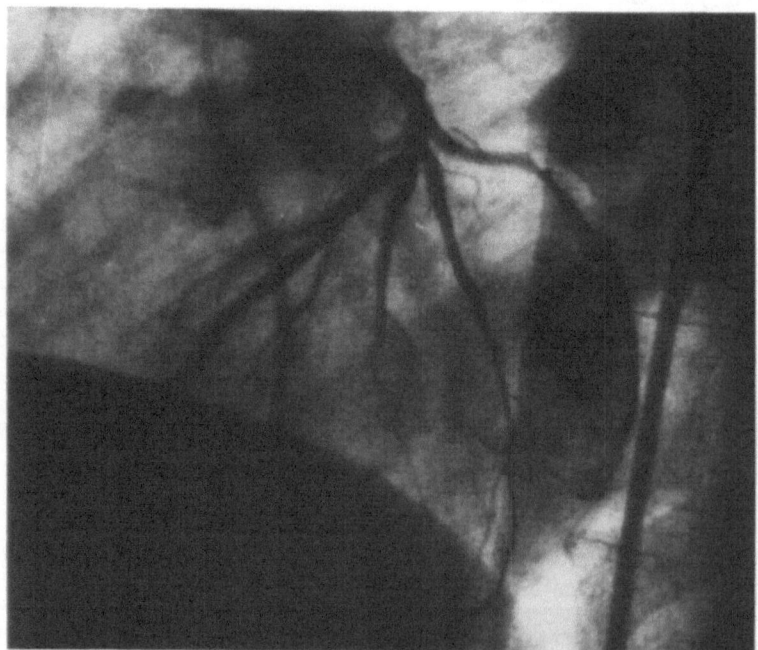

Figure 3. Angiogram of the LCA in a 53 year old male with severe angina pectoris and negative T-waves over the anterior wall. Only in this view some suspicion arises with respect to the trifunction of the LAD and both diagonal branches. From angiography alone, however, it is impossible to distinguish the culprit lesion. The intracoronary pressure recordings are shown in Figure 4.

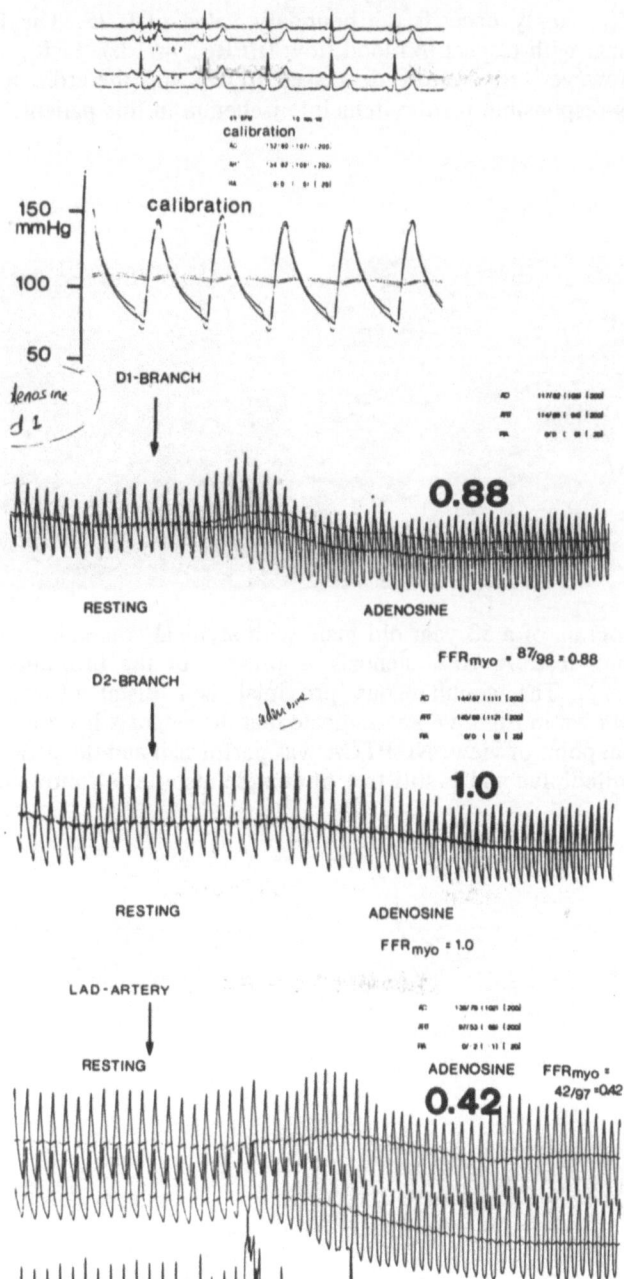

Figure 4. Pressure recordings during i.v. adenosine induced hyperemia in the ascending aorta and the 3 different coronary branches of the patient from Figure 3. As can be easily observed, fractional flow reserve of the myocardium, supplied by the first diagonal branch equals 0.88. Therefore, although some plaque must be present with some influence on maximum achievable blood flow to the myocardium of that branch, this branch cannot be responsible for the inducible ischemia in that

patient as FFR_{myo} amply exceeds the boundary value of 0.75. The D2 branch is completely normal with respect to blood flow ($FFR_{myo} = 1.0$). FFR_{myo} of the LAD-myocardium, however, is severely depressed (0.42) and therefore it is the LAD branch which is responsible for the inducible ischemia in this patient.

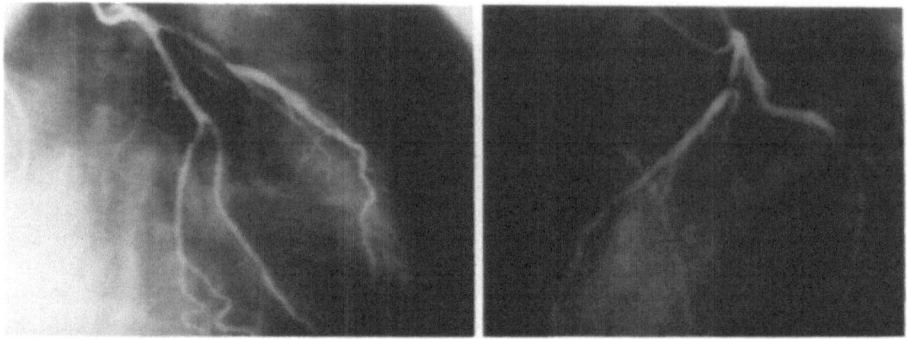

Figure 5. Angiogram of a 53 year old male with atypical complaints and a negative exercise Thallium test. A 70% stenosis is present in the proximal left anterior descending artery. The simultaneous proximal and distal hyperemic pressure recordings are shown in Figure 6 and indicate that the stenosis itself is not significant from a functional point of view. No PTCA was performed and the patient was treated by aspirin and nifedipine and is still free of complaints after a follow-up of almost 3 years.

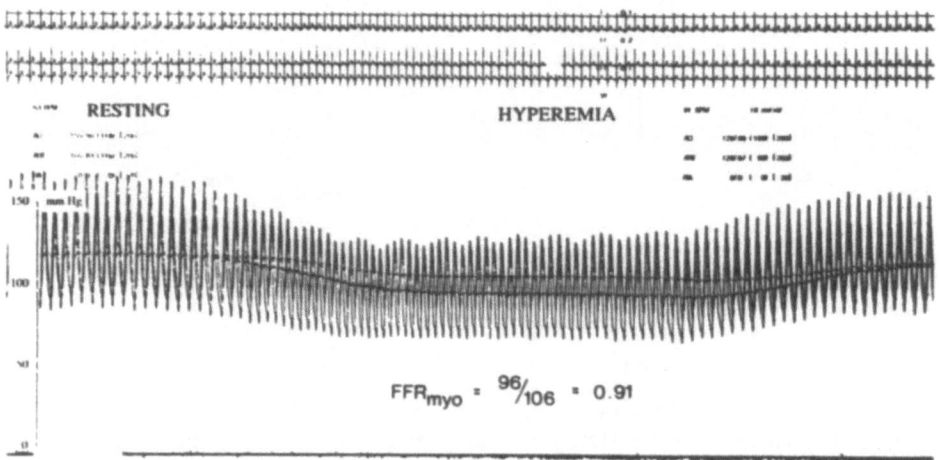

Figure 6. Simultaneous recording of arterial and transstenotic coronary pressure in the patient of Figure 5 at rest and at adenosine induced hyperemia. FFR_{myo} equals 96/106 = 0.91 indicating that the stenosis itself can not be responsible for ischemia.

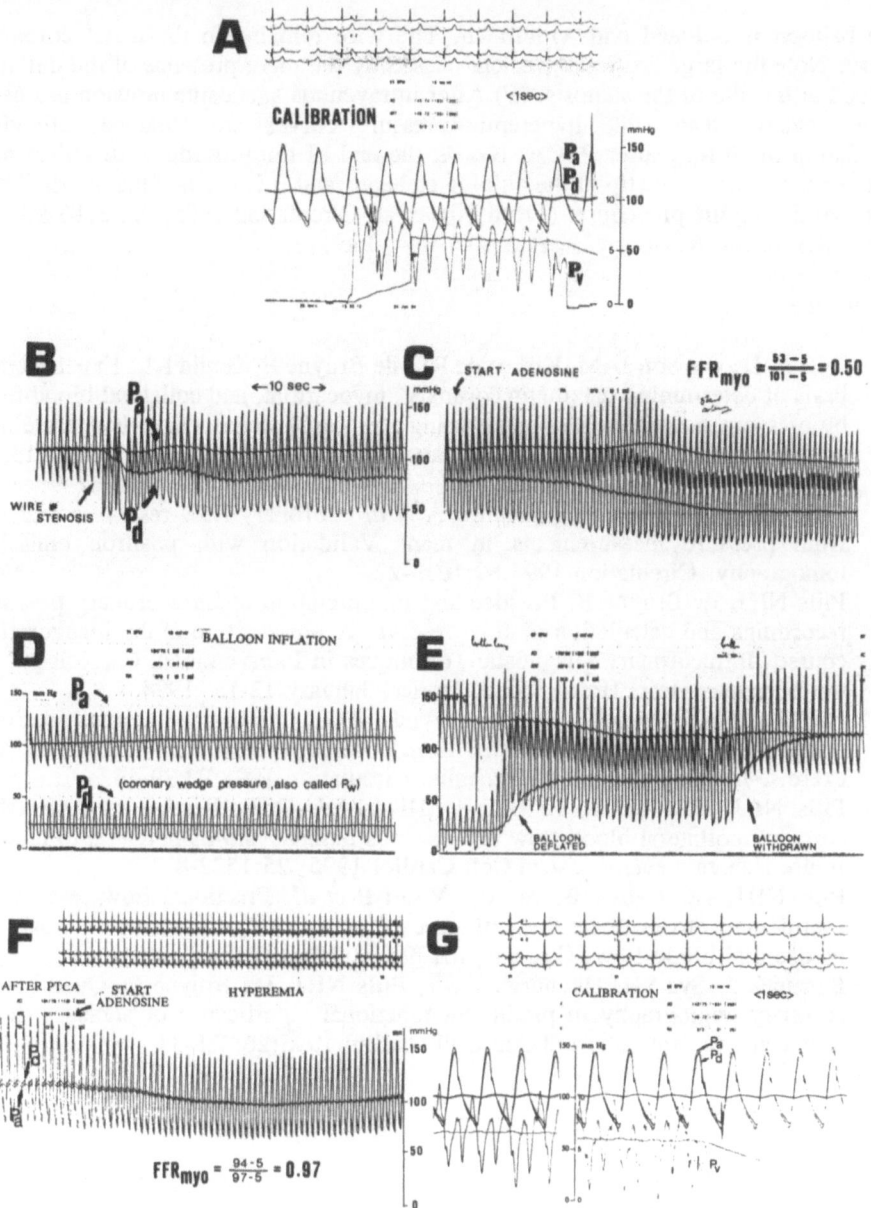

Figure 7. Tracings showing simultaneous phasic and mean recordings of P_a, P_d, and P_v before, during, and after PTCA of a left anterior descending coronary artery stenosis in a 59 year old woman. For clarity, P_v is not displayed in panels B through F. (A) Before the pressure wire is introduced into the coronary artery, the tip of the fiberoptic wire is at a location close to the tip of the guiding catheter, and equality of P_a and P_d at that point is verified. (B) The fiberoptic wire is advanced into the coronary artery and crosses the stenosis (#). (C) After start of intravenous adenosine infusion, steady-state hyperemic pressure curves are obtained, allowing calculation of FFR_{myo} before PTCA. (D) The balloon is advanced into the stenosis and inflated. (E)

The balloon is deflated and withdrawn. The wire remains in the distal coronary artery. Note the large artificial gradient caused by the mere presence of the deflated balloon at the site of the stenosis. (F) After intravenous adenosine infusion has been started again, steady-state hyperemic pressure curves are obtained, allowing calculation of FFR_{myo} after PTCA. (G) At the end of the procedure, the fiberoptic wire is withdrawn to the tip of the guiding catheter, and it is verified that no drift has occurred during the procedure. (From Pijls et al, Circulation 1995; 92: 3183-93, by permission of the American Heart Association, Inc.)

References

1. Pijls NHJ, van Son JAM, Kirkeeide RL, de Bruyne B, Gould KL. Experimental basis of determining maximum coronary, myocardial, and collateral blood flow by pressure measurements for assessing functional stenosis severity before and after percutaneous transluminal coronary angioplasty. Circulation 1993;87:1354-67.

2. De Bruyne B, Baudhuin T, Melin JA *et al*. Coronary flow reserve calculated from pressure measurements in man. Validation with positron emission tomography. Circulation 1994:89:1013-22.

3. Pijls NHJ, de Bruyne B. Practice and interpretation of intracoronary pressure recordings and calculation of flow reserve. A presentation at the inauguration course "Intracoronary Diagnostic Techniques in Interventional Cardiology" of the European Heart House, Nice, France, January 13-15, 1994.

4. De Bruyne B, Bartunek J, Sys SU, Heyndrick GR. Relation between myocardial fractional flow reserve calculated from coronary pressure measurements and exercise-induced myocardial ischemia. Circulation 1995;92:39-46.

5. Pijls NHJ, Bech GJW, El Gamal MIH *et al*. Quantification of recruitable coronary collateral blood flow in conscious humans and its potential to predict future ischemic events. J Am Coll Cardiol 1995; 25:1522-8.

6. Pijls NHJ, van Gelder B, van der Voort P *et al*. Fractional flow reserve. A useful index to evaluate the influence of an epicardial coronary stenosis on myocardial blood flow. Circulation 1995;92:3183-93.

7. Bartunek J, Sys SU, Heyndrickx GR, Pijls NHJ, De Bruyne B. Quantitative coronary angiography in predicting functional significance of stenoses in an unselected patient cohort. J Am Coll Cardiol 1995;26:328-34.

32. Functional assessment of stenosis significance after coronary arteriography; value of myocardial perfusion scintigraphy

ERNST E. VAN DER WALL & ALBERT V.G. BRUSCHKE

Summary

The angiographic severity of a coronary artery stenosis does not necessarily predict an abnormality in myocardial blood flow at rest or during exercise. A poor correlation has been observed between arteriographically defined stenosis and exercise capacity irrespective of whether the severity of the stenosis was assessed by visual or quantitative methods. Furthermore, the relative contribution of each coronary artery to global myocardial perfusion varies widely in any individual patient. The clinical application of coronary flow velocity measurements using the Doppler flow wire during cardiac catheterization represents a valuable means for providing immediate physiologic assessment of coronary artery lesion significance. Recent studies which addressed the correlations between translesional hemodynamics and noninvasive perfusion imaging have confirmed the accuracy and reliability of Doppler translesional flow velocity assessment. In this regard, myocardial perfusion scintigraphy can aid the clinician in interpreting the arteriographic information and in formulating a therapeutic regimen.

Introduction

Since the introduction of coronary arteriography in the 1960's, this invasive technique has become one of the foremost important diagnostic methods in the assessment of patients with coronary artery disease. Despite a relatively high interobserver and intraobserver variability by visual interpretation, coronary arteriography is still considered the gold standard for the assessment of physiological effects of coronary stenosis. In general practice, the assumption exists that there is a close correlation between arteriographic severity of stenosis of the coronary arteries and perfusion of the myocardium. This assumption implies that the decision as to whether to revascularize is predominantly based on the percent diameter stenosis found during coronary arteriography. However, several studies comparing arteriographic findings with postmortem findings have shown that coronary arteriography underestimates the severity of the lesion [1]. Overestimation of diameter stenosis may also occur due to for instance spasm of the coronary artery or insufficient filling with contrast medium.

A major drawback of using morphological changes as shown by coronary arteriography is the poor relation between stenosis severity and the functional significance of a stenosis. Also the length of the stenosis, the absolute cross-sectional luminal area of the segment, collateral circulation, and the presence or

411

J.H.C. Reiber and E.E. van der Wall (eds.), Cardiovascular Imaging, 411-423.
© 1996 *Kluwer Academic Publishers.*

absence of microcirculation are of major importance to the hemodynamic significance of the arterial lesion. Because of the abovementioned issues it seems obvious that assessment of functional significance of a certain coronary stenosis and assessment of myocardial perfusion should play an important role in the management of coronary artery disease. At present several methods are available for the functional assessment of lesion severity, in particular single-photon emission computed tomography (SPECT) using thallium-201 or technetium-99 labeled isonitriles, and positron emission tomography (PET) using oxygen-15 labeled water or nitrogen-13 ammonia.

In addition to the usefulness of myocardial perfusion scintigraphy in diagnosing and managing patients suspected for coronary artery disease, perfusion scintigraphy may also be useful in selecting patients for coronary angioplasty and in the management of patients who already underwent coronary revascularization. Several studies have revealed that perfusion scintigraphy may predict graft closure accurately following coronary artery bypass grafting. Therefore, myocardial perfusion scintigraphy may also be useful following coronary revascularization in identifying patients at high risk for graft occlusion.

In this chapter we will discuss the importance of assessment of myocardial perfusion by means of SPECT or PET imaging related to findings observed at coronary arteriography.

Myocardial perfusion

In normal coronary arteries myocardial blood flow is primarily regulated by the resistance of the arteriolar vessels. Epicardial arteries provide little resistance under physiological circumstances. However, in case of vessel stenosis a transstenotic pressure gradient develops which leads to arteriolar vasodilatation and subsequently results in normal flow to the myocardium distal from the stenosis. In animals, it has been reported that resting coronary blood flow can be maintained at normal levels if less than 90% of the cross-sectional area is obstructed. In case of increasing myocardial oxygen demand the distal arteriolar bed is unable to dilate further if there is an arterial cross-sectional obstructed area of more than 90% [2]. Coronary stenoses that are not able to maintain myocardial blood by arteriolar vasodilatation are considered to be physiologically significant. Under conditions of increased workload, vessel stenosis over 65% of the luminal cross-sectional area have shown to be of physiological significance.

Although other factors than cross-sectional diameter of the stenosis (e.g. length, exit and entrance angles, eccentricity) also have influence on coronary flow reserve, the capacity of normal animal vessels can accurately be predicted. Studies in humans have suggested that the relation between coronary stenosis and coronary flow reserve might be different due to the atherosclerotic nature of the obstruction instead of experimental constriction of a normal vessel. As myocardial blood flow is normal despite coronary stenoses, patients with stable coronary artery disease are frequently asymptomatic at rest. However, the insufficient coronary flow reserve may result in myocardial ischemia during periods of increased myocardial oxygen demand e.g. during exercise or during positive inotropic stimulation. Assessment of perfusion abnormalities by means of myocardial perfusion scintigraphy is based on this principle of transient flow inhomogeneity caused by increased workload.

Assessment of myocardial perfusion by radionuclide imaging

Various radionuclide tracers, imaging modalities, and protocols have been evaluated in order to achieve the best suitable protocol for the assessment of myocardial perfusion. At present the most widely used tracers for establishing myocardial perfusion are thallium-201 and technetium-99m labeled agents (sestamibi, tetrofosmin), and the currently accepted state-of-the-art imaging modality to assess myocardial perfusion is SPECT. A more sophisticated but less widely available imaging modality is PET, using oxygen-15 labeled water and nitrogen-13 ammonia as perfusion tracers. The characteristics of the perfusion tracers and the imaging modalities together with the appropriate imaging protocols are described in other chapters of this book and these aspects will therefore not be further discussed in this chapter.

Correlation of coronary arteriographic findings with functional measurements: initial findings

Coronary arteriography is still considered the gold standard for the diagnosis of coronary artery disease. However, the percent diameter of a stenosis is just one of the factors which determine whether a particular lesion will cause ischemia. Other important factors are the length of the lesion, the geometry, the minimum diameter of the lumen, the cross-sectional area of the lesion, the size of the vessel proximal and distal of the stenosis, vasoactivity of the lesion, the extent of the myocardium supplied by the particular artery, the degree of post-stenotic collateral support and myocardial oxygen demand.

Folland et al. [3] observed in 227 patients with >70% diameter stenosis in a single vessel by visual estimation a poor correlation between diameter stenosis and the functional significance of the stenosis. There was no consistent relationship between the arteriographically defined severity of the stenosis and the exercise capacity of the patient. Also, recently the importance of the coronary microcirculation has been demonstrated [4,5]. The arteries of the microcirculation can not be visualized by coronary arteriography whereas with perfusion imaging an indication for their functional status can be given. Since coronary arteriography only determines anatomical measures of a stenosis (for instance, minimal obstructive diameter, mean segmental diameter), these measures may not correlate well with the functional significance of a stenosis and myocardial perfusion scintigraphy will therefore be of additional value. This holds both for patients in the high risk groups in whom a careful risk-benefit analysis should be made and in patients with normal arteriograms and signs of ischemia on their exercise stress test. Gibson et al. [6] demonstrated in a prospective study comparing thallium scintigraphy to coronary arteriography and to submaximal exercise testing that thallium scintigraphy identified best the patients with a previous myocardial infarction who will subsequently have cardiac events.

Doppler flow measurements for assessment of coronary flow reserve

The assessment of coronary flow reserve (ratio of maximal hyperemic flow to resting or autoregulated flow) has been introduced as a reliable measure to determine the functional status of a coronary artery stenosis. White et al. [7] studied 39 patients with isolated, discrete coronary lesions in whom the reactive hyperemic responses were measured using a Doppler technique and who were subsequently compared to the cineangiogram. In these patients with lesions varying in severity from 10-95% stenosis, the percentage stenosis observed on the arteriogram did not significantly correlate with the reactive hyperemic response (Figure 1). Underestimation of the severity of the lesion occurred in 95% of the vessels with >60% diameter stenosis on coronary arteriography. Both overestimation and underestimation occurred in lesions with less than 60% stenosis. They concluded that the physiological effects of the majority of coronary stenoses cannot accurately be determined by means of coronary arteriography, indicating the need for better analytical methods to assess coronary stenosis such as coronary videodensitometry and improved radionuclide perfusion techniques.

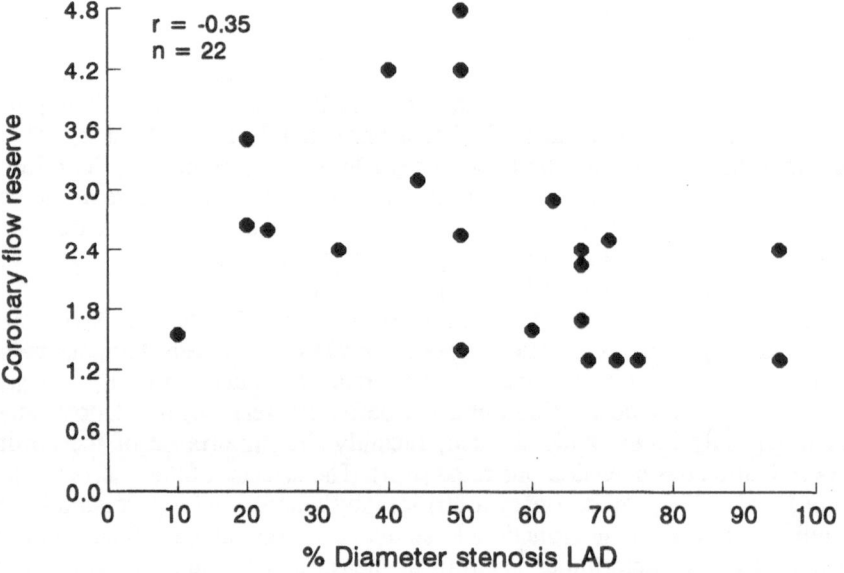

Figure 1. Relation between the coronary artery diameter stenosis and the coronary flow reserve in 22 patients with one discrete lesion in the left anterior descending coronary artery (LAD). (Modified from White et al., N Engl J Med 1984;310:819-24 [7])

Wilson et al. [8] performed a study on the prediction of the physiologic significance of coronary arterial lesions by quantitative lesion geometry in patients with limited coronary artery disease. They studied 50 patients with a single discrete coronary artery stenosis in only one (84%) or two vessels (16%)

and determined coronary flow reserve by the Doppler technique using papaverine as the vasodilating substance. In contrast to previous studies from their institution demonstrating a poor relationship between quantitative estimates of coronary luminal stenosis and intra-operative measurements of coronary flow reserve obtained in patients with multi-vessel coronary artery disease, the coronary flow reserve measured in patients with discrete limited coronary artery disease correlated closely with luminal stenosis determined precisely with quantitative coronary arteriography. Coronaries arteries with <70% area stenosis uniformly had normal coronary flow reserve (lower limit of normal 3.5) (Figure 2). Coronary arteries with >90% area stenosis were associated with a wide range of coronary flow reserves (1.0 to 2.8). They concluded that the evaluation of coronary flow reserve should facilitate the assessment of the physiological significance of coronary arterial lesions in the catheterization laboratory. It should, however be realized that in these studies [7,8] the Doppler probes were placed proximally to the coronary artery stenoses which may explain the relatively poor relation between stenosis severity and coronary flow reserve. In addition, the disappointing results may have been the result of the contaminating influence of hyperemic flow to summed proximal branch territories on the vasodilator reserve.

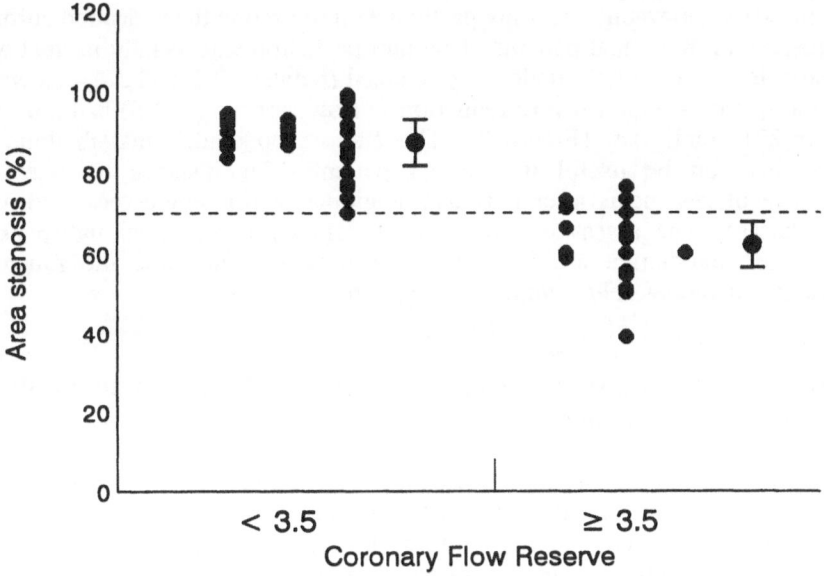

Figure 2. The percent area stenosis of lesions associated with normal (>3.5) and abnormal (≤3.5) coronary flow reserve. Coronaries arteries with <70% area stenosis uniformly had normal coronary flow reserve. (Modified from Wilson et al., Circulation 1987;75:723-32 [8])

Correlation between coronary flow reserve and myocardial perfusion imaging using videodensitometry

Zijlstra et al. [9] compared quantitative arteriographic analysis with measured coronary flow reserve and thallium-201 exercise perfusion scintigraphy using videodensitometric analysis. They studied 38 patients with single-vessel disease and the myocardial perfusion defects on thallium-201 scintigraphy were analyzed quantitatively and by visual interpretation. It was shown that both percent diameter stenosis and obstruction area generally correlated well with functional measurements of stenoses severity such as radiographically measured coronary flow reserve and thallium-201 scintigraphy. However, for individual patients the relation between pressure drop and coronary flow reserve was better than between obstruction area or percent diameter stenoses and coronary flow reserve. The hyperemic transstenotic pressure gradient was highly predictive ($>90\%$) of exercise thallium-201 results in patients with quantitative diameter stenoses of 6% to 75%, corresponding to arteriographic coronary flow reserve values of 5.5 to 0.4. This indicated that the calculated pressure drop over the stenosis was a more accurate anatomic description of the functional consequences of a coronary artery lesion. The pressure drop also served as a better variable to distinguish patients with normal and abnormally coronary flow reserve and predicted the results of thallium-201 scintigraphy more accurately. The authors further showed that thallium-201 scintigraphy was only partly useful to predict the measured coronary flow reserve in individual patients. Thallium perfusion was usually normal when coronary flow reserve was moderately reduced (between 2.5 and 3.4). However, almost all patients with a severe reduction in flow reserve (<2.5) had a positive thallium-201 scintigram (Figure 3). The authors concluded that thallium-201 scintigraphy can be useful in selected patients, for instance to assess the occurrence of restenosis after coronary angioplasty for single-vessel coronary artery disease. The assessment of coronary flow reserve is an indispensable addition to quantitative arteriography especially to determine the functional importance of moderately severe coronary artery lesions.

Correlation between intracoronary Doppler flow velocity measurements and myocardial perfusion imaging

Initial application of the Doppler technique required relatively large catheters that only provided access to the proximal coronary vasculature precluding the assessment of reliable correlations between stenosis morphology and function. To overcome this limitation, intracoronary angioplasty guide wires have been developed with a forward-directed Doppler crystal incorporated into the tip. Recent studies using intracoronary Doppler guide wire measurements showed a high concordance between stress SPECT perfusion data and the Doppler measurements of coronary flow reserve [10-12]. Joye et al. [10] showed a 84% concordance between stress thallium-201 findings and Doppler guide wire determination (using adenosine for inducing the hyperemic stimulus) in 30 patients with intermediate-severity stenoses. The sensitivity, specificity, and overall predictive accuracy of poststenotic coronary flow reserve were 94%,

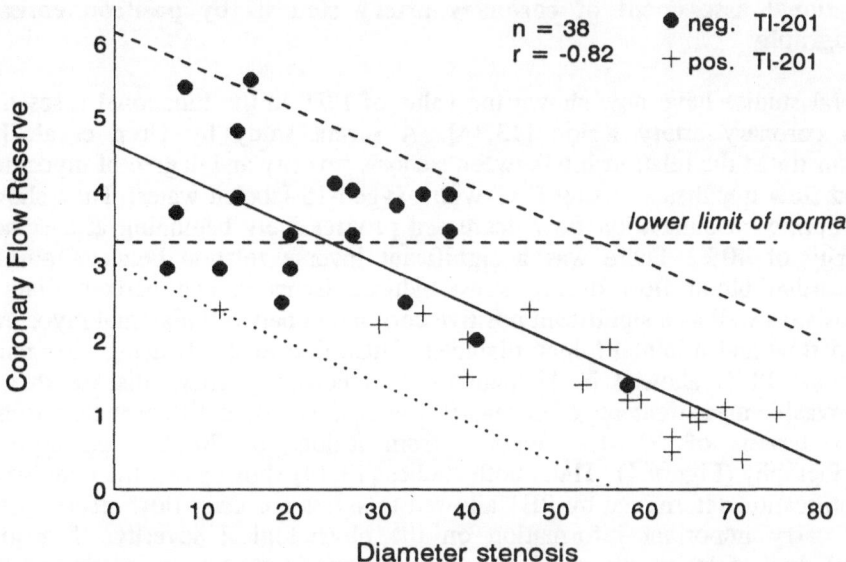

Figure 3. Relation between coronary flow reserve (CFR), thallium-201 scintigraphy and percent diameter stenosis (DS) in 38 patients. The dashed horizontal line is the lower limit of normal coronary flow reserve. The plusses represent 18 patients with a positive thallium scintigram. The closed circles represent 20 patients with a negative thallium scintigram. (Modified from Zijlstra et al., J Am Coll Cardiol 1988;12:686-91 [9])

95%, and 94%, respectively. They concluded that the Doppler procedure could be rapidly and safely performed during elective cardiac catheterization and may represent an alternative to ischemic stress testing. Deychak et al. [11], using Doppler guide wire measurements in 17 symptomatic patients with a positive stress thallium-201 SPECT scintigram, showed an excellent concordance between distal coronary flow reserve and diastolic/systolic flow-velocity ratio to thallium-201 scintigraphy. A coronary flow reserve of < 1.8 and a diastolic/systolic flow-velocity ratio of < 1.7 predicted reversible myocardial ischemia (concordance 96% and 88%, respectively). Similar findings have been observed with technetium-99m sestamibi SPECT imaging [12]. Miller et al. [12] showed a high correlation (89%) between an abnormal Doppler-derived poststenotic intracoronary flow reserve (≤2.0) and the presence of reversible defects at dipyridamole sestamibi perfusion imaging in 33 patients with intermediate-severity coronary artery disease. To summarize, the aforementioned studies [10-12] indicate that the evaluation of distal coronary flow indexes by intracoronary Doppler wire assessment may provide an alternative means of physiologic assessment of lesion severity during coronary arteriography.

Functional assessment of coronary artery stenosis by positron emission tomography

Several studies have now shown the value of PET in the functional assessment of a coronary artery lesion [13,14]. A recent study by Uren et al. [13] demonstrated the relationship between stenosis severity and degree of myocardial blood flow impairment using PET with oxygen-15 labeled water. They showed that during vasodilatation flow decreased progressively beginning at a stenosis severity of 40%. There was a significant inverse relation between absolute myocardial blood flow during stress-induced ischemia and percent diameter stenosis, as well as a significant positive correlation between maximal myocardial blood flow and minimal lumen diameter. DiCarli et al. [14], using nitrogen-13 ammonia PET, showed in 18 patients with coronary artery disease that the noninvasive measurements of coronary flow reserve could differentiate coronary artery lesions of 50-70% stenoses from lesions of 70-90% on coronary arteriography (Figure 4). Thus, both studies [13,14] showed that the noninvasive quantification determined by PET allowed to assess coronary flow reserve which may carry important information on the physiological severity of a given morphological lesion observed on coronary arteriography. Interestingly, both studies also showed that *resting* myocardial blood flow remained unchanged regardless of the severity of the stenosis.

Perfusion imaging in selecting patients for coronary angioplasty

The small risk to the patient and the substantial cost of cardiac catheterization make it desirable to restrict this examination to patients in whom the procedure is most likely to have therapeutic consequences. The selection of these high risk patients who need catheter intervention or bypass surgery is an important strength of perfusion imaging techniques. Numerous studies could demonstrate that perfusion imaging and coronary arteriography yield similar prognostic power in mildly symptomatic patients with coronary artery disease. However, the issue has not yet been settled whether coronary arteriography should not be performed and coronary angioplasty in patients with symptoms suggestive of coronary artery disease but a perfectly normal perfusion scintigram.

The evaluation of patients with multivessel disease for percutaneous transluminal coronary angioplasty raises the question: is incomplete revascularization an acceptable procedure in these patient, or does complete revascularization need to be performed, as in coronary artery bypass grafting? To provide an answer Breisblatt et al. [15] utilizes exercise thallium imaging as a guide to the performance of angioplasty in 85 patients with multivessel coronary disease. Pre-angioplasty exercise thallium-201 imaging helped to identify the primary stenosis ("culprit lesion") in 93% of patients.

Two weeks to one month after dilation of this lesion, repeated thallium-201 imaging identified two patients groups: Group 1, 47 patients with no evidence of ischemia in a second vascular distribution (no remote ischemia), and Group 2, 38 patients who needed further coronary angioplasty because of ischemia in another vascular territory (remote ischemia). In Group 2, 47% of patients had angioplasty

Myocardial blood flow (ml/min/g)

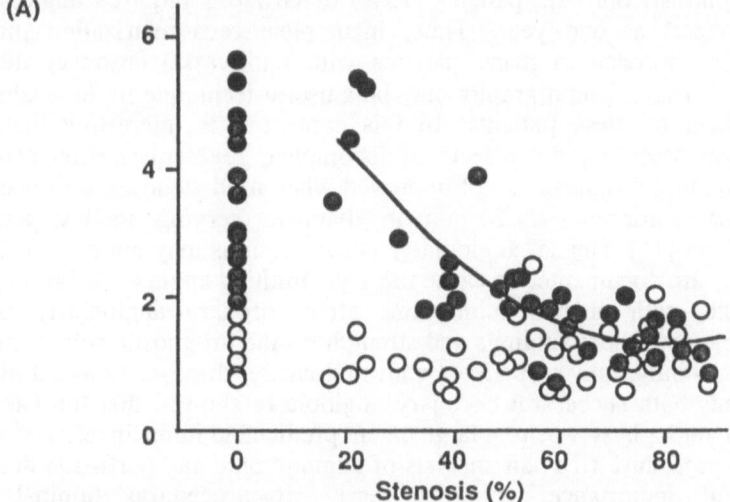

Myocardial blood flow (ml/min/g)

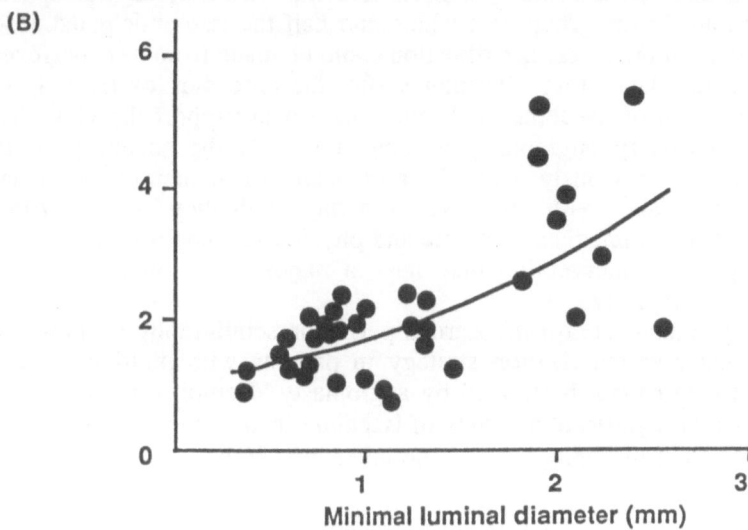

Figure 4. Myocardial blood flow versus severity as percent diameter stenosis (A) and as minimal lumen diameter (B). There was no significant correlation between blood flow in the 35 patients at base line (open circles) and the degree of their stenosis; flow during hyperemia (solid circles) however, was significantly impaired as stenosis severity increases. The values in the 21 controls are shown at 0% stenosis; some circles represent more than one control (A). There was a significant correlation between blood flow during hyperemia and the stenosis severity (B). (From Uren NG, et al., N Engl J Med 1994;330:1782-8 [13])

of a second vessel and 79% required multivessel angioplasty at one year follow-up. In contrast, only six patients (13%) of Group 1 required angioplasty of a second vessel at one year. Thus, incomplete revascularization may be an acceptable approach in many patients with multivessel coronary disease and thallium-201 stress scintigraphy may be a useful technique in the evaluation and management of these patients. In this context it is interesting that a recent publication assessing the effects of incomplete revascularization came to the conclusion that prognosis is not improved when mild stenoses are revascularized in coronary arteries ≥ 1.5 mm in diameter serving modest amounts of myocardium [16]. Hence, angioplasty in such lesions may not be justified except when they are documented to cause life-style limiting angina. The good prognosis in patients with normal scintigrams after coronary angioplasty is entirely compatible with these findings and strengthens the prognostic role of myocardial perfusion scintigraphy in patients with multivessel disease. Lewis et al. [17], in 59 patients with successful coronary angioplasty showed that the late result of coronary angioplasty was to a large extent predictable immediately and very early after the procedure from an analysis of angiographic and perfusion data at those times. Of importance, a larger early postprocedural luminal diameter accompanied by normal perfusion was associated with a significantly better late arteriographic result than was a better arteriographic (or normal perfusion) result alone. In these patients the restenosis rate was 20%, which was approximately half the rate for the group as a whole and half the rate anticipated according to current clinical practices. Stratification could be made from tests performed in the catheterization laboratory 30 minutes after the procedure or from data obtained before removal of the femoral sheath. These data support the view that the late result of coronary angioplasty depends more on the adequacy of the initial dilatation than previously realized, and that the assessment of the dilatation may not be complete with an arteriographic evaluation alone. Attention to comprehensive immediate anatomic and physiologic measurements regarding the adequacy of an intervention may have a major effect on the late result after coronary angioplasty.

Another potential role for myocardial perfusion scintigraphy is in the selection of the optimal revascularization strategy in patients with multivessel disease and vessels which cannot be treated by angioplasty. Demonstration of the presence or absence of significant amounts of ischemia in such vessels would either favor bypass grafting or angioplasty of the other vessel(s).

Assessment of coronary artery bypass graft patency

The assessment of patients following coronary artery bypass surgery differs significantly from that prior to revascularization. The diagnosis of coronary artery disease is no longer in question and the treatment options will not always be the same as in the initial assessment. Bypass surgery relieves angina in 60-90% of the patients with severe coronary artery disease. Symptomatic improvement after surgery is not only attributed to improvement of regional perfusion but also to perioperative infarction or a placebo effect. However, many patients have chest pain in the week following surgery despite a patent bypass. Since relief of symptoms is not a reliable indicator of graft patency and abolition of ischemic attacks, the evaluation of bypass patency by noninvasive methods may be important. Recurrence of ischemia after revascularization may be the result from incomplete revascularization, graft occlusion or disease, restenosis at the site of angioplasty, progression of coronary artery disease, perioperative myocardial infarction, or a combination of the aforementioned factors. Scintigraphic evaluation following revascularization may be useful in differentiating these conditions in a noninvasive manner.

Pfisterer et al. [18] performed a prospective study in 55 consecutive patients with a total of 154 grafts. At two weeks and one year after bypass surgery, thallium-201 rest and exercise scintigraphy and coronary angiography was performed for the evaluation of coronary bypass surgery. They found that the accuracy of noninvasive thallium scintigraphy to detect or exclude patients with bypass graft occlusion was 86%. They also found that thallium-201 imaging may be useful particularly in patients with asymptomatic chest pain following operation, and they concluded that thallium scintigraphy should be performed routinely in these patients after bypass surgery. Huikuri et al. [19] studied 60 consecutive patients following coronary artery bypass surgery and they concluded that abnormal myocardial perfusion due to stenosis or occlusion of bypass grafts was common in both symptomatic and asymptomatic patients. However, graft patency was significantly lower in asymptomatic patients with abnormal thallium perfusion compared to those with normal perfusion after bypass surgery. Overall accuracy for detecting one or more stenosed or occluded grafts was 77% in their study. In a recent study entitled CABADAS (Prevention of coronary artery bypass graft occlusion by aspirin, dipyridamole, and acenocoumarol/phenprocoumon study), Mulder et al. [20] showed that thallium-201 scintigraphy confirmed functionally the effects of medication on graft patency. Several other studies have shown similar accuracy of the predictive value of thallium scintigraphy in predicting graft patency following coronary artery bypass surgery.

Conclusions

The angiographic severity of a coronary artery stenosis does not necessarily predict an abnormality in myocardial blood flow at rest or during exercise. Although the vascular bed of the left anterior descending coronary artery is approximately twice that of the right or circumflex coronary arteries, the relative contribution of each coronary artery to global myocardial perfusion varies widely in any individual patient. Therefore, it is not surprising that a patient with triple vessel disease may do exceedingly well if there is no abnormality in myocardial perfusion during exercise or pharmacologic stress, whereas another patient with only single-vessel disease but a large ischemic perfusion defect may be at high risk for death or nonfatal infarction [21]. Excellent correlations have recently been observed between intracoronary Doppler flow measurements and myocardial perfusion scintigraphy. In this regard, perfusion scintigraphy can aid the clinician in interpreting the arteriographic information, in selecting patients for coronary angioplasty, and in assessing the results of coronary artery bypass graft surgery.

References

1. Arnett EN, Isner JM, Redwood DR *et al.* Coronary artery narrowing in coronary heart disease: comparison of cineangiographic and necropsy findings. Ann Intern Med 1979;91:350-6.
2. Gould KL. Noninvasive assessment of coronary stenoses by myocardial perfusion imaging during pharmacologic coronary vasodilation. I. Physiologic basis and experimental validation. Am J Cardiol 1978;41:267-78.
3. Folland ED, Vogel RA, Hartigan P *et al.* Relation between coronary artery stenosis assessed by visual, caliper and computer methods and exercise capacity in patients with single-vessel coronary artery disease. The Veterans Affairs ACME Investigators. Circulation 1994;89:2005-14.
4. James TN. The spectrum of diseases of small coronary arteries and their physiologic consequences. J Am Coll Cardiol 1990;15:763-74.
5. James TN, Bruschke AVG. Seminar on small coronary artery disease. Structure and function of small coronary arteries in health and disease. Introduction. J Am Coll Cardiol 1990;15:511-2.
6. Gibson RS, Watson DD, Craddock GB *et al.* Prediction of cardiac events after uncomplicated myocardial infarction: a prospective study comparing predischarge exercise thallium-201 scintigraphy and coronary angiography. Circulation 1983;68:321-36.
7. White CW, Wright CB, Doty DB *et al.* Does visual interpretation of the coronary arteriogram predict the physiologic importance of a coronary stenosis? N Engl J Med 1984;310:819-24.
8. Wilson RF, Marcus ML, White CW. Prediction of the physiologic significance of coronary arterial lesions by quantitative lesion geometry in patients with limited coronary artery disease. Circulation 1987;75:723-32.
9. Zijlstra F, Fioretti P, Reiber JHC, Serruys PW. Which cineangiographically assessed anatomic variable correlates best with functional measurements of stenosis severity? A comparison of quantitative analysis of the coronary cineangiogram with measured coronary flow reserve and exercise/redistribution thallium-201 scintigraphy. J Am Coll Cardiol 1988;12:686-96.
10. Joye JD, Schulman DS, Lasorda D, Farah T, Donohue BC, Reichek N. Intracoronary Doppler guide wire versus stress single-photon emission computed tomographic thallium-201 imaging in assessment of intermediate coronary stenoses. J Am Coll Cardiol 1994;24:940-7.
11. Deychak YA, Segal J, Reiner JS *et al.* Doppler guide wire flow velocity indexes measured distal to coronary stenoses associated with reversible thallium perfusion defects. Am Heart J 1995;129:219-27.
12. Miller DD, Donohue TJ, Younis LT *et al.* Correlation of pharmacological ^{99m}Tc-sestamibi myocardial perfusion imaging with poststenotic coronary flow reserve in patients with angiographically intermediate coronary artery stenoses. Circulation 1994;89:2150-60.
13. Uren NG, Melin JA, de Bruyne B, Wijns W, Baudhuin T, Camici PG. Relation between myocardial blood flow and the severity of coronary-artery stenosis. N Engl J Med 1994;330:1782-8.
14. DiCarli M, Czernin J, Hoh CK *et al.* Relation among stenosis severity, myocardial blood flow, and flow reserve in patients with coronary artery disease. Circulation 1995;91:1944-51.
15. Breisblatt WM, Barnes JV, Weiland F, Spaccavento LJ. Incomplete

revascularization in multivessel percutaneous transluminal coronary angioplasty: the role for stress thallium-201 imaging. J Am Coll Cardiol 1988;11:1183-90.

16. Cowley MJ, Vandermael M, Topol EJ *et al.* Is traditionally defined complete revascularization needed for patients with multivessel disease treated by elective coronary angioplasty? Multivessel Angioplasty Prognosis Study (MAPS) Group. J Am Coll Cardiol 1993;22:1289-97.

17. Lewis BS, Hardoff R, Merdler A *et al.* Importance of immediate and very early postprocedural angiographic and thallium-201 single photon emission computed tomographic perfusion measurements in predicting late results after coronary intervention. Am Heart J 1995;130:425-32.

18. Pfisterer M, Emmenegger H, Schmitt HE *et al.* Accuracy of serial myocardial perfusion scintigraphy with thallium-201 for prediction of graft patency early and late after coronary artery bypass surgery. A controlled prospective study. Circulation 1982;66:1017-24.

19. Huikuri HV, Ikäheimo MJ, Korhonen UR, Heikkilä J, Takkunen JT. Thallium scintigraphy in prediction of occlusion of bypass grafts in asymptomatic and symptomatic patients. Acta Med Scand 1987;222:311-8.

20. Mulder BJM, van der Doef RM, van der Wall EE *et al.* Effect of various antithrombotic regimens (aspirin, aspirin plus dipyridamole, anticoagulants) on the functional status of patients and grafts one year after coronary artery bypass grafting. Eur Heart J 1994;15:1129-34.

21. Mahmarian JJ, Pratt CM, Boyce TM, Verani MS. The variable extent of jeopardized myocardium in patients with single vessel coronary artery disease: quantification by thallium-201 single photon emission computed tomography. J Am Coll Cardiol 1991;17:355-62.

33. Blood flow measurements using 3D distance-concentration functions derived from digital x-ray angiograms

ALEXANDER M. SEIFALIAN, DAVID J. HAWKES, CHRISTOPHER
BLADIN, ALAN C. COLCHESTER & KENNETH E. HOBBS

Summary

We describe a method for measurement of velocity flow, absolute cross-sectional area and path length of identified arteries for high frame rate biplane x-ray angiograms. The system has been extensively validated with phantoms for vessel calibres from 3 to 6 mm and flow rates encompassing those expected "in-vivo". Mean volume flow agreed with electromagnetic flow meter readings to within 9% and peak flow agreed to within 10% for velocity flow below 1 m/sec when measuring a 150 mm length of artery at a framing rate of 25 frames per sec. Path lengths of bent wire were measured with an error of less than 2%. We present initial results using these measures to study the haemodynamics of the circulation from the arch of the aorta to the circle of Willis.

Introduction

The measurement of blood flow is important in understanding both normal physiology and disease processes as well as assessing the effects of therapeutic procedures such as angioplasty, shunting, bypass and transplantation. Currently no ideal method for measuring blood flow in humans is available [1,2]. Such a technique needs to be noninvasive, instantaneous, and repeatable [1,3]. Apart from the usefulness of such a technique as a basic physiologic and pathophysiologic tool, it will have great clinical importance. Such a technique will be useful before carotid endarterectomy, in the diagnosis of cerebral ischemia, in determining the prognosis in a comatose patient, and in treatment of stroke and brain injury [4,5].

Digital subtraction angiography (DSA) is a digital x-ray imaging technique used for the detection and assessment of vascular diseases [6,7]. By displaying the blood vessel image without background interference, DSA can provide an improved blood vessel image with a reduced amount of contrast injection in arterial angiography. The DSA routinely used is a safe, semi-invasive, inexpensive, outpatient graphic screening procedure of the entire vascular circulation [8-10]. DSA is routinely used as part of an interventional procedure such as angioplasty and stenting.

The new techniques described here require minimal change to existing acquisition protocols and therefore could be used without significant increase in radiation dose, volume of contrast material or time of procedures.

We have described a new digital x-ray angiographic method for determining

J.H.C. Reiber and E.E. van der Wall (eds.), Cardiovascular Imaging, 425-442.
© 1996 *Kluwer Academic Publishers.*

pulsatile flow waveform patterns from computer simulated dynamic x-ray angiographic data [11]. This method was validated further using the physical phantom and its clinical capability was demonstrated using the pre- and post-femoral artery percutaneous transluminal angioplasty [12]. When used to measure the blood flow waveform in the physical model, there was a close agreement between the flow waveforms measured by the electromagnetic and radiographic techniques. Thus, we were very interested in determining if we could extend this technique for use in measuring the absolute blood flow waveform in head and neck. Because the blood vessels in head and neck are tortuous and not parallel to the imaging plane, in addition we used a 3-dimensional (3D) reconstruction of a blood vessel centreline from biplane 2-dimensional (2D) angiograms [13-16], to determine the actual length and the vessel diameter of the blood vessel segment in the body. This requires accurate information concerning the x-ray magnification factor, as well as the orientation of the vessel segment relative to the image plane.

We describe here the experimental validation of the method and initial results of the clinical application of the technique in 3D. Phantom studies were used to compare simultaneous measurements of blood flow using x-ray angiographic data with measurements using an electromagnetic flowmeter (EMF).

Clinically the technique has been used to measure the cerebral blood flow in conjunction with routine cerebral angiography. Four patients with cerebrovascular disease have been studied and the blood flow waveforms of the internal carotid and vertebral arteries have been computed.

3D reconstruction of the vascular network

Theory

The relative position of a point in space can be computed if two x-ray images of the point are taken from different views. The principal behind this is that the x-ray imaging can be thought of as a perspective projection and by use of knowledge of the x-ray imaging geometry and the mathematics of projective transformations, the 3D coordinates of points in space can be obtained.

The transformation matrix

The geometric mathematics for reconstructing the centreline of vessels from biplanar x-ray angiograms using a cube with steel markers has been described [17]. This includes mathematical transformation from the object's coordination system to the two projected planes, as well as the principles of matching points in the two views. In general, perspective projection of a 3D object can be fully described in homogeneous coordinates by a 4*3 transformation matrix [13,15,18]:

$$(x, y, z, 1) * \mathbf{T} = S(u, v, 1) \tag{1}$$

where as x, y, z are the cartesian coordinates of a point in the object space, u, v are the image coordinates on the projected digital image of the above point, $\mathbf{T}$ is the

(4*3) matrix describing the transformation from 3D space to 2D projections and S is a scale factor depending on (x, y, z) and T.

Determination of the transformation matrix

By eliminating S in matrix equation (1), we obtain the following two equations:

$$x(t_{11}-t_{13}u) + y(t_{21}-t_{23}u) + z(t_{31}-t_{33}u) + t_{41}-t_{43}u = 0 \qquad (2)$$

$$x(t_{12}-t_{13}v) + y(t_{22}-t_{23}v) + z(t_{32}-t_{33}v) + t_{42}-t_{43}v = 0 \qquad (3)$$

If the 3D coordinates of points and their corresponding 2D coordinates on the two different projection planes are known, the elements $t(i,j)$ of the transformation matrix can be obtained from equations (2) and (3). Since the transformation matrix contains 11 elements, six control points of known coordinates (x_i, y_i, z_i) $(i=1, 2, 3, 4, 5, 6)$, and the 2D coordinates (u, v) of their projected points in two images are sufficient to establish the 12 simultaneous equations from (2) and (3), which are solved to obtain the transformation matrix. The obtained solutions, $t(i,j)$ values, are the characteristic parameters describing the projection of arbitrary points in 2D plane to the 3D space. Since, in practice, the available coordinates are never exact, the system of 12 equations may be solved by an approximation technique (such as least squares).

Reconstruction of 3D skeleton

The relationship between a 3D point of interest and its projected 2D points in two views, (u_1, v_1) and (u_2, v_2) is given by the following equations [from equations (2) and (3)]:

$$\begin{pmatrix} t_{11} & - & t_{13}u_1 \\ t_{12} & - & t_{13}v_1 \\ s_{11} & - & s_{13}u_2 \\ s_{12} & - & s_{13}v_2 \end{pmatrix} \begin{pmatrix} t_{21} & - & t_{23}u_1 \\ t_{22} & - & t_{23}v_1 \\ s_{21} & - & s_{23}u_2 \\ s_{22} & - & s_{23}v_2 \end{pmatrix} \begin{pmatrix} t_{31} & - & t_{33}u_1 \\ t_{32} & - & t_{33}v_1 \\ s_{31} & - & s_{33}u_2 \\ s_{32} & - & s_{33}v_2 \end{pmatrix} * \begin{pmatrix} x \\ y \\ z \end{pmatrix} = \begin{pmatrix} t_{43}u_1 & - & t_{41} \\ t_{43}v_1 & - & t_{42} \\ s_{43}u_2 & - & s_{41} \\ s_{43}v_2 & - & s_{42} \end{pmatrix} \qquad (4)$$

This matrix of four equations contains only three unknowns, x, y and z, and the least squares solution is found.

A perspex cube containing small steel balls at each corner and the centre of each face was constructed [13,15]. The cube has 14 steel markers of known relative position embedded at each corner and the centre of each side of a 60 mm cube. The cube is imaged just after the patient is examined with exactly the same x-ray gantry positions as those used for the patient. From the measured 2D coordinates on these two images and the known 3D coordinates of each steel marker, the projective transformation matrices for the biplanar angiograms are obtained.

Implementation of the technique

Using this principal, a System for Angiographic Reconstruction and Analysis (**SARA**) was implemented for digital biplanar x-ray angiographic images. SARA was programmed in 'C' on a SUN graphics workstation using the UNIX operating system, in the SUN View windowing environment, and applied to images of blood flow phantoms and DSA images from clinical investigations.

Image acquisition

All x-ray images were acquired on a Siemens Digitron II DSA system interfaced to an Ethernet LAN allowing transfer of images to a network of SUN Sparc workstations on which all software development and data processing was done. Images were obtained with a tube voltage of between 70 and 80 kVp, with a small focal spot in the pulsed x-ray exposure mode (18 msec per exposure). Digital images proportional to the logarithm of the x-ray image intensity were recorded. Careful calibration of our DSA system has confirmed this logarithmic relationship. For the phantom experiments the x-ray beam was filtered by an additional 1 mm of copper. The digital images were acquired on a 512 x 512 pixel matrix at 10 bits per pixel.

3D reconstruction of the arterial tree using SARA

The initial stage of the reconstruction involved the estimation of the transformation matrices relating a point in the 2D image plane to a point in 3D space. A corresponding pair of cube images was displayed and six or more steel ball markers on the cube were manually identified by a mouse-controlled cursor on the screen (Figure 1). The program SARA computes the centre of gravity of the ball-bearing markers in order to determine these points accurately. The average square error of selected points is displayed to confirm the identification of the right points.

Identification of corresponding points between two projection views

The 3D coordinates of a point can be found from two biplanar x-ray angiograms after computation of the transformation matrices by identifying the point on both views. A structure may be delineated by the identification of a set of corresponding points between the two projection views. If the structure under investigation is rather complex, then this identification is not an easy task. The operator can, however, obtain some program assistance with this. As soon as the operator indicates the projection of a point in one view, the program is able to draw an 'epipolar' line in the second view on which the projection of the point has to be positioned. The existence of such a line and its actual location can be derived from equations (4). These equations represent an overdetermined system of four equations and three unknowns. If one of the rows of equation (4) was eliminated, it would still be possible to solve for (x, y, z). In the 3D reconstruction of the vascular tree, the centreline is mapped out on a set of points: where the

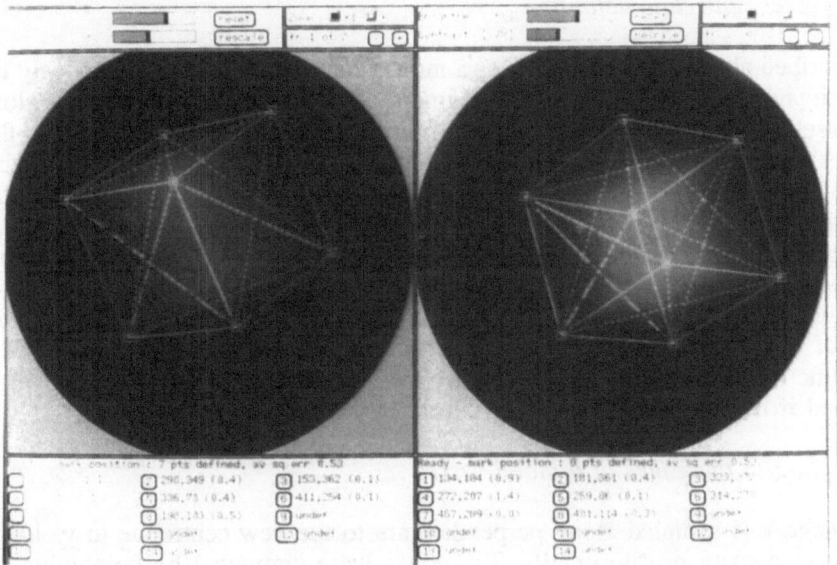

Figure 1. A pair of x-ray images of the cube with graphical su₋erimposition of the cube lines showing the generation of the transformation matrices.
(For colour plate of figure 1 see page 565)

vessel centreline point $Q_1(u_1,v_1)$ in the one projected view image corresponds ·to the vessel centreline point $Q_2(u_2,v_2)$ in the other projected image. In practice, using the epipolar line for the identification of the blood vessel has proved to be an extremely useful aid. This feature was implemented in SARA; indication of the projection of a landmark by the operator in one view is followed immediately by a program-identified epipolar line in the second view, along which the projection of the same landmark must lie. The operator is required to identify and track the projection of a stretch of artery in each of the two biplanar views and, as the landmark here is a length of artery, the identification of the points on the epipolar line is a fairly simple task. In SARA, corresponding points in the two tracked lines are determined as follows. Starting from the first point of the first line (u_1,v_1), an epipolar line in the second view is calculated. Subsequently, the intersection of this epipolar line with the drawn line in the second view is determined. This intersection is indicated by (u_2,v_2) in the second view. The matching 3D position of the point is then calculated according to equation (4) and the process is repeated for the second point in either the first or second view. This is continued until a complete series of 3D points is obtained, representing the structure of the identified artery. From the 3D location of points on the vessel centreline, the precise geometric magnification factor relating the vessel of interest to the computer image, the angle between the vessel long axis and the imaging plane, and the vascular path length between selected points were calculated by SARA.

Blood vessel centreline definition

As described above, an observer uses a mouse cursor to identify interactively the approximate centreline of the vessel segment of interest by defining points along the vessel segment. As the centreline definition needs only be approximate, this step may be performed rapidly. The system then joins successive points with a straight line. It also draws two lines parallel to this line that can be adjusted manually at the sides of the vessel to provide boundaries for calculation of the centreline and to search for the vessel edge. The system samples points perpendicular to each straight line and computes the centre of gravity of the grey level distribution. The updated position of the vessel centreline is taken as the locus of this centre of gravity. A smooth line is calculated to go through these centreline locations. The resulting centreline is displayed to the user and can be modified if necessary.

Calculation of the edges of a blood vessel

The image was sampled along perpendiculars to the new centreline to yield the transverse density profile (TDP). The edges were computed by combining the results of two edge operators, the first- and second-derivative of the TDP. Since the first-derivative operator tends to underestimate the actual edge position and the second-derivative operator tends to overestimate the actual edge position, it seems reasonable that a combination of the two operators would approximate the correct position. We chose the position where the sum of the moduli of the first- and second-derivatives of the TDP was a maximum [10] (Figure 2).

Cross-sectional area estimation

To compute volume flow from velocity the vessel cross-sectional area is required and to measure this we used a densitometric method we have described previously [19,20]. In brief, the technique is based on image densitometry in which the integral of image intensity a is computed along a profile perpendicular to the projection of the vessel axis. The true cross-section A is related to the densitometric measure a by:

$$A = a \left(\frac{\cos\theta}{M} \right) \left(\frac{1}{Kc} \right) \tag{5}$$

The x-ray magnification factor M and angle θ between the vessel axis and the x-ray axis are computed from the 3D reconstruction of the vascular configuration from two views. The remaining term is the product of the iodine concentration in the vessel c and a densitometric calibration constant K which relates the image grey value to the mass of iodine integrated along the x-ray path from x-ray focus to image. These were obtained from data generated from 3D reconstructions of biplanar x-ray angiographic data.

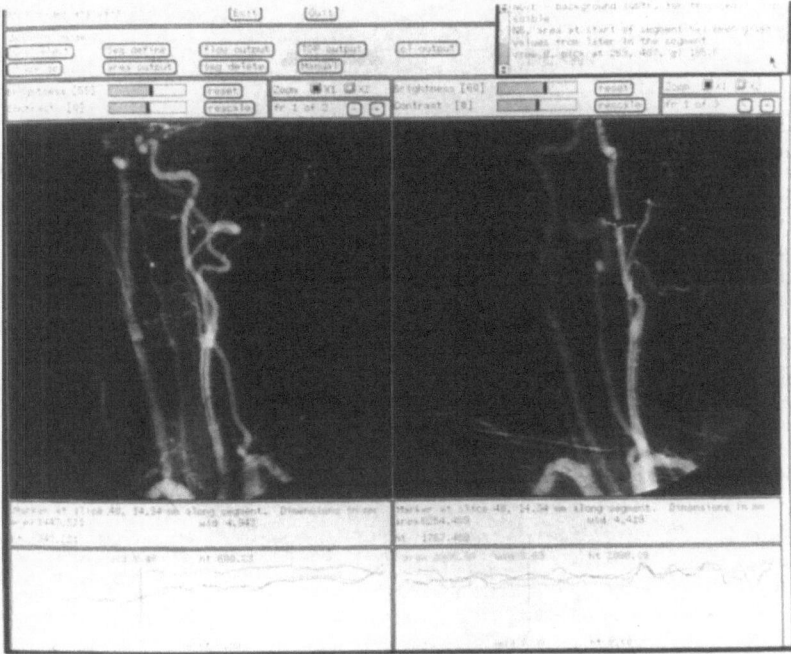

Figure 2. A biplanar digital x-ray angiogram of the aortic arch and the major arteries leading towards the head, with the detected edges superimposed on the angiograms (see Table 4, patient MB). (For colour plate of figure 2 see page 566)

Computation of flow velocity waveforms

We developed a new radiographic technique to measure the pulsatile flow pattern in a selected artery. In this technique, a parametric image of the product of the integral of the TDP and the factor $\cos(\Theta)$ was computed as a function of time and 3D distance along an identified vessel segment (Figure 3A). The image was resampled using linear interpolation to produce an image sampled at regular intervals along the vessel axis. At each point along the vessel segment the plot of the integral of the TDP versus time was normalised to peak opacification. This, in effect, produced an image proportional to image concentration in the vessel and had the effect of reducing artefact due to incomplete mask subtraction and beam hardening effects. This parametric image has been corrected for the x-ray magnification factor and angle of the blood vessel to the imaging plane using biplanar x-ray angiograms and the 3D reconstruction technique.

Adjacent plots of contrast concentration versus distance along the vessel segment were translated forwards or backwards along the distance axis until a match occurred. A match was defined as the shift, s, which yielded a minimum of the function Ψ_{js} for each j where:

$$\Psi_{js} = \frac{\left(\sum_{i-k,m} \left(\Phi_{i,j} - \Phi_{i+s,j+1}\right)^2\right)^{\frac{1}{2}}}{(m-k+1)} \qquad (5)$$

$\Phi_{i,j}$ = concentration of contrast material at position i and time j; $k=0$ for $s>0$ or $-s$ for $s\leq0$; $m=i_{max}$-s for $s>0$ or i_{max} for $s\leq0$. Note that $(i_{max}+1)$ is the total length of the vessel segment analyzed, divided by the sampling interval along the vessel segment.

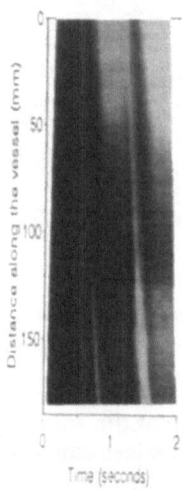

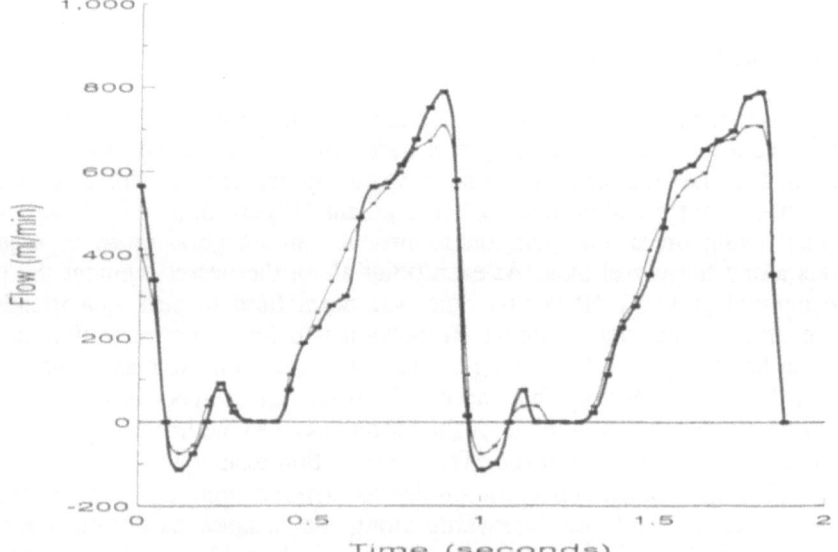

Figure 3. (A) Parametric image generated by 3D data processing for a 4.0 mm calibre with a mean blood flow of 271 ml/min. (B) Direct comparison of volume flow waveforms measured synchronously using the standard EMF (thin lines) and from the parametric image using our velocity computing algorithm (thick lines).

The shift, s, provides an estimate of the distance travelled by the bolus in the time interval j to $j+1$. The tracking procedure was constrained to a maximum rate of change of velocity and reset to zero velocity if the match was poor. Our software allowed concatenation of discrete segments of the same vessel to exclude image artifacts caused by crossing vessels or imperfect mask subtraction and, this allowed longer lengths of vessel to be studied.

Validation of SARA

The following phantoms were constructed for the validation of SARA: a) for validation of path length: three different lengths of bent wire in the shape of an 'S'; b) for cross-sectional area validation a vascular phantom was constructed from a 10 mm thick aluminium block. Seven holes were drilled through, with diameters ranging from 1 to 7 mm, to represent vessel length.

The phantoms were positioned at the isocentre of rotation of the x-ray gantry, with the maximum and minimum height setting 40 mm above and below this position. Biplanar x-ray angiograms were obtained of the phantoms with the corresponding cube images acquired with the x-ray equipment positioned as for the phantoms.

Phantom flow study

In order to assess the performance of the technique, a phantom was constructed to simulate pulsatile blood flow and hence to permit correlation of flow velocity derived from x-ray angiography with independent flow measurements using an EMF. The phantom consisted of a variable-speed pump (Bio Medicus, Bio-Medicus Inc., Minnetonka, MN 55343, USA), 7.00 m length of flexible plastic tubing, a tubular probe of an EMF (Nycotron Blood Flow Meter 376, Drammen, Norway) and a solenoid to simulate a pulsatile flow waveform, which includes reverse flow. Normal saline solution was used throughout the flow circuit. A catheter inserted upstream of the imaging site, by means of a Y-connector, was used to inject contrast material. Instantaneous flow rates were measured with a 9.5 mm calibre tubular flow probe placed in series, downstream of the imaging site, and a Nycotron EMF connected to a strip chart recorder. An ion chamber, to synchronise the EMF flow reading with x-ray exposure, was placed to one side of the tube. The ion chamber output was recorded on the same paper trace as the EMF reading. Synchronisation of the frame number of the angiographic run with the EMF trace was obtained by counting pulses derived from the ion chamber on the paper trace. Instantaneous blood flow was calculated at 0.04 sec intervals, corresponding to the x-ray framing rate, and compared with the output of the EMF flowmeter.

For phantom studies, Urografin 370 (370 mg of iodine/ml) was injected into the phantom via the catheter with a power injector (Simtrac C, Siemens, Erlangen, West Germany). The injector delivered contrast material at a rate of 3 ml/sec (a total volume of 9 ml per injection) during the image acquisition. The point of injection was 100 mm upstream from the imaged section of tubing. Five experiments were performed with the 3D phantom oriented at a 15° (for the 6.0 mm tube; internal diameter), 33° (for the tube with 4.0 mm internal diameter) and 35° (for tube with 3.0 mm internal diameter) angle to the imaging plane.

Clinical study

Four patients (one male and three females), with an age range from 57 to 68 years, were selected who were undergoing routine angiographic procedures for the investigation of cerebrovascular disease. All these patients had suffered a transient ischaemic attack (TIA). Symptoms of residual neurological damage were minimal, but a Doppler investigation, subsequent to hospital admission, had documented evidence of an extracranial vascular stenosis ($<50\%$ diameter reduction). These patients had been recommended for a routine DSA investigation to determine suitability for carotid endarterectomy. To allow for the quantification of the DSA run, a slight modification of the usual DSA procedure was required with one of the runs (neck) acquired at a rate of 25 frames/sec. Ethical Committee approval for the study protocol was obtained and all patients gave informed consent to the study.

For each patient biplanar images of the neck were obtained. For each pair of data acquisitions, the patient was aligned at the isocentre of the x-ray gantry and care was taken not to move the patient between each run. Each pair of runs consisted of biplanar x-ray angiography (LAO and RAO views at 45°). Each run was performed at 2 frames/sec apart from one of the neck view which was performed at 25 frames/sec for the flow analysis. To prevent patient movement during biplanar views, the patient's head was strapped to the table. The positions of the x-ray table and gantry, and the image intensifier height were recorded for each of the runs.

The magnification factor and the 3D orientation of a selected vessel were obtained after calibration of each x-ray view with a cube of known dimensions.

Statistical methods

All the data generated in this study were analysed using simple regression modelling with one predictor and one outcome variable. The degree of linearity between the two variables was expressed by the correlation coefficient with 1.00 indicating perfect linearity. The degree of agreement between the electromagnetic flowmeter and the angiographic technique was also analysed using the Bland and Altman technique [21].

Results

Measurement of the 3D path lengths and cross-sectional area

Table 1 shows the results of the three path length experiments. The discrepancies in path length measured with a ruler and computed from the 3D reconstruction were 2.2, 2.1 and 2.5 mm, which corresponded to an error of between 1.3 and

1.6%. There is a small systematic underestimation which was probably due to sampling effects along the tortuous wire. The accuracy is, nevertheless, more than adequate for our purposes.

The absolute cross-sectional areas of the vessels are compared with the true cross-sectional areas in Table 2, with $\pm$ SD for each mean value. As expected, the bigger the diameter the more accurate are the cross-sectional area measurements in percentage terms. The absolute error is independent of diameter and varies between 0 to 0.6 mm^2.

Table 1. Computation of 3D path length of bent wire.

Path length experiment	Length $\pm$ SD (mm) measured with ruler	from 3D reconstruction	No. of measurements	% error
I	140.1$\pm$0.2	142.3$\pm$0.7	7	-1.6
II	178.3$\pm$0.5	180.8$\pm$1.1	7	-1.4
III	159.8$\pm$0.7	161.9$\pm$1.4	7	-1.3

Phantom flow study

Using the 4.0 mm diameter tube, three experiments were performed with mean flow rates of 176, 271 and 689 ml/min, with corresponding peak velocities measured by the EMF of 647, 945 and 2337 mm/sec (Table 3). Figure 3B shows the flow waveforms produced from the x-ray angiographic technique in the experiments with a mean EMF flow rate of 271 ml/min. As is shown in the Figure 3B the flow waveform derived from the x-ray angiogram follows very closely that derived from the EMF with excellent correlation between the two instantaneous flow rates (Table 3). But, in the region of peak flows, the angiographic technique tends to overestimate by 4%. Similar results were obtained for 6.0 and 3.0 mm diameter tubes (Table 3).

Clinical study

Figure 4A shows a typical example of the parametric images generated for the right carotid artery of a 62-year-old female with minor right internal carotid stenosis and an aberrant left brachiocephalic artery (Figure 2). There were overlap and horizontal artifacts in all the parametric images and these were ignored during flow analysis. Figure 4B shows plots of the flow waveforms versus time extracted from the parametric images shown in Figure 4A. Also, in Doppler studies, the carotid arteries may normally show significant forward flow, but this is not the case with the angiographic data, which show that between each cardiac cycle the flow has fallen to zero, which could be due to lack of contrast material. Table 4 presents a summary of the results obtained for the four patients. As can be seen from Table 4 some data are missing, which is due to either vessels not being visible or being totally occluded.

Table 2. Table of the computation of the cross-sectional area A of holes drilled in aluminum block.

Diameter (mm)	Actual cross-sectional area (mm²)	Computed cross-sectional area A±SD (mm²)			No. of samples along image of hole	% error in A
		LAO view	RAO view	average		
7	38.5	34.0±1.1	41.8±1.2	37.9±0.8	160	1.6
6	28.3	27.4±0.6	28.5±0.8	28.0±0.5	160	1.1
5	19.6	18.1±1.0	21.0±0.6	19.6±0.6	160	0.0
4	12.6	12.9±0.9	13.2±0.6	13.1±0.5	160	-4.0
3	7.1	7.3±1.3	7.7±0.8	7.5±0.9	160	-5.6
2	3.1	3.1±0.6	3.5±0.6	3.3±0.4	160	-6.5
1	0.8	1.3±1.0	1.6±0.8	1.4±0.7	160	-75.0

Table 3. Summary of results of 3D flow phantom experiments.

Experiment	Vessel internal diameter (mm)	Mean flow (ml/min)		Peak Velocity (mm/sec)		Correlation coefficient (r)	No. of cardiac cycles
		EMF	angiographic	EMF	angiographic		
I	3.0	229	209	1232	1471	0.857	2
II	4.0	271	266	945	1050	0.990	3
III	4.0	689	703	2337	2820	0.955	1
IV	4.0	176	181	647	700	0.955	3
V	6.0	586	591	763	800	0.986	4

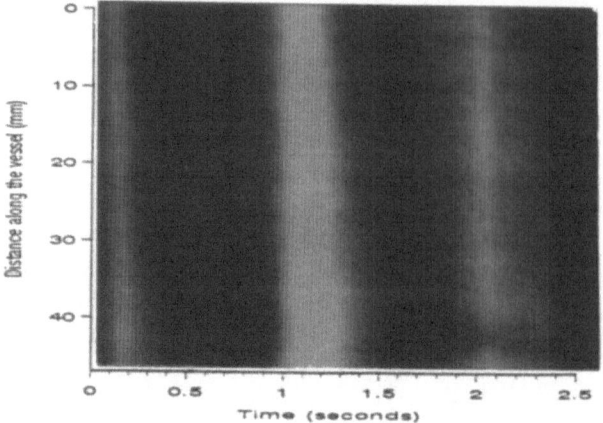

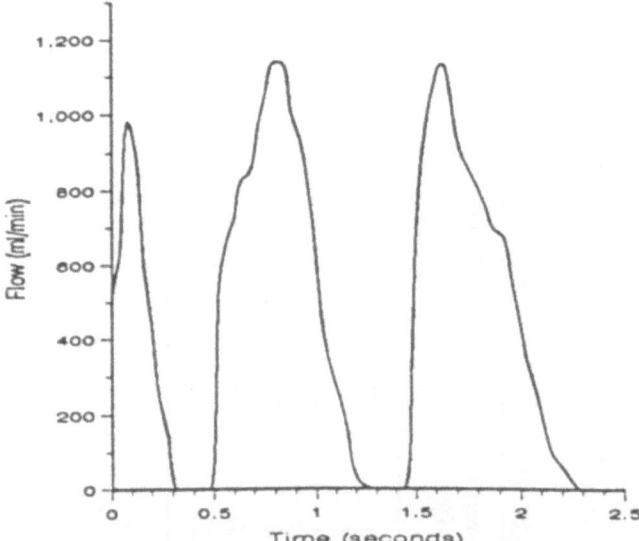

Figure 4. A clinical example of (A) parametric image showing contrast medium concentration (grey scale) at different positions down the right common carotid (RCC), the vertical axis and at different times (the horizontal axis). (B) Plots of the volume flow velocity waveforms extracted from the parametric image shown in (A).

Table 4. Summary of results from quantitative digital x-ray angiographic studies in patients who have undergone head and neck DSA examinations. The table shows mean velocity V in mm/sec, cross-sectional area A in mm^2 and flow F in ml/min. The results have been computed for the left common carotid (LCC), right common carotid (RCC), left internal carotid (LIC), right internal carotid (RIC), left vertebral (LVE) and right vertebral (RVE) arteries.

Patient →	A			B			C			D		
Artery	V	A	F	V	A	F	V	A	F	V	A	F
LCC	359	19.7	425	259	24.4	380	374	24.9	558	350	19.2	403
RCC	453	18.2	494	412	25.2	623	301	26.5	478.6		Occluded	
LIC	480	10.2	293		Occluded			Not visible		520	10.5	327
RIC	415	13.3	331	396	18.3	435		Not visible			Occluded	
LVE	590	10.6	376	442	3.7	98		Not visible		470	11.3	319
RVE	504	4.5	136	287	22.5	387		Not visible			Occluded	

Discussion

Our technique for estimating flow velocity is based upon an integration of contrast medium across the vessel lumen at any point along the vessel. We therefore do not retain any information about the transverse distribution of flow velocity across the lumen. Such information is in any case limited by the fact that only a 2D projection of the 3D distribution can be retrieved from a single x-ray view. In some vessels, the flow may be nearly laminar with a parabolic distribution of flow velocities across the lumen. At the leading edge of a bolus, this will mean that the more central high velocity streamlines are overrepresented and velocity will be overestimated. However, the opposite will occur at a later stage of the passage of the bolus, and provided measurements are also made from all phases of bolus transit, the errors will tend to balance.

Our procedure for computing the shift, s, of the bolus along the axis of the vessel at each frame interval is simple but effective. However, it can fail in the presence of artefacts or a low contrast concentration gradient along the vessel. Reliability would be improved by recording no value (rather than zero flow), when the distance-concentration gradient was lower than a threshold value. In Figure 4B the zero flow values recorded from the angiographic data at the beginning of systole should not be treated as measurements at all and could have been identified as phases when no valid flow data were retrievable.

The technique of 3D reconstruction is robust and accurate. The information about vessels from x-ray angiography could thus be combined with other functional and anatomical studies [22,23] so that, for example, tissue perfusion from nuclear medicine studies could be related to measurements of vascular supply. There is a payoff between the maximum measurable blood velocity, vessel path length imaged and framing rate. If the bolus of contrast material imaged in one frame has moved completely from the field of view in the next frame then the method will fail. In practice our phantom work has shown that a frame-to-frame overlap of about 50% provides adequate data to match distance concentration functions. Hence at 25 frames/sec we require about 80 mm of vessel length to measure instantaneous flow velocities of up to 1 m/sec. Within this constraint our phantom work predicts that we can measure mean and peak flow rates to within about 10% of that measured using an EMF.

The human brain receives its vascular supply from four main arteries, the carotids and the vertebrals. In most studies dealing with cerebral ischaemia, quantitative information about the state of these arterial systems is lacking, especially for the vertebral arteries. The reason for this is that the lack of any adequate technique that works well enough to estimate vertebral artery blood flow. Other technique such as Doppler ultrasound cannot measure vessel with a relatively deep course overlaid by other arteries or bone.

Gold standards are unavailable in the clinical setting which make the accuracy of the results difficult to gauge, but assessment of the results with regard to patient history and radiological interpretation of the x-ray images showed good correlation in most cases. Normal velocities obtained using duplex Doppler ultrasound in the carotid arteries are usually between 600 and 1000 mm/sec; however, they can range from less than 300 to 1200 mm/sec [24]. There is normally no significant increase in velocity as one progresses from the common carotid artery into the internal carotid artery, but there may be a slight decrease in peak systolic velocity. The values obtained using the angiographic method are consistent with these values.

One of the problems of our technique is the presence of stenosis along the blood vessel imaged. When matching contrast concentration profiles, we assume that axial flow velocity is independent of position along the vessel. By normalising each row of the parametric image to peak opacification we, in effect, convert parametric images to concentration rather than mass. This will partially compensate for any effect that small stenoses might have on the matching technique, but in long or more severe stenoses, this region will have to be excluded from the matching procedure.

In conclusion, we have described and validated a robust method for the computation of volume flow which utilises a 3D representation of a vascular segment reconstructed from calibrated biplane views. The technique can be incorporated into the clinical routine with minimal change to conventional image acquisition protocols. The calibration procedure is technically straightforward, can take place after the procedure has been completed and is rapid to perform. Although the technique requires high frame rate angiograms (25 frames/sec in the work described here) most commercial DSA systems permit rapid summation of images acquired with a low dose per frame at high framing rates to generate images of better contrast but at a lower effective framing rate. Thus there should be little or no radiation dose penalty or increase in iodine contrast administered as compared with routine clinical practice.

References

1.   Seifalian AM, Stansby GP, Hobbs KE, Hawkes DJ, Colchester AC.

Measurement of liver blood flow: a review. HPB Surg 1991;4:171-86.

2. Seifalian AM. The computation of blood flow waveforms from digital x-ray angiographic data [Ph.D. Thesis]. London University, 1993.

3. Posner JB. Newer techniques of cerebral blood flow measurement. Stroke 1972;3:227-37.

4. Jennett WB, Harper AM, Gillespie FC. Measurement of regional cerebral blood flow during carotid ligation. Lancet 1966;2:1162-3.

5. Harper AM. Measurement of cerebral blood flow by radioisotopes and its value in clinical practice. Practitioner 1971;207:291-300.

6. Pond GD, Osborne RW, Capp MP *et al.* Digital subtraction angiography of peripheral vascular bypass procedures. AJR Am J Roentgenol 1982;138:279-81.

7. Guthaner DF, Wexler L, Enzmann DR *et al.* Evaluation of peripheral vascular disease using digital subtraction angiography. Radiology 1983;147:393-8.

8. Turnipseed WD, Sackett JF, Strother CM, Crummy A, Mistretta CA, Kruger RA. Computerized arteriography of the cerebrovascular system: its use with intravenous administration of contrast material. Arch Surg 1981;116:470-3.

9. Reiber JHC, Serruys PW editors. State of the art in quantitative coronary angiography. Dordrecht: Martinus Nijhoff, 1986.

10. Reiber JHC, Kooijman CJ, Slager CJ. Computer assisted analysis of the severity of obstructions from coronary cineangiograms: a methodological review. Automedica 1984;5:219-38.

11. Seifalian AM, Hawkes DJ, Colchester ACF, Hobbs KEF. A new algorithm for deriving pulsatile blood flow waveforms tested using stimulated dynamic angiographic data. Neuroradiology 1989;31:263-9.

12. Seifalian AM, Hawkes DJ, Hardingham CR, Colchester ACF, Reidy JF. Validation of a quantitative radiographic technique to estimate pulsatile blood flow waveforms using digital subtraction angiographic data. J Biomed Eng 1991;13:225-33.

13. Mackay SA, Potel MJ, Rubin JM. Graphics methods for tracking three-dimensional heart wall motion. Comput Biomed Res 1982;15:455-73.

14. Reiber JHC, Gerbrands JJ, Troost GJ *et al.* 3-D reconstruction of coronary arterial segments from two projections. In: Heintzen PH, Brennecke R, editors. Digital imaging in cardiovascular radiology. Stuttgart: Thieme, 1983:151-63.

15. Hawkes DJ, Colchester ACF, Mol CR. The accurate 3-D reconstruction of the geometric configuration of vascular trees from x-ray recordings In: Guzzardi R. editor. Physics and engineering of medical imaging. Dordrecht: Martinus Nijhoff, 1987:250-8.

16. Colchester ACF, Hawkes DJ, Brunt JNH, du Boulay GH, Wallis A. Pulsatile blood flow measurements with the aid of 3-d reconstruction from dynamic angiographic recordings. In: Bacharach SL, editor. Information processing in medical imaging. Dordrecht: Martinus Nijhoff, 1986:247-65.

17. Kim HC, Min BG, Lee TS, Lee SJ, Park JH, Han MC. Three-dimensional digital subtraction angiography. IEEE Trans Med Imaging 1982;MI-1:152-8.

18. Rogers DF, Adams JA. Mathematical elements for computer graphics. 2nd ed. New York: McGraw-Hill, 1990:101-33.

19. Colchester ACF, Brunt JNH. Measurement of vessel calibre and volume blood flow by dynamic quatitative digital angiography: An initial application showing variation of cerebral artery diameter with PaCo2. J Cereb Blood Flow Metab 1983;3:S640-1.

20. Hawkes DJ, Colchester ACF, de Belder MA *et al.* The measurement of absolute

lumen cross sectional area and lumen geometry in quantitative angiography. In: Todd-Pokropek AE, Viergever MA, editors. Medical images: formation, handling and evaluation. Heidelberg: Springer-Verlag, 1992:609-26.

21. Bland JM, Altman D. Statistical methods for assessing agreement between two methods of clinical measurement. Lancet 1986;1:307-10.

22. Hill DLG, Hawkes DJ, Crossman JE *et al*. Registration of MR and CT images for skull base surgery using point-like anatomical features. Br J Radiol 1991;64:1030-5.

23. Hill DL, Hawkes DJ, Harrison N *et al*. A strategy for automated multimodality image registration incorporating anatomical knowledge and imager characteristics. Lecture Notes Comput Sci 1993;687:168-81.

24. Robinson ML. Duplex sonography of the carotid arteries. Semin Roentgenol 1992;27:17-27.

34. On-line assessment of myocardial flow reserve

MARTIN J.SCHALIJ, PIETER M.J. van der ZWET, MARIKEN J. GELDOF & JOHAN H.C. REIBER

Summary

Myocardial blood flow is determined by two variables, namely, the resistance of the myocardial perfusion bed and the perfusion pressure. Maximal myocardial flow at any given pressure is a function of the total cross-sectional area of the coronary resistance vessels. Myocardial flow reserve at any given pressure is thus a function of the resistance of the myocardial perfusion bed. Because flow reserve depends, among others, on perfusing pressure and basal coronary flow, it is variable and a large range of normal values have been reported. Therefore, MFR measurements in patients must be interpreted cautiously. Despite these limitations, it may be useful to calculate myocardial flow reserve in individual patients to evaluate the severity of coronary artery stenoses in addition to routine selective coronary arteriography, to study microvascular pathology in patients with evidence of small vessel disease and to evaluate the effects of left ventricular hypertrophy on myocardial perfusion. In this paper a radiographic technique for assessing regional coronary blood flow, based on the indicator dilution theory is described. Relative flow was represented by the ratio of maximal contrast density and appearance time of contrast. By computing the ratio of hyperemic flow and basal flow, myocardial flow reserve can be determined. Until recently the densitometric assessment of MFR was a time-consuming technique which included several potential sources of errors. A major problem concerned the difficulties in controlling the densitometric aspects which are related to the use of cinefilm. The introduction of digital image processing techniques enables the on-line assessment of myocardial flow reserve in routine clinical practice and eliminates the potential photographic source of error. Despite the theoretical limitations inherent to the method, at this time densitometric flow measurement is still one of the most useful techniques to study regional myocardial perfusion. The results of our validation study corroborate this perception.

Introduction

In patients with coronary artery disease selective coronary arteriography plays a pivotal role in clinical decision making. Coronary arteriography is unsurpassed in its ability to show the morphology of coronary arteries, however, it has since long been recognized that no simple relation exists between the visually or quantitatively estimated severity of coronary artery disease and its effects on regional myocardial perfusion [1,2]. Furthermore, due to inherent limitations of cardiac image acquisition systems, only the larger epicardial coronary vessels with sizes of more than 0.5 mm can be studied [3]. To express in a convenient manner the capacity of the coronary vascular system to increase flow, Gould [4]

443

J.H.C. Reiber and E.E. van der Wall (eds.), Cardiovascular Imaging, 443-459.
© 1996 *Kluwer Academic Publishers.*

introduced the concept of myocardial flow reserve (MFR, defined as the ratio between maximal coronary blood flow and basal flow [4]), that has been accepted as a functional index of the severity of disturbances of the coronary circulation [5]. Despite several theoretical limitations, in clinical practice MFR measurements can be used to determine the significance of coronary artery stenosis provided the microcirculation is normal or conversely, to evaluate myocardial microcirculation in the presence of normal epicardial arteries [6].

A number of noninvasive and invasive techniques are available to measure MFR in experimental and clinical settings. Noninvasive imaging techniques such as cine computed tomography, contrast echocardiography and magnetic resonance imaging can be used to study coronary flow and transmural flow distribution. Until now it is not clear to what extent these techniques can be introduced in routine clinical practice. The most promising noninvasive technique presumably is positron emission tomography (PET) which enables repeated measurements of regional myocardial perfusion. A widespread introduction of this method is still hampered by the almost prohibitive financial consequences.

Invasive techniques such as intravascular Doppler ultrasound and digital subtraction angiography have been subject to extensive research for many years [7-13].

A direct method to obtain relative myocardial flow in patients became available with the introduction of the intravascular Doppler guide wire [7], using Doppler flow velocity spectra to assess relative coronary blood flow. The earlier wires had a diameter of at least 0.9 mm (3 F) which affected coronary blood flow significantly, thereby limiting the usefulness of this technique. However, steerable Doppler wires with a diameter of only 0.46 mm have become available. In several studies high correlation coefficients between flow velocity measurements by these Doppler probes and absolute flow measurements were demonstrated [13]. With this technique, myocardial flow reserve can be assessed by comparing hyperemic and basal flow velocity values. However, only flow velocity in larger epicardial vessels can be measured, and consequently only limited and indirect information about regional myocardial perfusion can be derived. Furthermore, changes in the position of the Doppler flow velocity may affect the measured flow velocity values unpredictably.

Based on the principles of the indicator dilution theory, Rutishauser [8,9] introduced, more than 20 years ago, a radiographic technique for assessing regional coronary blood flow. The transit time of contrast agent at two sequential locations was determined and after calculation of the volume of the coronary segment absolute flow could be derived. Based on these principles, Vogel [10,11] developed a digital arteriographic method to measure myocardial flow reserve. Relative flow was represented by the ratio of maximal contrast density and appearance time of contrast. By computing the ratio of hyperemic flow and basal flow, myocardial flow reserve can be determined. Although, as discussed by Pijls et al. [12], several theoretical problems exist, densitometric assessment of relative flow can be used to obtain information about the severity of coronary artery disease. Until recently densitometric assessment of MFR was a time-consuming technique which included several potential sources of errors. A major problem concerned the difficulties in controlling the densitometric aspects which are related to the use of cinefilm. The introduction of digital image processing

techniques enables the on-line assessment of myocardial flow reserve in routine clinical practice and eliminates the potential photographic source of error.
In this overview some of the advantages and limitations of the densitometric assessment of myocardial flow reserve will be discussed.

Basic principles

The measurements of flow in coronary arteries, and perfusion of the myocardium are based on measuring arrival time values of contrast agent. The contrast agent is injected into the selected coronary artery, and by measuring appearance time of the contrast agent at a certain point in the coronary system, the (average) flow at that point can be calculated.
These assumptions are based on the indicator-dilution theory, which states that flow (Q) can be calculated as:

$$Q = V/T_{mean},$$

where V is the combined volume of epicardial vessels and myocardial bed, and T_{mean} is the mean transit time of the indicator at a certain position in the myocardial bed. However, the volume cannot be measured directly from the densitometric data. For the determination of the myocardial perfusion, the maximally reached density (D_{max}) of contrast agent is used as a parameter for the volume of the myocardial bed: it is assumed to be proportional to the absolute volume value. The calculation of mean transit time requires the acquisition of runs of a sufficiently long length. In clinical practice however, this is often not feasible. Therefore, the arrival time of contrast agent (T_{arr}) has often been used as a substitute for the mean transit time. A relative value for flow therefore can be defined as:

$$Q_{rel} = D_{max}/T_{arr}.$$

Since it is not possible to measure absolute flow values directly from densitometric data, the calculated flow values can only be interpreted by comparing them to calculated flow values in other parts of the image, or to flow values at the same point in the image, that have been acquired under different conditions. When, in the last case, hyperemic and basal flow states are compared, the myocardial flow reserve can be calculated as:

$$Q_{hyp}/Q_{basal} = (D_{maxhyp}/T_{arrhyp}) / (D_{maxbasal}/T_{arrbasal}).$$

The most promising technique that satisfies these conditions has been published by Vogel [10,11]. Using electrocardiographically gated power injection of contrast agent at a rate assumed to be sufficiently rapid to achieve complete replacement of blood, an image subtraction technique is applied that allows determination of myocardial time/density curves before and during coronary vasodilation. In each cycle, one image is selected, preferably the enddiastolic image. This technique measures the contrast appearance time and the maximum density value for each pixel in the entire image sequence. By performing this procedure at baseline flow state as well as at hyperaemia, induced by intracoronary administration of a drug dilating the myocardial bed, MFR can be defined for each pixel or for a user-defined region-of-interest (ROI) on the myocardial muscle.

Over the last few years, modifications of this approach have been reported by van der Werf et al. [17] and Pijls et al. [12]. They developed a technique for synchronizing the heart rate with the x-ray frequency (apparent cardiac arrest), which minimizes any possible mismatch between the mask image and the subsequent contrast image. Furthermore, they concluded that changes in myocardial perfusion can be accurately assessed by calculating the mean transit time [12], instead of the appearance time. This assessment is strictly according to the original principles of the indicator dilution theory. Another difference of this approach is that it is only applied to two maximum flow states, for example before and after a coronary intervention.

Despite the simplicity of the perfusion model, clinical application of densitometric measurements has been limited due to a number of problems. First of all, the baseline flow values have been shown to be unreliable since the baseline level depends on a large number of parameters, which cannot be controlled completely. Furthermore, in many cases the mask-mode subtraction technique shows a large number of artifacts. During the acquisition of the image sequences it is required that the patient holds his/her breath and lies perfectly still for a long time (± 10 seconds). As a result, due to movement of the patient during acquisition of the run, up to 30% of the acquired studies cannot be used. In these cases regions in the mask image do not correspond to the same regions in the subsequent densitometric images, and perfusion discrepancies occur. This impedes the clinical application of perfusion measurements.

Videodensitometry

A technique that is based on the principles of measuring contrast arrival times requires acquisition of a series of images. The first image (the mask) is used as an estimation for the background of the image: it is subtracted from the other acquired images. In theory this technique (called mask-mode subtraction or Digital Subtraction Angiography, DSA) creates images, whose differences in grey values are caused by the presence of contrast agent. To allow the calculation of contrast density, a relation must be found between the grey values and the mass density of contrast agent at that point. For digitized cinefilms this relation cannot be obtained easily. The grey value of cinefilm does not only depend on the mass density of the contrast agent and the background structures, but also on the development process of the film, the light settings of the cinevideoconverter and the characteristics of the frame grabber, that actually digitizes the video signal. These parameters are difficult to control and can easily lead to large errors in the flow reserve measurements.

With the emergence of digital cardiac imaging systems, the problems related to film processing and digitization disappeared. The optical signal from the image intensifier is directly digitized, and the digitized images are stored on large disks. The relation between grey value and mass is now much better defined.

Since the attenuation of x-rays through a body is inversely related to the exponent of the radiated mass, mask-mode subtraction can be achieved by subtracting the logarithm of the grey value of the mask from the logarithm of the other images. The resulting grey values are then linearly proportional to the mass of the contrast agent at that point and thus to the volume of blood, if a homogeneous concentration of contrast is assumed.

Clearly, a good subtraction can only be obtained when the regions in the mask image correspond exactly to the same regions in the subsequent images. If this is not the case, subtraction artifacts will be created, that will influence the validity of the measurements.

Acquisition protocol

After the cannulation of left coronary artery, an optimal x-ray projection separating left anterior descending artery (LAD) and the left circumflex branch (LCx) has to be chosen. The image intensifier has to be set into the 7 or 9 inch mode. Flow is measured at baseline and during hyperaemia, induced by the intracoronary administration of 12.5 mg HCl-papaverine. Measurements are made 30 seconds after injection of papaverine. To limit contrast related flow effects, the time interval between each pair of data measurements must be at least 10 minutes.

Angiographic flow measurements

Data acquisition is performed in the "lock-in" acquisition mode, fixing the kilovoltage of the x-ray system and at 25 frames/sec [16]. Acquisition is started two or three cardiac cycles before contrast agent injection to stabilize the imaging system and to allow selection of an appropriate background image at the time of analysis. To minimize the effects of contrast on the coronary flow, a non-ionic contrast medium should be used. Images are obtained after power injection of 5 to 7 ml contrast agent (at a flow rate of 5 to 7 ml/s).

During data acquisition the hearts are artificially stimulated just above the intrinsic sinus rhythm synchronized with the DCI x-ray pulses to simulate apparent cardiac arrest [17]. Image acquisition is stopped when venous return becomes visible.

After image acquisition end-diastolic images are selected for analyzing purposes. The selected consecutive end-diastolic frames in an angiographic run represent one run. The combination of basal and hyperemic runs are denoted a run-pair. Typically a run consisted of 8 (maximum 11) end-diastolic frames. Next, a logarithmic mask mode subtraction is carried out. Finally, the basal and hyperemic phase-matched logarithmical mask-subtracted images are stored in a temporary file for subsequent analysis.

The data from this temporary file are used to obtain a functional image. Both from the hyperemic and the basal run two parametric images are generated, a contrast medium arrival picture (CMAP) and a maximal density picture. The contrast medium arrival picture is obtained by determining for each pixel how much time has passed before its density exceeded a threshold level of 50% of the maximal density. In the maximal density image each pixel is assigned the maximal value obtained over all end-diastolic images which are part of the run. From these CMAP and maximal density pictures a relative flow image is computed by dividing for each pixel the maximal density value by the CMAP value. This is done for both the baseline and the hyperemic images. Finally the ratio between the maximal relative flow and baseline flow images is expressed as the myocardial flow reserve image. Before determining the final results in manually drawn regions-of-interest (ROI's) a background correction is performed. Due to this correction the original mask-mode background subtracted images were recalculated. Background correction is necessary to compensate for slow-varying image parameters that change the acquired images after the mask image. To calculate regional MFR values, ROI's can be drawn over the distal myocardial perfusion bed. The program defines for each ROI the number of valid pixels. A pixel is valid when the grey value in both density images (hyperemic and basal) is above a certain threshold. The number of valid pixels (non-zero pixels, or NZP) is given as a percentage on the video output. Normally, when the acquisition protocol is carefully followed, NZP values of 95 to 100 percent are easily achievable. The mean myocardial flow reserve and the standard deviation of the MFR within each ROI are calculated, using only the valid, nonzero, pixels. Finally, the resulting mean MFR, the standard deviation and the number of valid pixels are displayed on the video monitor. By using a special software package, implemented on a MS-DOS PC system, the corresponding time-density curves of each of the ROI's can be viewed and analyzed. This has been an valuable tool to judge the quality of the acquired images.

Validation studies

To study the applicability of the MFR package, an animal study was performed, to compare the results of the MFR package, as it is implemented on the available digital angiographic imaging systems (DCI-SX, Philips Medical Systems, Best, The Netherlands) with absolute flow and flow reserve values.

Mongrel dogs (n = 15) were anesthesized with intravenous fentanyl (0.05 mg/kg/hr) and nembutal (7.5 mg/kg/hr) after premedication with nesdonal (25 mg/kg). Respiration was supported mechanically using a mixture of oxygen and room air after endotracheal intubation.

The actual flow and flow reserve values were measured by placing two perivascular ultrasonic flow probes around the proximal parts of the left anterior descending coronary artery (LAD) and left circumflex branch (LCx). These Doppler flow probes enable precise measurement of coronary blood flow [14,15]. Coronary artery stenoses were produced during continuous flow monitoring by tightening a ligature that was placed just distal to the flow probes. In several dogs multiple sets of coronary and MFR measurements were carried out, at different vules of the severity of the stenosis.

Results

Effect of contrast agent injection on coronary flow

Contrast agent injection resulted in a reproducible triphasic change of coronary blood flow [2,20]. Figure 1 shows the effects of contrast agent injection (6 ml, flow rate: 6 ml/sec) on mean coronary blood flow. Although both basal flow and hyperemic flow were influenced, the time courses of the effects were different. A short initial increase in flow (coinciding with the passage of contrast material) was followed by a sharp decrease. The nadir was reached after 4.2 sec ($\pm$0.8) at baseline and after 2.4 sec ($\pm$0.7) during hyperemia (p < 0.005). Basal flow decreased by 66% ($\pm$9.2) and hyperemic flow by 57% ($\pm$0.5, p < 0.005). Basal flow returned to normal after 7.9 sec ($\pm$2.0), whereas hyperemic flow was restored after 6.2 sec ($\pm$2.0, p < 0.05). After normalization a long lasting (more than 20 seconds) hyperemic period followed. Even during papaverine induced hyperemia, an additional hyperemic response was observed in all experiments. These different effects of contrast medium injection on basal flow and hyperemic flow may hamper a straightforward application of densitometric techniques for the assessment of myocardial flow reserve.

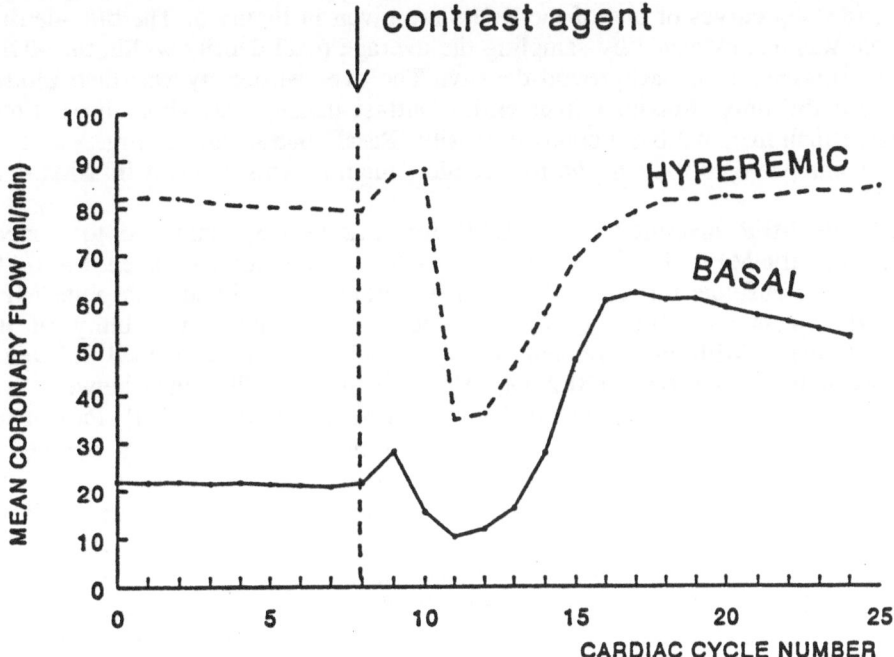

Figure 1. The triphasic response caused by contrast agent injection was observed in all experiments. Both basal flow and hyperemic flow were influenced; however, the time course of the effects was different. A short initial increase of flow (coinciding with the passage of contrast) was followed by a sharp decrease. After normalization a longlasting (more than 20 seconds) hyperemic period follows. Even during papaverine induced hyperemia an additional hyperemic response was observed.

Densitometric myocardial flow reserve

All images were acquired during apnoea and almost motionless images could be obtained in all experiments.

A typical example of such an experiment is given in Figure 2. Panels A, C, E, demonstrate the image acquired during basal flow, corresponding maximal contrast density picture and the contrast medium arrival time picture respectively,. The corresponding hyperemic pictures are displayed in panels B,D and F. A clear difference in contrast density exists between the basal maximal density image and the hyperaemic maximal density image. In Figure 3 the computed MFR image is given. In Figure 4 the ultimate results for each of the regions of interest are displayed together with the basal and hyperemic flow images. Regions-of-interest were placed over the peripheral myocardial perfusion bed and the corresponding MFR-values are shown (lower right panel). The corresponding MFR-image is also given (lower left panel). The MFR-value of each ROI, the standard deviation and the number of nonzero pixels are given as well. The number of nonzero pixels is a reflection of the quality of the image and should be 100.

For each of the ROI's a basal and hyperemic time versus density curve was reconstructed to reassure the quality of the acquired data. The corresponding time-density curves of one of the ROI's are given in Figure 5. The time-density curve was reconstructed by sampling the average pixel density within the ROI's after subtraction of background density. The average density was then plotted against the time. Maximal hyperemic contrast density was about three times higher than maximal basal contrast density. Basal contrast arrival time was 1.22 beats compared to 0.82 in the hyperemic situation. This resulted in a MFR of 3.87.

Absolute MFR measured in the LAD was 3.2 (± 1.5) compared to a mean densitometric MFR of 3.6 (± 1.0, n = 20). The correlation coefficient was 0.70. The mean absolute difference between densitometric MFR and absolute MFR measurements was -0.6 (± 1.4). Short-term (10 minutes) variability of the densitometric MFR measurements was good with an average signed difference between the two series of 0.2 (± 0.9). The average difference between two consecutive series of absolute MFR measurements was -0.1 (± 1.4). Part of the difference between consecutive MFR measurements was caused by changes in basal flow. The average difference between two basal flow measurements was 6.0, whereas the average difference between two consecutive hyperemic flows measurements was only 1.0. Absolute MFR measured in the LCx was 2.8 (± 1.0, n=20) and the corresponding densitometric LCx MFR was 3.5 (± 1.7, n=20). The correlation coefficient was 0.78. The average difference between these two series of measurements was -0.7 with a standard deviation of 1.0. Again, the short-term variability of the densitometric MFR measurements was good with an average difference between the two different series of 1.0 (± 0.7). The average difference between two absolute MFR measurements was 1.1 (± 0.6). The variability was again caused by changes in basal flow. The correlation between absolute flow measurements and densitometric relative flow measurements was significant but lower than expected. The difference may in part be explained by the effects of collateral circulation on regional myocardial

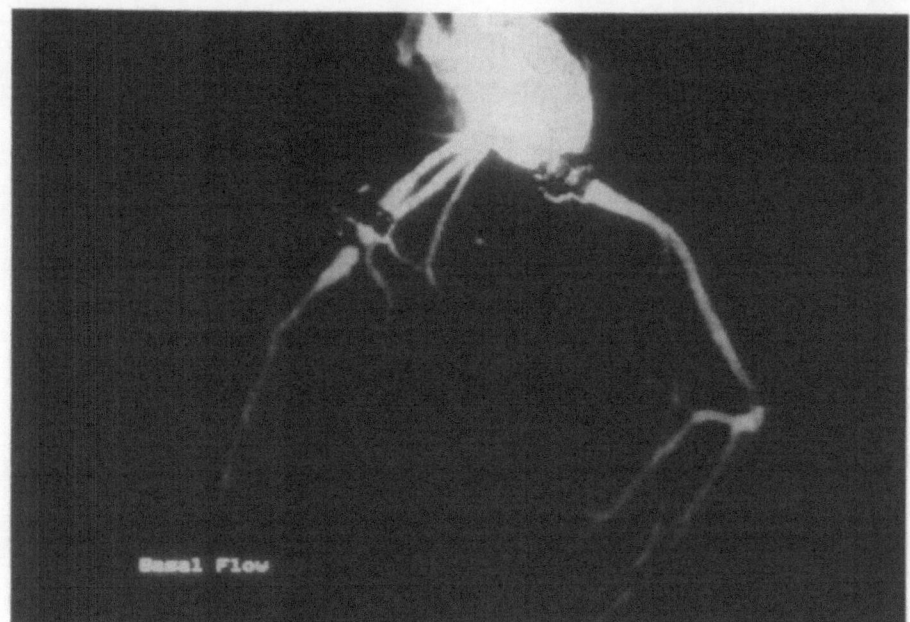

a

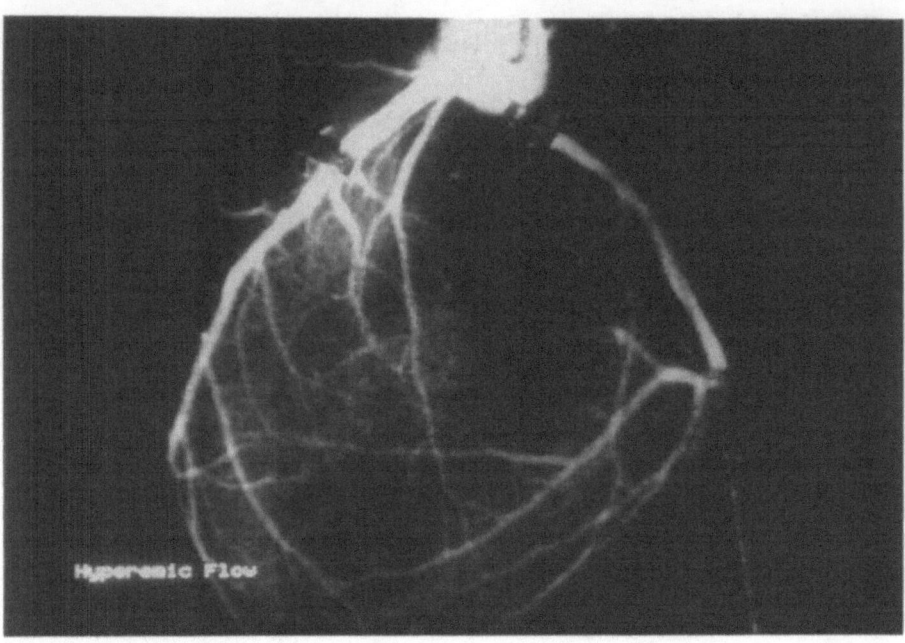

b

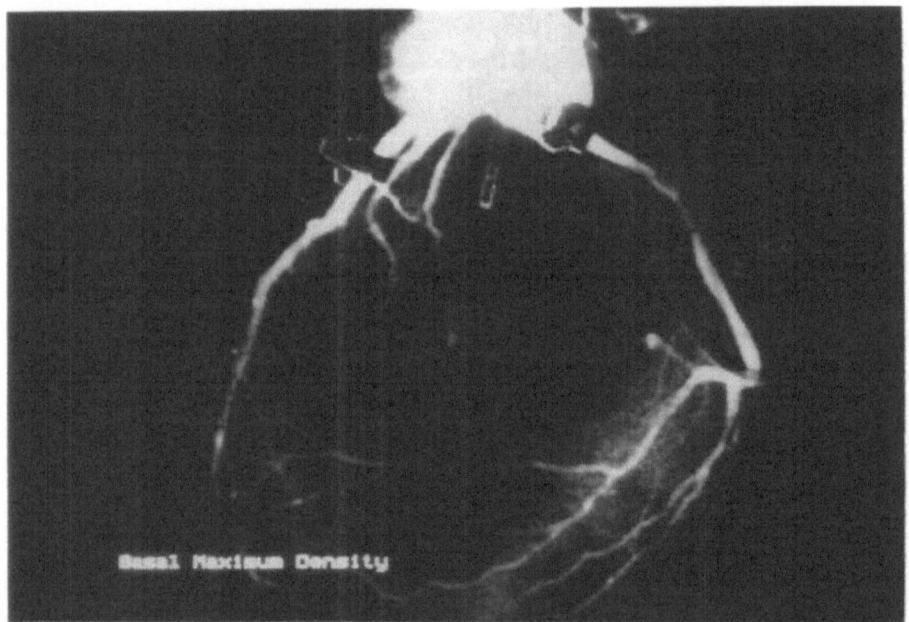

c

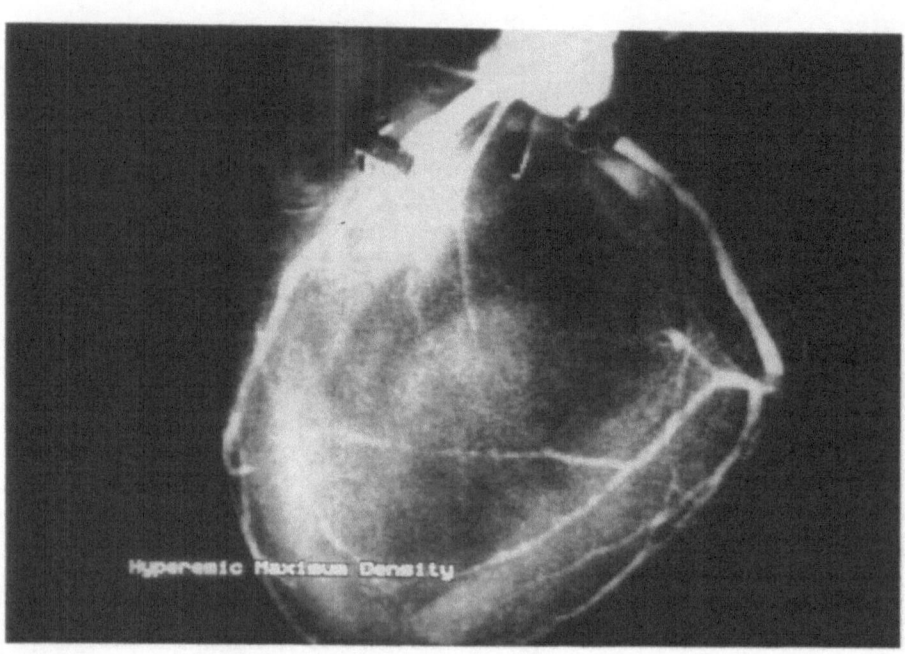

d

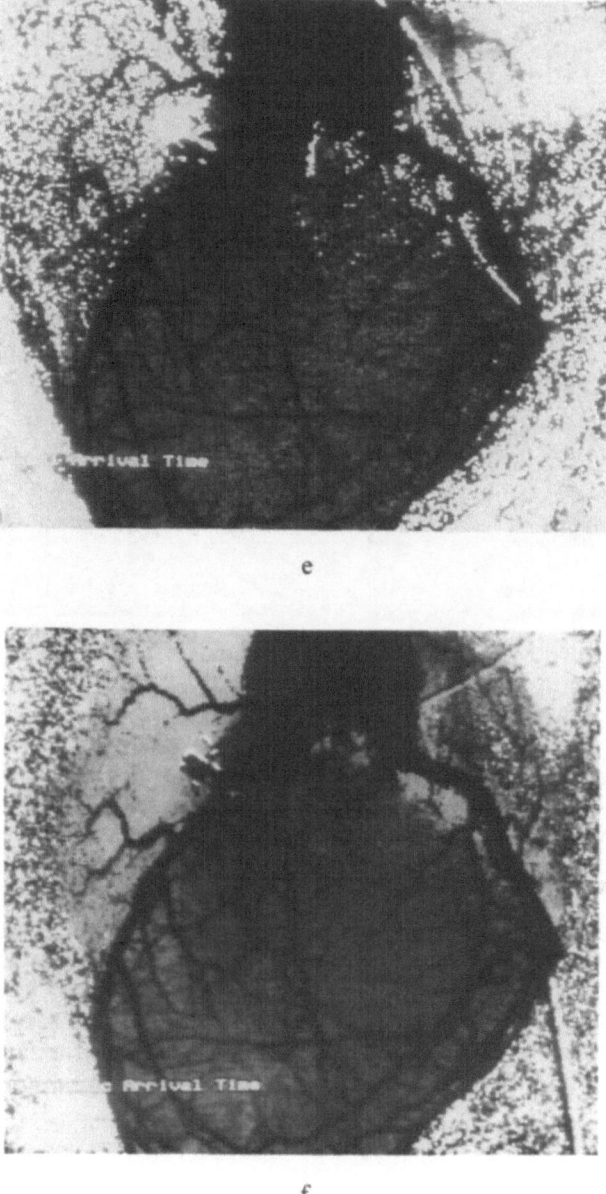

e

f

Figure 2. Typical example of densitometric assessment of myocardial flow reserve. Panels (A), (C), (E), respectively, give the image acquired during basal flow, the corresponding maximal contrast density picture and the contrast medium arrival time picture. The corresponding hyperemic pictures are displayed in panels (B), (D) and (F). There is a clear difference in contrast density between the basal maximal density image and the hyperemic maximal density image.

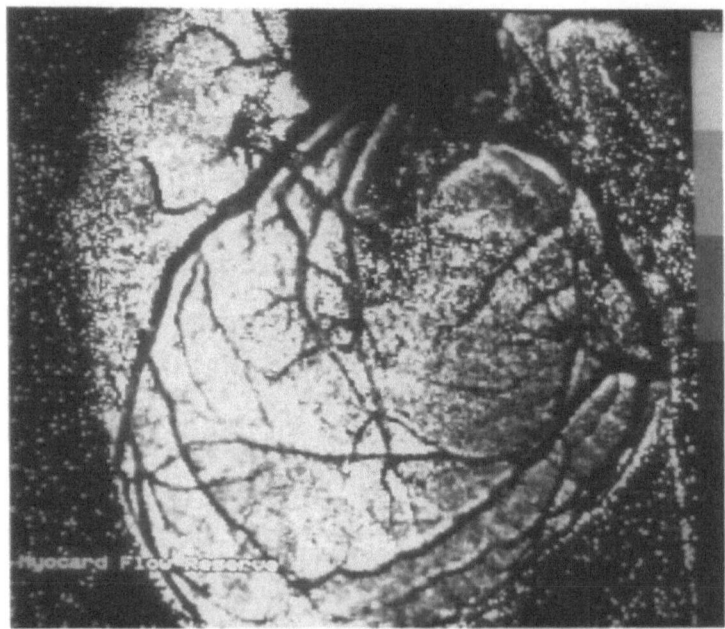

Figure 3. Computed Myocardial Flow Reserve image. This image is computed from the data displayed in Figure 2.

blood flow. Figure 6 shows an example of collateral coronary circulation. After banding the proximal LAD (arrow), the LAD flow was reduced, and large collaterals between the LAD and LCx became apparent. Flow measured by the transonic flow probe decreased by more than 50%, whereas still a densitometric myocardial flow reserve of 2.5 was still measured over the distal LAD perfusion bed. Therefore, part of the weak correlation between absolute flow measurements and densitometric flow measurements could be explained by taking into account the variable and unknown contribution of collateral coronary circulation. Since densitometric measurements were made over the distal myocardial perfusion bed, these were affected by the collateral circulation to a greater extent than absolute flow measurements, obtained proximal in the large epicardial arteries.

Human studies

Until now a number of different studies have been performed in patients. More than 60 patients were studied to evaluate the severity of coronary artery stenosis. Data acquisition was possible in all patients; however 20% of the studies could not be analyzed completely due to movement artifacts. No procedure related complications were encountered. Another study was performed in patients with acute anterior wall myocardial infarctions. In this group of patients (n=30) baseline flow was measured 5 times during the first hour after mechanical reperfusion, starting 10 minutes after reperfusion. By comparing these 5 consecutive runs with each other, changes in relative flow could be calculated.

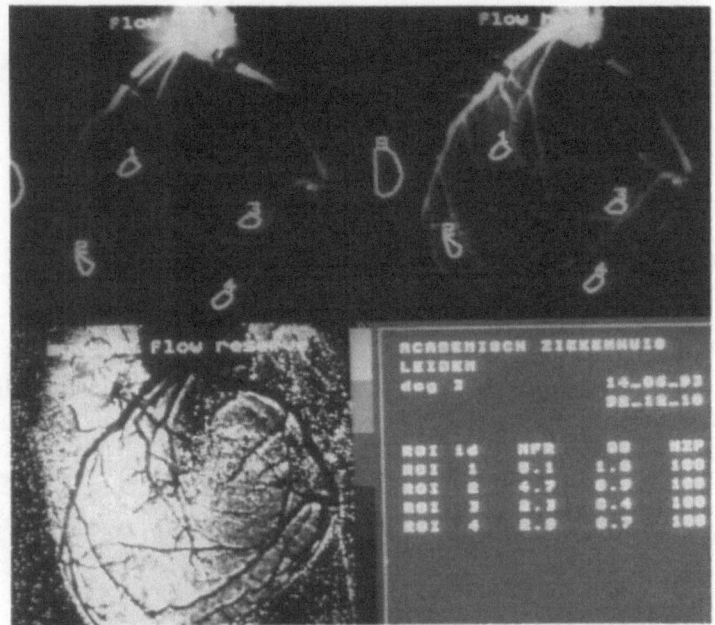

Figure 4. The ultimate results for each of the regions-of-interest are displayed together with the basal and hyperemic flow images (upper two panels). Regions-of-interest were placed over the peripheral myocardial perfusion bed and the corresponding myocardial flow reserves are given (lower right panel). The corresponding myocardial flow reserve image is also given (lower left panel). Besides the myocardial flow reserve of each ROI the standard deviation and the number of nonzero pixels are given. The number of nonzero pixels is a reflection of the quality of the image and should be 100(%).

Although it was possible to acquire images in all patients, again about 20% of thestudies could not be analyzed mainly due to motion artifacts. No procedure related complications were encountered.

Discussion

Myocardial blood flow is determined by two variables, namely, the resistance of the myocardial perfusion bed and the perfusion pressure [19]. Maximal myocardial flow at any given pressure is a function of the total cross-sectional area of the coronary resistance vessels. Myocardial flow reserve at any given pressure is thus a function of the resistance of the myocardial perfusion bed. Because flow reserve depends, among others, on perfusing pressure and basal coronary flow, it is variable and a large range of normal values have been reported. Therefore, MFR measurements in patients must be interpreted cautiously. Despite these limitations, it may be useful to calculate myocardial flow reserve in individual patients to evaluate the severity of coronary artery

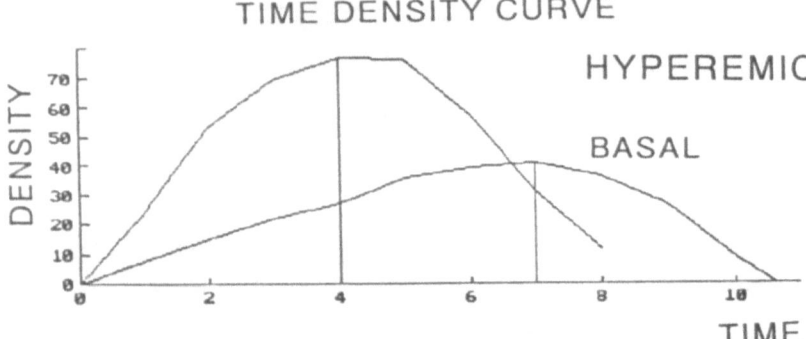

Figure 5. Time versus density curve reconstructed to reassure the quality of the acquired data. The time-density curve was reconstructed by sampling the average pixel density within the ROI's after subtraction of background density. The average density was then plotted against the time. Maximal hyperemic contrast density was about three times larger than maximal basal contrast density. Basal contrast arrival time was 1.22 compared to 0.82 in the hyperemic situation. This resulted in a MFR of 3.87.

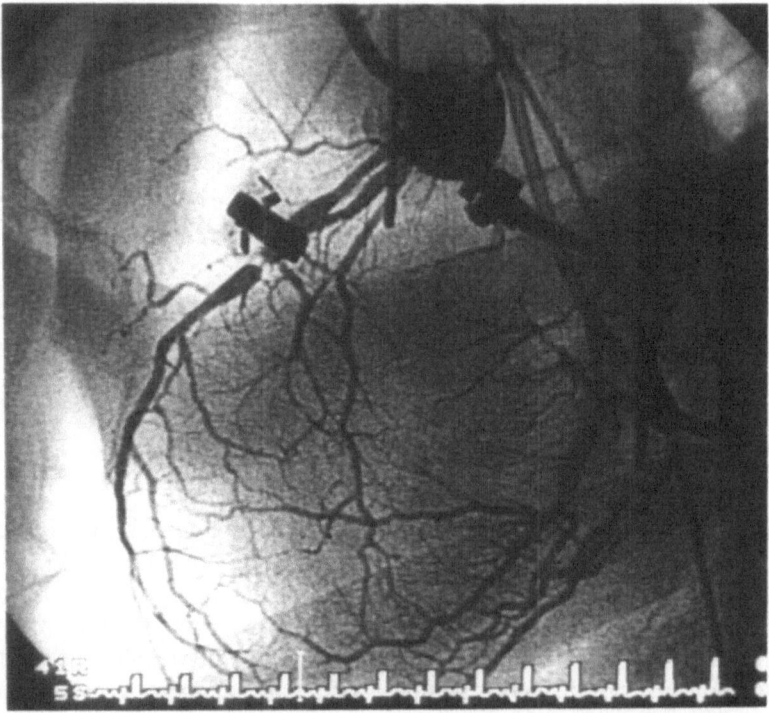

Figure 6. After banding of the proximal LAD (Arrow), extensive collaterals between LCx and LAD became apparant.

stenoses in addition to routine selective coronary arteriography, to study microvascular pathology in patients with evidence of small vessel disease and to evaluate the effects of left ventricular hypertrophy on myocardial perfusion. Until now routine clinical application was hampered by time consuming off-line analysis or technical limitations.

Densitometric assessment of myocardial flow reserve

One of the disadvantages of Rutishauser's original technique was that only the flow in proximal epicardial arteries could be measured. Therefore, Vogel and co-workers [10,11] developed a different approach derived from the indicator dilution theory enabling relative flow measurements in the distal myocardial perfusion bed. Arrival time of contrast was used as a flow parameter and by computing the ratio between hyperemic and basal arrival times myocardial flow reserve could be derived. To improve the results maximal contrast density was used to account for changes in vascular volume.

Theoretical problems limit this straightforward application of the indicator dilution theory [12,18]. One of the premises of the indicator dilution theory is that the dye (contrast agent) does not affect flow. As demonstrated by several investigators and confirmed by the results of this study, contrast agent does affect coronary flow [2,18]. Flow was reduced by more than 50% after contrast agent injection in all experiments. Furthermore, the time course of the effects was found to be significantly different in the basal and hyperemic conditions. These different effects on coronary circulation compounds the interpretation of densitometric flow measurements. Another premise of the indicator dilution theory is that the vascular volume remains constant. This is not the case. To overcome this problem, Cusma [20] used changes in contrast density to represent changes in vascular volume assuming complete exchange of blood by contrast, but this approach is open to criticism [12]. The use of arrival time of contrast instead of mean transit time is a simplification which may introduce a certain error. Therefore, Pijls et al. developed a method using mean transit time of contrast to compare hyperemic flow before and after interventions. This technique has distinct advantages; however, it does not allow MFR measurements.

Despite the theoretical limitations inherent to the method, at this time densitometric flow measurement is still one of the most useful techniques to study regional myocardial perfusion.

The results of our validation study corroborate this perception. A significant but rather low correlation was observed between absolute flow measurements and relative flow measurements. Besides the methodological explanations, this may be explained by the different levels at which the measurements were performed. Absolute flow is measured in the proximal portion of large coronary arteries, whereas densitometric flow is measured over the distal myocardial perfusion bed. As demonstrated, the presence of an extensive collateral network affects peripheral flow measurements to a larger extent than it does proximal flow measurements. Therefore, densitometric flow measurements may provide a better index of regional myocardial perfusion than absolute flow measurements [18]. However, it still is a complex technique with several theoretical limitations which warrant further clinical research.

Conclusion

Digital densitometry enables on-line regional relative flow measurements and despite the theoretical limitations, it may be the most practical technique to study regional myocardial perfusion. Further research is needed to determine its value in clinical decision making.

References

1. Harrison DG, White CW, Hiratzka LF *et al*. The value of lesion cross-sectional area determined by quantitative coronary angiography in assessing the physiologic significance of proximal left anterior descending coronary arterial stenoses. Circulation 1984;69:1111-9.
2. Klocke FJ. Measurements of coronary blood flow and degree of stenosis: current clinical implications and continuing uncertainties. J Am Coll Cardiol 1983;1:31-41.
3. Bruschke AVG, Padmos I, Buis B, van Benthem A. Arteriographic evaluation of small coronary arteries. J Am Coll Cardiol 1990;15:784-9.
4. Gould KL, Libscomb K, Hamilton GW. Physiologic basis for assessing critical coronary stenosis. Instantaneous flow response and regional distribution during coronary hyperaemia as measures of coronary flow reserve. Am J Cardiol 1974;33:87-94.
5. Gould KL. Quantification of coronary artery stenosis in vivo. Circ Res 1985;57:341-53.
6. Hoffman JIE. Maximal coronary flow and the concept of coronary vascular reserve. Circulation 1984;70:153-9.
7. Wilson RF, Laughlin DE, Ackell PH *et al*. Transluminal, subselective measurement of coronary artery blood flow velocity and vasodilator reserve in man. Circulation 1985;72:82-92.
8. Rutishauser W, Simon H, Stucky JP, Schad N, Noseda G, Wellauer J. Evaluation of roentgen cine densitometry for flow measurement in models and in the intact circulation. Circulation 1967;36:951-63.
9. Rutishauser W, Bussman WD, Noseda G, Meier W, Wellauer J. Blood flow measurement through single coronary arteries by roentgen densitometry. I. A comparison of flow measured by a radiologic technique applicable in the intact organism and by electromagnetic flowmeter. AJR Am J Roentgenol Radium Ther Nucl Med 1970;109:12-20.
10. Vogel R, LeFree M, Bates E *et al*. Application of digital techniques to selective coronary arteriography: use of myocardial contrast appearance time to measure coronary flow reserve. Am Heart J 1984;107:153-64.
11. Vogel RA. The radiographic assessment of coronary blood flow parameters. Circulation 1985;72:460-5.
12. Pijls NHJ, Uijen GHJ, Hoevelaken A *et al*. Mean transit time for the assessment of myocardial perfusion by videodensitometry. Circulation 1990;81:1331-40.
13. Doucette JW, Corl PD, Payne HM *et al*. Validation of a Doppler guide wire for intravascular measurement of coronary artery flow velocity. Circulation

1992;85:1899-911.

14. Drost CJ, Dobson A, Sellers AF, Barnes RJ, Comline RS. An implantable transit time ultrasonic flowmeter for long term measurement of blood volume flow. [Abstract] Fed Proc 1984;43:538.

15. Vatner SF, Franklin D, Vangitters RL. Simultaneous comparison and calibration of the Doppler and electromagnetic flowmeters. J Appl Physiol 1970;29:907-10.

16. Reiber JHC, Koning G, van der Zwet PMJ *et al*. Assessment of myocardial flow reserve with the DCI. Medica Mundi. In press.

17. Van der Werf T, Heethaar RM, Stegehuis H, Meijler FL. The concept of apparent cardiac arrest as a prerequisite for coronary digital subtraction angiography. J Am Coll Cardiol 1984;4:239-44.

18. Geldof MJA, Schalij MJ, Manger Cats V *et al*. Comparison between regional myocardial perfusion reserve and coronary flow reserve in the canine heart. Eur Heart J 1995;16:1860-71.

19. Spaan JAE. Coronary blood flow mechanics, distribution, and control. Dordrecht: Kluwer Academic Publishers 1991:333-61.

20. Cusma JT, Toggart EJ, Folts JD *et al*. Digital subtraction angiographic imaging of coronary flow reserve. Circulation 1987;75:461-72.

35. Intravenous myocardial contrast echocardiography for myocardial perfusion

STEPHANIE COULTER, & MICHAEL H. PICARD

Summary

Since the earliest applications of echocardiography, contrast has been used to identify cardiac structures and localize abnormalities. Recently, new gas-filled microbubble preparations have been developed for use as echocardiographic contrast agents. These agents can be detected by ultrasound by the increase in reflected signal from the blood pool. Since these microbubbles are smaller than the diameter of pulmonary capillaries, they travel and are detected in the left heart when injected through peripheral veins and can be detected in the coronary circulation. Using such agents, direct injections have demonstrated the ability to delineate myocardial perfusion territories by echocardiography. This technique has the potential for combining the in-vivo assessment of myocardial perfusion with simultaneous evaluations of cardiac structure and function and to do it noninvasively. Applications include assessment of: blood flow, myocardial blood volume, microvascular integrity, myocardial viability, area at risk for myocardial ischemia/infarction (location, extent and degree), success of acute reperfusion techniques (including thrombolysis), the influence of collateral circulation, bypass graft function and as an adjunct perfusion imaging agent during stress echo. Current challenges include improving our understanding of the factors responsible for bubble stability and optimizing techniques to deliver adequate concentrations of bubbles to the coronary circulation from a peripheral injection. As our understanding of the factors influencing microbubbles is translated into the development of new agents, and as our echocardiographic imaging technique are modified, the prospect of noninvasive, bedside assessment of myocardial perfusion appears closer.

Introduction

Since the earliest applications of echocardiography, contrast has been used to identify cardiac structures [1], localize intracardiac shunts [2], quantitate valvular regurgitation [3] and assess diastolic function [4]. While invasive angiographic methods enable an assessment of the anatomy of the coronary circulation, their ability to quantitate myocardial perfusion territory is more challenging. For that reason, the concept of visualizing and quantitating myocardial perfusion at the bedside with echocardiography combined with the injection of air filled microbubbles has generated continued interest. The goal of this evolving technique is to track myocardial perfusion by intravenous injection of microbubbles which are small enough to pass through the right heart, and pulmonary circulation thus appearing in the left heart and coronary circulation. When properly constructed, the microbubbles reflect sound and thus their

J.H.C. Reiber and E.E. van der Wall (eds.), Cardiovascular Imaging, 461-472.
© 1996 *Kluwer Academic Publishers.*

appearance in cardiac chambers and myocardium can be easily identified by an increased signal during standard transthoracic echocardiography. This technique has the potential for combining the in-vivo assessment of myocardial perfusion with simultaneous evaluation of cardiac structure and function. The recent development of nontoxic microbubbles with mean diameters less than that of pulmonary capillaries now makes this goal attainable.

Microbubble effects

Microbubbles are composed of gases surrounded by a liquid. These microbubbles are strong reflectors of sound due to the large difference in acoustic impedance between the gas entrapped within the bubble and the liquid (blood). Because bubbles are spherical, the intensity of their reflections are independent of the direction of the ultrasound source. The amplitude or strength of the reflected signal from the bubble varies linearly with the 6th power of a bubble's radius [5]. The reflected signal is also influenced by the resonance of bubbles. The resonant frequency is the frequency that results in the greatest amount of reflected signal and is a function of bubble size and intra-cavitary pressure [6].

Microbubble stability

The clearance of microbubbles occurs in capillary networks which entrap microbubbles with diameters greater than the capillaries. Here they are broken into fragments with release of their gaseous core. Pulmonary capillaries range in size from 1 to 16 micron with the majority of capillaries in the 4 to 8 micron range [7]. Thus the passage of bubbles is a function of size and they must be smaller than 8 micron to consistently pass through the pulmonary capillary bed to reach the left heart. Microbubbles also slowly shrink in size as their gaseous core diffuse into the surrounding undersaturated blood [8]. This rate of bubble dissolution is related to the solubility and diffusivity of the gas. In the past, most contrast agents were composed of air-filled microbubbles but recently gases with lower solubility and/or diffusivity have been used to improve persistence and stability. These gases include helium, nitrogen, perfluoropropane, sulfur hexafluoride and emulsions of dodecafluoropentane [9,10]. The rate of bubble dissolution is also a function of bubble size since the smaller bubbles, by virtue of higher surface tension, have a higher internal pressure which facilitates outward gas diffusion and encourages bubble dissolution. Surfactant properties of viscous liquids decrease the surface tension of the bubbles in solution and therefore prolong bubble life.

Bubble stability is also a function of the surrounding pressure, frequency of the sound used for imaging and the motion of the bubble inside the liquid [11-15]. Clinical studies have suggested and experimental studies have confirmed that for some agents there is a disappearance of the contrast effect in the left ventricle during systole [12,16]. The video intensity of the contrast decreases significantly faster when microbubbles are exposed to high systemic pressures and this effect appears most prominent for smaller bubbles (Figure 1). Potential explanations for this phenomenon include accelerated breakage of the bubbles, accelerated diffusion of gas out of the bubbles and transient compression of bubbles [11,12]. An additional effect of pressure on microbubbles is observed during exposure to ultrasound. The ultrasound pulses used for clinical transthoracic echocardiography can generate acoustic pressure waves which can result in local pressures of over 10,000 mmHg and affect bubble stability.

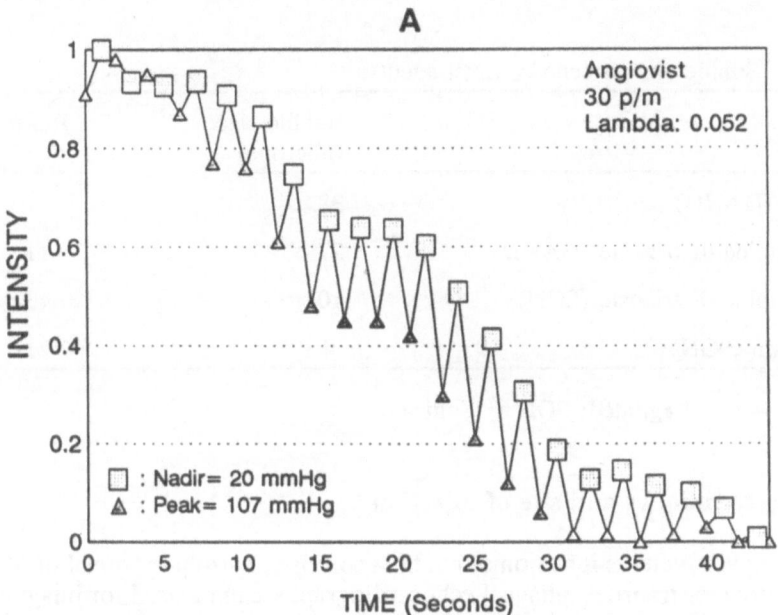

Figure 1. Example of pressure sensitivity of contrast effect. Hand agitated meglumine diatrizoate was exposed to pulsatile pressures of 107/20 mmHg in a closed chamber. A pulsatile alteration in videointensity is noted - with a decrease in intensity during the peak pressure and a partial recovery of intensity during the nadir pressure. In addition a more gradual decay in video intensity is observed. (From Padial et al., J Am Soc Echocardiogr 1995;8:285-92)

Thus the challenge in contrast echocardiography is to gain a full understanding of the factors which influence bubble stability and to construct bubbles that allow excellent backscatter and survival. Larger bubbles act as more effective scatterers of sound and have the potential for a longer survival before dissolution, yet the bubbles must be small enough to pass through capillaries.

Microbubble production

Microbubble size is a function of the method of production. Sonication results in bubbles of smaller size and a narrower range of diameters than hand agitation (Table 1). The earliest agents were composed of sterile saline but the poor surfactant properties resulted in survival times too short to allow adequate time for imaging. Angiographic contrast agents (meglumine diatrizoate), indocyanine green, lipids and gelatin possess surfactant properties which provide longer stability and all have been used in experimental studies [17-19]. Sonication of human serum albumin results in a microbubble with a 30-50 nm shell. This shell reduces backscatter but results in increased stability and bubble life long enough for systemic and intracardiac transit. This approach yields bubbles of 4-5 micron which have rheologic properties similar to red blood cells [20-22].

Table 1. Bubble size of echo contrast agents.

Agent	Bubble size (microns)	Ref.#
Saline (HAND)	38	11
Meglumine diatrizoate (HAND)	27	11
Meglumine diatrizoate (SON)	10	43
Albumin (SON)	4.9	21

HAND = Hand agitated; SON = Sonicated

Imaging techniques and site of injection

Following intravenous injection of contrast solution, two-dimensional or M-mode transthoracic or transoesophageal echocardiography can be used for imaging. The specific imaging planes are dictated by the purpose of the contrast study: LV cavity opacification, endocardial border detection, Doppler signal enhancement or myocardial enhancement. Parasternal short axis and apical views can be used to assess myocardial perfusion (Figure 2). Short axis planes allow tomographic images which mirror histologic sections used to quantitate infarct size and area at risk [23]. Apical four chamber views on the other hand allow for simultaneous visualization of all cardiac chambers which may be helpful to assess transit time, global ventricular function and the base to apex extent of myocardial perfusion. With current agents where microbubble survival is a limiting factor, the site of microbubble injection determines the chamber with optimal contrast enhancement. Right sided ventricular opacification is easily obtained with venous injections. Invasive or intra-arterial injections (left atrium, left ventricle, coronary artery, aortic root) presently provide the best left-sided contrast enhancement for myocardial perfusion. Detection of myocardial perfusion from intravenous injections of sonicated albumin using standard echocardiography has been limited. Uptake in the septum has been demonstrated using transoesophageal echocardiography [24]. Others have detected contrast enhancement of the myocardium by transthoracic echocardiography [25,26]. Most approaches to date have required the additional use of coronary vasodilators to expand the coronary-myocardial blood and contrast volume. Modifications to image acquisition have improved the ability to detect contrast in the myocardium following intravenous injection. For example, interrupted or triggered imaging, results in only one

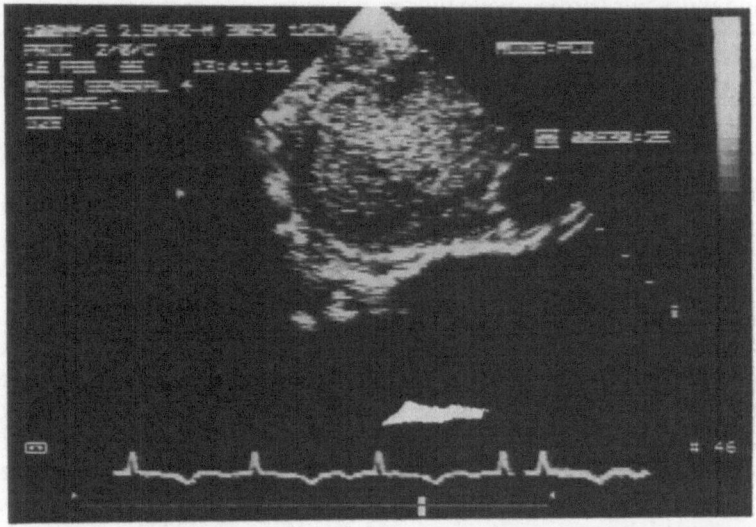

a

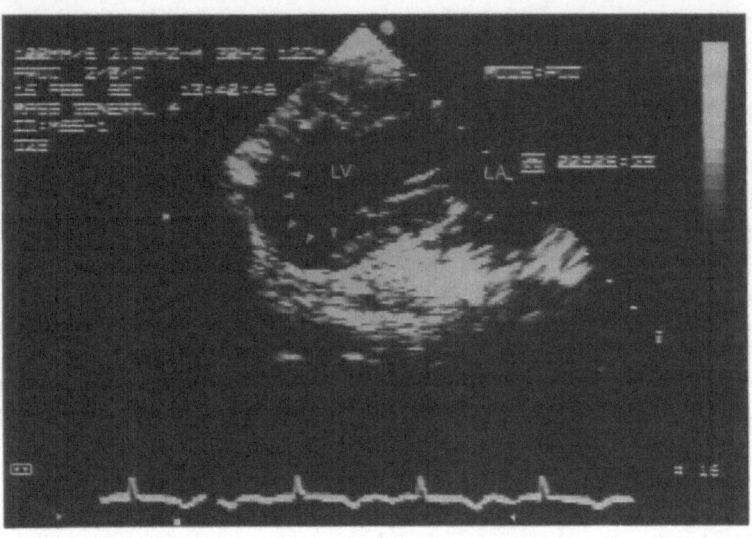

b

Figure 2. (A) Modified transthoracic echocardiographic long axis view demonstrating appearance of sonicated albumin microbubbles in the left ventricle after intravenous injection in an ovine model 28 days after ligation of left anterior descending coronary artery. (B) After passage of contrast from left ventricle into the coronary circulation, an increase in video intensity is observed in the more basal portions of the myocardium with a resultant defect in perfusion in the apex (arrows). This defect corresponds to the infarcted region of myocardium. LV - left ventricle; LA - left atrium.

ultrasound pulse per cardiac cycle thus reducing bubble destruction and increasing the delivery to the myocardium [14]. Second harmonic imaging which takes advantage of bubble specific resonant properties also results in improved visualization of myocardial contrast from intravenous injection [27,28].

Experimental and clinical studies

Invasive contrast echocardiography

Direct injection of echocardiographic contrast at the level of the coronary arteries, left atrium, left ventricle or aortic root has the potential to improve the assessment of: blood flow, myocardial blood volume, microvascular integrity, myocardial viability, myocardial ischemia/infarction (location, extent and degree), the influence of collateral circulation and bypass graft function. Prior to investigations of the intravenous injection technique, most studies utilized a left sided injection. This has allowed the study of contrast echo under conditions where contrast delivery is optimized and therefore should demonstrate the true accuracy of the technique.

One of the most promising uses of contrast echocardiography via invasive injection has been in the setting of acute myocardial infarction for the assessment of area at risk, infarct size, and viability during coronary occlusion. This has clinical importance since the area at risk is the most important determinant of ultimate infarct size. Early experimental studies using renografin have demonstrated the ability of this contrast technique to accurately delineate the area subtended by an occluded artery and in jeopardy of necrosis [29]. In contrast to normally perfused myocardial zones, during coronary occlusion the regions supplied by the occluded artery will not opacify (Figure 2). In addition, during successful reperfusion and repeat contrast injection, improved myocardial blood flow can result in improvement in myocardial opacification. The quantification of the area at risk by intra-arterial myocardial contrast echo has been compared to technetium autoradiography and other histopathologic measures. Early studies by Kaul demonstrated an excellent correlation ($r=0.96$) of in-vivo contrast and the post-mortem "gold standard" [29]. In such studies using short axis planes the only region of the left ventricular myocardium incompletely assessed is the true apex. Indirect markers of the area at risk such as hemodynamic indices and left ventricular performance (cardiac output, LV ejection fraction, mean arterial pressure) have also been compared to intra-arterial myocardial contrast measurement in the coronary occlusion model. In such experimental studies a risk area of greater than 25-40% was required to produce significant hemodynamic changes. Normalized cardiac output and left ventricular ejection fraction were inversely related to the area at risk [30]. In such investigations the relationship between area at risk and infarct size detected at post-mortem was linear and dependent on the duration of coronary occlusion.

Quantitation of myocardial perfusion is based on the assumption that the microbubbles travel in concert with the surrounding blood through the epicardial coronary arteries and into the capillary networks unimpeded. If microbubbles are not destroyed during transit they can act as intravascular tracers since they remain in the myocardial circulation. These tracers then concentrate in myocardial regions relative to myocardial blood flow. If one assumes constant myocardial blood volume and that the concentration of bubbles exiting the region of interest is identical to that which entered this region, a change in microbubble transit time (as assessed by the video-intensity time relation within the myocardium) should correlate with regional myocardial blood flow [31]. Quantitation of flow has been a challenge since many factors influence the stability of the injected bolus of contrast. For this reason, at present, most quantitation of myocardial blood flow and blood volume is performed via direct coronary injection to insure that a predictable and reproducible bolus of contrast can be delivered to the region of interest. An additional limitation to simple methods to quantitate flow based on the time-video intensity relationship of the contrast effect is that the relation between bubble concentration and video intensity must be linear and this is not necessarily the case for most echocardiographic instruments for the range of concentrations utilized in clinical practice. To overcome this limitation, more complex functions can be used to quantitate flow or the processing variables of the echocardiographic instrument can be modified for each contrast agent.

The use of myocardial contrast echo to predict myocardial salvage following thrombolysis has attracted much interest. Ito and colleagues investigated 39 patients with first acute anterior myocardial infarction undergoing acute reperfusion [32]. Sonicated angiographic contrast was injected directly into the left and then the right coronary systems before and after either intracoronary thrombolysis or PTCA. Although the reperfusion was graded as successful in all angiographic methods, the myocardial contrast echo method defined two groups following reperfusion: those with persistent myocardial opacification defects ("no reflow") and those without defects (successful reflow). Follow-up wall-motion and ejection fractions were compared on days 1 and 28 following MI. In those with successful reperfusion by contrast echo, improvement in both regional and global function occurred during the first month post-MI. In contrast, the degree of improvement especially in wall motion score and extent of dysfunction was markedly less or absent for those with evidence of no reflow. Thus myocardial contrast echo has the potential to provide early prognostic information about the success of coronary reperfusion.

A most important observation from this study is that in a subgroup of patients whose reperfusion was deemed successful by coronary angiography, a lack of adequate myocardial perfusion was noted by the contrast echo technique. This highlights the difference in the two techniques and a potential advantage of contrast echo since the strength of contrast angiography is in the assessment of the epicardial arteries and the strength of contrast echo is its assessment of perfusion territory. This report by Ito also provides clinical support for the earlier observation of the no reflow phenomenon in an experimental model of coronary occlusion and thrombolysis by Kloner and colleagues [33]. Extensive myocardial necrosis, myocardial edema and microcirculatory damage have been hypothesized as the causes of an impeded microcirculatory flow. Subsequent clinical studies using intracoronary contrast echo have demonstrated adverse effects of no reflow with a higher incidence of post-MI ventricular dilatation, symptomatic heart failure and mortality compared to similarly treated infarct patients with successful reflow [34].

The assessment of collateral flow in humans has been hampered by the ability of current methods to resolve the small collateral vascular channels. Myocardial enhancement from contrast echocardiography has been demonstrated to result from flow via collateral vessels [35]. Experimental studies have shown that this contrast effect can be detected with collateral flows lower than 0.3 cc/min/gm which is the flow rate necessary to preserve myocardial function [36]. Invasive contrast echocardiography has been utilized to demonstrate in patients with acute and subacute myocardial infarction, that collateral circulation can maintain perfusion and function but that restoration of anterograde flow is necessary for a consistent improvement in regional function [37]. Using intracoronary injections of contrast echo to document the presence or absence of collaterals, it has been demonstrated that successful reperfusion up to five weeks following coronary occlusion can improve regional function in areas with preserved collateral flow [38].

Contrast echocardiography has utility in the operating room to determine the most effective route and adequacy of cardioplegia. This has been accomplished by examining perfusion patterns obtained by aortic root and coronary sinus injections [39]. Quantitation of relative contrast intensity in the myocardium after direct injection into bypass grafts has been used to predict late improvement in recovery of myocardial function in patients undergoing CABG after myocardial infarction [40].

Intravenous studies

The prospect of detection of myocardial perfusion from an intravenous injection of echocardiographic contrast agents has been the major force responsible for the development of this field. Potential applications include the bedside assessment of the success of reperfusion therapy, the outpatient diagnosis of significant coronary artery disease, assessment of the physiologic significance of coronary collateral vessels, assessment of myocardial perfusion before and after interventions, and as an adjunct to stress echocardiography to relate coronary anatomy and physiology to ventricular structure and function. To date, the available contrast agents approved for clinical use have limited ability to assess myocardial perfusion using standard transthoracic echocardiographic instruments and partial success with newer imaging techniques such as second harmonic imaging [27]. New investigational agents, however, have been demonstrated to opacify the myocardium from intravenous injections [41].

Villaneuva and colleagues correlated area at risk and infarct size by contrast echo using right heart injections of sonicated albumin to technetium sestamibi autoradiography in a canine model of left anterior descending coronary artery occlusion and reperfusion. With the adjunctive use of adenosine and/or dobutamine, optimal images of myocardial opacification were achieved from right atrial injections in 65% compared with 89% of left atrial injections. Comparable linear relations between the two methods for area at risk and infarct size were noted for both the right atrial and left atrial injections [42,23]. In addition, transmural myocardial blood flow during reperfusion, measured by radioactive microspheres, was inversely correlated with the myocardial contrast echo area at risk. These data suggest that right sided injections of echocardiographic contrast can detect, in vivo, infarct size or area at risk in the setting of myocardial infarction and reperfusion. When these findings are combined with those from left atrial and intracoronary injections, it would appear that intravenous myocardial contrast echo, particularly when combined with pharmacologic agents to enhance coronary delivery, has the potential to distinguish viable from infarcted myocardium. Recently, Grayburn et al. [41] reported similar results from peripheral venous injections utilizing a dodecafluoropentane emulsion.

Limitations

With currently available agents, a major limitation has been the inability to image the myocardium in the far field due to attenuation of the signal from the contrast in the left ventricular cavity. This can be overcome by utilizing multiple imaging planes. In addition attenuation appears to be minimized with the newest investigational agents especially those whose effect persists in the myocardium after ventricular opacification has resolved. Another limitation as discussed above, is that a greater understanding of the relation of video intensity and bubble concentration is necessary for all echocardiographic instruments and all contrast agents before quantitation of blood flow and blood volume can be routinely accomplished. Additionally, the instruments and images must be optimized for each agent without sacrificing the quality of the noncontrast images. Lastly, due to an inability to deliver a high enough concentration of bubbles to the myocardium from a peripheral intravenous injection, at present most applications of myocardial contrast echocardiography for perfusion are with direct, invasive injections.

In the current era of health care reform additional challenges to the clinical application of contrast echocardiography arise. These include minimizing the cost of these agents, simplifying the delivery of the agents, and establishing the cost effectiveness of the technique.

Numerous studies using a range of contrast agents have demonstrated the safety, utility and potential of contrast echocardiography. The assessment of myocardial perfusion by echocardiography from intravenous injections requires agents that can be reproducibly delivered to the left heart in concentrations large enough to opacify the myocardium. As our understanding of the factors influencing microbubbles is translated into the development of new agents, and as imaging parameters are optimized and echocardiographic instruments are improved, the prospect of noninvasive, bedside assessment of myocardial perfusion appears closer.

References

1. Gramiak R, Shah PM. Echocardiography of the aortic root. Invest Radiol 1968;3:356-66.
2. Valdes-Cruz LM, Sahn DJ. Ultrasonic contrast studies from the detection of cardiac shunts. J Am Coll Cardiol 1984;3:978-85.
3. Reid CL, Kawanishi DT, KcKay CR, Elkayam U, Rahimtoola SH, Chandraratna PA. Accuracy of evaluation of the presence and severity of aortic

and mitral regurgitation by contrast 2-dimensional echocardiography. Am J Cardiol 1983;52:519-24.

4.   Williams MJA, McClements BM, Picard MH. Improvement of transthoracic pulmonary venous flow Doppler signal with intravenous injection of sonicated albumin. J Am Coll Cardiol 1995;26:1741-6.

5.   Powsner SM, Keller MW, Saniie J, Feinstein SB. Quantitation of echo-contrast effects. Am J Physiol Imaging 1986;1:124-8.

6.   De Jong N, ten Cate FJ, Lancée CT, Roelandt JRTC, Bom N. Principles and recent developments in ultrasound contrast agents. Ultrasonics 1991;29:324-30.

7.   Hogg JC, Neutrophil kinetics and lung injury. Physiol Rev 1987;67:1249-95.

8.   Epstein PS, Plesset MS. On the stability of gas bubbles in liquid-gas solutions. J Chem Phys 1950;18:1505-9.

9.   Porter TR, Xie F. Visually discernible myocardial echocardiographic contrast after intravenous injection of sonicated dextrose albumin microbubbles containing high molecular weight, less soluble gases. J Am Coll Cardiol 1995;25:509-15.

10. DeMaria AN, Dittrich H, Kwan OL, Kimura B. Myocardial opacification produced by peripheral venous injection of a new ultrasonic contrast agent [abstract]. Circulation 1993;88(4 pt 2):I-401.

11. Vuille C, Nidorf M, Morrissey RL, Newell JB, Weyman AE, Picard MH. Effect of static pressure on the disappearance rate of specific echocardiographic contrast agents. J Am Soc Echocardiogr 1994;7:347-54.

12. Padial LR, Chen MH, Vuille C, Guerrero JL, Weyman AE, Picard MH. Pulsatile pressure affects the disappearance of echocardiographic contrast agents. J Am Soc Echocardiogr 1995;8:285-92.

13. Mor-Avi V, Shroff SG, Robinson KA et al. Effects of left ventricular pressure on sonicated albumin microbubbles: evaluation using an isolated rabbit heart model. J Am Coll Cardiol 1994;24:1779-85.

14. Porter TR, Xie F. Transient myocardial contrast after initial exposure to diagnostic ultrasound pressures with minute doses of intravenously injected microbubbles. Circulation 1995;92:2391-5.

15. Rovai D, Lombardi M, Ghelardi G et al. Discordance between responses of contrast echo intensity to increased flow rate in human coronary circulation and in vitro. Am Heart J 1992;124:398-404.

16. Shapiro JR, Reisner SQA, Lichtenberg GS, Meltzer RS. Intravenous contrast echocardiography with the use of sonicated albumin in humans: systolic disappearance of left ventricular contrast after transpulmonary transmission. J Am Coll Cardiol 1990;16:1603-7.

17. Feinstein SB. Myocardial perfusion imaging: contrast echocardiography today and tomorrow [editorial]. J Am Coll Cardiol 1986;8:251-3.

18. Unger EC, Lund PJ, Shen DK, Fritz TA, Yellowhair D, New TE. Nitrogen-filled liposomes as a vascular US contrast agent: preliminary evaluation. Radiology 1992;185:453-6.

19. Meltzer RS, Klig V, Teichholz LE. Generating precission microbubbles for use as an echocardiographic contrast agent. J Am Coll Cardiol 1985;5:978-82.

20. Reisner SA, Ong LS, Lichtenberg GS et al. Myocardial perfusion imaging by contrast echocardiography with use of intracoronary sonicated albumin in humans. J Am Coll Cardiol 1989;14:660-5.

21. Keller MW, Segal SS, Kaul S, Duing BR. The behavior of sonicated albumin microbubbles in the microcirculation: a basis for their use during myocardial

contrast echo. Circ Res 1989;65:458-67.

22. Keller MW, Glasheen WP, Kaul S. Albunex a safe and effective commercially produced agent for myocardial contrast echo. J Am Soc Echocardiogr 1989;2:48-52.

23. Villaneuva FS, Glasheen WP, Sklenar J, Kaul S. Assessment of risk area during coronary occlusion and infarct size after reperfusion with myocardial contrast echocardiography using left and right atrial injections of contrast. Circulation 1993;88:596-604.

24. Voci P, Bilotta F, Merialdo P, Agati L. Myocardial contrast enhancement after intravenous injection of sonicated albumin microbubbles: a transoesophageal echocardiography dipyridamole study. J Am Soc Echocardiogr 1994;7:337-46.

25. Villaneuva FS, Glasheen WP, Sklenar J, Jayaweera AR, Kaul S. Successful and reproducible myocardial opacification during two-dimensional echocardiography from right heart injection of contrast. Circulation 1992;85:1557-64.

26. Saunders W, Cheirif J, Desier R et al. Contrast opacification of left ventricular myocardium following intravenous administration of sonicated albumin microspheres. Am Heart J 1991;122:1660-5.

27. Feinstein S, Pascoe R, Picard M et al. Harmonic imaging in patients following intravenous contrast injections: preliminary data [abstract]. Circulation 1995;92(Suppl.I):I-463.

28. De Jong N, ten Cate FJ, Lancée CT, Roelandt JRTC, Bom N. Principles and recent developments in ultrasound contrast agents. Ultrasonics 1991;29:324-30.

29. Kaul S, Pandian NG, Okada RD, Pohost GM, Weyman AE. Contrast echocardiography in acute myocardial ischemia: I. in vivo determination of total left ventricular "area at risk". J Am Coll Cardiol 1984;4:1272-82.

30. Kaul S, Glasheen W, Ruddy TD, Pandian NG, Weyman AE, Okada RD. The importance of defining left ventricular area at risk in vivo during acute myocardial infarction: an experimental evaluation with myocardial contrast two-dimensional echocardiography. Circulation 1987;75:1249-60.

31. Skyab DM, Jayaweera AR, Goodman NC, Ismail S, Camarano G, Kaul S. Quantification of myocardial perfusion with myocardial contrast echocardiography during left atrial injection for contrst: implications fro venous injection. Circulation 1994;90:1513-21.

32. Ito H, Tomooka T, Sakai N et al. Lack of myocardial perfusion immediately after successful thrombolysis. Circulation 1992;85:1699-1705.

33. Kloner RA, Ganote CE, Jennings RB. The 'no re-flow' phenomenon after temporary coronary occlusion in the dog. J Clin Invest 1974;54:1496-1508.

34. Ito H, Maruyama A, Iwakura K et al. Clinical implications of the 'no reflow' phenomenon: a predictor of complications and left ventricular remodelling in reperfused anterior wall myocardial infarction. Circulation 1996;93:223-8.

35. Kemper AJ, O'Boyle JE, Sharma S et al. Hydrogen peroxide contrast-enhanced two-dimensional echocardiography: real-time in vivo delineation of regional myocardial perfusion. Circulation 1983;68:603.

36. Cheirif JB, Narkiewicz-Jodko JB, Hawkins HK, Bravenac JS, Quinones MA. Myocardial contrast echocardiography: relation of collateral perfusion to extent of injury and severity of contractile dysfunction in a canine model of coronary thrombosis and reperfusion. J Am Coll Cardiol 1995;26:537-46.

37. Ragosta M, Camarano G, Kaul S, Powers ER, Sarembock IJ, Gimple LW. Microvascular integrity indicates myocellular viability in patients with recent myocardial infarction: new insights using myocardial contrast echocardiography.

Circulation 1994;89:2562-9.

38. Sabia PJ, Powers ER, Ragosta M, Sarembock IJ, Burwell LR, Kaul S. An association between collateral blood flow and myocardial viability in patients with recent myocardial infarction. N Engl J Med 1992;327:1825-31.

39. Wei K, Omran AS, Ikonomidis J et al. Optimizing myocardial perfusion during coronary bypass - a contrast echo study. J Am Soc Echocardiogr 1995;8:341.

40. Hirata N, Shimazaki Y, Nakano S, Sakai K, Sakaki S, Matsuda H. Evaluation of regional myocardial perfusion in areas of old myocardial infarction after revascularization by means of intraoperative myocardial contrast echocardiography. J Thorac Cardiovasc Surg 1994;108:1119-24.

41. Grayburn P, Erickson JM, Escobar J, Womack L, Velasco CE. Peripheral intravenous myocardial contrast echocardiography using a 2% dodecafluoropentane emulsion: identification of myocardial risk area and infarct size in the canine model of ischemia. J Am Coll Cardiol 1995;26:1340-7.

42. Villaneuva FS, Glasheen WP, Sklenar J, Jayaweera AR, Kaul S. Successful and reproducible myocardial opacification during two-dimensional echocardiography from right heart injection of contrast. Circulation 1992;85:1557-64.

43. Feinstrein SB, Ten Cate FJ, Zwehl W et al. Two-dimensional contrast echocardiography. I. in vitro development and quantitative analysis of echo contrast agents. J Am Coll Cardiol 1984;3:14-20.

36. Newer imaging techniques in contrast echocardiography

SHARON L. MULVAGH

Summary

Newer imaging techniques in contrast echocardiography are rapidly evolving concurrent with the development of newer contrast agents able to produce left ventricular cavity and myocardial opacification after an intravenous injection. Harmonic imaging and noncontinuous ultrasound transmission are such developments in the application of ultrasound technology. Harmonic imaging is a new approach to the detection of echocardiographic contrast agents which exploits the nonlinear response of microbubbles when exposed to ultrasound energy. Microbubbles resonating in an acoustic field generate sub and supra harmonic emissions which occur at multiples of the insonifying frequency. Since tissues that do not contain contrast agent do not produce such a response, the identification of contrast in perfused structures is enhanced by detection of higher harmonic signals. Blood pool cavities, vascularized tissue and coronary vessels have been clearly defined during harmonic imaging of contrast agents. Early observations in patients have demonstrated the potential of harmonic imaging alone, or in combination with transient suspension of ultrasound, to achieve enhanced noninvasive assessment of ventricular function and myocardial perfusion.

Introduction

Contrast echocardiography has evolved rapidly, due to major recent advances in both contrast agent development and ultrasound equipment technology. Transpulmonary passage of intravenously administered contrast agents and resultant left ventricular opacification has been demonstrated in humans [1,2]. Newer agents, containing various stabilizing gases, produce both left ventricular and myocardial opacification after intravenous injection in animal models during normal and altered perfusion states [3-9]. Experimental human studies indicate similar findings [10,11] suggesting enormous potential for the clinical application of these new agents. However, the myocardial contrast effect is variably detected when imaged with standard commercially available ultrasound equipment, and if higher doses are utilized to improve detectability, attenuation from within the ventricles frequently interferes with complete visualization of the myocardium. Harmonic ultrasound imaging is a method to enhance the detection of ultrasound contrast agents within blood-containing cavities and vascularized tissue [12,13]. This novel ultrasonic detection method is enabled by the nonlinear emission of harmonics by resonant microbubbles pulsating in an ultrasonic field [14,15]. Prototype ultrasound systems currently under investigation employing this principle utilize specialized transducers and software to transmit ultrasound at the

473

J.H.C. Reiber and E.E. van der Wall (eds.), Cardiovascular Imaging, 473-484.
© 1996 *Kluwer Academic Publishers.*

fundamental frequency (*f*) and receive ultrasound at a multiple of this frequency (i.e. 2*f*, 3*f*, etc). For example, to detect the second harmonic of ultrasound transmitted at 2.5 MHz, the system would receive signals at 5 MHz. Detection of sub-harmonics in addition to supra-harmonics is theoretically possible, although preclinical and clinical evaluations to date have focussed upon detection of the second harmonic (2*f*). Contrast containing structures are enhanced relative to the surrounding noncontrast filled structures, thereby increasing the strength of the "signal" relative to the background "noise". This has significant implications for clinical detection of myocardial perfusion by contrast echocardiography. The basic principles of harmonic imaging during continuous and transient ultrasound delivery will be reviewed, followed by preclinical and clinical experience with various gas-filled microbubbles demonstrating promising potential applications.

Harmonic ultrasound imaging

Traditionally, the most important property of ultrasonic contrast agents has been their capacity to enhance the backscatter signal by creating numerous small reflective surfaces and produce 2-dimensional images of greater definition. Free or encapsulated gas bubbles have been considered superior to colloidal suspensions, emulsions or aqueous solutions in their ability to enhance backscatter [16]. However, bubbles additionally exhibit properties more complex than other scatterers. When placed in an ultrasound field, the bubbles oscillate in a complicated manner dependent upon the size and composition of the bubble, the nature of the surrounding medium, and the ultrasound frequency [14]. This oscillation of bubbles results in the emission of sound waves with a wide range of frequencies, a feature which is termed "nonlinear behaviour". The emission of ultrasound is greatest when the bubbles are insonified at their optimal resonant "first" harmonic, or "fundamental" frequency. In this case, higher harmonic (2*f*, 3*f*, 4*f*, etc.) signals will be emitted very efficiently and their amplitude may be greater than the signals at the insonifying frequency. Imaging of these harmonic ultrasound signals is undergoing intensive investigation and development. Second harmonic ultrasound imaging of newer contrast agents has been shown to provide improved detection of left ventricular contrast agent intensity and duration in animal and human studies [17,18]. Myocardial perfusion has been demonstrated noninvasively in animal studies during intravenous injection of perfluorocarbon contrast agents imaged with harmonic ultrasound [9,19,20].

The first theoretical description of the behavior of bubbles exposed to an external pressure field was established by Lord Rayleigh in 1917 through simple observations of a boiling tea kettle [21], and served as the basis for extensive complex numerical and in vitro investigations exploring the nonlinear behavior of small gas bubbles in an ultrasonic field [22-25]. Tucker and Welsby proposed that the detection of second harmonic ultrasound signals was a very sensitive indicator for the presence of intravascular bubbles in subjects being monitored for decompression sickness [26]. Characterization of the nonlinear second harmonic emissions from resonant bubbles was done in vitro by Miller [15] and was shown to be related to bubble size, with a smaller bubble size producing a more profound second harmonic response.

Experimental in-vitro studies have suggested that the detection of nonlinear ultrasound contrast agents within blood containing cavities and vascularized tissue could provide the capability to allow real-time imaging of flowing blood and, ultimately, organ perfusion with ultrasound [12,13,27]. Myocardial blood perfusion has been historically difficult to quantify because of the characteristically slow movement of red blood cells through the capillaries, and the small amount of blood contained within a perfused volume. Thus the overwhelming tissue signal obscures detection of the blood signal. However, tissue artifact and inadequate blood signal intensity can be overcome by studying the second harmonic component of the backscattered echo, which is much greater in magnitude for the contrast agent than for the tissue. This enables detection of slow, small volume blood flow in the presence of the more prevalent tissue, whose reflection at the fundamental frequency overwhelms the signal from the blood. Harmonic imaging theoretically should allow measurement of relative changes in blood perfusion, permitting the echocardiographic assessment of myocardial perfusion to determine regions of inadequate or absent blood supply. Indeed, we have been able to demonstrate the detection and measurement of coronary blood flow during transthoracic harmonic imaging of nonlinear contrast agents in the canine model [20]. Similarly, detection of myocardial tissue contrast in preclinical and early clinical studies during harmonic imaging confirm the dramatic improvement in signal-to-noise ratio when using this technique, although best results have been obtained when transmission of ultrasound is intermittently suspended [28,29].

Noncontinuous ultrasound delivery

The novel approach of intermittent insonification by R-wave triggered acquisition of cardiac images, a method which has been coined "transient response imaging" or TRI [28,29] , has only recently been described. The reduced ultrasound exposure, in contrast to real-time imaging, results in increased intensity and persistence of contrast effect within the left ventricular cavity, and more notably, in the myocardium. We have observed that the combination of reduced acoustic power with TRI enables much improved detection of contrast microbubbles within the myocardium, improving the potential for noninvasive perfusion imaging [30]. Preliminary clinical studies suggest the combination of second harmonic imaging, and TRI may provide enhanced detection of myocardial perfusion [29]. The theories as to why transient suspension of ultrasound enhances contrast effect include the possibilities of reduced microbubble destruction or, conversely, transient cavitation and release of ultrasound energy.

Contrast agent interactions with newer ultrasound imaging techniques

Recent advances in contrast agent development have resulted in the development of free or coated microbubbles (i.e. albumin, galactose, phospholipids, surfactants) containing inert, relatively heavy, poorly soluble gases (i.e.

perfluorocarbons, sulfur hexafluoride). These microbubbles range in size between 1 and 10 μm and persist in the circulation for up to several minutes.

The myocardial contrast effect of these new agents is variably detectable depending upon the agent and imaging technique. If higher doses are utilized to increase the myocardial microbubble concentration, attenuation from within the right and left ventricles frequently interferes with complete visualization of the myocardium. Harmonic imaging can enhance microbubble detection, enabling the utilization of lower doses of contrast agent, thereby reducing the problem of attenutation.

The resonance phenomenon resulting in the generation of harmonic signals is dependent not only upon the bubble radius, which determines the resonant frequency, but also the interrelated factors of acoustic pressure and velocity of the wavefront, the characteristics of the surrounding medium, and the composition and viscoelastic properties of the microbubble shell [14]. The second harmonic potential of many of these new contrast agents has been demonstrated [17] and a multitude of clinical applications are evolving (see below). Fortunately, the resonant frequency of the microbubbles utilized in contrast echocardiography (median size less than 6 μm), coincides with the range of ultrasound routinely employed during transthoracic echocardiography (2 to 4 MHz). Transmission of ultrasound at or near the resonant frequency of the contrast microbubbles enhances the harmonic signals and improves the detection of contrast agent by second harmonic imaging during clinical cardiac ultrasound examinations. Most contrast agents are composed of microbubbles with a range of sizes rather than a single uniform dimension. This feature may be an additional clinical advantage for second harmonic imaging, as the ultrasound transducers may not need to be precisely tuned to the bubbles, but can employ a broad bandwidth and still reliably produce harmonic effects.

Newer ultrasound equipment technology

In addition to having a contrast agent capable of harmonic resonance, second harmonic imaging requires echocardiographic equipment capable of exploiting this phenomenon. Several ultrasound manufacturers are now developing or modifiying existing transducers and imaging systems to permit harmonic imaging. Although laboratory measurements of harmonic signals have employed separate transducers for transmission and reception, this is not practical for clinical imaging. Instead, clinical systems utilize broad band transducers which are driven at a low frequency (usually 1.8 to 2.5 MHz) and receive across a wide range of frequencies (usually 3.6 to 5.0 MHz) permitting detection of the second harmonic. Electronic signal processing is then employed to process and display the harmonic frequencies. Because there is overlap between the actual transmitted frequency range and the second harmonic signals which are processed, the images usually contain some higher frequency fundamental image data. This results in the display of the background tissues, which theoretically do not emit significant harmonic signals. The background tissues are relatively weakly displayed compared to signal from the contrast agent so the theoretical advantage of "improved signal to background noise" of second harmonic imaging is maintained, and the fundamental tissue image provides an orienting reference when contrast is not present, facilitating clinical imaging. Second harmonic principles have been implemented not only for gray scale imaging, but also for color flow, pulsed wave and continuous wave Doppler. While these other modalities have been less extensively evaluated than gray scale imaging, their sensitivity and specificity for contrast agents appear to be improved with in vivo gains of more than 30 dB demonstrated [31].

Experimental observations and potential clinical applications of newer imaging techniques in contrast echocardiography

Very recent and ongoing experimental studies have demonstrated that the harmonic signals generated by oscillating microbubbles improve the identification of contrast agents within the left ventricular blood pool, myocardial tissue and coronary vasculature. Transient suspension of ultrasound delivery may further enhance contrast effect.

Left ventricular blood pool cavity enhancement by second harmonic contrast echocardiography

Left ventricular opacification can be utilized in general echocardiography as well as in special imaging situations such as stress echocardiography. In canine studies evaluating various intravenously injected contrast agents we have shown that second harmonic ultrasound imaging results in a 15-70 % increase in left ventricular cavity contrast intensity, as well as increased duration of detection [32]. Qualitative and quantitative assessment of left ventricular opacification during second harmonic imaging of peripherally injected contrast agents has recently been done in humans, and has demonstrated improved left ventricular cavity enhancement compared to fundamental contrast enhanced imaging. DeMaria and coworkers have reported a seven times increase in the ratio of left ventricular cavity to myocardial intensity in five patients undergoing second harmonic imaging compared to standard transthoracic echocardiography during injections of Levovist[R] (Schering AG, Berlex USA) [18]. Similarly, we have found a 35 to 105 % increase in the background-subtracted pixel intensity within the left ventricular cavity in ten patients undergoing stress echocardiography and peripheral injections of Levovist® [33] (Figure 1). Similar objective increases in pixel intensity during second harmonic imaging have been observed with Albunex® (Mallinckrodt Medical, USA) in patients undergoing pharmacologic stress echocardiography [34] (Figure 2), confirming the visual impression of improved left ventricular cavity delineation with second harmonic imaging when compared to fundamental contrast echocardiography. We have currently studied 14 patients referred for diagnostic echocardiography with MRX-115 (Aerosomes®, ImaRx Pharmaceutical Corp., USA) an intravenously injected perfluorocarbon containing contrast agent composed of microbubbles contained within a liposomal membrane, and have noted markedly persistent and intense detection of contrast effect within the left ventricular cavity during second harmonic imaging, long after the contrast is no longer detected using fundamental imaging (Figure 3).

Importantly, no adverse hemodynamic effects or symptoms have been observed when using this agent.

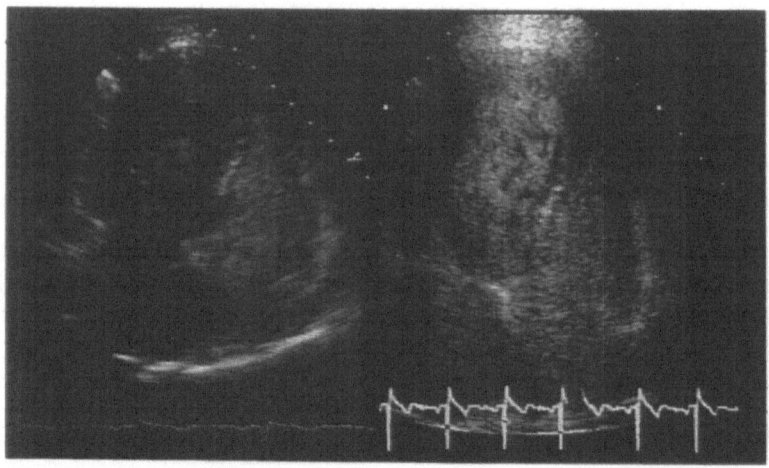

Figure 1. Transthoracic apical 4-chamber images (left ventricle on left, apex up) obtained after intravenous injection of Levovist® (Berlex, USA) 3.2 g in a 63 year old female. Left: Fundamental imaging (Hewlett-Packard (HP) Sonos 1500). Right: second harmonic imaging (2.5 MHz transmit, 5.0 MHz receive; Acuson prototype).

Myocardial   perfusion   detection   during   second   harmonic   contrast echocardiography

Newer contrast agents containing stabilizing gases, primarily composed of perfluorcarbons, have been demonstrated to produce both left ventricular and myocardial opacification after intravenous injection during normal and altered perfusion states during [3-11]. Our experience with second harmonic imaging of these agents during continuous delivery of ultrasound has revealed the presence of an inhomogenous distribution of myocardial contrast consistent with delineation of intramyocardial coronary vessels [20] (see below).

Very recent preclinical and preliminary clinical studies suggest that the combination of second harmonic imaging, and intermittent triggered acquisition, or transient-response imaging (TRI), provides enhanced detection of myocardial perfusion using intravenously injected perfluororcarbon-exposed sonicated dextrose albumin [28,29]. We have made similar observations in the cohort of patients described above that have received intravenous injections of Aerosomes® (Figure 4). Intensive clinical investigation in this area is ongoing as the newer generation of contrast agents is progressing through developmental studies. Preliminary data indicate that myocardial perfusion detection using second harmonic imaging of intravenously injected contrast agents may be reliably achieved in humans, especially when the physical properties of the transmitted ultrasound are optimized to reduce destruction and enhance detection of the

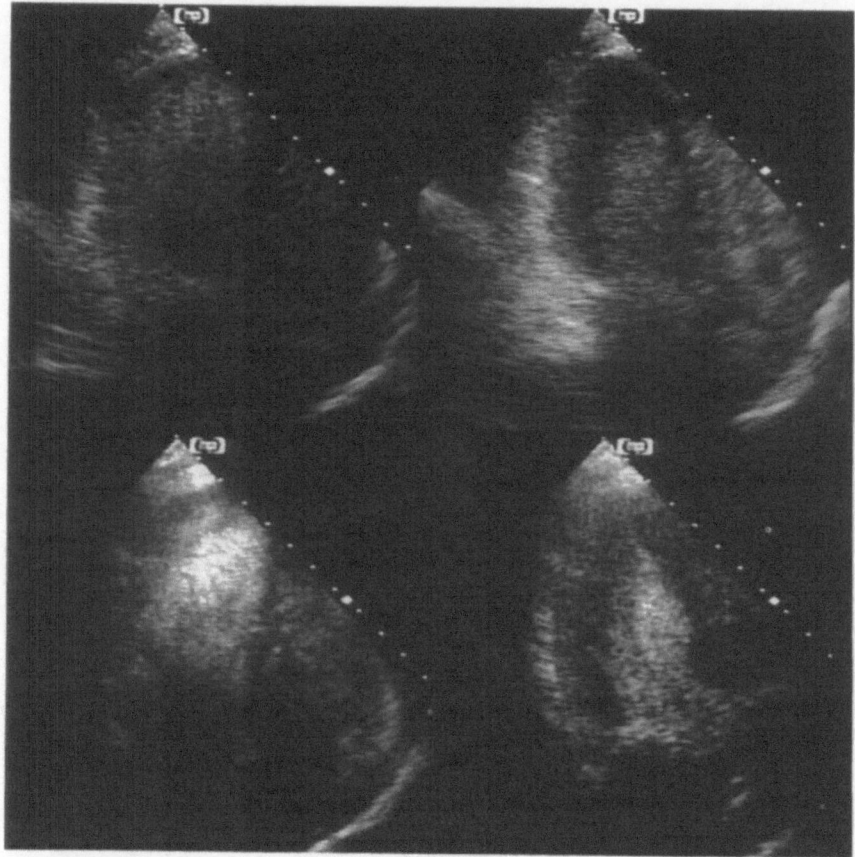

Figure 2. End-diastolic (left panels) and peak systolic (right panels) transthoracic apical long-axis images (left ventricle on left, apex up) obtained during dobutamine infusion (30 ug/kg/min) and 10 ml intravenous Albunex* in a 65 year old female. Upper panels: fundamental imaging (HP Sonos 2500, 2.5 MHz). Lower panels: second harmonic imaging (HP Sonos 2500, 1.8 MHz transmit, 3.6 MHz receive).

microbubbles. Post-processing techniques applying colorization schema to improve differentiation of gray levels, as utilized in the nuclear cardiology laboratory, may enhance the detection and evaluation of regional myocardial blood flow abnormalities.

Coronary visualization and blood flow measurements during second harmonic contrast echocardiography

We have noninvasively demonstrated [20] myocardial blood flow in intramyocardial coronary arteries during second harmonic ultrasound imaging in the closed chest dog during intravenous injections of the perfluorocarbon contrast agent AF0145 (Imagent*US, Alliance Pharmaceutical Corp., USA). The novel

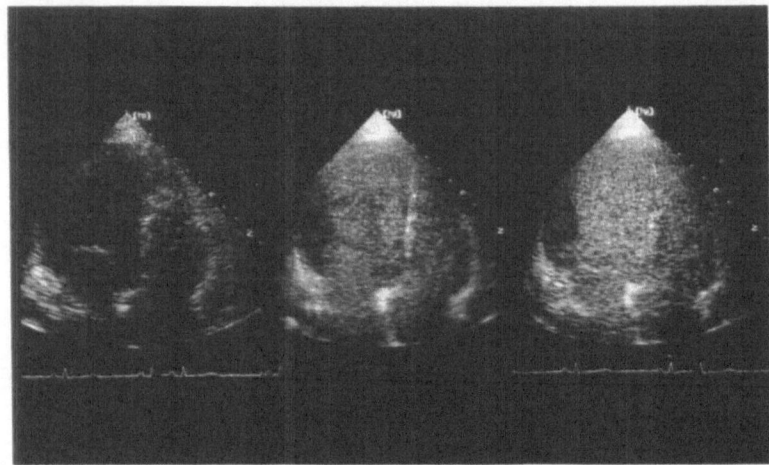

Figure 3. Transthoracic apical 4-chamber images (left ventricle on left, apex up) before (left), 30 sec after (center), and 5 minutes after (right), intravenous Aerosomes® in a 62 year old female. Left and center images with fundamental (HP Sonos 1500, 2.5 MHz) and right image with second harmonic imaging (HP Sonos 2500, 1.8 MHz transmit, 3.6 MHz receive).

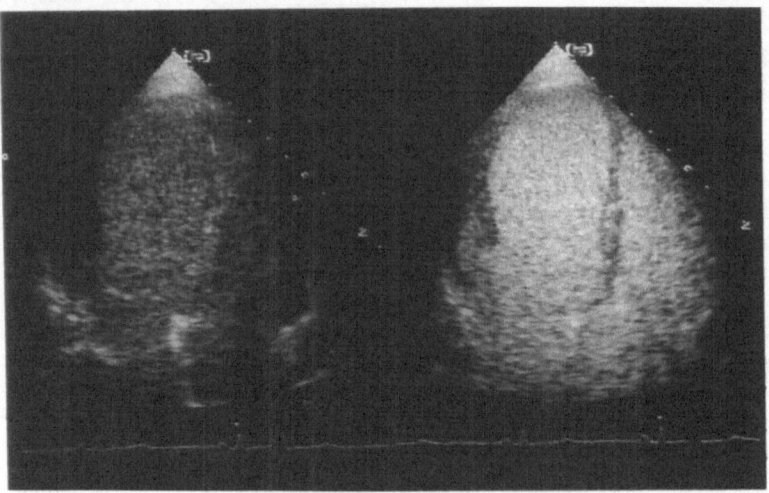

Figure 4. Second harmonic transthoracic images (HP Sonos 2500, 1.8 MHz transmit, 3.6 MHz receive) 6 minutes after Aerosomes® (same patient and orientation as figure 3). Left: Single end-diastolic frame during continuous ultrasound transmission. Right: Single end-diastolic frame after 5 cardiac cycles of intermittent (R-wave only) ultrasound transmission. Note the myocardial opacification.

appearance of heterogeneous, linear branching opacificied structures within the myocardium was confirmed to represent coronary arterial vascular arcades by comparison with simultaneous coronary Doppler flow signals measured using an intracoronary wire. The Doppler signals were measured at baseline and during adenosine administration; the coronary vasodilator reserve ratio determined using the noninvasive harmonic contrast Doppler and invasive Doppler flow wire methodologies were similar, suggesting that the noninvasive assessment of coronary vasculature and measurement of coronary vasodilator reserve is possible using second harmonic contrast echocardiography. These observations have yet to be extended into the clinical arena, but preliminary data appear promising.

Conclusions

Contrast echocardiography has become a clinical reality with the immediate and pending commercial availability of intravenously injected agents capable of transpulmonary passage and left ventricular cavity opacification with improved endocardial border detection. Preliminary studies indicate a potential application of echocardiographic contrast agents in stress echocardiography, where enhancement of regional wall motion abnormality analysis and left ventricular systolic function assessment has been observed. Early experiences indicate that second harmonic imaging further improves the left ventricular cavity contrast effect during pharmacologic stress echocardiography, enabling more confident assessments of regional wall motion abnormalities when compared with fundamental imaging. Newer perfluorocarbon-containing echocardiographic contrast agents appear to have the potential to provide myocardial perfusion assessment in the cardiac patient population, particularly when second harmonic and intermittent, rather than continuous, ultrasound delivery are combined. The application of three-dimensional echocardiographic epicardial acquisition techniques utilizing these principles has demonstrated enhanced delineation of myocardial perfusion defects in open-chest canines [35].

These new agents and technologies are currently undergoing intensive preclinical and clinical investigation [36]. Early preliminary results appear promising, especially for the detection of coronary artery disease and the evaluation of acute myocardial infarction both before and after attempted reperfusion, but have yet to be rigorously compared to current methods of myocardial perfusion assessment. Clinical implications of such a completely noninvasive, nonionizing, portable, relatively inexpensive technique yielding immediate results and capable of serial investigations would have major impact upon the diagnosis, evaluation and treatment of both acute and chronic coronary ischemic syndromes.

References

1.	Feinstein SB, Cheirif J, Ten Cate FJ *et al*. Safety and efficacy of a new transpulmonary ultrasound contrast agent: initial multicenter clinical results. J Am Coll Cardiol 1990;16:316-34.
2.	Schlief R, Schurmann R, Niendorf HP. Blood-pool enhancement with SHU 508

A. Results of phase II clinical trials. Invest Radiol 1991;(Suppl.1):S188-9.

3. Porter TR, Xie F. Visually discernible myocardial echocardiographic contrast after intravenous injection of sonicated dextrose albumin microbubbles containing high molecular weight, less soluble gases. J Am Coll Cardiol 1995;25:509-15.

4. Grayburn PA, Erikson JM, Escobar J, Womack L, Velasco CE. Peripheral intravenous myocardial contrast echocardiography using a 2% dodecafluoropentane emulsion: identification of myocardial risk area and infarct size in the canine model of ischemia. J Am Coll Cardiol 1995;26:1340-47.

5. Dittrich HC, Bales GL, Kuvelas T, Hunt RM, McFerran BA, Greener Y. Myocardial contrast echocardiography in experimental coronary artery occlusion with a new intravenously administered contrast agent. J Am Soc Echocardio 1995;8:465-74.

6. Porter TR, Feng X, Kricsfeld A, Kilzer K. Noninvasive identification of acute myocardial ischemia and reperfusion with contrast ultrasound using intravenous perfluoropropane-exposed sonicated dextrose albumin. J Am Coll Cardiol 1995;26:33-40.

7. Ismail S, Jayaweera AR, Goodman NC, Camarano GP, Skyba DM, Kaul S. Detection of coronary stenoses and quantification of the degree and spatial extent of blood flow mismatch during coronary hyperemia with myocardial contrast echocardiography. Circulation 1995;91:821-30.

8. Grauer S, Pantely GA, Xu J et al. Aerosomes MRX-115: echocardiographic and hemodynamic characteristics of new echo contrast agent that produces myocardial opacification after intravenous injection in pigs [abstract]. Circulation 1994;90(pt2):I-556.

9. Mulvagh SL, Foley DA, Aeschbacher BC, Klarich KW, Seward JB. A new intravenous perfluorochemical echocardiographic contrast agent, Imagent® US: imaging characteristics and hemodynamic profile [abstract]. J Am Soc Echocardio 1995;8:345.

10. Sutherland GR, Grauer SE, Moran C, Ishii M, Sahn DJ. Aerosomes MRX-115 echo contrast agent demonstrates myocardial opacification after intravenous injection in humans, without significant side effects, in a phase I clinical trial [abstract]. Circulation 1995;92:I-463.

11. Dittrich HC, Kuvelas T, Dadd K et al. Safety and efficacy of the ultrasound contrast agent FS069 in normal humans: results of a phase I trial [abstract]. Circulation 1995;92:I-464.

12. Schrope BA, Newhouse VL, Uhlendorf V. Simulated capillary blood flow measurement using a nonlinear ultrasonic contrast agent. Ultrasonic Imaging 1992;14:134-58.

13. Schrope BA, Newhouse VL. Second harmonic ultrasonic blood perfusion measurement. Ultrasound in Med & Biol 1993;19:567-79.

14. De Jong N, ten Cate FJ, Lancee CT, Roelandt JR, Bom N. Principles and recent developments in ultrasound contrast agents. Ultrasonics 1991;29:324-30.

15. Miller DL. Ultrasonic detection of resonant cavitation bubbles in a flow tube by their second-harmonic emissions. Ultrasonics 1981;19:217-24.

16. Ophir J, Parker KJ. Contrast agents in diagnostic ultrasound. Ultrasound Med Biol 1989;15:319-33.

17. Foley DA, Mulvagh SL, Aeschbacher BC, Klarich KW, Seward JB. Second harmonic imaging of echocardiographic contrast agents: unique features and promising characteristics [abstract]. J Am Coll Cardiol 1995;16A.

18. Mahmud E, Cotter B, Kimura B *et al*. Second harmonic imaging enhances contrast echocardiography in patients with cardiac disease: demonstration of feasibility [abstract]. J Am Coll Cardiol 1995;25:39A.

19. Walker KW, Grauer SE, Ge J, Giraud GD, Pantely GA, Powers J. Second harmonic mode imaging of intravenously injected Aerosomes MRX-115 increases myocardial echo contrast opacification at lower doses. Circulation 1995;92:I-193.

20. Mulvagh SL, Foley DA, Aeschbacher BC, Klarich KW, Seward JB. Second harmonic imaging of intravenously administered echocardiographic contrast: visualization of coronary arteries and measurement of coronary blood flow. J Am Coll Cardiol 1996. In press.

21. Lord Rayleigh. On the pressure developed by a liquid during the collapse of a spherical cavity. Philos Mag 1917;34:94-8.

22. Eatock BC, Nishi RY. Numerical studies of the spectrum of low intensity ultrasound scattered by bubbles. J Acoust Soc Am 1985;77:1692-701.

23. Lauterborn W. Numerical investigations of nonlinear oscillations of gas bubbles in liquids. J Acoust Soc Am 1976;59:283-93.

24. Prosperetti A. Nonlinear oscillations of gas bubbles in liquids: steady-state solutions and the connection between subharmonic signal and cavitation. J Acoust Soc Am 1974;56:878-85.

25. de Jong N, Cornet R, Lancée CT. Higher harmonics of vibrating gas-filled microspheres. Part one: simulations. Part two: measurements. Ultrasonics 1994;32:447-59.

26. Tucker DG, Welsby VG. Ultrasonic monitoring of decompression (letter). Lancet 1968;1:1253.

27. Burns PN. Ultrasound contrast agents in radiological diagnosis. Radiol Med 1987;1-5:71-82.

28. Porter TR, Xie F. Transient myocardial contrast after initial exposure to diagnostic ultrasound pressures with minute doses of intravenously injected microbubbles. Cirulation 1995;92:2391-5.

29. Porter TR, Armbruster R, Holdeman K, Xie F. Second harmonic transient response imaging with intravenous perfluorocarbon-exposed sonicated dextrose albumin in patients with previous myocardial infarction: initial clinical experience [abstract]. J Am Coll Cardiol 1996;27:76A.

30. Foley DA, Mulvagh SL, Villarraga HR *et al*. Optimization of echocardiographic contrast: ultrasound equipment and microbubble interactions. Advances in Echocardiography, Chicago, Illinois. October 12-13, 1995.

31. Burns PN, Powers JE, Hope-Simpson D *et al*. Harmonic power mode Doppler using microbubble contrast agents: an improved method for small vessel flow imaging. Institute for Electronics Engineers 1994;3:1547-50.

32. Villarraga HR, Foley DA, Pellikka PA *et al*. Second harmonic imaging of myocardial contrast agents: qualitative and quantitative observations from animal and human studies. Workshop on: Second Harmonic Technology in Cardiac Ultrasound. Costa Mesa, CA, November 11th, 1995.

33. Allen MR, Pellikka PA, Villarraga MR, Foley DA, Pumper GM, Mulvagh SL. Second harmonic enhancement of echocardiographic contrast intensity and duration in patients [abstract]. J Am Soc Echocardiography 1996. Submitted.

34. Villarraga HR, Pumper GM, Foley DA, Pellikka PA, Mulvagh SL. Enhancement of left ventricular opacification by Albunex° using second harmonic imaging during dobutamine stress echocardiography [abstract]. J Am

Soc Echocardiography 1996. Submitted.
35. Cao QL, Masani N, Delabays A *et al*. Harmonic imaging and single frame "triggered mode" data acquisition enhance delineation of myocardial perfusion defects by volume-rendered 3-dimensional echocardiography [abstract]. J Am Coll Cardiol 1996:27;21A.
36. Villarraga HR, Foley DA, Mulvagh SL. Contrast Echocardiography 1996: A Review. Texas Heart J 1996. In press.

37. Myocardial perfusion and function by MR imaging techniques

ALBERT de ROOS, ERNST E. van der WALL, ROB van der GEEST & JOHAN H.C. REIBER

Summary

Magnetric resonance (MR) imaging techniques are currently under development to assess various aspects of ischemic heart disease. Qualitative assessment of myocardial perfusion can be accomplished using MR contrast agents as perfusion marker. The MR perfusion technique is still somewhat limited due to the limited number of slices which are obtainable with currently available fast imaging methods. Further development is required in this area to improve the speed of acquisition methods which may encompass the entire left ventricle during first-pass of the MR contrast agent.

MR imaging techniques are well suited to evaluate both regional and global ventricular function. Full coverage of the entire left ventricle in multiple imaging sections can now be accomplished in relative short imaging times during breath-hold. The functional MR technique is well adapted for high-speed evaluation of function both at rest and under stress conditions. Tools for image analysis are now readily available to extract the functional data in a time-efficient manner.

MR imaging may become a cost-effective technique for the evaluation of patients with coronary artery disease, when perfusion and functional data can be acquired and analyzed from the entire left ventricle both at rest and under stress in a time-efficient manner.

Introduction

The combined evaluation of myocardial perfusion and function may be helpful to diagnose ischemic heart disease and to differentiate various ischemic heart syndromes. Alterations in both regional perfusion and function are early markers of ischemic heart disease. Myocardial perfusion imaging is important to evaluate the functional significance of coronary artery disease. This information is also useful for risk stratification in patients with ischemic heart disease. Furthermore, regional contraction abnormalities of the myocardium may signify the presence of underlying coronary artery disease. Depending on the severity of the underlying coronary artery disease, abnormalities in function and/or perfusion may become manifest only under stress conditions.

Reversible ischemia, infarcted myocardium, stunned myocardium and hibernating myocardium can be further characterized by a match or mismatch between perfusion and functional abnormalities both at rest and under stress. Radionuclide scintigraphy and echocardiography are time-honored tests to evaluate ischemic myocardial disease. However, when using traditional methods a number of separate tests is required to characterize the ischemic syndromes. Magnetic

485

J.H.C. Reiber and E.E. van der Wall (eds.), Cardiovascular Imaging, 485-497.
© 1996 *Kluwer Academic Publishers.*

resonance (MR) imaging is emerging as a potential useful modality to assess function and perfusion in one comprehensive imaging session. Although, MR imaging may ultimately allow the combined assessment of function and perfusion in a time-efficient and reliable manner there are still notable technical limitations. In this chapter, issues related to the evaluation of myocardial function and perfusion using MR techniques will be discussed.

Myocardial perfusion imaging

Assessment of the area at risk distal to coronary artery stenoses requires the use of contrast media. Gadolinium-based compounds (e.g. Gadolinium-DTPA, Gadolinium-DOTA, etc) have been most widely used in clinical studies. These extracellular agents can be safely used in patients with ischemic heart disease. Early studies were performed during the equilibrium phase using relative slow imaging techniques, which do not allow to capture the first transit of the agent through the myocardium. Infarcted myocardium is visualized using this approach as a relative 'hot spot' owing to the delayed accumulation of gadolinium compounds in the infarcted region.

More recently, ultrafast MR imaging has provided the opportunity to acquire dynamic information related to the passage of gadolinium compounds through the myocardium and thus provides an indirect measure of myocardial perfusion. Ultrafast MR imaging consists of a 180° inversion pulse followed by a gradient-echo sequence with very short repetition times and echo times to obtain a T1-weighted image in a fraction of the cardiac cycle [1,2]. Initially, feasibility studies demonstrated the first-pass transit of gadolinium compounds through the cardiac compartments and left ventricular myocardium after peripheral bolus injection of the contrast medium.

A limitation of the ultrafast technique is that only one or a few tomographic sections are obtained during first-pass perfusion. Myocardial perfusion studies both at rest and under stress will become clinical useful whenever images can be obtained reliably in a multislice mode.

Perfusion quantification

Although attempts are made to quantify perfusion in absolute terms, the accurate assessment of relative perfusion may provide clinical useful information. Absolute quantification of myocardial perfusion is hampered by several prerequisites which have to be fulfilled, including: (a) complete and uniform mixture of the contrast medium with the blood; (b) the volume of the contrast medium is negligible to the volume of the vasculature; (c) the indicator does not affect the hemodynamics of flow; (d) the indicator does not affect the vascular equilibrium; (e) the relationship between the change in signal intensity and the concentration of the indicator is known; (f) recirculation is negligible; and (g) there is no extravascular loss of the indicator during first pass [3].

Normal and ischemic myocardium differ in perfusion or instantaneous blood volume, which will result in a difference in the local concentration of the contrast medium between normal and abnormal tissue [4]. Fast gradient-echo or echo-planar MR techniques can be used to monitor the passage of contrast media through the central circulation and to follow the first pass through the myocardium as a marker for regional blood volume or perfusion. Signal intensity-versus-time curves during the first passage of contrast media can be constructed as an estimate of regional myocardial blood flow. However, the use of extracellular agents like Gadolinium-DTPA is not optimal for myocardial perfusion imaging, because these agents are not confined to one tissue compartment. As a consequence, the accumulation of Gadolinium-DTPA and other extracellular contrast agents in the myocardium will not only depend on tissue blood volume and blood flow but also on the intravascular and interstitial distribution volumes and the permeability of the capillaries [5]. It is estimated that approximately 50 percent of the injected dose of Gadolinium-DTPA is cleared from the capillaries during the first pass through the myocardium. Unfortunately, there is no simple relationship between myocardial signal intensity after administration of extracellular contrast media and the concentration of the contrast agent, limiting the possibilities for absolute perfusion quantification. In addition, first pass myocardial perfusion studies require a rapid bolus injection within 2 sec and an imaging sequence with a high temporal resolution of at least one image per heart beat to capture the transit of the contrast agent through the myocardium, thereby avoiding problems caused by recirculation of the contrast medium [5]. A potential confounding factor that may preclude reliable myocardial perfusion imaging is the methodology of contrast medium administration. It has been noted that the ventricular signal intensity versus time curves depend on the injection site (peripheral bolus injection versus injection through a catheter placed in the right atrium) and bolus concentration [6].

Potential applications

Despite a number of limitations, MR perfusion imaging has successfully been applied in patients with healed myocardial infarcts to identify the scar as a relative perfusion defect [7] and also for detecting perfusion-related abnormalities in the myocardium distal to coronary artery stenoses with more than 80 percent luminal narrowing [8]. Time-versus-intensity curves reveal lower peak signal intensity and lower upslope of signal increase distal to significant coronary artery stenoses as compared to normally perfused myocardium. These perfusion abnormalities may restore to normal after successful reperfusion therapy [8].

Stress MR perfusion

Dipyridamole stress can be applied to reveal perfusion defects distal to coronary artery stenoses which may not be detected under resting conditions [5]. Dipyridamole acts as a coronary vasodilator particularly by its effect at the level of the small resistance arterioles [9]. Its dilating action has not been fully elucidated, but appears to be related to the increased plasma level of endogenous adenosine, a potent coronary arteriolar vasodilator. In patients with significant coronary artery stenosis, the vascular bed distal to the stenosis is somewhat dilated to promote normal resting flow. Therefore, the coronary vasodilator reserve is limited and severe stenoses will result in an exhausted flow reserve.

When dipyridamole is administered in these patients, no significant further vasodilatation will occur distal to the stenosed vessel and subendocardial flow will not increase. In contrast, the normal coronary arteries possess their full capacity to vasodilate. Hence, a regional flow heterogeneity or perfusion maldistribution between normal and ischemic myocardium may become evident. Pennell et al. [10] were the first to report the results of dipyridamole stress MR imaging in patients with coronary artery disease. Reversible wall motion abnormalities were detected in only 67 percent of patients with reversible thallium perfusion defects, indicating that dipyridamole is not ideally suited to induce wall motion abnormalities. Several studies have shown the feasibility of dipyridamole stress MR imaging for detecting perfusion abnormalities related to coronary artery disease with a sensitivity, specificity and accuracy of 65, 76 and 74 percent, respectively [11,12]. Matheijssen et al. [12] used double-level MR perfusion imaging in patients with documented single-vessel coronary artery disease using Gadolinium-DTPA as perfusion marker before and after dipyridamole infusion. A good correlation between MR-defined perfusion defects during dipyridamole hyperemia and tomographic technetium-99m SestaMIBI imaging (SPECT) was found. Quantitative analysis of signal intensity-versus-time curves obtained with MR imaging revealed that the signal intensity increase after bolus injection of Gadolinium-DTPA using a linear fit and the slope of the curve correctly identified perfusion abnormalities.

Regional myocardial function

Gradient-echo MR imaging is well suited to detect myocardial ischemia by analysis of global and regional cardiac function [13]. Both abnormal wall motion and more specifically abnormal wall thickening indicate diminished regional myocardial function [14]. The capability of gradient-echo MR imaging to provide functional information about the state of pathologically altered myocardium in combination with assessment of diastolic wall thickness and systolic wall thickening makes it suitable for identification of myocardial viability [15,16]. In a recent study, Baer et al. [17] compared low-dose dobutamine MR imaging with positron emission tomography in 35 patients with myocardial infarction (>4 months old). They showed that MR imaging was very accurate in assessing myocardial viability. Viable myocardium was characterized by preserved end-diastolic wall thickness and a dobutamine-inducible contraction reserve, suggesting that both parameters should be taken into account to maximize the sensitivity of MR imaging for the detection of myocardial viability. Viability was defined by MR imaging when a segment that was akinetic at baseline revealed an end-diastolic wall thickness of more than 5.5 mm (i.e. the mean wall thickness in a normal control group minus 2.5 standard deviations) and evidence of systolic wall thickening of more than 1 mm under low dose (10 microgram per min per kg) dobutamine stress. Recovery of wall thickening under dobutamine stress appeared to be the best predictor of viability as compared to positron emission tomography. These findings are supported by Perrone-Filardi et al. [18,19] using positron emission tomography with fluorine-18-fluorodeoxyglucose. In most regions with reduced end-diastolic wall thickness and absent wall thickening absence of metabolic activity was shown, indicating the suitability of MR imaging in the evaluation of myocardial viability.

Viability demonstrated by MR imaging as a contraction reserve in akinetic myocardium reveals the potential functional competence of the myocardium and may therefore be more predictive of recovery after revascularization than the detection of myocardial glycolytic activity by positron emission tomography. Positron emission tomography may detect metabolic activity in myocardium with severe impairment of function with only small remnants of viable tissue, which will not show recovery of function during stress or after revascularization [17].

Stress MR imaging

In recent years, pharmacologic stress has been applied during MR imaging for detection of functional abnormalities in patients with coronary artery disease, because physical exercise during MR imaging is difficult to perform due to motion artifacts and space restriction. Dobutamine stress may be more reliable than dipyridamole stress for inducing wall motion abnormalities in patients with coronary artery disease, whereas dipyridamole stress should be reserved for myocardial perfusion imaging. Dobutamine is a synthetic catecholamine with relatively selective positive inotropic stimulation. The onset of action occurs within 2 minutes after administration and the maximal effect occurs after 10 to 14 minutes. Pharmacologic stress using dobutamine has a number of advantages, including the ease of administration by a peripheral vein, the close resemblance to physical exercise, the short half-life of the drug, high tolerance and safety and the extensive clinical experience with the agent [9]. Dobutamine increases myocardial oxygen consumption by augmenting contractility and heart rate. Hence, a marked imbalance between myocardial oxygen demand and supply may occur, resulting in myocardial ischemia. Under dobutamine stress wall motion abnormalities may occur as an early manifestation of myocardial ischemia. The occurrence of ventricular arrhythmias is an infrequent, but potentially serious side-effect of dobutamine administration.

Pennell et al. [20] studied 22 patients with coronary artery disease both by dobutamine MR imaging and thallium tomography. Comparison of perfusion defects and wall motion abnormalities during stress showed 90% agreement, and dobutamine infusion was well-tolerated in all patients. Van Rugge et al. [21] in 23 healthy volunteers, identified wall motion dynamics and provided calculations of segmental wall thickening and hemodynamic parameters using dobutamine stress imaging. In 37 patients with coronary artery disease, van Rugge et al. [22] showed an overall sensitivity of 81 percent and a specificity of 100 percent when using dobutamine MR imaging; in patients with single-, double-, and triple-vessel disease the sensitivity values were 75, 80 and 100 percent, respectively. In a subsequent study, comprising 39 consecutive patients with clinically suspected coronary artery disease referred for coronary arteriography and in 10 normal subjects, it was shown that dobutamine-stress MR imaging identified wall motion abnormalities by quantitative analysis using the centerline method [23]; the sensitivity, specificity, and accuracy were 91, 80, and 90 percent, respectively. These findings were corroborated by Baer et al. [23], who studied 28 patients with dobutamine MR imaging and found an overall sensitivity of 87 percent and a specificity of 100 percent for the detection of coronary artery disease. In another study, Baer et al. [24] compared the findings of dobutamine MR imaging with dobutamine-stress technetium-99m MIBI tomographic imaging in 35 patients with coronary artery disease; a high concordance between the two imaging modalities was found with respect to the detection of a dobutamine ischemic response. These studies illustrate the feasibility to perform MR stress imaging and to detect the functional sequelae of reversible myocardial ischemia.

In summary, determination of wall motion and wall thickening by cardiac MR imaging may play an important role in the accurate detection and functional characterization of patients with suspected or known coronary artery disease. Dynamic gradient-echo MR imaging using pharmacologic stress may constitute a new modality to detect coronary artery disease. Using the centerline method for analysis, accurate quantitative information can be obtained from regions that show reduced wall thickness and thickening caused by stress-induced myocardial ischemia (Figure 1). However, further technical developments are required before pharmacologic stress MR imaging becomes a serious challenge to pharmacologic stress radionuclide perfusion imaging or to two-dimensional echocardiography.

Global ventricular function

Introduction

The evaluation of global ventricular function is of significant value in the management of patients with chronic coronary artery disease using serial measurements, after acute myocardial infarction and for evaluating effects of reperfusion therapy after acute infarction. The depression in resting ejection fraction is probably the most significant determinant of prognosis in patients after acute myocardial infarction. Mortality rates increase progressively as ejection fraction decreases in patients with chronic stable angina. Resting left ventricular function appears to be one the most significant determinants of long-term prognosis in those patients. Serial assessment of left ventricular function in patients with chronic ischemic heart disease may be helpful to identify the evolvement from low-risk to high-risk patient groups.

Global ventricular function refers to the effectiveness of the heart as a pump. This pumping function is dependent on the interaction between preload, afterload and myocardial contractility. The definitions of preload, afterload and ejection fraction underscore the relevance of measuring ventricular volumes and myocardial mass for accurate determination of global ventricular function. The time-honored methods used for evaluating ventricular function are not free of risk and discomfort to the patient (cardiac catheterization and radionuclide imaging), rely on geometric assumptions (x-ray contrast ventriculography, echocardiography) or may be hampered by the dependency on adequate acoustic windows and operator skill (echocardiography). In contrast, MR imaging is potentially well suited to assess ventricular function, as exemplified by its non-invasiveness, lack of radiation exposure, its indepency of geometric assumptions, operator independency and high accuracy and reproducibility [25-27]. A stack of MR images that encompass the entire heart provide a intrinsically three-

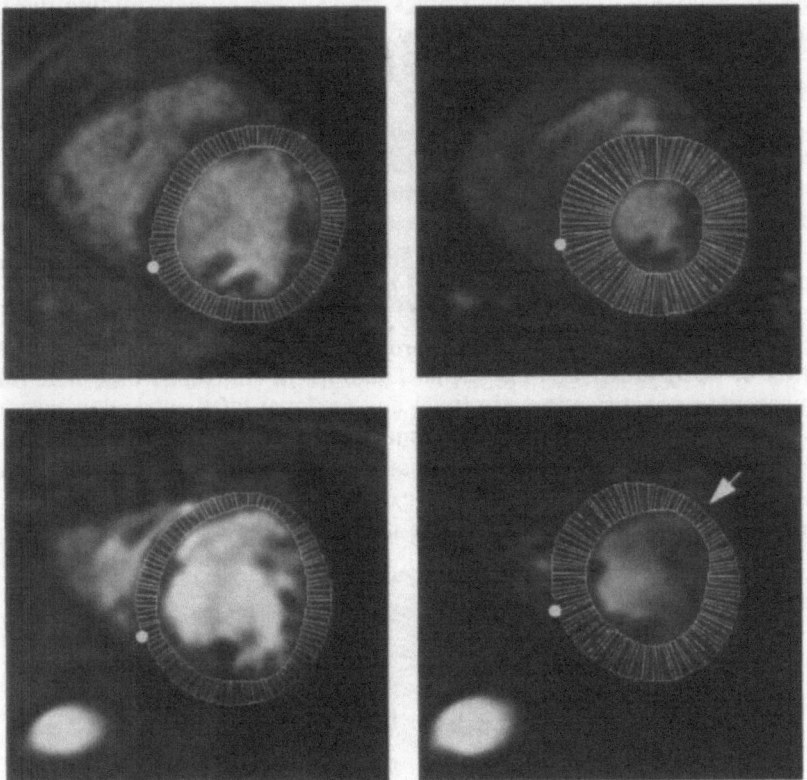

Figure 1. Illustration of the application of the centerline method for quantifying wall motion dynamics. End-diastolic (upper left panel) and end-systolic (upper-right panel) mid-ventricular MR images in normal subject show homogeneous contraction around the circumference of the left ventricle. End-diastolic (lower left panel) and end-systolic (lower right panel) MR images demonstrate diminished contraction during systole in the anterior wall of the left ventricle in a patient who suffered from a recent anterior wall infarction.

dimensional data set from which systolic and diastolic ventricular function can be extracted without the need to rely on geometric assumptions (Figure 2). In addition to volume measurements, the MR data set can also be used to measure ventricular mass. Thus, MR imaging fulfills many prerequisites for optimal assessment of cardiac performance and for evaluating serial changes in cardiac function before and after interventions [28].

Left ventricular volumes and mass

Absolute cavity volumes of the left ventricle can readily be measured by drawing endocardial contours in contiguous MR imaging sections and by adding up the enclosed blood pool areas. Summation of blood pool areas from the end-diastolic and end-systolic time frames provides the end-diastolic volume and end-systolic

volume, respectively. These time frames are selected by determining the largest
and smallest cavity volume, respectively.

Recent technological developments have resulted in a significant reduction in the
acquisition times and improvements in image quality. However, the required
manual tracing of myocardial contours is a time-consuming and tedious
procedure, which introduces observer bias and remains a major limitation in the
clinical use of cardiovascular MRI for the quantative evaluation of left ventricular
function. The clinical value of cardiovascular MRI would significantly improve
if the process of contour detection and subsequent quantitative analysis could be
automated and integrated in a dedicated software package.

Towards these goals the MASS (MR Analytical Software System) software
package was developed at our institution [29]. This package offers automated
detection of endocardial and epicardial contours in short-axis cine MR imaging
and subsequent quantification of global and regional left ventricular parameters.
The accuracy of in vitro measurements obtained by MR imaging has been
established by imaging ventricular casts of known volume [30]. In vivo MR
measurements have been validated less extensively and rigidly. A major problem
for in vivo validation is the choice of a universally accepted 'gold standard' for

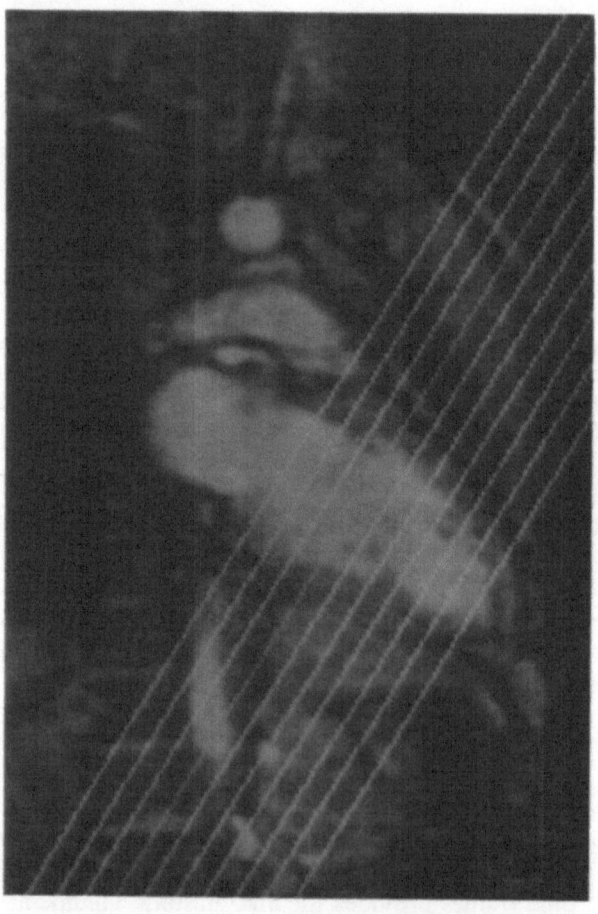

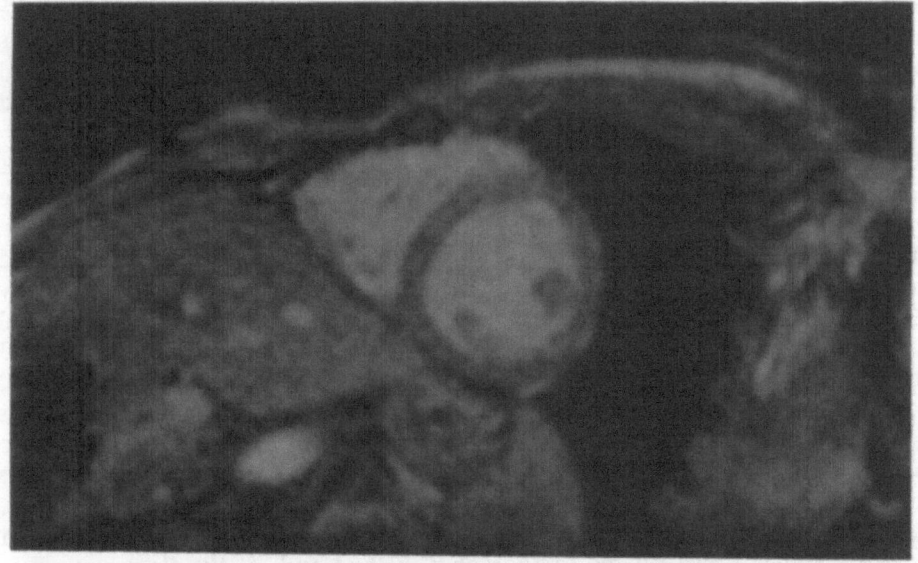

b

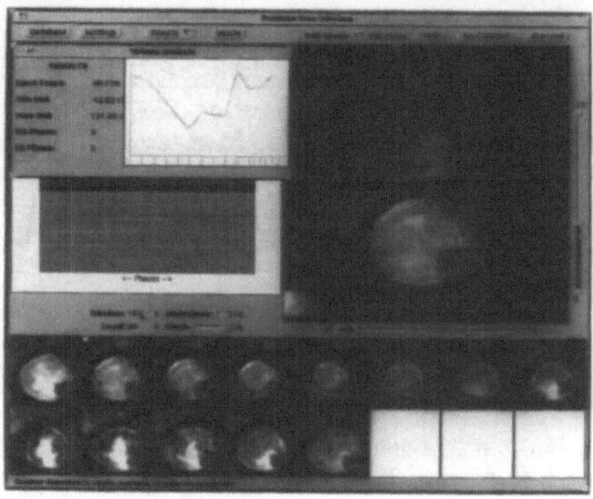

c

Figure 2. Illustration of the set-up (A) for the acquisition of MR images encompassing the entire left ventricle in the short-axis orientation. Midventricular short-axis MR image at the level of the papillary muscles is illustrated in B. The volumetric data set of the left ventricle is analyzed semi-automatically to extract systolic and diastolic function using the MASS-software developed in our institution (C) [29].

measuring cavity volumes in the beating heart. The ideal gold standard would assess ventricular volumes simultaneously with MR imaging, because the end-diastolic and end-systolic volumes may vary from heartbeat to heartbeat. In practice, no realistic gold standard is available, with the possible exception of the accurate but cumbersome intraventricular balloon method. To date, measurements based on in vivo MR imaging of absolute ventricular volumes have been validated with non-simultaneously performed x-ray contrast ventriculography. Good correlation has been found between these two methods for measuring end-diastolic and end-systolic volumes in over 35 patients with correlation coefficients ranging from .84 to .98. [31,32]. While it is difficult to validate absolute ventricular volumes, validating measurements of stroke volume and ejection fraction is relatively straightforward. Left ventricular ejection fraction measured from MR images agrees well with that measured with x-ray ventriculography [31,33,34] and radionuclide ventriculography [35,36] as evaluated in several studies involving over 130 patients with correlation coefficients ranging from .83 to .98. Left ventricular stroke volumes determined by MR imaging agree well with the results of an indicator dilution method as evaluated in various studies involving over 40 subjects [37,38]. Left ventricular stroke volumes have also been validated against MR flow measurements in the ascending aorta, which is an intrinsically different approach than measurements based on volume calculations [39,40]. Good correlations were determined between left ventricular stroke volumes based on the tomographic method and on the flow method in more than 20 subjects with correlation coefficients between .96 and .98. These reports provide ample evidence that the MR-derived measurements of absolute left ventricular volumes, stroke volumes and ejection fraction are indeed correct and highly accurate. To date, no clinical outcome studies have been performed based on MR measurements of left ventricular function. It is of vital importance to demonstrate the prognostic significance of MR-based measurements of ventricular function after myocardial infarction in terms of cardiac events (mortality, repeat myocardial infarction, unstable angina, development of angina or heart failure, or need for angioplasty or surgery). This information should become available to justify the routine use of MR imaging in various patient categories with chronic coronary artery disease or acute myocardial infarction in a cost-effective manner.

References

1. Atkinson D, Burstein D, Edelman RR. First-pass cardiac perfusion: evaluation with ultrafast MR imaging. Radiology 1990;174:757-62.
2. van Rugge FP, Boreel JJ, van der Wall EE et al. Cardiac first-pass and myocardial perfusion in normal subjects assessed by subsecond Gd-DTPA enhanced MR imaging. J Comput Assist Tomogr 1991;15:959-65.
3. Wood AM, Hoffmann KR, Lipton MJ. Cardiac function: quantification with magnetic resonance and computed tomography. Rad Clin North Am 1994:553-79.
4. Higgins CB, Saeed M, Wendland M et al. Contrast media for cardiothoracic MR imaging. J Magn Reson Imaging 1993;3:265-76.
5. Wilke N, Simm C, Zhang J et al. Contrast-enhanced first pass myocardial perfusion imaging: correlation between myocardial blood flow in dogs at rest and during hyperemia. Magn Reson Med 1993;29:485-97.

6. Keijer JT, van Rossum AC, van Eenige MJ *et al.* Semiquantitation of regional myocardial blood flow in normal human subjects by first-pass magnetic resonance imaging. Am Heart J 1995;130:893-901.

7. Van Rugge FP, van der Wall EE, van Dijkman PRM, Louwerenburg HW, De Roos A, Bruschke AVG. Usefulness of ultrafast magnetic resonance imaging in healed myocardial infarction. Am J Cardiol 1992;70:1233-7.

8. Manning WJ, Atkinson DJ, Grossman W, Paulin S, Edelman RR. First-pass nuclear magnetic resonance imaging studies using gadolinium-DTPA in patients with coronary artery disease. J Am Coll Cardiol 1991;18:959-65.

9. Van Rugge FP, van der Wall EE, Bruschke AVG. New developments in pharmacologic stress imaging. Am Heart J 1992;124:468-85.

10. Pennell DJ, Underwood SR, Longmore DB. Detection of coronary artery disease using MR imaging with dipyridamole infusion. J Comput Assist Tomogr 1990;14:167-70.

11. Eichenberger AC, Schuiki E, Kochli VD, Amann FW, McKinnon GC, von Schulthess GK. Ischemic heart disease: assessment with gadolinium-enhanced ultrafast MR imaging and dipyridamole stress [see comments]. J Magn Reson Imaging 1994;4:425-31.

12. Matheijssen NAA, Louwerenburg HW, van Rugge FP *et al.* Comparison of Ultrafast Dipyridamole Magnetic Resonance Imaging with Dipyridamole SestaMIBI SPECT for Detection of Perfusion Abnormalities in Patients with One-Vessel Coronary Artery Disease: Assessment by Quantitative Model Fitting. Magn Reson Med 1996;35:221-8.

13. Meese RB, Spritzer CE, Negro-Vilar R, Bashore T, Herfkens RJ. Detection, characterization and functional assessment of reperfused Q-wave acute myocardial infarction by cine magnetic resonance imaging. Am J Cardiol 1990;66:1-9.

14. Matheijssen NAA, De Roos A, Doornbos J, Reiber JHC, Waldman GJ, van der Wall EE. Left ventricular wall motion analysis in patients with myocardial infarction using magnetic resonance imaging. Magn Reson Imaging 1993;11:485-92.

15. Ryan T, Tarver RD, Duerk JL *et al.* Distinguishing viable from infarcted myocardium after experimental ischemia and reperfusion by using nuclear magnetic resonance imaging. J Am Coll Cardiol 1990;15:1355-64.

16. Vliegen HW, de Roos A, Bruschke AV, van der Wall EE. Magnetic resonance techniques for the assessment of myocardial viability: clinical experience. [Review]. Am Heart J 1995;129:809-18.

17. Baer FM, Voth E, Schneider CA, Theissen P, Schicha H, Sechtem U. Comparison of low-dose dobutamine-gradient-echo magnetic resonance imaging and positron emission tomography with [18F]fluorodeoxyglucose in patients with chronic coronary artery disease. A functional and morphological approach to the detection of residual myocardial viability. Circulation 1995;91:1006-15.

18. Perrone-Filardi P, Bacharach SL, Dilsizian V *et al.* Metabolic evidence of viable myocardium in regions with reduced wall thickness and absent wall thickening in patients with chronic ischemic left ventricular dysfunction. J Am Coll Cardiol 1992;20:161-8.

19. Perrone-Filardi P, Bacharach SL, Dilsizian V, Maurea S, Frank JA, Bonow RO. Regional left ventricular wall thickening. Relation to regional uptake of 18fluorodeoxyglucose and 201Tl in patients with chronic coronary artery disease and left ventricular dysfunction. Circulation 1992;86:1125-37.

20. Pennell DJ, Underwood SR, Manzara CC *et al*. Magnetic resonance imaging during dobutamine stress in coronary artery disease. Am J Cardiol 1992;70:34-40.

21. Van Rugge FP, Holman ER, van der Wall EE, de Roos A, van der Laarse A, Bruschke AVG. Quantitation of global and regional left ventricular function by cine magnetic resonance imaging during dobutamine stress in normal human subjects. Eur Heart J 1993;14:456-63.

22. Van Rugge FP, van der Wall EE, de Roos A, Bruschke AV. Dobutamine stress magnetic resonance imaging for detection of coronary artery disease. J Am Coll Cardiol 1993;22:431-9.

23. Van Rugge FP, van der Wall EE, Spanjersberg SJ *et al*. Magnetic resonance imaging during dobutamine stress for detection and localization of coronary artery disease. Quantitative wall motion analysis using a modification of the centerline method. Circulation 1994;90:127-38.

24. Baer FM, Voth E, Theissen P, Schneider CA, Schicha H, Sechtem U. Coronary artery disease: findings with GRE MR imaging and Tc-99m-methoxyisobutyl-isonitrile SPECT during simultaneous dobutamine stress. Radiology 1994;193:203-9.

25. Buser PT, Auffermann W, Holt WW *et al*. Noninvasive evaluation of global left ventricular function with use of cine nuclear magnetic resonance. J Am Coll Cardiol 1989;13:1294-300.

26. Cranney G, Lotan CS, Dean L, Baxley W, Bouchard A, Pohost GM. Left ventricular volume measurement using cardiac axis nuclear magnetic resonance imaging. Circulation 1990;82:154-63.

27. Pattynama PMT, Lamb HJL, van der Velde EA, van der Wall EE, De Roos A. Left ventricular measurements with cine and spin-echo MR imaging: a study of reproducibility with variance component analysis. Radiology 1993;187:261-8.

28. Fujita N, Hartiala J, O'Sullivan M *et al*. Assessment of left ventricular diastolic function in dilated cardiomyopathy with cine magnetic resonance imaging: effect of an angiotensin converting enzyme inhibitor, benazepril. Am Heart J 1993;125:171-8.

29. Van der Geest RJ, Jansen E, Buller VGM, Reiber JHC. Automated detection of left ventricular epi- and endocardial contours in short-axis MR images. Comp Cardiol; 1994:33-6.

30. Longmore DB, Underwood SR, Hounsfield GN *et al*. Dimensional accuracy of magnetic resonance in studies of the heart. Lancet 1985;i:1360-62.

31. MacMillan RM, Murphy JL, Kresh JY, Chandrasekaran K, Muhr WF, Haskin ME. Left ventricular volumes using cine-MRI: Validation by catheterization ventriculography. Am J Card Imaging 1990;4:79-85.

32. Just H, Holubarsch C, Friedburg H. Estimation of left ventricular volume and mass by magnetic resonance imaging: comparison with quantitative biplane angiocardiography. Cardiovasc Intervent Radiol 1987;10:1-4.

33. Van Rossum AC, Visser FC, Sprenger M, van Eenige MJ, Valk J, Roos JP. Evaluation of magnetic resonance imaging for determination of left ventricular ejection fraction and comparison with angiography. Am J Cardiol 1988;62:628-33.

34. Edelman RR, Thompson R, Kantor H, Brady TJ, Leavitt M, Dinsmore R. Cardiac function: Evaluation with fast-echo MR imaging. Radiology 1987;162:611-5.

35. Møgelvang J, Thomsen C, Mehlsen J, Bulow J, Kelbaek H, Hendriksen O. Left

ventricular ejection fraction determined by magnetic resonance imaging and gated radionuclide ventriculography. Am J Noninvasive Cardiol 1987;1:278-83.

36. Gaudio C, Tanzilli G, Mazzarotto P. Comparison of left ventricular ejection fraction by magnetic resonance imaging and radionuclide ventriculography in idiopathic dilated cardiomyopathy. Am J Cardiol 1991;67:411-5.

37. Markiewicz W, Sechtem U, Kirby R, Derugin N, Caputo GC, Higgins CB. Measurement of ventricular volumes in the dog by nuclear magnetic resonance imaging. J Am Coll Cardiol 1987;10:170-7.

38. Culham JA, Vince DJ. Cardiac output by MR imaging: an experimental study comparing right ventricle and left ventricle with thermodilution. Can Assoc Radiol J 1988;39:247-9.

39. Kondo C, Caputo GR, Semelka R, Foster E, Shimakawa A, Higgins CB. Right and left ventricular stroke volume measurements with velocity-encoded cine MR imaging: in vitro and in vivo validation. AJR 1991;157:9-16.

40. Rebergen SA, Ottenkamp J, Doornbos J, van der Wall EE, Chin JGJ, De Roos A. Postoperative pulmonary flow dynamics after Fontan surgery: assessment with nuclear magnetic resonance velocity mapping. J Am Coll Cardiol 1993;21:123-31.

38. Myocardial perfusion imaging by SPECT

ERNST E. VAN DER WALL

Summary

Over the last decade, substantial advancements in the field of myocardial perfusion scintigraphy have markedly improved the diagnosis and subsequent evaluation of patients with coronary artery disease (CAD). These improvements have mainly originated from the transition of planar imaging to single-photon emission computed tomography (SPECT). In addition, several new technetium-99m (^{99m}Tc) based radiopharmaceuticals have entered the clinical arena which are very suitable for SPECT imaging. Lastly, new pharmacological stress agents have been developed. In this era of continuing cost containment, myocardial perfusion scintigraphy using SPECT imaging has emerged as a highly cost-effective noninvasive modality for guiding patient management.

This chapter will concentrate on the merits of SPECT imaging, the use of the appropriate SPECT imaging protocols both for thallium-201 (^{201}Tl) and ^{99m}Tc-labeled agents, and the application of pharmacologic stress in myocardial perfusion SPECT imaging.

Planar versus SPECT imaging

Planar myocardial perfusion scintigraphy is a time-honored technique for diagnosing patients with CAD and is widely available, simple to perform, allows accurate quantitative analysis, and requires less quality control than SPECT imaging [1]. However, with planar imaging there is significant overlap of normally and abnormally perfused myocardium which limits its overall diagnostic accuracy. Myocardial imaging with SPECT, an inherently three-dimensional technique, can overcome many of the limitations of planar imaging and is more accurate for the overall detection and localization of coronary artery stenoses [2]. The introduction of triple-head cameras has opened new avenues for myocardial perfusion SPECT imaging.

SPECT quantification

A well-recognized advantage of SPECT is the ability to accurately quantify the global extent of left ventricular hypoperfusion and the percent of myocardial scar and ischemia. Although different software packages are currently available, all are based principally on a circumferential profile technique whereby pixel count activity is determined along radii from the left ventricular endocardium to epicardium over the entire 360° of each stress and redistribution (or rest) short-axis slice from cardiac apex to base. The count activity for each radius is normalized to the radius with the highest activity in each of the initial stress and

J.H.C. Reiber and E.E. van der Wall (eds.), Cardiovascular Imaging, 499-512.
© 1996 *Kluwer Academic Publishers.*

delayed short axis slices. Two-dimensional polar maps of the three-dimensional myocardial radionuclide activity are then computer-generated (bull's eye reconstruction) and statistically compared to a normal patient data bank. Quantification with SPECT has been validated in models of experimental infarction, and also in clinical trials comparing scintigraphic infarct size to enzymatic estimates of myocardial infarction [3]. The unique ability of SPECT to quantify the extent of myocardial scar and ischemia is now recognized to confer important prognostic information.

Reproducibility of SPECT

In large multicenter trials, mean patient data are used to assess the efficacy of different therapeutic regimens, but in clinical practice individual efficacy becomes the critical issue. In order to define what constitutes a real change in myocardial perfusion beyond technique variability, the reproducibilities of both planar and SPECT imaging have recently been investigated [4]. The intra- and interobserver reproducibility of SPECT for quantifying perfusion defects proved to be excellent with correlation coefficients of $r = .99$ and $r = .98$, respectively, $(p < .0001)$. Furthermore, the inter-study reproducibility was equally high.

Perfusion tracers for SPECT imaging

Over the past 5 years, several myocardial perfusion agents labeled with ^{99m}Tc have become commercially available. One of them, ^{99m}Tc-sestamibi (Cardiolite) has already been in clinical use in several countries around the world [5]. Another agent, ^{99m}Tc-teboroxime (Cardiotec), has been approved for clinical use but has had much less clinical utilization. The newest ^{99m}Tc-labeled perfusion agent that has undergone clinical evaluation is ^{99m}Tc-tetrofosmin (Myoview) [6]. The advent of these compounds occurred 15-20 years after the introduction of myocardial perfusion scintigraphy in 1976 as a clinical tool using ^{201}Tl as a tracer. In the coming years, the new ^{99m}Tc-labeled agents will in all likelihood radically change the ways one performs myocardial perfusion scintigraphy. Because of the constraints imposed by the physical characteristics of ^{201}Tl - such as the low emission energies (68 to 80 keV) resulting in severe photon attenuation, the long half-life (73 hours) limiting the maximal injected dose to only a few millicuries (megabecquerels), and the need to be produced in a cyclotron, ^{201}Tl has been considered a relatively poor perfusion tracer when imaged with single-crystal gamma cameras. Consequently, nuclear medicine physicians and cardiologists have searched for other tracers such as ^{99m}Tc, which is a much more favorable agent for the current generation of SPECT gamma cameras (half-life 6 hours, emission energy 140 keV). At present, there are convincing data that all the prognostic indicators, which have been extensively validated with respect to ^{201}Tl scintigraphy, will also apply to the ^{99m}Tc-labeled agents [7].

Myocardial SPECT imaging with ^{201}Tl

Thallium-201 perfusion imaging has been used with excellent clinical results for almost 20 years. Since 1977 the traditional exercise-delayed imaging protocol has been used in millions of patients. According to the traditional imaging protocol the patient performs symptom-limited exercise on a treadmill or bicycle. At peak exercise 2-3 mCi (75-110 MBq) of ^{201}Tl is injected intravenously. The patient is encouraged to continue to exercise for 1 to 2 more minutes. The patient is then positioned as soon as possible under the gamma camera (within 5-10 minutes after termination of exercise). Delayed redistribution imaging is performed 2-4 hours after injection of ^{201}Tl.

Several new imaging protocols have been recently proposed in ^{201}Tl myocardial perfusion imaging. It has been shown that, with the above-described conventional ^{201}Tl imaging protocol, the reversibility of exercise-induced perfusion defects, and thus myocardial viability, may be underestimated. Depending on the population studied, 40-60% of patients with fixed defects may have viable myocardium in the defect area. The traditional 2-4 hour delay is apparently too short for complete redistribution of ^{201}Tl to occur. To circumvent this limitation, a number of alternative protocols have been developed for the combined assessment of perfusion and viability.

A first protocol uses late redistribution imaging to be performed 24 hours after injection of ^{201}Tl in patients with fixed defects on conventional 2-4 hour delayed imaging [8]. This modification requires no additional injection of ^{201}Tl. However, the count density is usually low 24 hours after injection, resulting in suboptimal images. Compared with imaging after a rest reinjection, less defect reversibility is detected [9].

In a subsequent more efficient protocol, for the first time described by Dilzisian et al. in 1990 [10], ^{201}Tl is reinjected at rest as soon as 3-4 hour redistribution SPECT imaging is completed (classical reinjection protocol). Imaging is started 30 to 45 minutes after rest reinjection and complete evaluation by ^{201}Tl imaging is achieved in one day. Despite the relatively long imaging procedure of 5-6 hours, the standard stress-redistribution-reinjection protocol has been accepted as a routine procedure in many nuclear medicine laboratories [11].

A newly proposed elegant imaging protocol is the so-called stress-immediate reinjection procedure, initially proposed by Van Eck-Smit et al. in 1993 [12], whereby ^{201}Tl is reinjected at rest as soon as exercise imaging is completed. Delayed rest imaging is performed 1 hour after the rest injection. The total procedure is much shorter (2.5 hours) than the conventional ^{201}Tl imaging protocol or the classical reinjection protocol. In a quantitative comparative analysis of the stress-stress-redistribution-reinjection approach versus the stress-immediate reinjection approach in the same patient, excellent agreement existed for perfusion defect size and defect reversibility [13]. Another variation of this modification involves the administration of 20 mg isosorbide dinitrate orally after exercise before ^{201}Tl reinjection [14].

A last ^{201}Tl SPECT imaging protocol is the so-called rest-redistribution imaging, first described by Ragosta et al. in 1993 [15]. In contrast to the ^{201}Tl exercise protocols, the rest-4-hour redistribution procedure is mainly reserved for identifying viable tissue in patients with moderate to severe ischemic left ventricular dysfunction and can predict functional recovery after coronary bypass procedures.

Although each of the aforementioned approaches has its own merits, the most practical approach for exercise ^{201}Tl SPECT imaging is, in my opinion, to follow the stress-immediate reinjection protocol because of its time-saving and patient-convenient aspects. Besides, this approach provides at least similar information on myocardial perfusion and viability in patients with ischemic heart disease as the more established protocols [16,17]. Quantitative analysis of exercise and rest defect size by SPECT bulls-eye analysis enhances the confidence to distinguish patients with truly fixed defects from those with defect reversibility. Figure 1 shows the currently established protocols for ^{201}Tl myocardial perfusion imaging.

Myocardial SPECT imaging with ^{99m}Tc-sestamibi

One of the essential hallmarks of ^{99m}Tc-sestamibi is its lack of significant washout (or redistribution). The high photon flux it produces can advantageously be used for SPECT imaging. Myocardial SPECT images are usually of higher quality than those produced by ^{201}Tl scintigraphy. Because of the initially high liver uptake, which clears rapidly, the images are optimally acquired after 1 hour following ^{99m}Tc-sestamibi injection. Since ^{99m}Tc-sestamibi concentrates in the myocardium and does not undergo redistribution, two separate injections are required to distinguish stress-induced defects from resting defects.

The rest and stress images are ideally acquired on two different days to allow the decay of the initial activity to occur prior to the second injection [18]. This 2-day protocol allows the injection of 20-30 mCi (750-1100 MBq) ^{99m}Tc-sestamibi during each of the 2 days. Alternatively, rest and exercise images may be acquired in the same day, using an initial dose of 10 mCi (370 MBq) followed by a second dose of 20 mCi (750 MBq). Taillefer et al. [19] have suggested that when two images acquired on the same day, the rest-stress protocol is somewhat superior to the stress-rest sequence, because some defects may appear to be reversible (ischemic) in the former protocol but fixed (scar) in the latter. However, when they compared the rest-stress with the stress-rest protocol, a concordance of 92% among normal, ischemic, or scarred segments was found; a discrepancy was observed in less than 8% of the myocardial segments analyzed. On the other hand, the advantage of performing the stress ^{99m}Tc-sestamibi images first is that of these stress images are normal, the rest images may not be necessarily, thus reducing in time for the study, the radiation dosimetry to the patient, and the cost of the study. The "ideal" protocol for ^{99m}Tc-sestamibi imaging will almost certainly need to be tailored to the individual institution's particular needs. For example, in an institution where patients with low likelihood of coronary artery disease are imaged frequently, a protocol beginning with the stress image first may be more cost- and time-effective, since many of these patients will have a normal study, thus rendering the rest study redundant. If the stress studies are abnormal, a rest study ideally should be obtained on a separate day or several hours after the first injection.

The relative high dose of ^{99m}Tc can be used for the assessment of global and regional left ventricular function. With a rapid bolus injection of ^{99m}Tc-sestamibi,

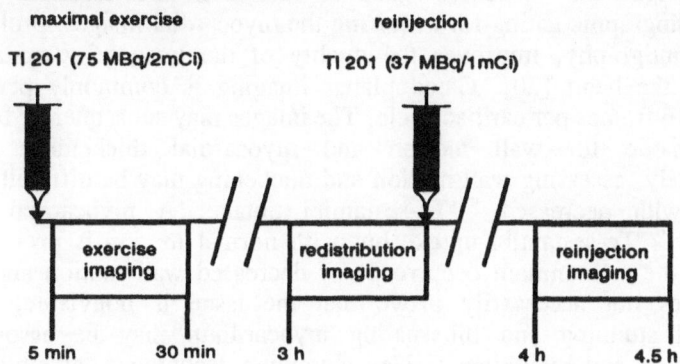

REINJECTION IMAGING
(Dilsizian N Engl J Med '90)

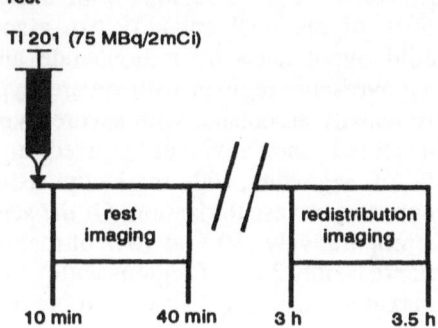

REST/REDISTRIBUTION IMAGING
(Ragosta et al., Circulation 1993)

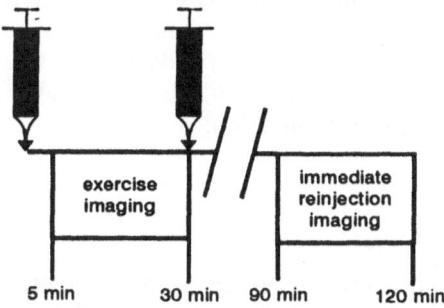

IMMEDIATE REINJECTION IMAGING
(van Eck-Smit J Nucl Med'93)

Figure 1. Currently established protocols for ^{201}Tl myocardial SPECT imaging in the detection of perfusion and viability.

first pass studies can be performed at rest and during exercise with specially designed high-count sensitive gamma cameras. The feasibility of using electrocardiographic gating for acquiring the myocardial images, preferably with SPECT scintigraphy, improves the quality of the images by minimizing the motion of the heart [20]. Gated planar imaging is commonly performed by acquiring 16 frames per cardiac cycle. The images may subsequently be displayed in cine mode for wall motion and myocardial thickening assessment. Unfortunately, assessing wall motion and thickening may be difficult, especially in\ areas with decreased ^{99m}Tc-sestamibi uptake. A myocardial wall with diminished ^{99m}Tc-sestamibi uptake but with normal motion is probably viable. However, the concomitant occurrence of decreased wall motion and decreased uptake does not necessarily prove that the issue is nonviable, since both myocardial stunning and hibernating myocardium may be associated with hypoperfusion and hypokinesis. New computer techniques, albeit in the early stages of development, hold promise to quantitatively assess wall motion and thickening on sestamibi images.

Comparison of segmental perfusion by resting ^{99m}Tc-sestamibi images and wall motion by radionuclide angiography has been used recently to characterize myocardial viability [21]. In this study 77% of regions with normal or only mildly decreased perfusion (>50% of maximal uptake) were associated with either normal wall motion or mild hypokinesis by radionuclide angiography, indicating myocardial viability. Conversely, regions with severe hypoperfusion (<50% of maximal uptake) were usually associated with severe hypokinesis or akinesis, and hence were considered indicative of scarred myocardium. Furthermore, in this study 61% of segments with markedly reduced ^{99m}Tc-sestamibi uptake improved after coronary revascularization. Of the segments with mild to moderate hypoperfusion preoperatively (50% to 70% of maximal counts) 80% improved postoperatively, whereas only 39% of regions with ^{99m}Tc-sestamibi uptake less than 50% of maximal had significant improvement after revascularization.

In conclusion, best imaging results with ^{99m}Tc-sestamibi are obtained with the 2-day imaging protocol because the count density of these images are usually excellent. From a more practical point of view a same-day protocol is preferred whereby stress imaging is performed first. The last option is more convenient for nuclear medicine laboratories, although one should be aware of relative low counts in the stress images. For simultaneous assessment of left ventricular perfusion and function, ^{99m}Tc labeled agents are the imaging agents of choice. It can be anticipated that computer software will be developed that allows for quantitative assessment of myocardial perfusion, regional wall motion, and ejection fraction with one single image acquisition.

Dual-isotope SPECT imaging

In 1993, dual isotope imaging has been proposed as an alternative means for detecting CAD by Berman et al. [22]. With this approach, ^{201}Tl is given at rest and ^{99m}Tc-sestamibi during stress. The protocol is a 1-day study whereby the patient is first injected at rest with 2.5-3.5 mCi (90-130 MBq) ^{201}Tl followed by imaging 15 minutes later. Immediately after completion of the rest imaging, stress imaging is performed with administration of 20-30 mCi ^{99m}Tc-sestamibi at peak exercise followed by imaging 30 minutes later. As this approach is significantly shorter than the same-day ^{99m}Tc-sestamibi protocols, this protocol was primarily designed to improve patient throughput. Although attractive from a practical point of view, disadvantages of the dual-isotope SPECT imaging protocol are the use of ^{201}Tl at rest and the use of two tracers with different physical characteristics, affecting count density and imaging quality.

Myocardial SPECT imaging with ^{99m}Tc-teboroxime

The agent ^{99m}Tc-teboroxime is unique among myocardial perfusion agents because it has been shown to be a much better tracer of myocardial blood flow than ^{201}Tl or ^{99m}Tc-sestamibi [23]. However, the biokinetics of ^{99m}Tc-teboroxime are markedly different from those of ^{201}Tl and ^{99m}Tc-sestamibi in that it has a very rapid clearance from the myocardium. This characteristic of ^{99m}Tc-teboroxime precludes the acquisition of consistently good quality images, in particular when using SPECT imaging. Unless one employs specially designed fast-imaging protocols [24,25], clinical imaging with ^{99m}Tc-teboroxime is disappointing and the agent is therefore not widely used at the present time.

Myocardial SPECT imaging with ^{99m}Tc-tetrofosmin

Technetium-99m tetrofosmin is one of the most recently developed agents for myocardial perfusion SPECT imaging. Similar to ^{99m}Tc-sestamibi, ^{99m}Tc-tetrofosmin shows a very slow clearance from the myocardium allowing serial imaging during several hours. The ^{99m}Tc-tetrofosmin stress imaging protocol is based on a same-day or a separate day imaging protocol (Figure 2), similar to the known ^{99m}Tc-sestamibi SPECT imaging protocols [26]. With a same-day imaging protocol, 7 mCi (250 MBq) ^{99m}Tc-tetrofosmin is administered at rest followed by imaging 1 hour later. The stress dosage (20 mCi, 750 MBq) is given 3 hours after the rest injection, and stress imaging is performed 30 minutes following injection of the radionuclide. In this way performed, the imaging procedure results in a total investigation time of around 4 hours. With a separate-day imaging protocol, at peak stress 14 mCi (370 MBq) ^{99m}Tc-tetrofosmin is injected and imaging is started 30 minutes following termination of exercise. On a separate day, 14 mCi (500 MBq) is administered at rest followed by imaging 1 hour later. The period between injection and imaging is required because of liver activity and its subsequent clearance, which takes more time when administered at rest compared to exercise. Similar to ^{99m}Tc-sestamibi, the use of ^{99m}Tc-tetrofosmin allows the acquisition of first pass and gated SPECT studies. At present there is only limited clinical experience with ^{99m}Tc-tetrofosmin, but initial results are very promising [6,27].

99mTc-tetrofosmin same-day rest-stress protocol

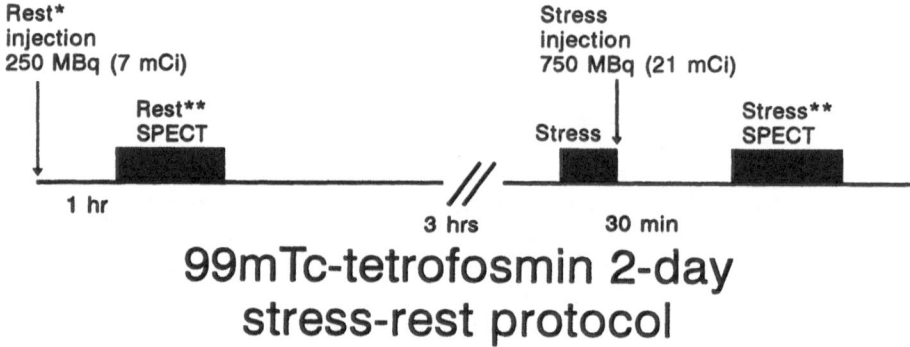

99mTc-tetrofosmin 2-day stress-rest protocol

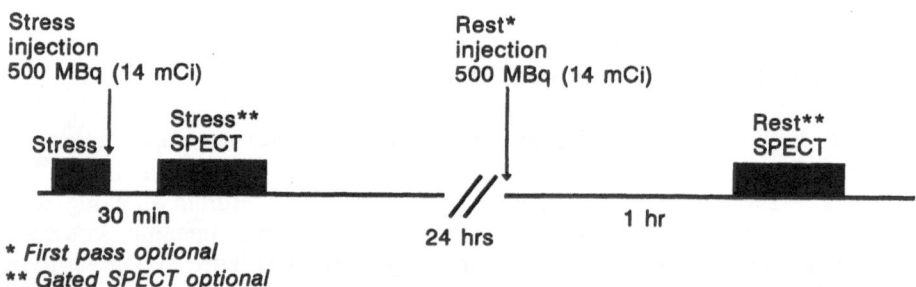

* First pass optional
** Gated SPECT optional

Figure 2. Currently established protocols for ^{99m}Tc-tetrofosmin myocardial perfusion SPECT imaging.

Detection of coronary artery disease

A pooled analysis of the six largest studies evaluating ^{201}Tl exercise SPECT imaging for the detection of CAD has recently been reported [28]. Coronary angiography was used as the reference standard for assessing the sensitivity of SPECT with a >50% stenosis considered significant. Specificity was based on whether patients had normal coronary arteriograms or a low predicted risk (<5%) for CAD. The overall sensitivity of SPECT for detecting CAD was 90% (range 81-98%) for the 1.042 patients analyzed - 99% in those patients with, and 85% in those without, prior infarction. Most patients with single vessel (83%) and virtually all patients with double (93%) and triple (95%) vessel disease were detected. Furthermore, two-thirds of patients with multivessel involvement were correctly identified as having multivessel disease. Of the 1.328 abnormal coronary arteries, 79% were detected, with sensitivity increasing to 88% for arteries with ≥70% stenosis.

The specificity of SPECT was 70% for the 239 patients with normal arteriograms, but increased to 89% for those with low predicted risk. The lower specificity in patients with normal arteriograms is related to post-test referral bias since, in general, more patients with abnormal images undergo coronary angiography. The high specificity (84%) of SPECT for detecting the 1.468 angiographically normal coronary arteries in this series, is consistent with the 89% specificity observed in patients with low predicted risk. When comparing the diagnostic power of ^{201}Tl to that of ^{99m}Tc-sestamibi, similar sensitivities and specificities have been found when planar imaging was used [29]. When SPECT imaging was used, similar sensitivities and only a trend to higher specificities with ^{99m}Tc-sestamibi were observed [30]. However, because of its superior imaging qualities compared to ^{201}Tl, one could make a strong case for using ^{99m}Tc-sestamibi SPECT in obese patients and in women with massive breast tissue. As with any technique, strict quality control is necessary to obtain good results. When performed properly, exercise SPECT is highly accurate for detecting the presence, extent and location of CAD in patients referred for evaluation of chest pain syndromes.

Role of pharmacologic stress

Despite the wide clinical utility of exercise perfusion scintigraphy, 25-30% of patients referred for imaging cannot perform adequate exercise which may significantly reduce sensitivity. This is particularly true in patients who terminate exercise early for noncardiac reasons, such as claudication from peripheral vascular disease or dyspnea from a primary pulmonary condition. Furthermore, even in patients who do develop transient perfusion abnormalities during submaximal exercise, the extent of the jeopardized myocardial risk zone may be significantly underestimated. In order to broaden the clinical availability of perfusion scintigraphy, the pharmacologic vasodilators, adenosine and dipyridamole, and more recently, dobutamine, have steadily gained acceptance as alternatives to exercise stress. As with exercise scintigraphy, SPECT is notably better for detecting and localizing CAD than planar imaging.

Adenosine has been studied in well over 1.000 patients at doses of 140 mcg/kg/min. The reported sensitivity and specificity of adenosine SPECT imaging are 90% and 89%. respectively, with excellent comparability to exercise [31]. Although the experience with dobutamine scintigraphy is limited, Hays et al. [32] reported a sensitivity and specificity of 86% and 90%, respectively, at a maximal dobutamine dose of 40 mcg/kg/min. Marwick et al. [33] compared dobutamine and adenosine echocardiography to ^{99m}Tc-sestamibi SPECT in 97 consecutive patients without prior infarction. Adenosine and dobutamine were infused up to peak doses of 180 and 40 mcg/kg/min, respectively. In this trial, adenosine and dobutamine SPECT imaging had equivalent sensitivity (86% and 80%, respectively), and specificity (71% and 74%, respectively), whereas the sensitivity of adenosine echocardiography was inferior to SPECT with either stressor (58%, p < 0.001). The sensitivity of dobutamine echocardiography, however, was comparably high at 85% with a specificity of 82%. Similar reports from other investigators indicate that dobutamine is a more rational choice with echocardiography than pharmacologic coronary vasodilators, whereas all three major pharmacologic stressor agents can be combined successfully with SPECT imaging.

Assessment of prognosis

Myocardial perfusion imaging is invaluable for assessing risk in a wide spectrum of patients. A negative perfusion scan for ischemia has been consistently shown to predict a very low annual risk ($<1\%$) for death or non-fatal infarction when combined with either exercise or pharmacologic stressors [34,35]. Conversely, patients with scintigraphically assessed ischemia are at considerably higher risk, which increases with the extent to hypoperfused myocardium. As shown in a recent study using quantitative exercise ^{201}Tl SPECT, patients with perfusion defects significantly increased risk for death or non-fatal infarction (25%) compared to those with smaller defects (5%, $p < 0.001$) [36]. Furthermore, defect size contributed most to overall risk when compared to angiographic or treadmill data. Similar data have now been reported for ^{99m}Tc sestamibi SPECT imaging, which showed a benign long-term prognosis in patients with a normal cardiac perfusion image [7].

Exercise scintigraphy can accurately risk stratify patients after myocardial infarction and is of greater relative value than routine coronary angiography or submaximal exercise testing for discriminating low from high risk patients. This has also been shown using dipyridamole or adenosine stress. With adenosine SPECT a very low one year cardiac event rate in patients with small ($<20\%$) nonischemic perfusion defects is observed. Conversely, risk progressively increases with larger perfusion defects and relatively greater ischemia. Thus, there is mounting evidence that defect size and the extent of ischemia accurately predict risk in a wide spectrum of patients with CAD. At the present time, precise risk analyses based on the extent of left ventricular involvement have only been reported using myocardial perfusion scintigraphy.

Evaluation of the effects of therapy

Sequential myocardial perfusion scintigraphy has been successfully used to assess the efficacy of anti-anginal medications both in patients with coronary artery spasm and, more recently, in those with fixed obstructive CAD. Agents that improve coronary blood flow will diminish exercise-induced ischemia, limit heterogeneity in myocardial perfusion and thereby reduce scintigraphic defects. It has been observed that calcium-antagonists can significantly reduce exercise-induced scintigraphic ischemia compared to placebo (Figure 3). In fact, over one-third of patients randomized to active therapy may show a $>10\%$ reduction in their absolute perfusion defect size over a one week treatment period. If the total extent of jeopardized myocardium defines risk, it is logical to assume that by reducing or eliminating perfusion defects prognosis should improve. Prospective randomized trials are still needed to prove this hypothesis.

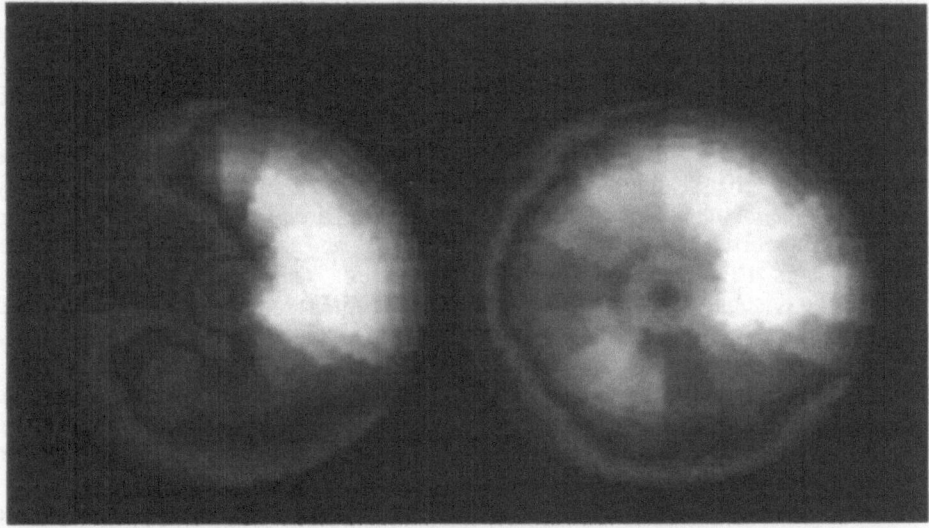

Figure 3. Bull's eye plot of ^{99m}Tc-tetrofosmin images obtained during stress before (*left*) and during diltiazem medication (*right*). Before medication the anteroseptal area shows a significant perfusion defect which is almost completely resolved during diltiazem therapy. (For colour plate of figure 3 see page 567)

Conclusions

Myocardial perfusion scintigraphy using SPECT, by virtue of its extensive clinical validation and versatility, is presently the technique of choice for evaluating patients with known or suspected CAD. Precise quantification of perfusion defects with SPECT has further improved risk stratification and can provide an accurate serial assessment of patients following therapeutic interventions. The development of new perfusion tracers has considerably widened our scope in order to further explore the physiologic mechanisms of myocardial perfusion and viability. In conjunction with the application of vasodilatory substances, myocardial stress perfusion scintigraphy is now virtually accessible to all patients referred for cardiac evaluation. In this era of continuing cost containment, myocardial perfusion SPECT imaging emerges as a highly cost-effective noninvasive modality for guiding patient management.

References

1. Verzijlbergen JF, Van Oudheusden D, Cramer MJ *et al*. Quantitative analysis of planar technetium-99m Sestamibi myocardial perfusion images. Clinical application of a modified method for the subtraction of tissue crosstalk. Eur Heart J 1994;15:1217-26.
2. Kiat H, Berman DS, Maddahi J. Comparison of planar and tomographic

exercise thallium-201 imaging methods for the evaluation of coronary artery disease. J Am Coll Cardiol 1989;13:613-6.

3.   Mahmarian JJ, Pratt CM, Borges-Neto S, Cashion WR, Roberts R, Verani MS. Quantification of infarct size by 201Tl- single-photon emission computed tomography during acute myocardial infarction in humans. Comparison with enzymatic estimates. Circulation 1988;78:831-9.

4.   Mahmarian JJ, Pratt CM, Nishimura S, Abren A, Verani MS. Quantitative adenosine 201Tl single-photon emission computed tomography for the early assessment of patients surviving acute myocardial infarction. Circulation 1993;87;1197-210.

5.   Wackers FJ, Berman DS, Maddahi J et al. Technetium-99m hexakis 2-methoxyisobutyl isonitrile: human biodistribution, dosimetry, safety, and preliminary comparison to thallium-201 for myocardial perfusion imaging. J Nucl Med 1989;30:310-11.

6.   Zaret BL, Rigo P, Wackers FJT et al. Myocardial perfusion imaging with ^{99m}Tc tetrofosmin. Comparison to ^{201}Tl imaging and coronary angiography in a phase III multicenter trial. Tetrofosmin International Trial Study Group. Circulation 1995;91:313-9.

7.   Berman DS, Hachamovitch R, Kiat H et al. Incremental value of prognostic testing in patients with known or suspected ischemic heart disease: a basis for optimal utilization of exercise technetium-99m sestamibi myocardial perfusion single-photon emission computed tomography. J Am Coll Cardiol 1995;26:639-47.

8.   Kiat H, Berman DS, Maddahi J et al. Late reversibility of tomographic myocardial thallium-201 defects: an accurate marker of myocardial viability. J Am Coll Cardiol 1988;12:1456-63.

9.   Kayden DS, Sigal S, Soufer R, Mattera J, Zaret BL, Wackers FJT. Thallium-201 for assessment of myocardial viability: quantitative comparison of 24-hour redistribution imaging with imaging after reinjection at rest. J Am Coll Cardiol 1991;18:1480-6.

10. Dilsizian V, Rocco TP, Freeman NMT, Leon MB, Bonow RO. Enhanced detection of ischemic but viable myocardium by the reinjection of thallium after stress-redistribution imaging. N Engl J Med 1990;323:141-6.

11. Kuijper AFM, Vliegen HW, van der Wall EE et al. The clinical impact of thallium-201 reinjection scintigraphy for detection of myocardial viability. Eur J Nucl Med 1992;19:783-99.

12. Van Eck-Smit BLF, van der Wall EE, Kuijper AFM, Zwinderman AH, Pauwels EKJ. Immediate thallium-201 reinjection following stress imaging: a time-saving approach for detection of myocardial viability. J Nucl Med 1993;34:737-43.

13. Wackers FJ, Pieri PL, McMahon M et al. Quantitative reproducibility of repeated planar thallium stress imaging [abstract]. J Nucl Med 1993;34(5 Suppl):44P.

14. He ZX, Darcourt J, Guignier A et al. Nitrates improve detection of ischemic viable myocardium by thallium-201 reinjection SPECT. J Nucl Med 1993;34:1472-7.

15. Ragosta M, Beller GA, Watson DD, Kaul S, Gimple LW. Quantitative planar rest-redistribution ^{201}Tl imaging in detection of myocardial viability and prediction of improvement in left ventricular function after coronary bypass surgery in patients with severely depressed left ventricular function. Circulation 1993;87:1630-41.

16. Van Eck-Smit BLF, van der Wall EE, Zwinderman AH, Pauwels EKJ. Clinical value of immediate thallium-201 reinjection imaging for the detection of ischaemic heart disease. Eur Heart J 1995;16:410-20.

17. Van Eck-Smit BLF, van der Wall EE. Reinjection of thallium for detection of viable myocardium: why not do it immediately? Br Heart J 1995;74:101-2.

18. Taillefer R, Laflamma L, Dupras G, Picard M, Phaneuf DC, Léveille J. Myocardial perfusion imaging with ^{99m}Tc-methoxy-isobutyl-isonitrile (MIBI): comparison of short and long time intervals between rest and stress injection. Preliminary results. Eur J Nucl Med 1988;13:515-22.

19. Taillefer R. Technetium-99m sestamibi myocardial imaging: same-day rest stress studies and dipyridamole Am J Cardiol 1990;66:80E-84E.

20. Verzijlbergen JF, Suttorp MJ, Ascoop CAPL *et al.* Combined assessment of technetium-99m sestamibi planar myocardial perfusion images at rest and during exercise with rest-exercise left ventricular wall motion studies evaluated from gated myocardial perfusion studies. Am Heart J 1992;123:59-68.

21. Rocco TP, Dilsizian V, Strauss HW, Boucher CA. Technetium-99m isonitrile myocardial uptake at rest. II. Relation to clinical markers of potential viability. J Am Coll Cardiol 1989;14:1678-84.

22. Berman DS, Kiat H, Friedman JD *et al.* Separate acquisition rest thallium-201/stress technetium-99m sestamibi dual-isotope myocardial perfusion single photon emission computed tomography: a clinical validation study. J Am Coll Cardiol 1993;22:1455-64.

23. Seldin DW, Johnson LL, Blood DK *et al.* Myocardial perfusion imaging with technetium SQ30217: comparison with thallium-201 and coronary anatomy. J Nucl Med 1989;30:312-9.

24. Hendel RC, McSherry B, Karimeddini M, Leppo JA. Diagnostic value of a new myocardial perfusion agent, teboroxime (SQ 30,217), utilizing a rapid planar imaging protocol: preliminary results. J Am Coll Cardiol 1990;16:855-61.

25. Chua T, Kiat H, Germano G *et al.* Rapid back to back adenosine stress/rest technetium-99m teboroxime myocardial perfusion SPECT using a triple-detector camera. J Nucl Med 1993;34:1485-93.

26. Jain D, Wackers FJ, Mattera J, McMahon M, Sinusas AJ, Zaret BL. Biokinetics of technetium-99M-tetrofosmin: myocardial perfusion imaging agent: implications for a one-day imaging protocol. J Nucl Med 1993;34:1254-9.

27. Sridhara BS, Braat S, Rigo P, Itti P, Cload P, Lahiri A. Comparison of myocardial perfusion imaging with technetium-99m-tetrofosmin versus thallium-201 in coronary artery disease. Am J Cardiol 1993;72:1015-9.

28. Mahmarian JJ, Pratt CM, Boyce TM, Verani MS. The variable extent of jeopardized myocardium in patients with single vessel coronary artery disease: quantification by thallium-201 single photon emission computed tomography. J Am Coll Cardiol 1991;17:355-62.

29. Verzijlbergen JF, Cramer MJ, Niemeyer MG, Ascoop CA, van der Wall EE, Pauwels EK. 99Tcm-SESTAMIBI for planar myocardial perfusion imaging;not as ideal as the physical properties. Nucl Med Commun 1991;12:381-91.

30. Cramer MJ, Verzijlbergen JF, van der Wall EE *et al.* Head-to-head comparison between technetium-99m-sestamibi and thallium-201 tomographic imaging for the detection of coronary artery disease using combined dipyridamole-exercise-stress. Coron Artery Dis 1994;5:787-91.

31. Nishimura S, Mahmarian JJ, Boyce TM, Verani MS. Quantitative thallium-201 single-photon emission computed tomography during maximal pharmacologic

coronary vasodilation with adenosine for assessing coronary artery disease. J Am Coll Cardiol 1991;18:736-45.

32. Hays JT, Mahmarian JJ, Cochran AJ, Verani MS. Dobutamine thallium-201 tomography for evaluating patients with suspected coronary artery disease unable to undergo exercise or vasodilator pharmacologic stress testing. J Am Coll Cardiol 1993;21:1583-90.

33. Marwick T, Willemart B, D'Hondt AM *et al*. Selection of the optimal nonexercise stress for the evaluation of ischemic regional myocardial dysfunction and malperfusion. Comparison of dobutamine and adenosine using echocardiography and ^{99m}Tc-MIBI single photon emission computed tomography. Circulation 1993;87:345-54.

34. Brown KA. Prognostic value of thallium-201 myocardial perfusion imaging. A diagnostic tool comes of age. Circulation 1991;83:363-81.

35. Oosterhuis WP, Breeman A, Niemeyer MG *et al*. Patients with a normal exercise thallium-201 myocardial scintigram: always a good prognosis? Eur J Nucl Med 1993;20:151-8.

36. Iskandrian AS, Chae SC, Heo J, Stanberry CD, Wasserleben V, Cave V. Independent and incremental prognostic value of exercise single-photon emission computed tomographic (SPECT) thallium imaging in coronary artery disease. J Am Coll Cardiol 1993;22:665-70.

39. Myocardial blood flow quantitation with positron emission tomography

WILLIAM WIJNS, ANNE BOL & JACQUES A. MELIN

Summary

Dynamic Positron Emission Tomography (PET) with the use of appropriate tracers is the only technique available thus far that permits quantitation of regional myocardial blood flow (MBF) in absolute terms, i.e. ml/min/g of tissue. This review discusses some of the contributions of PET measurements of MBF to the understanding of the pathophysiology of coronary artery disease.

Quantitation of MBF by PET depends on its unique performance in terms of instrumentation physics, tracer kinetics and on the applicability of appropriate protocols for data acquisition. True tissue tracer concentrations are obtained by correction for attenuation and finite resolution effects. Both $^{13}NH_3$ and $H_2^{15}O$ can be used as flow tracers together with validated models. From the MBF values obtained during baseline conditions as well as during pharmacologically induced hyperaemia, MBF reserve can be computed.

Mean values in normal volunteers range between 0.8 ± 0.2 and 1.2 ± 0.3 ml/min/g at rest, 2.7 ± 0.9 and 4.6 ± 1.6 ml/min/g during hyperaemia. The MBF reserve ranges between 2.9 ± 1.0 and 4.4 ± 1.2. This wide range for normalcy represents biological heterogeneity. Hyperaemic MBF and MBF reserve decrease above 60 years of age.

In stable patients with coronary stenosis and normal myocardial contraction, baseline MBF does not decrease despite increasing stenosis severity. Hyperaemic MBF and MBF reserve decrease progressively when stenosis reaches 40 % in diameter. In some patients, MBF provided through collaterals is able to maintain nearly normal MBF reserve.

Very few quantitative data are available on the effects of mechanical revascularisation by bypass surgery or balloon dilatation. After balloon angioplasty, MBF reserve was shown to increase only gradually despite immediate enlargement of the epicardial coronary lumen. A transient disturbance in the microcirculation, perhaps through endothelial dysfunction, was postulated. Indeed, PET measurements of MBF and MBF reserve are sensitive to changes in lipid profile and risk factor modification.

PET studies of MBF can be used prospectively to evaluate the impact of various interventions on the coronary circulation. Ongoing attempts to refine the technique are directed towards the measurement of the transmural gradient in MBF and to the quantitation of perfusion to healthy myocardium remaining within areas of permanent ischemic damage.

J.H.C. Reiber and E.E. van der Wall (eds.), Cardiovascular Imaging, 513-529.

Introduction

Nutrient perfusion to the myocardium at the tissue level depends on a cascade of interactions between a number of factors among which the net driving perfusion pressure, the state of the epicardial conduits and the function of the large microcirculatory compartment. Regulation in health and disorders caused by disease can affect any or a combination of these three main determinants of myocardial perfusion. Various techniques were developed over the last decades to interrogate myocardial blood flow (MBF) and flow distribution [1,2]. The ability to accurately measure the perfusion pressure in humans only became available recently with the development of pressure and flow velocity monitoring guide wires [3-5]. Data obtained in subjects without overt epicardial disease have confirmed that these conduits do not represent a significant obstacle to flow until they become severely narrowed by atheromatous plaque accumulation [5]. Other techniques including coronary angiography and its quantitation [6-8], or intravascular ultrasound are precisely confined to the anatomic and functional evaluation of the epicardial vessels (the "capacitance" compartment). The "resistance" compartment has been studied using several invasive and noninvasive imaging techniques, none of which could provide reliable measurements of nutrient flow [8,9]. Their impossibility to quantitate tissue perfusion depends on the intrinsic physical constraints of the imaging systems as well as on the physiological limitations of the compounds used as flow tracers. Both issues were eventually solved by the long-lasting refinements of the Positron Emission Tomography (PET) technique, as will be outlined briefly below [10]. The basic concept is that the absolute level of tissue perfusion in ml/min/100 g is a net measurement which represents the integrated response of the entire coronary circulation to all factors intervening at any level. Interpretation of the results is greatly enhanced by the knowledge of the basic hemodynamics and the coronary anatomy, such that the cause(s) of reduced perfusion can be easily localized.

Coronary artery disease (CAD) and atherosclerosis certainly represent the main cause of disturbances in myocardial perfusion in western countries and this chapter will be limited to this topic. A more extensive review of the new information derived from PET measurements of flow in others cardiac disorders can be found elsewhere [11].

Methodological issues

The physical properties of PET including its high sensitivity coupled to the principle of coincidence detection and attenuation correction can largely overcome the intrinsic limitations of other imaging devices [10,12]. These quantitative capabilities of PET were recognized from the onset back in the late seventies, but it is only recently that adequate quantitative measurements became available albeit in a small number of laboratories including ours [13]. It should be remembered that imaging the heart is particularly demanding considering the cyclic changes in cavity size and wall thickness, the thin myocardial walls (on average 10 to 15 mm), the presence of four adjacent chambers and the superimposed respiratory motion [14]. High resolution tomographs permitting rapid acquisition of sequential data in a dynamic mode only became available since the early nineteen's together with the development of appropriate tracers and well-validated tracer kinetics models [15]. These models now include corrections for the underestimation of true radiotracer concentration due to the partial volume effect and spillover from the left ventricular chamber into the myocardial regions of interest [16-19]. The methodological steps that are required (Table 1) were summarized by Bol et al. [13,16] in previously published reviews. Methodological issues that remain imperfectly dealt with include correction for scattered radiation, spillover from the right ventricular chamber to the interventricular septum, time shifts between the input function and the tissue response particularly when the atrial blood pool is used, and quantification of tracer uptake in pathological regions containing mixed tissue types, i.e., myocardial scar [20].

Table 1. MBF quantitation with PET.

LEVEL 1 :	Obtain quantitative regional tissue radioactivity from images
ISSUES :	a. High count rates and dead-time losses b. Scattered radiation c. Photon attenuation d. Finite resolution effects
LEVEL 2 :	Translate regional tissue radioactivity in terms of biological parameters i.e. MBF in ml/min/g
ISSUES :	a. Tracer input b. Tissue response c. Combined time-activity curves d. Metabolite correction when applicable e. Tracer kinetic model

Another equally important component of the tedious quantification procedure is the choice of an appropriate tracer. Among the various positron-labelled tracers that have been evaluated, $^{13}NH_3$ and $H_2^{15}O$ are currently the only ones that have undergone validation in animal studies [21]. PET measurements indeed showed to be comparable to flow estimates obtained by radioactive microspheres over a large range of values. The accuracy of measurements obtained with $^{13}NH_3$ (physical half life 9.8 min) was confirmed despite the fact that tracer extraction is flow-dependent. Modelling based on the use of a compartmental model separating the first-pass extraction of the tracer from its metabolic trapping permits to correct for the decreasing $^{13}NH_3$ retention fraction with increasing flow [22]. Later metabolic trapping in the glutamine pool makes this tracer particularly suited for high contrast imaging. At the opposite, $H_2^{15}O$ is an inert agent which easily permits repetitive measurements due to its very short physical half life (2.1 min). The tracer can be administered intravenously as labelled water or inhaled as $C^{15}O_2$, which results in the rapid labelling of lung water by carbonic anhydrase. The kinetic models are based on a constant partition coefficient of $H_2^{15}O$ between tissue and blood as well as on free tracer diffusion [23-25]. An example of left ventricular (tracer input) and myocardial (tissue response) time-activity curves is shown on Figure 1. The choice between one or the other tracer depends on local experience, availability, dosimetry and convenience.

PET measurements of MBF are usually performed during baseline conditions and repeated after pharmacological hyperaemia. The rationale behind this approach has been extensively validated: by reducing resistances in the microvasculature to a minimum, the maximally achievable flow is reached which linearly depends on perfusion pressure [26-30]. To this end, various physiologic and pharmacological stimuli have been used. Currently either intravenous infusion of adenosine (140 μg/kg/min) or dipyridamole (0.56 to 0.84 mg/kg over 4 to 10 min, respectively) are used in most of the published studies. Both drugs are known to cause selective vasodilatation of the small coronary vessels less than 150 μm in diameter [31-33]. The degree of coronary dilatation achievable in humans seem to be comparable with both agents [34]. Unlike maximal flow, baseline flow is strongly coupled to the cardiac work and oxygen demand. Normalization of the measured value to the prevailing hemodynamics at the time of data acquisition is necessary, for instance with the use of the rate-pressure product [11]. The ratio of hyperaemic over baseline flow values can then be computed on a regional basis as the absolute blood flow reserve in the different myocardial segments.

Normal values and physiological variations

The normal values (mean and standard deviation) for absolute baseline and hyperaemic MBF are given in Figure 2. The data are taken from 12 published series in a total of 179 normal volunteers, mostly male [24,25,34-42]. The baseline values are adjusted for the mean rate-pressure product of the group. The normal absolute MBF reserve thus ranges between 3.0 and 4.5. A number of points can be made:

1. MBF values measured with $^{13}NH_3$ or $H_2^{15}O$ appear identical. Confirmation by direct measurements using both tracers in the same subjects has not yet been published in length.
2. Hyperaemic MBF values obtained using either dipyridamole or adenosine appear identical. Chan et al. [34] used both agents in the same subjects and found similar results, although the response to adenosine tended to be less variable than the response to dipyridamole.
3. The spread of normal baseline and hyperaemic MBF is quite large. For instance, a baseline value as low as 0.5 ml/min/g remains within the physiological range. This finding likely represents true biological heterogeneity rather than measurement variability as similar observations were made in dogs using microspheres [43] and in humans using intracoronary flow velocity sampling [3]. However, data on the reproducibility of MBF measurements should be determined in each laboratory from repeated PET studies in the same subjects.

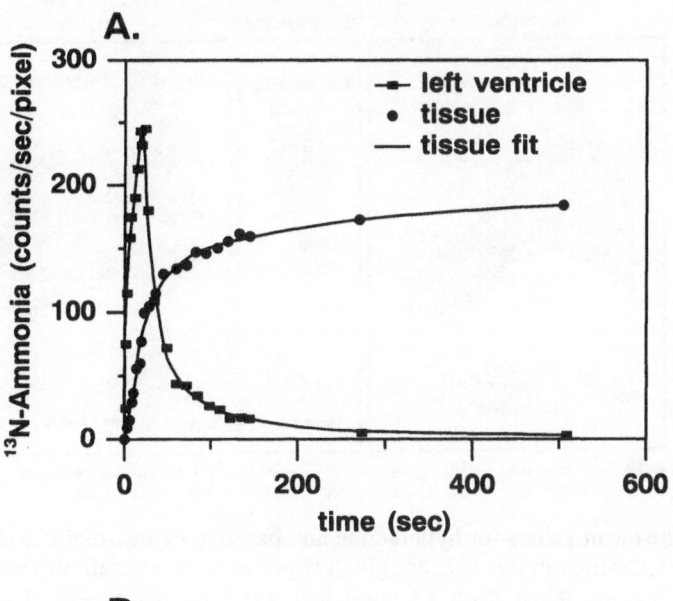

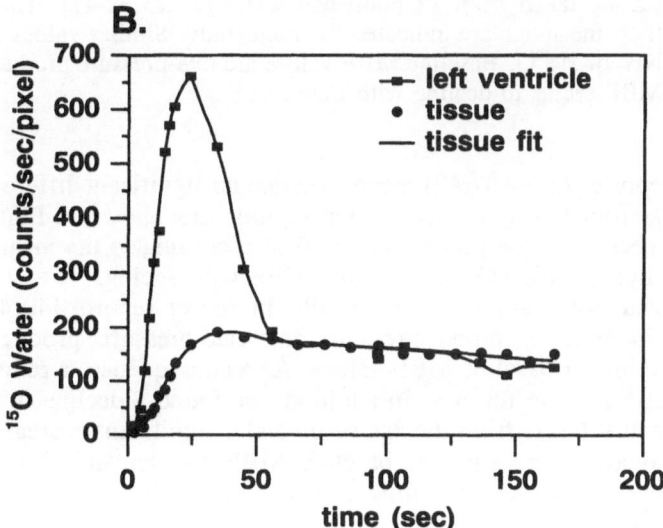

Figure 1. Panel A: The tracer input and the tissue response curves following the intravenous administration of $^{13}NH_3$ are plotted as activity in counts/sec/pixel (vertical axis) versus time in seconds (horizontal axis). The fit through the data is shown as well (solid line). Small regions of interest were drawn in the left ventricular cavity and in the myocardium. Delayed tracer retention in tissue long after blood pool clearance allows to obtain high contrast images with favorable signal-to-background ratio. Panel B: Data are shown in the same format following the intravenous administration of $H_2^{15}O$. Note the different scale for time and activity as well as the low signal-to-background ratio which explain the less than ideal image quality obtained with this tracer. Modified with permission from Bol et al. [13].

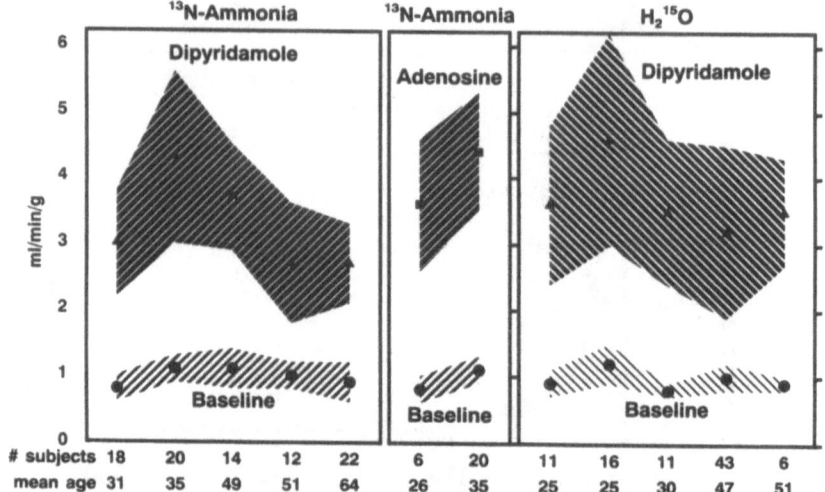

Figure 2. The mean values for hyperaemic and baseline myocardial blood flow (MBF in ml/min/g) obtained in normals are given together with standard deviations (shaded area). The data are taken from 12 published series [24,25,34-42]. The number of subjects and their mean age are indicated for each study. Similar values are obtained with either $^{13}NH_3$ or $H_2^{15}O$. Baseline MBF values are rate-pressure product corrected. Hyperaemic MBF seems to decline with increasing age.

4. Several reports [22,34-37,42] mentioned that no significant difference in MBF values was found between myocardial regions (not shown in Figure 2).
5. From inspection of the pooled data ranked according to the mean age of the subjects, hyperaemic MBF seems to decline with ageing.

The latter issue was addressed specifically in recent reports [40,42,44]. The progressive increase in blood pressure and rate-pressure product with age translates into higher baseline MBF values. As a consequence, a reduction in the calculated MBF reserve follows. In addition, we found a decline in hyperaemic MBF in normal subjects from the age of 60 and a significant decrease in reserve thus persisted after correction of baseline MBF for demand (Figure 3). The subjects in our study were carefully selected on the basis of normal history, physical examination, resting and exercise electrocardiogram and were part of a prospective study of several physiological aspects of ageing [40]. Advanced age resulted in a significant increase in minimum total coronary resistance, as calculated from the ratio between MBF and perfusion pressure during hyperaemia (Figure 3). These findings underscore the importance of comparing data obtained in patient populations with age-matched controls.

Myocardial blood flow in chronic ischemic heart disease

The obvious consequence of the presence of a severe coronary stenosis is to generate a pressure gradient at the epicardial level thereby reducing the distal

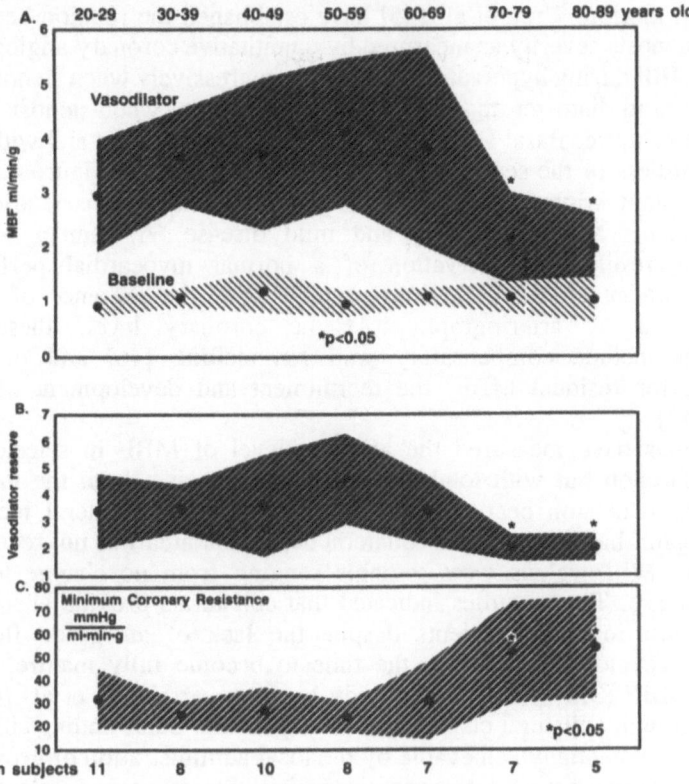

Figure 3. The effect of ageing on vasodilator and baseline MBF (panel A), vasodilator reserve (panel B) and minimum coronary resistance (panel C) is summarized for deciles from 20-29 up to 80-89 years old. Baseline MBF values were corrected for the rate-pressure product. The number of normal subjects studied in each decile is indicated. The significantly reduced MBF reserve beyond 70 years of age results from an absolute decrease in hyperaemic MBF. Modified with permission from Uren et al. [40].
* p < 0.05

perfusion pressure to the myocardium. This creates an additional pathological resistance to flow at a level which normally behaves as a capacitance. The seminal work by Gould et al. [26] has described the relation between epicardial stenosis and coronary flow in terms of fluid dynamics. Based on these early observations obtained in acute dog experiments, it was assumed that the increasing accumulation of atherosclerotic plaque within the coronary arteries of patients with CAD will progressively exhaust the MBF reserve and eventually reduce baseline MBF. In a group of 35 patients with single vessel disease and normal wall motion, Uren et al. [45] have established the relation between PET MBF and stenosis severity as measured by quantitative coronary angiography. As expected, MBF during hyperaemia decreased progressively when stenosis severity reached 40 % in diameter and MBF reserve was absent when stenosis was 80 % in diameter or more. Basal MBF, however, remained constant and within normal values regardless of the severity of stenosis as illustrated in Figure 4. The latter findings explain why accumulation of plaque within coronary arterial walls usually remains a well tolerated and mild disease. A number of adaptive mechanisms result in preservation of a normal myocardial perfusion and contraction under resting conditions, even despite the presence of sometimes severe disease by arteriography. At the coronary level, these adaptive mechanisms include compensatory wall remodelling [46] and of particular importance for residual MBF, the recruitment and development of collateral channels [47].

A few studies have measured the absolute level of MBF in selected patients without infarction but with total coronary occlusion in whom the myocardium distal to the occlusion becomes entirely dependent on collateral blood supply [48,49]. Again, basal flow to the collateral dependent area was not reduced. After hyperaemia, MBF values were variable ranging from no change to a nearly normal increase. These studies indicated that collaterals provide adequate blood supply at rest in stable patients despite the lack of antegrade flow. When sufficiently developed and given the time to become fully mature, a sizeable reserve in MBF (3.0 ± 0.6 in the study by Vanoverschelde et al. [48] can be provided through collateral channels in some patients. Such findings illustrate the benefit that is potentially achievable by the local administration of growth factors stimulating angiogenesis, a therapeutic option that is perhaps close to initial clinical evaluation [50,51]. It also explains why patients with seemingly comparable extent and severity of CAD by angiography may have a markedly different prognosis based on functional stress testing, as demonstrated by numerous noninvasive studies [52,53]. In the low-risk patient, a good response to stress reveals that the residual MBF (provided either through the native circulation or through collaterals) still permits a normal heart function despite the progressive accumulation of atherosclerotic plaque. Conversely, an abnormal stress result indicates a reduced level of residual myocardial perfusion and/or contraction reserve, thereby alerting to the presence of large areas of the myocardium that are potentially jeopardized.

Effect of therapeutic interventions

In patients with symptomatic CAD, mechanical revascularization by coronary artery bypass surgery or percutaneous transluminal coronary angioplasty (PTCA) is recommended [54,55]. The proven benefits include relief of symptoms, improved quality of life and prolonged survival, the latter particularly when the left ventricular function was depressed preoperatively. These beneficial effects are likely achieved by the restoration of a normal MBF reserve. Surprisingly very few quantitative data on the effects of revascularization on MBF are available and in particular none after bypass surgery.

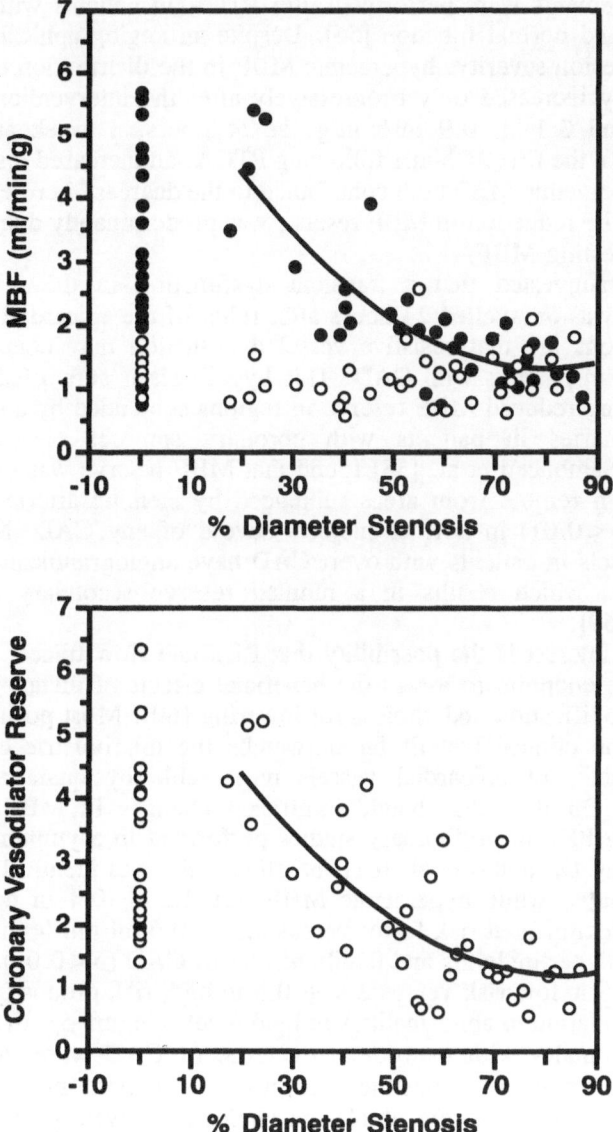

Figure 4. There is a significant impact of stenosis severity assessed by quantitation of percent diameter stenosis on hyperaemic MBF (top panel) and coronary vasodilator reserve (bottom panel). Top panel: normal values for baseline MBF (open circles) and hyperaemic MBF (filled circles) are plotted at 0 % diameter stenosis and not included in the regression. Note that baseline MBF does not decline despite increasing stenosis severity. The curvilinear relationship (r= 0.83) between hyperaemic MBF (filled circles) and % diameter stenosis is as follows: y = 6.7 - 0.1 x + 8.4 x² (n = 35). Bottom panel: the curvilinear relationship (r= 0.77) between coronary vasodilator reserve (open circles) and % diameter stenosis is as follows: y = 6.7 - 0.1 x + 7.8 x² (n = 35). Normal values are plotted at 0 % diameter stenosis and not included in the regression. Modified with permission from Uren et al. [45].

Serial measurements were performed after PTCA in patients with stable single vessel CAD and normal function [56]. Despite an angiographically satisfactory reduction in lesion severity, hyperaemic MBF in the distribution territory of the lesioned artery increased only progressively after the intervention: 2.1 ± 0.8, 2.3 ± 0.7 and 3.1 ± 0.9 ml/min/g, at 24 hours, 1 week and 3 months, respectively. In the first 24 hours following PTCA, an increased resting MBF and a reduced hyperaemic MBF both contributed to the decrease in reserve. At 7 days after PTCA, the reduction in MBF reserve was predominantly due to a sustained elevation of resting MBF.

The authors suggested that a transient dysfunction in the microcirculatory compartment was unravelled 24 hours after relief of the epicardial stenosis [56]. The implications are that resistive vessel dysfunction may contribute to flow dysregulation in patients with CAD. This hypothesis is supported by a number of data showing reduced MBF reserve in regions subtended by angiographically normal coronaries in patients with coronary stenoses elsewhere [57,58]. Forinstance, Sambuceti et al. [58] found that MBF reserve was only 2.3 ± 0.8 in myocardium remote from areas subtended by stenotic arteries compared to 3.6 ± 0.9 ($p < 0.01$) in normal subjects devoid of any CAD. Most likely all coronary vessels in patients with overt CAD have angiographically undetectable atherosclerosis which results in a blunted reserve secondary to endothelial dysfunction [59].

Of particular interest is the possibility that PET and flow tracers could be used as a surrogate endpoint to assess the beneficial effects of dietary interventions, risk factor modification and cholesterol lowering [60]. Most positive trials have shown that the clinical benefit far outweighs the micrometric changes in the luminal diameter of epicardial vessels measurable by quantitative coronary angiography. On the other hand, significant changes in MBF reserve were observed with PET in preliminary studies performed in asymptomatic subjects. In the study by Dayanikli et al. [61], baseline MBF was identical in low versus high risk groups, while hyperaemic MBF was 2.6 ± 0.4 in normal subjects without any documented risk factor versus 2.2 ± 0.6 ml/min/g in asymptomatic subjects with hyperlipidemia and family history of CAD ($p < 0.05$). MBF reserve was 4.3 ± 0.5 in low risk versus 2.9 ± 0.9 in high risk groups ($p < 0.001$) and decreased in relation to abnormalities in lipid levels (Figure 5). In another study, asymptomatic males with or without evidence of CAD were submitted for 6 weeks to a program of moderate cardiovascular conditioning also including dietary changes and lowering of plasma cholesterol levels [62]. MBF reserve improved through both a reduction in basal and an increase in hyperaemic MBF. Exercise capacity increased from 10 ± 3 to 14 ± 3.6 METS at follow-up ($p < 0.01$). These encouraging results obtained in small groups of subjects support the use of PET measurements of absolute MBF in prospective secondary and primary prevention trials.

Future directions

The quantitative measurement of MBF with PET permits an integrated assessment of the coronary circulation which incorporates adaptive and pathological changes

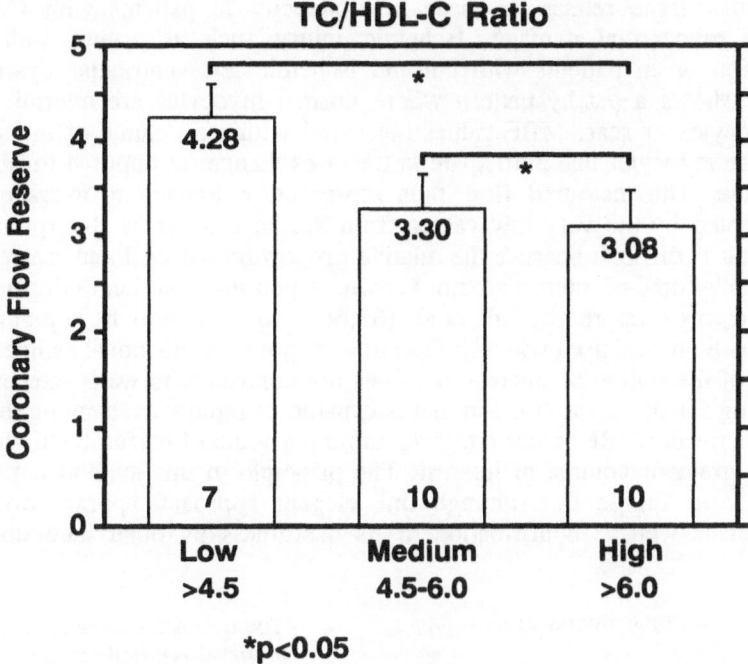

Figure 5. Coronary flow reserve in asymptomatic subjects decreases significantly as the abnormalities in serum lipid profile are more severe. Three risk categories for coronary artery disease (low, medium, high) are defined based on the ratio between total cholesterol (TC) and HDL cholesterol (HDL-C). The number of subjects in each group is indicated. Adapted with permission from Dayanikli et al. [61].
* p < 0.05.

acting at any level from the coronary ostium through the microcirculatory network. MBF values, particularly those obtained following application of hyperaemic stimuli, represent the net tissue perfusion that is maximally achievable, i.e. the main determinant of tissular function and outcome in patients with CAD. Therefore MBF measurements with PET are the ideal endpoint for future studies on mechanical interventions, regression trials and studies on angiogenesis.

There are, however, two major limitations. Flow to the subendocardial layers of normal myocardium is greater than to the subepicardium and the subendocardium is also more sensitive to ischemia [63]. Therefore, it would be of great interest to be able to measure the transmural MBF gradient. Unfortunately, this has only been possible in individuals with thickened myocardial walls, such as the septum in patients with hypertrophic cardiomyopathy [36,64]. In patients with CAD, the presence of subendocardial ischemia has not been demonstrable directly. Whether this limitation will be overcome by the introduction of the next generation of PET cameras with even higher spatial resolution (3-4 mm full width at half maximum) remains to be evaluated.

The second issue relates to tissue heterogeneity in patients with CAD and ischemic myocardial damage. Ischemic injury such as occurs with infarct reperfusion or in patients with chronic ischemic left ventricular dysfunction, typically shows a patchy pattern where normal myocytes are intermixed with fibromyocytes or scar. MBF values measured within a volume of interest only depend on myocytes that participate in tracer exchange, as opposed to fibrous or scar tissue. The measured flow thus represents a transmural average that is contaminated by the very low values from the necrotic areas. Interpretation of such result is difficult because the relative proportions of vital and scarred tissue within the volume of interest are not known. A possible solution to this important limitation was proposed by Iida et al. [65,66]. These authors have modified the tracer kinetic model used with $H_2^{15}O$ as to incorporate a functional estimate of the fraction of the region of interest that does not contribute to water exchange. By accounting for the tissue fraction that is capable of rapidly exchanging the freely diffusible tracer, MBF values are given in ml per gram of perfusable tissue rather than per gram of volume of interest. The principle of this method is presented intuitively in Figure 6. Although this elegant approach appears promising, validation as well as confirmation of its usefulness by other laboratories are awaited.

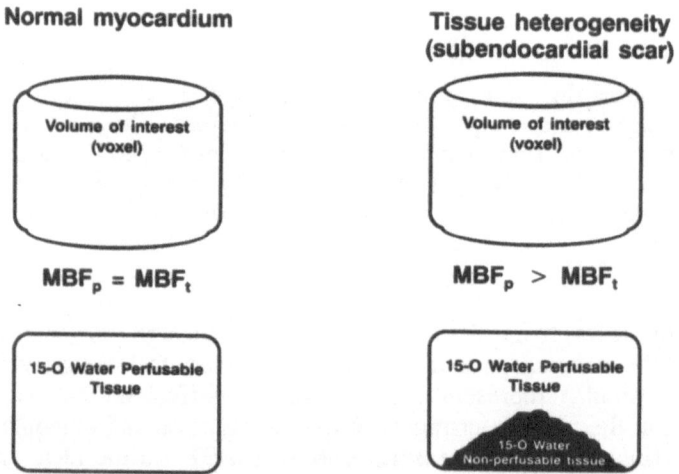

Figure 6. The problem of myocardial tissue heterogeneity and the concept of water perfusable tissue is illustrated. In the absence of scar within the myocardial region (left panels), MBF values measured per gram of volume of interest (MBF_t) or per gram of perfusable tissue (MBF_p) are identical. This is because in normal myocardium, the tissue fraction that is capable of rapidly exchanging water is close to 1. In the presence of subendocardial necrosis (right panels), MBF_t appears reduced. However, the measured flow represents an average value which is contaminated to an unknown extent by the very low flow in the scar tissue (not capable of rapidly exchanging $H_2^{15}O$). Using the modified tracer kinetic model allows to functionally separate the water perfusable from the nonwater perfusable fraction of the volume of interest. Therefore MBF_p predominantly measures flow to the residual normal myocardium. Modified with permission from Iida et al. [65].

References

1. Marcus ML, Wilson RF, White CW. Methods of measurement of myocardial blood flow in patients: a critical review. Circulation 1987;76:245-53.
2. Levine AB, Baim DS. Evaluation of myocardial blood flow and metabolism. In: Grossman W, Baim DS, editors. Cardiac catheterization, angiography and intervention, 4th ed. Philadelphia: Lea & Febiger, 1991:343-62.
3. Donohue TJ, Kern MJ, Aguirre FV *et al*. Assessing the hemodynamic significance of coronary artery stenoses: analysis of translesional pressure-flow velocity relationship in patients. J Am Coll Cardiol 1993;22:449-58.
4. De Bruyne B, Bartunek J, Sys SU, Heyndrickx GR. Relation between myocardial fractional flow reserve calculated from coronary pressure measurements and exercise-induced myocardial ischemia. Circulation 1995;92:39-46.
5. Pijls NHJ, Van Gelder B, van der Voort P *et al*. Fractional flow reserve. A useful index to evaluate the influence of an epicardial coronary stenosis on myocardial blood flow. Circulation 1995;92:3183-93.
6. Brown BG, Bolson E, Frimer M, Dodge HT. Quantitative coronary angiography: estimation of dimensions, hemodynamic resistance and atheroma mass of coronary artery lesions using the arteriogram and digital computation. Circulation 1977;55:329-37.
7. Goldstein RA, Kirkeeide RL, Demer LL *et al*. Relation between geometric dimensions of coronary artery stenoses and myocardial perfusion reserve in man. J Clin Invest 1987;79:1473-8.
8. Kirkeeide RL, Gould KL, Parsel L. Assessment of coronary stenoses by myocardial perfusion imaging during pharmacologic coronary vasodilatation. VII. Validation of cornary flow reserve as a single integrated functional measure of stenosis severity reflecting all its geometric dimensions. J Am Coll Cardiol 1986;7:103-13.
9. L'Abbate A, Maseri A. Xenon studies of myocardial blood flow: theoretical, technical, and practical aspects. Semin Nucl Med 1980;10:2-16.
10. Hoffman EJ, Phelps ME. Positron emission tomography: Principles and quantitation. In: Phelps ME, Mazziotta JC, Schelbert HR, editors. Positron emission tomography and autoradiography: principles and applications for the brain and the heart. New York: Raven Press, 1986:237-86.
11. Camici PG, Gropler RJ, Jones T *et al*. The impact of myocardial blood flow quantitation with PET on the understanding of cardiac diseases. Eur Heart J 1996;17:25-34.
12. Spinks TJ, Jones T, Gilardi MC, Heather JD. Physical performance of the latest generation of commercial positron scanner. IEEE Trans Nucl Sci 1988;35:721-5.
13. Bol A, Wijns W, Melin JA. Methodological issues in regional myocardial perfusion imaging with positron emission tomography. In: van der Wall EE, Blanksma PK, Niemeyer MG, Paans AMJ, editors. Cardiac positron emission tomography. Dordrecht: Kluwer Academic Publishers, 1995:211-20.
14. Schelbert HR, Schwaiger M. PET studies of the heart. In: Phelps ME, Mazziotta JC, Schelbert HR, editors. Positron emission tomography and autoradiography: principles and applications for the brain and heart. New York: Raven Press, 1986:581-662.
15. Huang SC, Phelps ME. Principles of tracer kinetic modeling in positron

emission tomography and autoradiography. In: Phelps ME, Mazziotta JC, Schelbert HR, editors. Positron emission tomography and autoradiography. Principles and applications for the brain and heart. New York: Raven Press, 1986:287-346.

16. Bol A, Michel C, Melin JA, Wijns W. Requisites to modelling of tracer kinetics in the heart using positron emission tomography. In: Beckers C, Goffinet A, Bol A, editors. Positron emission tomography in clinical research and clinical diagnosis. Dordrecht: Kluwer Academic Publishers, 1989:249-62.

17. Hoffman EJ, Huang SC, Phelps ME. Quantitation in positron emission tomography: 1. Effect of object size. J Comput Assist Tomogr 1979;3:299-308.

18. Parodi O, Schelbert HR, Schwaiger M, Hansen H, Selin C, Hoffman EJ. Cardiac emission computed tomography: underestimation of regional tracer concentrations due to wall motion abnormalities. J Comput Assist Tomogr 1984;8:1083-92.

19. Bacharach S, Douglas M, Carson R et al. Three-dimensional registration of cardiac positron emission tomography attenuation scans. J Nucl Med 1993;34:311-21.

20. Herrero P, Hartman JJ, Senneff MJ, Bergmann SR. Effects of time discrepancies between input and myocardial time-activity curves on estimates of regional myocardial perfusion with PET. J Nucl Med 1994;35:558-66.

21. Bol A, Melin JA, Vanoverschelde J-LJ et al. Direct comparison of ^{13}N-ammonia and ^{15}O-water estimates of perfusion with quantification of regional myocardial blood flow by microspheres. Circulation 1993;87:512-25.

22. Hutchins GD, Schwaiger M, Rosenspire KC, Krivokapich J, Schelbert H, Kuhl DE. Noninvasive quantification of regional blood flow in the human heart using N-13 ammonia and dynamic positron emission tomographic imaging. J Am Coll Cardiol 1990;15:1032-42.

23. Iida H, Kanno I, Takahashi A et al. Measurement of absolute myocardial blood flow with $H_2^{15}O$ and dynamic positron emission tomography. Strategy for quantification in relation to the partial-volume effect. Circulation 1988; 78: 104-115

24. Bergmann SR, Herrero P, Markham J, Weinheimer CJ, Walsh MN. Noninvasive quantitation of myocardial blood flow in human subjects with oxygen-15 labelled water and positron emission tomography. J Am Coll Cardiol 1989;14:639-52.

25. Araujo LI, Lammertsma AA, Rhodes CG et al. Noninvasive quantification of regional myocardial blood flow in coronary artery disease with oxygen-15-labeled carbon dioxide inhalation and positron emission tomography. Circulation 1991;83:875-85.

26. Gould KL, Lipscomb K, Hamilton GW. Physiologic basis for assessing critical coronary stenosis. Instantaneaous flow response and regional distribution during coronary hyperemia as measures of coronary flow reserve. Am J Cardiol 1974;33:87-94.

27. Gould KL. Noninvasive assessment of coronary stenoses by myocardial perfusion imaging during pharmacologic coronary vasodilation. I. Physiologic principles and experimental validation. Am J Cardiol 1978;41:267-78.

28. Gould KL, Westcott JR, Albro PC, Hamilton GW. Noninvasive assessment of coronary stenoses by myocardial imaging during pharmacologic vasodilation. II. Clinical methodology and feasibility. Am J Cardiol 1978;41:279-89.

29. Hoffman JIE. Maximal coronary flow and the concept of coronary vascular

reserve. Circulation 1984;70:153-9.

30. Klocke FJ. Measurements of coronary flow reserve: defining pathophysiology versus making decisions about patient care. Circulation 1987;76:1183-9.

31. Kanatsuka H, Lamping KG, Eastham CL, Dellsperger KC, Marcus ML. Comparison of the effects of increased myocardial oxygen consumption and adenosine on the coronary microvascular resistance. Circ Res 1989;65:1296-305.

32. Rossen JD, Simonetti I, Marcus ML, Winniford MD. Coronary dilation with standard dipyridamole and dipyridamole combined with handgrip. Circulation 1989;79:566-72.

33. Christensen CW, Rosen LB, Gal RA, Haseeb M, Lassar TA, Port SC. Coronary vasodilator reserve. Comparison of the effects of papaverine and adenosine on coronary flow, ventricular function and myocardial metabolism. Circulation 1991;83:294-303.

34. Chan SY, Brunken RC, Czernin J *et al*. Comparison of maximal myocardial blood flow during adenosine infusion with that of intravenous dipyridamole in normal men. J Am Coll Cardiol 1992;20:979-85.

35. Geltman EM, Henes CG, Senneff MJ, Sobel BE, Bergmann SR. Increased myocardial perfusion at rest and diminished perfusion reserve in patients with angina and angiographically normal coronary arteries. J Am Coll Cardiol 1990;16:586-95.

36. Camici P, Chiriatti G, Lorenzoni R *et al*. Coronary vasodilation is impaired in both hypertrophied and nonhypertrophied myocardium of patients with hypertrophic cardiomyopathy: a study with nitrogen-13 ammonia and positron emission tomography. J Am Coll Cardiol 1991;17:879-86.

37. Sambuceti G, Parodi O, Marcassa C *et al*. Alteration in regulation of myocardial blood flow in one vessel coronary artery disease determined by positron emission tomography. Am J Cardiol 1993;72:538-43.

38. Merlet P, Mazoyer B, Hittinger L *et al*. Assessment of coronary reserve in man: comparison between positron emission tomography with oxygen-15 labeled water and intracoronary Doppler technique. J Nucl Med 1993;34:1899-904.

39. Muzik O, Beanlands R, Wolfe E, Hutchins GD, Schwaiger M. Automated region definition for cardiac nitrogen-13-ammonia PET imaging. J Nucl Med 1993;34:336-44.

40. Uren NG, Camici PG, Melin JA *et al*. Effect of aging on myocardial perfusion reserve. J Nucl Med 1995;36:2032-6.

41. Radvan J, Camici PG, Marwick T, Boyd H, Sheridan DJ. Physiological hypertrophy does not affect coronary flow reserve in man [abstract]. Circulation 1993;88(4 pt 2):I-214.

42. Czernin J, Muller P, Chan S *et al*. Influence of age and haemodynamics on myocardial blood flow and flow reserve. Circulation 1993;88:62-9.

43. Austin RE Jr, Aldea GS, Coggins DL, Flynn AE, Hoffman JIE. Profound spatial heterogeneity of coronary reserve. Discordance between patterns of resting and maximal myocardial blood flow. Circ Res 1990;67:319-31.

44. Senneff MJ, Geltman EM, Bergmann SR. Noninvasive delineation of the effects of moderate aging on myocardial perfusion. J Nucl Med 1991;32:2037-42.

45. Uren NG, Melin JA, De Bruyne B, Wijns W, Baudhuin T, Camici PG. Relation between myocardial blood flow and the severity of coronary artery stenosis. N Engl J Med 1994;330:1782-8.

46. Glagov S, Weisenberg E, Zarins CK, Stankunavicius R, Kolettis GJ.

Compensatory enlargement of various human atherosclerotic coronary arteries. N Engl J Med 1987:316:1371-5.

47. Schaper W, Schaper J, editors. Collateral circulation. Heart, brain, kidney, limbs. Boston: Kluwer Academic Publishers, 1993.

48. Vanoverschelde J-LJ, Wijns W, Depre C *et al.* Mechanisms of chronic regional postischemic dysfunction in humans. New insights from the study of non-infarcted collateral-dependent myocardium. Circulation 1993;87:1513-23.

49. McFalls EO, Araujo LI, Lammertsma A *et al.* Vasodilator reserve in collateral-dependent myocardium as measured by positron emission tomography. Eur Heart J 1993;14:336-43.

50. Takeshita S, Pu L-Q, Stein LA *et al.* Intramuscular administration of vascular endothelial growth factor induces dose-dependent collateral artery augmentation in a rabbit model of chronic limb ischemia. Circulation 1995;90:II-228-34.

51. Asahara T, Bauters C, Zheng LP *et al.* Synergistic effect of vascular endothelial growth factor on angiogenesis in vivo. Circulation 1996;92:II-365-71.

52. Gohlke H, Samek L, Betz P, Roskamm H: Exercise testing provides additional prognostic information in angiographically defined subgroups of patients with coronary artery disease. Circulation 1983;68:979-85.

53. Wijns W, Musschaert-Beauthier E, Van Domburg R *et al.* Prognostic value of symptom limited exercise testing in men with a high prevalence of coronary artery disease. Eur Heart J 1985;6:939-45.

54. Detre K, Peduzzi P, Murphy M *et al.* Effect of bypass surgery on survival in patients in low- and high-risk subgroups delineated by the use of simple clinical variables. Circulation 1981;63:1329-38.

55. Mark DB, Nelson CL, Califf RM *et al.* Continuing evolution of therapy for coronary artery disease. Initial results from the era of coronary angioplasty. Circulation 1994;89:2015-25.

56. Uren NG, Crake T, Lefroy DC, De Silva R, Davies GJ, Maseri A. Delayed recovery of coronary resistive vessel function after coronary angioplasty. J Am Coll Cardiol 1993;21:612-21.

57. Uren NG, Marraccini P, Gistri R, De Silva R, Camici PG. Altered coronary vasodilator reserve and metabolism in myocardium subtended by normal arteries in patients with coronary artery disease. J Am Coll Cardiol 1993;22:650-8.

58. Sambuceti G, Parodi O, Marcassa C *et al.* Alteration in regulation of myocardial blood flow in one vessel coronary artery disease determined by positron emission tomography. Am J Cardiol 1993;72:538-43.

59. Zeiher AM, Drexler H, Wollschlager H, Just H. Endothelial dysfunction of the coronary microvasculature is associated with coronary blood flow regulation in patients with early atherosclerosis. Circulation 1991;84:1984-92.

60. Waters D: Plaque stabilization: a mechanism for the beneficial effect of lipid-lowering therapies in angiographic studies. Prog Cardiovasc Dis 1994;37:107-20.

61. Dayanikli F, Grambow D, Muzik O, Mosca L, Rubenfire M, Schwaiger M. Early detection of abnormal coronary flow reserve in asymptomatic men at high risk for coronary artery disease using positron emission tomography. Circulation 1994;90:808-17.

62. Czernin J, Barnard J, Sun KT *et al.* Effect of cardiovascular conditioning and low fat diet on myocardial blood flow and flow reserve. Circulation 1995;92:197-204.

63. Hoffmann JIE. Transmural myocardial perfusion. Prog Cardiovasc Dis

1987;29:429-64.

64. Camici PG, Cecchi F, Gistri R *et al*. Dipyridamole-induced subendocardial underperfusion in hypertrophic cardiomyopathy assessed by positron emission tomography. Coron Artery Dis 1991;2:837-41.

65. Iida H, Rhodes CG, De Silva R *et al*. Myocardial tissue fraction: correction for partial volume effects and measure of tissue viability. J Nucl Med 1991;32:2169-75.

66. Yamamoto Y, De Silva R, Rhodes CG *et al*. A new strategy for the assessment of viable myocardium and regional myocardial blood flow using ^{15}O-water and dynamic positron emission tomography. Circulation 1992;86:167-78.

40. What is the current role of ultrafast CT in coronary imaging?

BRUCE H. BRUNDAGE

Summary

There is a great need for noninvasive imaging of the coronary arteries. The development of successful treatments for arresting or even reversing the atherosclerotic process makes it mandatory that we develop simple, safe and inexpensive ways to identify early coronary artery disease before acute myocardial infarction or sudden death occurs. Ultrafast computed tomography (UFCT) shows great promise as a method for imaging the coronary arteries with and without contrast medium enhancement. Numerous studies have now demonstrated that the identification and quantification of coronary artery calcium deposits by UFCT is simple to perform and accurate. The amount of coronary calcium present strongly correlates with the amount of plaque burden in the arteries and this correlates with the risk for the presence of obstructive disease and clinical events. Furthermore, early pilot studies indicate that coronary arterial lumens can be well visualized by the use of intravenous contrast enhancement and three-dimensional reconstruction. Clearly, UFCT will continue to play an important role in the imaging of coronary arteries.

Introduction

Coronary artery disease is the most important cause of death and disability in the western world. Major advances in diagnosis and treatment in the last 25-30 years have resulted in a significant increase in longevity of both men and women in the industrialized world. Imaging of the coronary arteries has played a significant role in advancing our diagnostic and treatment abilities. However while coronary angiography has been and still is an extremely useful technique, it is invasive, expensive, associated with some risks and two dimensional. Recent advances in both magnetic resonance imaging and ultrafast computed tomography (UFCT) have given rise to the possibility of the development of noninvasive three-dimensional coronary artery imaging. Such a development would likely revolutionize our approach to the diagnosis of coronary artery disease as much as Sones' development of selective coronary angiography and would also likely lead to further advances in the treatment of coronary disease.

Technical aspects of coronary artery imaging with UFCT

Ultrafast CT, also known as electron beam computed tomography (EBCT), was developed in the early 1980's. Briefly, images are created by generating a powerful electron beam which is swept across a series of semi-circular tungsten

J.H.C. Reiber and E.E. van der Wall (eds.), Cardiovascular Imaging, 531-544.
© 1996 *Kluwer Academic Publishers.*

targets to create a fan beam of x-rays which traverse the patients thorax and then strike a detector array. The electron beam can be steered across each tungsten target in as little as 50 msec creating a virtually motion free image (Figure 1). Detailed descriptions of the technology are described elsewhere [1]. To image the coronary arteries scans are acquired in 100 msec. The scans are gated to the electrocardiogram so the images are acquired at 80% of the R-R interval, a time when cardiac motion is minimal.

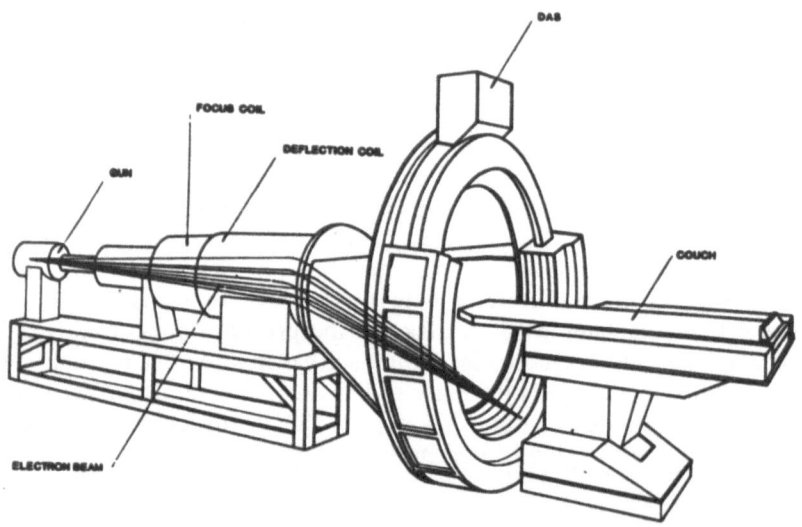

Figure 1. A cut-away diagram of ultrafast CT scanner depicts the path of the electron beam from the cathode (gun) to the anodes. DAS = digital acquisition system.

Coronary arteries are imaged with and without the use of iodinated contrast medium. Imaging the coronary arteries to detect the presence of coronary calcium (indications will be discussed later) does not require contrast medium. The coronary arteries are surrounded by fat which acts as a natural contrast agent allowing the definition of the external surface of the coronary artery (Figure 2). Calcium pyrophosphate, the deposit associated with coronary atherosclerosis, is very dense and therefore easily detected by UFCT (Figure 3). The heart is imaged from the base, just above the take-off of the left coronary artery to the apex. This requires 40 three mm adjacent scans which are acquired in one breath-hold. Some centers obtain only 30 scans because >95% of all coronary calcium is deposited in the proximal portions of the coronary vessels.

Iodinated contrast medium is required to image the lumens of coronary arteries by UFCT. Contrast is injected in a superficial antecubital vein at a rate of 4 ml/sec. Images are acquired in 100 msec and are gated to the electrocardiogram. Usually 60 three mm adjacent scans are required to image the entire length of the coronary arterial tree because the scanner couch is only incremented 2 mm with each scan to provide for a 1 mm overlap of adjacent scans which enhances the spatial resolution of the three-dimensional reconstructed

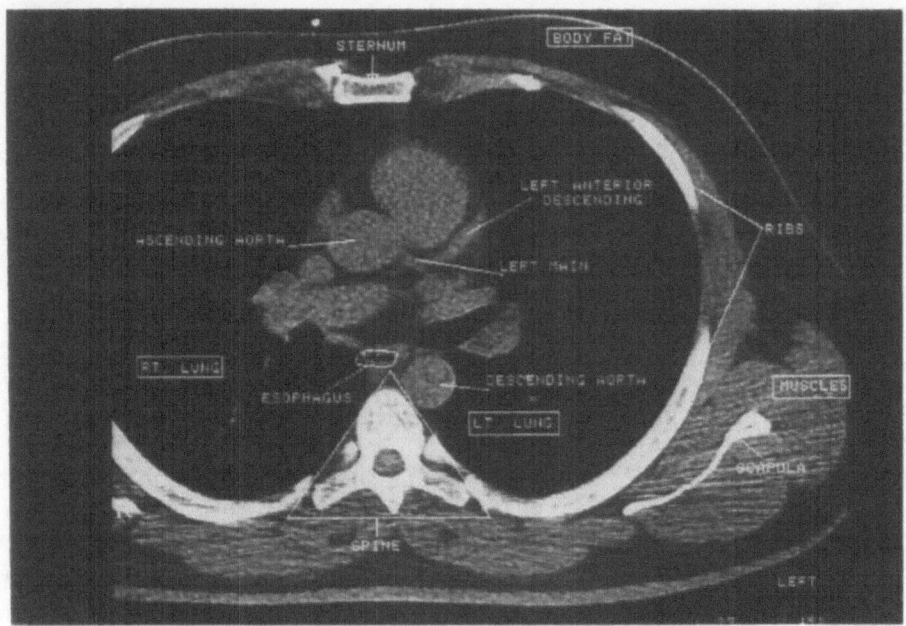

Figure 2. This unenhanced UFCT scan defines the origin of a normal left coronary artery.

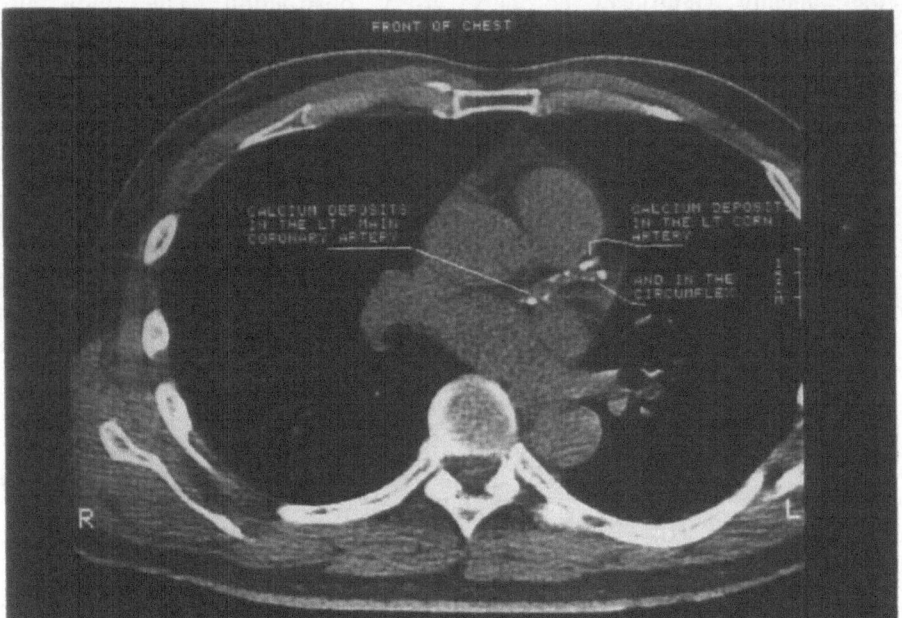

Figure 3. This unenhanced UFCT scan demonstrates left coronary calcium deposits typically seen with coronary atherosclerosis.

images. Three mm by 1 mm and 1.5 mm by 1 mm imaging protocols are also employed but require 50% more images. The radiation dose of each scan slice is less than one Gy.

Calcium detection by UFCT

Blankenhorn demonstrated the strong relationship between coronary calcium and coronary atherosclerosis. The presence of calcium always means that atherosclerosis is present [2]. Many investigators have tried to exploit this relationship by employing fluoroscopy to detect coronary artery calcium and using it as a surrogate for the presence of coronary artery disease [3]. While this approach had shown some promise, it never received wide clinical acceptance, primarily because of limited sensitivity and specificity. The development of UFCT resulted in a method for very sensitive detection of coronary calcification and provided a means for quantifying its amount which, as will be discussed later, greatly improved specificity for detecting significant coronary disease.

A number of studies have been performed showing the relationship between coronary angiographic evidence of obstructive coronary artery disease and the presence of coronary calcium [4-6]. These studies have evaluated patients undergoing clinically indicated coronary angiography and thereby largely a symptomatic population. Recently, a large multicenter study of 710 patients who had a coronary angiogram and an UFCT within three months was published [7]. This study demonstrated that the presence of any amount of coronary calcium was highly sensitive (95%) for detecting patients in the cohort who had angiographically significant coronary artery obstruction. The study also demonstrated that this sensitivity increased to over 99% for patients 50 years of age and older. There were only 23 false negative studies in the entire 710 patients and 83% of these patients had only single vessel disease. There were only 3 false negative studies in patients over the age of 50. This study however, found the detection of any calcium was not very specific (44%) for obstructive coronary disease, but if the number of coronary vessels containing calcium were taken into account, the specificity was markedly improved. The specificity rose to 96% if all three coronary arteries and the left main had calcification (Figure 4). Furthermore the study demonstrated an increasing specificity with increased amounts of calcium as measured by UFCT. Probability tables as to the risk for multivessel obstructive coronary artery disease for men and women based on the total amount of coronary calcium and the number of calcified vessels were devised (Figure 5).

This study and others have demonstrated that the detection and quantification of coronary calcium by UFCT can be a very sensitive and specific test for predicting the presence of obstructive disease in symptomatic patients. Another recent report from Japan indicates the detection of coronary calcium in symptomatic patients has a diagnostic accuracy at least equal to exercise thallium stress testing [8].

We have recently completed an angiographic study of asymptomatic patients who had large amounts of coronary calcium on UFCT scans. Somewhat surprisingly, there was a strong linear correlation ($r=0.85$) between the worst angiographic stenosis and the square root of the calcium score [9]. A coronary artery score of 1600 predicted a worst coronary stenosis of 40% diameter reduction. Therefore,

Prediction of Obstructive Angiographic Disease by Number of Calcified Vessels on UFCT

No. of Calcified Vessels	Sensitivity	Specificity	Positive Predictive Value	Negative Predictive Value
1-Vessel calcification	92%	54%	84%	71%
2-Vessel calcification	76%	78%	90%	55%
3-Vessel calcification	56%	88%	93%	43%
4-Vessel calcification	20%	98%	96%	31%

UFCT indicates ultrafast computed tomography. Four-vessel disease represents coronary calcification in the left anterior descending, right coronary, left main, and circumflex arteries.

Figure 4. The table indicates that as the number of calcified coronary vessels increases the likelihood of detecting angiographically significant coronary disease increases. Published with permission of authors and the American Heart Association. Circulation 1996; 93: 900.

the evidence in both symptomatic and asymptomatic patients strongly indicates the more coronary calcium detected the worse the coronary artery disease. Given the ease with which the UFCT can be performed to detect coronary calcium and its relatively low cost (US$ 350-400), the test may begin to rival exercise electrocardiographic stress testing as the initial diagnostic evaluation in patients with suspected coronary artery disease.

The true value of a screening test for coronary artery disease in asymptomatic individuals can only be determined by long-term outcome measured by hard clinical endpoints, such as death and acute myocardial infarction. We have followed over 1400 asymptomatic patients for nearly five years after determining the presence or absence of coronary calcium by digital subtraction fluoroscopy. After only one year, the group with coronary calcium had a four fold higher incidence of acute myocardial infarction than the group without coronary calcium. They also had a higher incidence of coronary revascularization and the development of angina as determined by the Rose questionnaire [10]. All surviving cases had an ultrafast CT scan between year 2 and 3 of follow-up. Analysis of these data confirm a continued 4 to 5 fold increase in the incidence of myocardial infarction in the calcium group. The UFCT data also show a four fold increase in the incidence of death in this group. Further analysis of these data indicate that the greater the amount of coronary calcium the greater the risk for death and acute myocardial infarction [11]. The extended follow-up data also continue to show a significant increase in the development of angina and the need for coronary revascularization in the coronary calcium group.

Over 15 years ago, Margolis et al. [12] reported that the presence of coronary calcium detected by fluoroscopy imparted an increase risk for death during a 8 year follow-up in a group of 800 patients undergoing coronary angiography for clinical indications. Surprisingly, the presence of coronary calcium was more

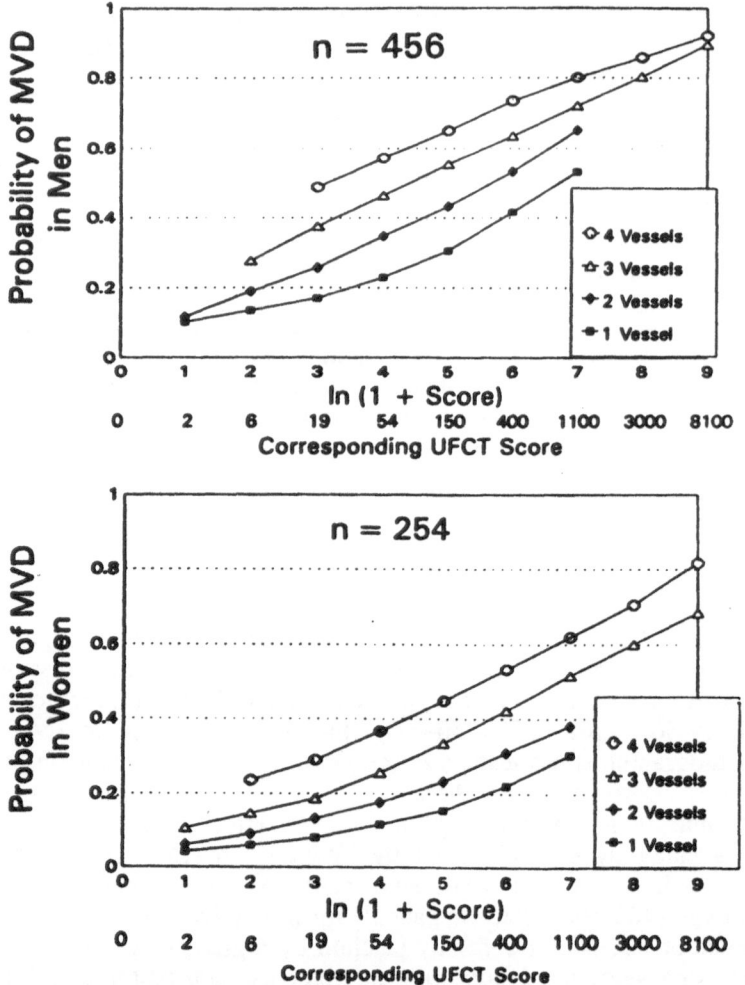

Figure 5. These graphs demonstrate the relationship between the amount of coronary calcium (UFCT score) and the probability of finding multivessel coronary disease (MVD) on the coronary angiogram for men and women. Published with permission of the authors and the American Heart Association. Circulation 1996; 93: 902.

predictive of subsequent death than the amount of angiographic coronary disease. Our research group recently repeated this study in 491 patients who had coronary angiography for clinical indications and UFCT assessment for coronary calcification [13]. We also demonstrated reduced survival in patients with coronary calcium. Again the detection of coronary calcium by UFCT was a better predictor of survival than the amount of angiographic coronary artery disease (Figure 6A,6B). Furthermore the greater the amount of calcium measured by UFCT the greater the risk of death rising from 2% in the lowest quartile to 18% in the highest quartile, a 9 fold increase (Figure 7).

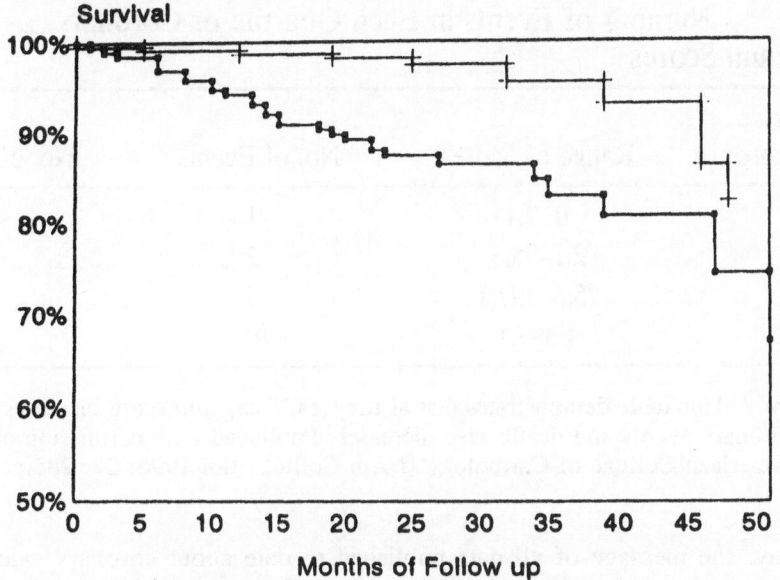

Figure 6A. All cause survival distribution for patients with UFCT calcium scores < 100 (+) and > 100 (□).

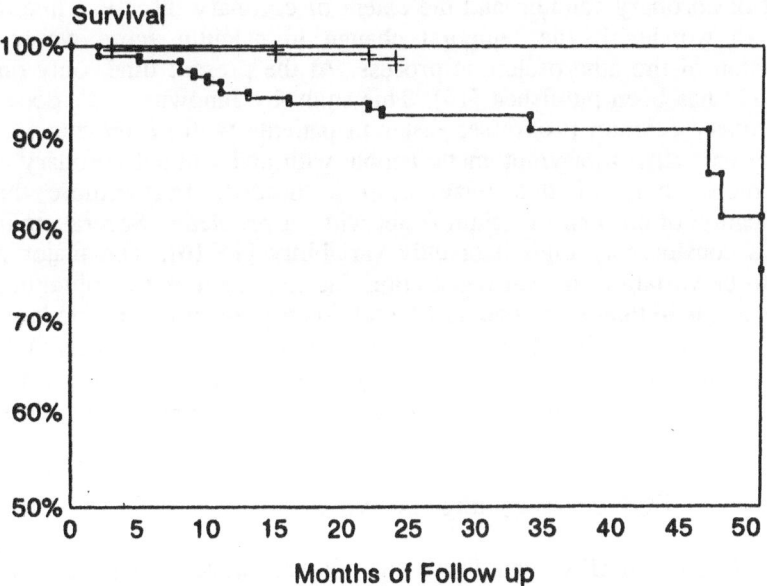

Figure 6B. All cause survival distribution for patients without significant coronary angiographic disease (< 50% stenosis)(+) and with significant disease (> 50% stenosis)(□). Published with permission of authors and American College of Cardiology. J Am Coll Cardiol 1996; 27: 288-289.

Number of Events in Each Quartile of Coronary Calcium Scores

Quartile of Score	Range of Scores	No. of Events	No. of Deaths
1	0–2.1	1	3
2	2.1–75.3	2	4
3	75.3–397.1	8	9
4	>397.1	10	22

Figure 7. This table demonstrates that as the UFCT calcium score increases, the risk for coronary events and deaths also increases. Published with permission of authors and American College of Cardiology. J Am Coll Cardiol 1996; 27: 288.

Clearly, the message of all data published to date about coronary calcification strongly indicates that the greater the amount of coronary calcium the greater the amount of coronary atherosclerosis and therefore the greater the risk for obstructive disease, acute myocardial infarction and death. These observations hold for both asymptomatic as well as symptomatic individuals.

Both pathologic and angiographic studies show a strong correlation between the amount of coronary calcium and the extent of coronary disease. Therefore it is logical to wonder if the temporal change in calcium score would predict progression of the atherosclerotic process. At the present time, only one small pilot study has been published [14]. This study by Janowitz et al. does suggest that coronary calcium progresses faster in patients with symptomatic coronary artery disease than in asymptomatic people with and without coronary calcium. Much more study of this relationship is needed. Furthermore the serial quantification of coronary calcium is not without problems. Several studies have shown a considerably high interstudy variability [15,16]. The major problem seems to be variation in scan registration due to patient and diaphragm motion. Improvements in total scan time may largely rectify this problem and longitudinal studies of changes in coronary calcium may prove extremely helpful in understanding the progression of coronary artery disease and the impact of risk factor control, such as with the use of new powerful lipid-lowering drugs.

Intravenous UFCT coronary angiography

Recent advances in UFCT hardware and software have stimulated new interest in employing this technology to image coronary artery lumens. The ability to image once every heart cycle and to obtain slice thicknesses as small as 1.5 mm offers the opportunity to define small coronary arterial branches. The development of software that permits three-dimensional reconstruction of the UFCT data on personal computers has further stimulated interest.

We recently designed a study to test the spatial resolution of currently available technology [17]. We imaged 12 hearts removed at autopsy after selectively injecting the coronary arteries with a barium sulfate solution (Figure 8). The images were reconstructed three-dimensionally and reviewed by a cardiologist to identify significant coronary obstructions. These results were compared to the coronary lesions identified by the pathologist when sectioning the arteries. Lesions were classified by both observers in the following categories: 0-49%, 50-74%, 75-99% and 100%. There was 86% agreement within one category for the 38 vessels analyzed. These preliminary results are promising and indicate that with further improvements in hardware and software, that clinically useful intravenous UFCT coronary angiography is possible.

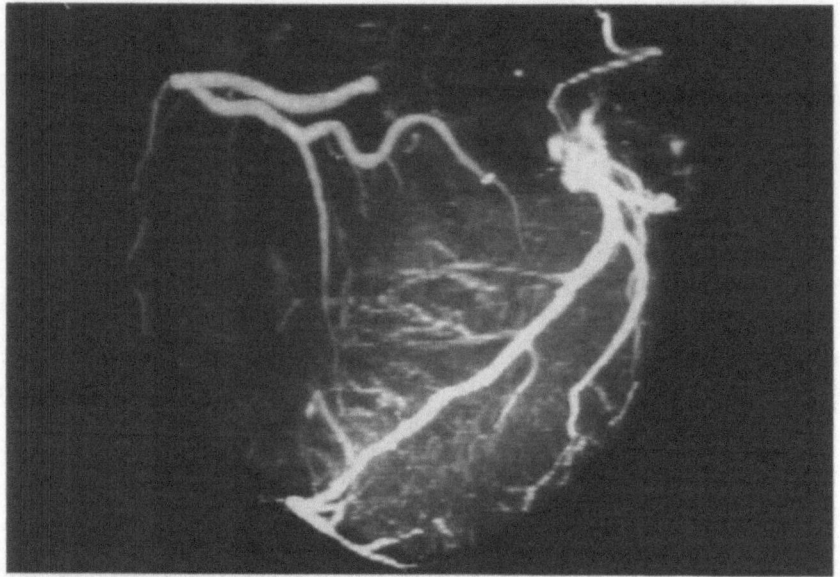

Figure 8. A single view of a 3-dimensional reconstruction of normal coronary arteries from UFCT scans of a postmortem heart. The arteries were selectively injected with a barium sulfate solution.

Encouraged by these findings and the report of others [18], we have begun imaging the coronary arteries with UFCT by intravenous contrast enhancement of patients also undergoing invasive coronary arteriography to determine how good current technology is. In most cases the proximal coronary arteries are well visualized (Figure 9). In some cases, distal coronary branches are reasonably well seen (Figure 10), however further development appears necessary before widespread clinical utility can be expected. Based on our early experience further improvements in temporal resolution, total image acquisition time, contrast medium density and spatial resolution appear to be necessary. Shorter scan times, pharmacologic increases in heart rate, more central injection of contrast medium, improved reconstruction algorithms, more scanner detectors and increased x-ray

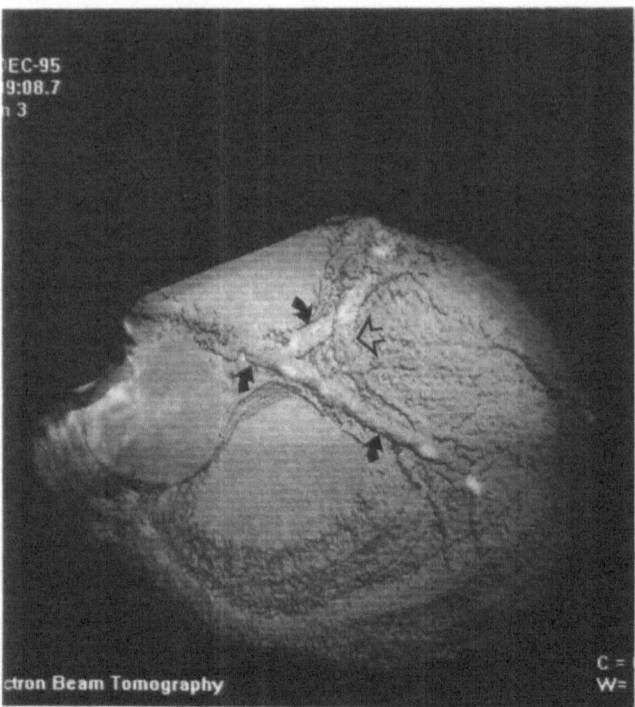

Figure 9. A top-down view of a 3-dimensional reconstruction of the left main, circumflex and left anterior descending coronary arteries (solid arrows) and cardiac vein (open arrow). White areas are calcium deposits in the coronary arteries.

dose need to be evaluated as potential solutions.

These early results suggest that even with current technology, clinically useful applications of intravenous UFCT coronary angiography are possible. The rapidly increasing use of the transarterial placement of intracoronary stents for the treatment of coronary artery obstruction have increased the need for a simple method to corroborate stent patency. The current spatial resolution of UFCT seems sufficient to determine coronary stent patency as these are usually placed in the proximal portions of the coronary arteries. The widespread use of thrombolytic therapy for the treatment of acute myocardial infarction and the increasing acceptance of the open artery hypothesis raise the possibility of using intravenous UFCT coronary angiography to determine post-thrombolysis infarct vessel patency in a relatively simple and minimally invasive manner. This idea would seem to be fruitful area for future investigation.

Recent reports from the magnetic resonance imaging literature have described successful identification of anomalous origins of coronary arteries with this imaging technique. We too have found UFCT as a useful technique for defining

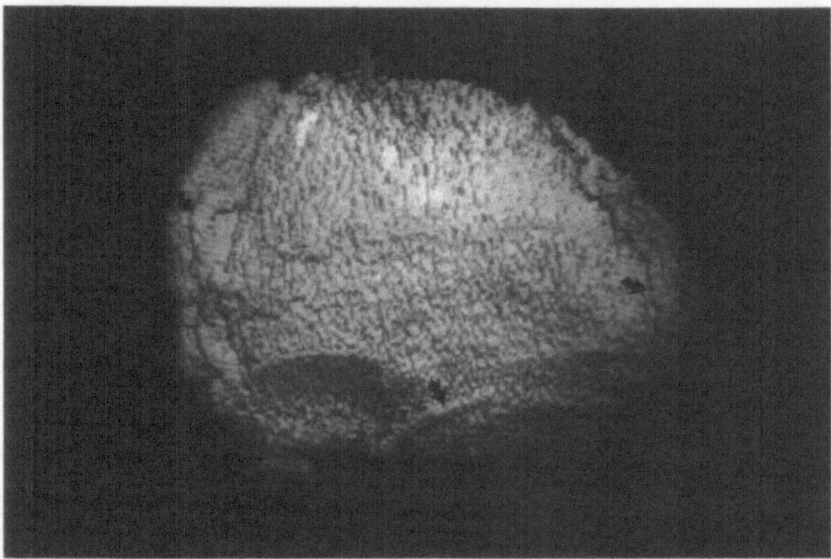

Figure 10. An underneath, right-sided view of a 3-dimensional reconstruction of the coronary arterial tree demonstrates portions of the mid right coronary, distal left anterior descending and posterior descending coronary arteries (arrows).

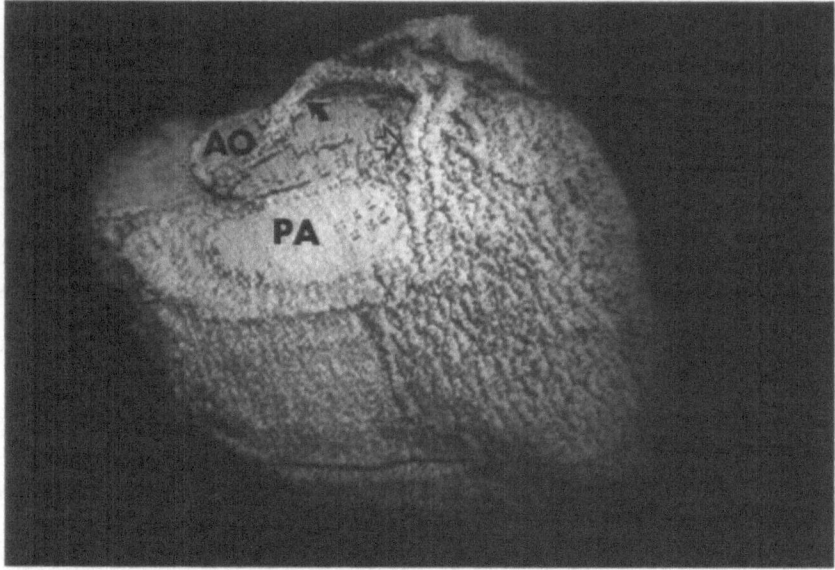

Figure 11. A selected view of a 3-dimensional reconstruction of the coronary arteries demonstrates the abnormal origin of the right coronary artery (solid arrow) from the left anterior descending coronary artery (open arrow) and its course between the pulmonary artery (PA) and aorta (AO).

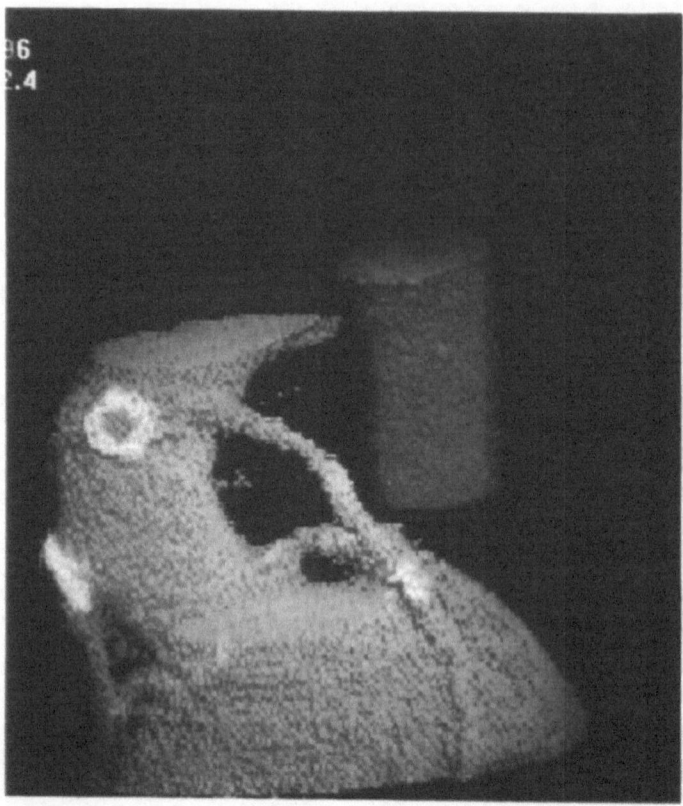

Figure 12. A selected view of a 3-dimensional reconstruction of the ascending aorta and base of the heart demonstrates patent saphenous vein grafts to the left anterior descending and right coronary arteries. Radio-opaque markers identify the aortic anastomoses.

the origin of anomalous arteries (Figure 11). It is likely that UFCT will be an alternative method for identifying the aortic origin of coronary arteries.

Finally, many years ago we first reported the use of x-ray transmission computed tomography to determine coronary artery bypass graft patency [19]. Now with the development of three-dimensional reconstruction software and the improved resolution of UFCT, this use of UFCT needs to be revisited. Preliminary studies in our institution have suggested that intravenous coronary bypass graft angiography with UFCT may have significant clinical utility (Figure 12).

Imaging the coronary arteries with UFCT has many potentially useful clinical applications. Substantial data indicate that the detection and quantification of coronary calcification by UFCT is clinically useful and well likely be put into widespread use for screening purposes. With further technological development, intravenous three-dimensional coronary angiography with UFCT may also have clinical utility.

References

1. McCullough CH, Robb RA. Ultrafast computed tomography: principles and instrumentation. In: Skorton DJ, Schelbert HR, Wolf GL, Brundage BH, editors. Marcus' cardiac imaging. 2nd ed. Philadelphia: W. B. Saunders, 1996.
2. Blankenhorn DH. Coronary artery calcification, a review. Am J Med Sci 1961;242:1-10.
3. Gianrossi R, Detrano R, Colombo A, Froelicher V. Cardiac fluoroscopy for the diagnosis of coronary artery disease: a meta analytic review. Am Heart J 1990;120:1179-88.
4. Tanenbaum SR, Kondos GT, Veselik KE, Prendergast MR, Brundage BH, Chomka EV. Detection of calcific deposits in coronary arteries by ultrafast computed tomography and correlation with angiography. Am J Cardiol 1989;63:870-2.
5. Breen JF, Sheedy PF 2nd, Schwartz RS *et al.* Coronary artery calcification detected with ultrafast CT as an indication of coronary artery disease. Radiology 1992;185:435-9.
6. Fallavollita JA, Brody AS, Bunnell IL, Kumar K, Canty JM Jr. Fast computed tomography detection of coronary calcification in the diagnosis of coronary artery disease. Comparison with angiography in patients < 50 years old. Circulation 1994;89:285-90.
7. Budoff MJ, Georgiou D, Brody A, *et al.* Ultrafast computed tomography as a diagnostic modality in detection of coronary artery disease: a multicenter study. Circulation 1996;93:898-904.
8. Kajinami K, Seki H, Takekoshi N, Mabuchi H. Noninvasive prediction of coronary atherosclerosis by quantification of coronary artery calcification using electron beam computed tomography: comparison with electrocardiographic and thallium exercise stress test results. J Am Coll Cardiol 1995;26:1209-21.
9. Guerci AD, Spadaro LA, Popma J *et al.* Electron beam tomography of coronary arteries: Relationship of coronary calcium score to arteriographic findings in asymptomatic and symptomatic adults [abstract]. Am J Card Imaging 1995;9(Suppl.1):5.
10. Detrano RC, Wong ND, Tang W, *et al.* Prognostic significance of cardiac cinefluoroscopy for coronary calcific deposits in asymptomatic high-risk subjects. J Am Coll Cardiol 1994;24:354-8.
11. Detrano R, Tang W, Wong N *et al.* Coronary calcium predicts myocardial infarction in asymptomatic subjects after two years of follow-up [abstract]. J Am Coll Cardiol 1995;25(Special Issue):13A.
12. Margolis JR, Chen JT, Kong Y, Peter RH, Behar VS, Kisslo JA. The diagnostic and prognostic significance of coronary artery calcification. A report of 800 cases. Radiology 1980;137:609-16.
13. Detrano R, Hsiai T, Wang S *et al.* Prognostic value of coronary calcification and angiographic stenoses in patients undergoing coronary angiography. J Am Coll Cardiol 1996;27:285-90.
14. Janowitz WR, Agatston AS, Viamonte M Jr. Comparison of serial quantitative evaluation of calcified coronary artery plaque by ultrafast computed tomography in persons with and without obstructive coronary artery disease. Am J Cardiol 1991;68:1-6.
15. Kaufmann RB, Sheedy PF 2nd, Breen JF *et al.*: Detection of heart calcification with electron beam CT: interobserver and intraobserver reliability for scoring

quantification. Radiology 1994;190:347-52.

16. Shah V, Claudio J, Wolfkiel CJ, Rich S, Devries SR. Reproducibility of coronary artery calcium scoring with ultrafast CT [abstract]. J Am Coll Cardiol 1992;19(Suppl.A):189A.

17. Cutrone J, DeVito A, Lin S, Bakhsheshi H, Zalace C, Brundage B. Ultrafast CT 3-D coronary angiography: imagine the possibilities [abstract]. Am J Card Imaging 1994;9(Suppl):12.

18. Moshage WEL, Achenbach S, Seese B, Bachmann K, Kirchgeorg M. Coronary artery stenoses: three-dimensional imaging with electrocardiographically triggered, contrast agent-enhanced, electron beam CT. Radiology 1995;196:707-14.

19. Brundage BH, Lipton MJ, Herfkens RJ *et al.*: Detection of patent coronary bypass grafts by computed tomography. A preliminary report. Circulation 1980;61:826-31.

41. Assessment of the coronary arteries with electron beam computed tomography

AXEL SCHMERMUND, DIETRICH BAUMGART, GÜNTER GÖRGE,
RAINET SEIBEL*, DIETRICH GRÖNEMEYER, RAIMUND ERBEL

Summary

Coronary artery disease (CAD) is one of the leading causes of mortality and morbidity in the western industrialized countries. Recent studies demonstrate the feasibility of successful primary and secondary prevention. However, the detection of early stages of CAD is an unresolved issue. Whereas sensitivity and specificity of traditional risk factor assessment and stress tests are limited, the analysis of coronary calcification allows one to obtain a direct sign of coronary atherosclerosis. This concept has been applied using fluoroscopy and conventional computed tomography (CT). However, the exact localization and quantification of coronary calcification only became possible with the advent of electron beam CT (EBCT). This new method showed a high prevalence of coronary calcification in the asymptomatic population. With the definition of a standardized 'calcium score' the normal age-specific distribution and amount of coronary calcification was investigated. EBCT proved to be more sensitive in the diagnosis of both nonobstructive and obstructive CAD than risk factor analysis and stress testing, respectively. Obstructive CAD, however, cannot yet be predicted with high enough accuracy. A close correlation of EBCT coronary calcification was found to exist with: a) the total coronary plaque volume defined by histo-pathology; b) intracoronary ultrasound findings; c) the number of coronary risk factors; and d) the coronary prognosis. Using EBCT, a reliable noninvasive identification of persons at risk was obtained for the first time. Guidelines for the use of EBCT in the early diagnosis and treatment of CAD are being developed.

Introduction

In the western industrialized countries, cardiovascular diseases, especially coronary artery disease (CAD), are the leading causes of death. Although in the USA the incidence of coronary events has constantly been reduced over the past 25 years, still about 20 % of American males develop CAD before the age of 60 [4]. The early detection of CAD is difficult: the disease usually is not accompanied by warning symptoms in its earlier stages. In most cases, a myocardial infarction occurs without preceding typical symptoms [23]. Coronary risk factors known from epidemiologic studies increase the statistic probability of cardiac events, but considering their inadequate sensitivity and specificity, they can be used to justify aggressive intervention only in the highest percentiles of risk [32]. The stress tests established in clinical practice today (treadmill stress ECG, single photon emission CT, stress echocardiography) do not have the potential to detect early stages of CAD with nonobstructing stenoses. Even in

545

J.H.C. Reiber and E.E. van der Wall (eds.), Cardiovascular Imaging, 545-558.
© 1996 *Kluwer Academic Publishers.*

stenoses ≥ 50 %, sensitivity and specificity are limited [10]. Additionally, the experience with ultrasound examinations of the carotid arteries has been somewhat disappointing: the correlation of carotid intima-media thickness with CAD seems to be rather weak [1].

With the use of coronary angiography it became evident that even nonobstructive coronary artery disease with luminal diameter narrowing < 50 % is associated with a significantly increased mortality [34]. Nonobstructive plaques were shown to rupture and to induce thrombus formation, myocardial infarction, and sudden cardiac death [14,28]. On the other hand, recent studies have demonstrated impressive reductions of CAD morbidity and mortality with the use of 3-hydroxy-3-methylglutaryl-coenzyme A reductase inhibitors. In patients with known CAD with a median follow-up period of 5.4 years, coronary mortality was reduced by 42 % (p = 0.00001), and mortality of all causes by 30 % (p = 0.0003) [46]. Of even greater importance, the new class of drugs was shown to allow successful primary prevention in 45 - 64-year old males with mild hypercholesterolemia [43]. Whereas in an untreated group of 3293 males, 248 coronary events were observed within 5 years, only 174 events were seen among 3302 males treated with a 3-hydroxy-3-methylglutaryl-coenzyme A reductase inhibitor. Thus, the rate of coronary events was reduced by 31 % (p < 0.001). Mortality of all causes was reduced by 22 % (p = 0.051). With regard to these results, the identification of asymptomatic persons who are likely to benefit most from primary prevention measures ('targeted prevention') seems to be of great interest [12].

Coronary calcification

Coronary calcification is almost invariably associated with coronary atherosclerosis and plaque formation [17,31,36]. Its quantity reflects the overall extent of coronary atherosclerosis. Often, calcium formation results from complex plaque formation with hemorrhage and necrosis. In an acute thrombotic occlusion, it may not be present [31]. The time period required for calcification of an arteriosclerotic plaque is unknown. However, smaller amounts of calcium have been shown to be present in noncomplex, lipid rich and fibromuscular plaques [31]. According to the classification of Stary, who evaluated coronary atherosclerotic plaque development from childhood to middle age in almost 600 hearts, calcium is already present in plaques seen in adolescents ('Stary type III plaque') [45]. Calcification is earliest found in the proximal segment of the left anterior descending artery, especially at the site of bifurcation of the left main stem. Its distribution involves mainly proximal coronary segments, and in the left coronary artery, calcification is hardly ever found at distal sites when not present in proximal segments [31,47]. Recent investigations suggest an active role for calcification in atherogenesis rather than resulting from a degenerative process. Local factors known from osteogenesis are secreted by activated pericytes ('calcifying vascular cells'), and histologic features comparable to bone matrix formation are seen in the arterial wall [13].

Assessment of coronary calcification

Coronary calcification is mainly assessed by three methods: fluoroscopy, conventional/helical CT, and electron beam CT (EBCT). Although associated with a higher radiation exposure, fluoroscopy does not reach the sensitivity of the tomographic methods, because various structures are overimposed. Coronary calcification can only be distinguished from underlying or overimposed structures with cardiac motion. This is especially difficult in women and obese subjects. Calcification localized in proximal coronary segments may be missed. Although the procedure largely depends on the operator's skill, inter- and intraobserver variability have never been tested. Even with the use of digital substraction fluoroscopy, only about 50% - 60% of the calcified lesions detected by EBCT are seen [2]. Lesions cannot be quantified, and documentation of the study results on hard disks is difficult.

Conventional computed tomography allows the identification of coronary calcification with a sensitivity superior to that of fluoroscopy [35]. Image acquisition times of at least 600 msec, however, lead to motion artifacts and volume averaging and decrease the sensitivity for detection of small calcified lesions. Moreover, calcium burden cannot be quantified precisely.

Electron beam CT

By avoiding mechanical movement of the x-ray source and the detector system, EBCT allows scanning times of 50 - 100 msec and freezing cardiac motion [21]. X-rays are produced by an electron beam that is steered by electromagnets. It is focused on the curved tungsten target that forms an arc of 210° centered below the patient (Figure 1). The tungsten target consists of four parallel rings, of which either all four or only one are activated. Of the two detector rings, one consists of 432 elements, the other of 864, thus allowing to choose between a 256 x 256 or a 512 x 512 pixel matrix. Two modes of operation are possible: a single slice mode with activation of only one target ring and the high resolution detector, or a multi-slice mode using all four target rings and both detectors. For the assessment of coronary calcification, the single slice mode with a section thickness of 3 mm is usually preferred. It yields a spatial resolution of about 0.2 mm^2 ($>$ 6 line pairs/mm) [21]. This allows an increased precision in diagnosing and especially quantifying coronary calcification compared to conventional helical CT [6]. Depending on the examination protocol, the radiation exposure to the thorax measures 0.5 to 5 mSv and thus is comparably low [3].

With the introduction of a standardized algorithm for the quantification of coronary calcification assessed by EBCT ('Agatston calcium score', Figure 2) [2], the results of EBCT examinations became internationally comparable. Inter- und intraobserver variability were reported to be neglectable [2,26]. In an investigation of the repeatability of the EBCT protocol, 256 subjects underwent two sequential EBCT examinations within a period of some minutes [8]. Small lesions with a CT density $>$ 130 Hounsfield Units (HU) were seen in the second examination in $>$ 50 % if the area of the hyperattenuating focus was $>$ 2 mm^2, and in $>$ 75 % if the area was $>$ 3 mm^2.

In 109 patients with known CAD, calcium scores were significantly higher than

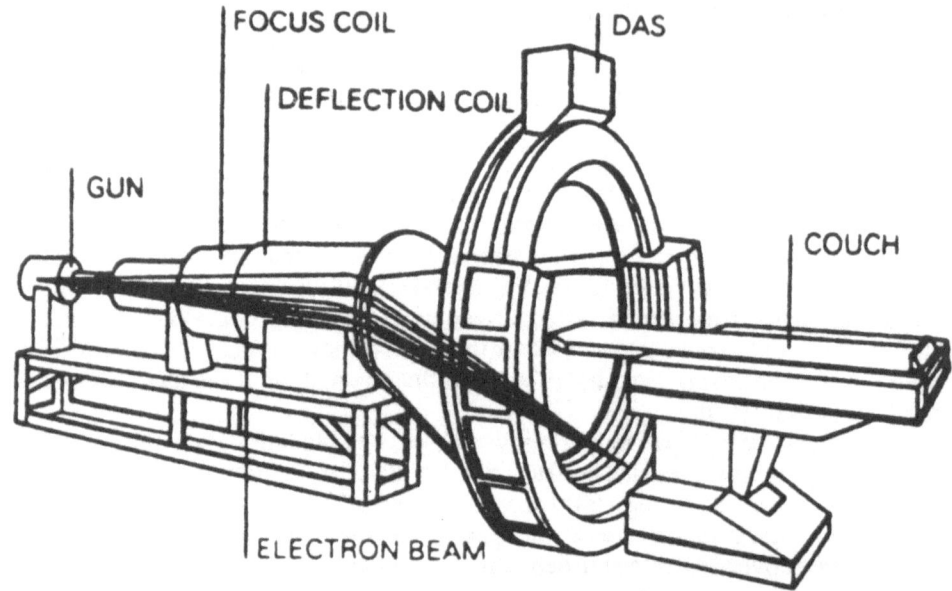

Figure 1. Schematic drawing of an electron beam CT scanner. The electron beam is steered and focused by electromagnets, being swept along a curved tungsten target that surrounds the patient. X-rays are produced where the electron beam strikes the tungsten. This allows a scan acquisition time of 50 - 100 msec. DAS = Detector Array System.

in 475 asymptomatic persons without a history of CAD [2]. With this background, a study was undertaken to define a normal range of the Agatston calcium score in apparently healthy subjects in different age groups [25]. Asymptomatic subjects with higher than 'normal' scores or scores comparable to those found in patients with known CAD might then be suspected to carry an increased risk for CAD. In order to define the calcium score range, 1898 asymptomatic subjects (1396 males and 502 females) were examined with EBCT [25] (Table 1). Corresponding to the natural history of coronary atherosclerosis, coronary calcification was seen roughly 10 years earlier in males than in females with an almost ubiquitous finding in the elderly. In the age group of 30 - 39 years, 21 % of the males and 11 % of the females showed coronary calcification, but 85 % of the males and 67 % of the females in the age group of 60 - 69 years. When coronary calcification was found in subjects aged 30 - 39 years, low calcium scores were seen with a mean score of 8 in males and 2 in females [25] (Table 1).

Histopathologic correlative studies

Histopathologic correlative studies showed a positive correlation of coronary calcification analysis with EBCT and luminal narrowing caused by atherosclerotic

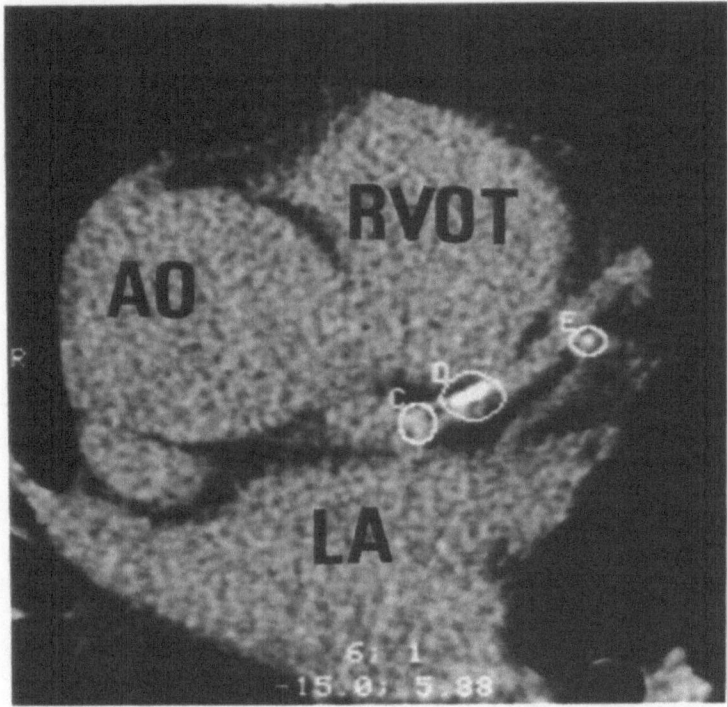

Figure 2. Calculation of the Agatston calcium score using the electron beam CT scan. Depicted is a transversal slice (3 mm thickness) at the level of the left main coronary artery. Left main coronary artery (LMCA) and left anterior descending artery (LAD) can be identified. Areas with a CT density > 130 Hounsfield Units (HU) are encircled and marked with the letters C, D, and E. Lesion C is situated at the junction of LMCA and LAD, D in the proximal LAD, and E in the very proximal portion of a diagonal branch. In the scan, a cardiac vein that is running parallel to the LAD can be seen below the LAD. Using the Agatston calcium score, the peak density and the area of the encircled lesion is being considered. According to the CT density of a given lesion, a 'maximal CT number' (MCTN) is attributed. For lesion C (151 HU) the MCTN is 1, for lesion D (631 HU) it is 4, and for lesion E (257 HU) it is 2. The MCTN is multiplied with the area of the lesion. Thus, lesion D yields a calcium score of 4 x 16.7 mm^2 = 66.8, and lesion E of 2 x 2.3 mm^2 = 4.6. AO = Aorta, LA = left atrium, RVOT = right ventricular outflow tract.

Table 1. Prevalence of coronary calcification as assessed by electron beam CT and Agatston calcium score (mean ± SEM) in 1898 asymptomatic subjects [25].

	Asymptomatic males				Asymptomatic females		
Age (years)	Number	Prevalence of coronary calcification	Mean Agatston calcium score	Age (years)	Number	Prevalence of coronary calcification	Mean Agatston calcium score
0 - 29	73	11 %	0.5 ± 0.35	0 - 29	17	6 %	0.06 ± 0.05
30 - 39	283	21 %	8 ± 2.1	30 - 39	63	11 %	2 ± 1.3
40 - 49	534	44 %	28 ± 4.5	40 - 49	124	23 %	11 ± 4.1
50 - 59	312	72 %	140 ± 18.3	50 - 59	117	35 %	63 ± 45.0
60 - 69	65	85 %	239 ± 46	60 - 69	56	67 %	122 ± 36.6
70 - 79	32	94 %	425 ± 74.6	70 - 79	45	89 %	243 ± 49.5
80 - 89	5	100 %	468 ± 161.9	80 - 89	4	100 %	249 ± 68

plaque formation [37,44]. The predictive value for individual lesions, however, was low: a given Agatston calcium score was found to correspond to obstructing as well as to nonobstructing stenoses. On the other hand, the abscence of calcification in the EBCT examination yielded a high negative predictive value, precluding luminal diameter narrowing > 50 % in 97,5 % [44]. In the hearts of 50 male persons aged 30 - 69 years and deceased with various symptoms of CAD, calcification determined with EBCT was compared to calcification determined with histomorphometry [29,30]. A close correlation of the calcium quantities determined with the two methods was found (r = 0,96) [29]. The prevalence of calcification detected with histomorphometry increased steadily with the degree of stenosis [30] (Table 2).

Altogether, the correlation of calcification to the degree of stenosis is limited, because the external diameter of coronary arteries can increase with an enlarging plaque area ('compensatory remodeling') [19]. Only when the plaque area exceeds 40 - 45 % of the coronary artery area, luminal narrowing becomes evident [18]. In a recent histopathologic study, EBCT coronary calcium area accordingly was correlated to coronary plaque area rather than to coronary luminal narrowing [39]. It showed a strong relation of EBCT calcium area to coronary atherosclerotic plaque area of the whole heart (r = 0.93, p < 0.001), the major coronary arteries, and coronary artery segments. EBCT calcium area precisely determined the plaque area of the coronary arteries, their 'plaque burden'. It was suggested that the EBCT calcium area represented about one fifth of the total coronary plaque area [39].

Table 2. Prevalence of histomorphometric coronary calcification in coronary stenoses of different severity [30].

Grade of stenosis	0 - 25 %	26 - 50 %	51 - 75 %	76 - 100 %
Prevalence of histomorpho-metric calcification	4 %	28 %	61 %	93 %

Comparison to coronary angiography

The accuracy of CAD-diagnosis by determining EBCT coronary calcification depends on the standard method used for comparison. It is above 80% for angiographically detectable CAD ($\geq$ 10% diameter narrowing) as well as for angiographically obstructive disease ($\geq$ 50% diameter narrowing) [27]. Accuracy is similar in men and in women [38]. Calcium score increases significantly with the number of angiographically diseased vessels [3]. However, there is a wide overlap of calcium scores in patients with and without obstructive CAD, and these two groups cannot accurately be distinguished [16]. The abscence of coronary calcification, however, seems to be of high negative predictive value (> 95%) [9]. An Agatston calcium score < 10 ruled out (obstructive) CAD in 92 % and a calcium score < 2 in 95 %. The abscence of EBCT calcification precluded (obstructive) CAD in 98 % [7].

Comparison to intracoronary ultrasound studies

Considering the weaknesses of coronary angiography as a silhouette method with visualization only of the coronary lumen and not of the vessel wall, EBCT was compared to intracoronary ultrasound (ICUS). (Figure 3) In 52 patients, the relation of EBCT calcification to plaques assessed with ICUS was found to be very close when calcium deposits were seen with ICUS [40]. EBCT allowed the identification of calcified plaques with a sensitivity of 94 %. Interestingly, noncalcified plaques assessed by ICUS were represented as hyperattenuating EBCT foci in > 45 %. In 30 patients with normal coronary angiogram but detection of early coronary plaque formation with ICUS, EBCT identified calcified and noncalcified plaques with a sensitivity of 100 % and 60 %, respectively, and thus showed a better sensitivity for early atherosclerotic lesions than coronary angiography [20].

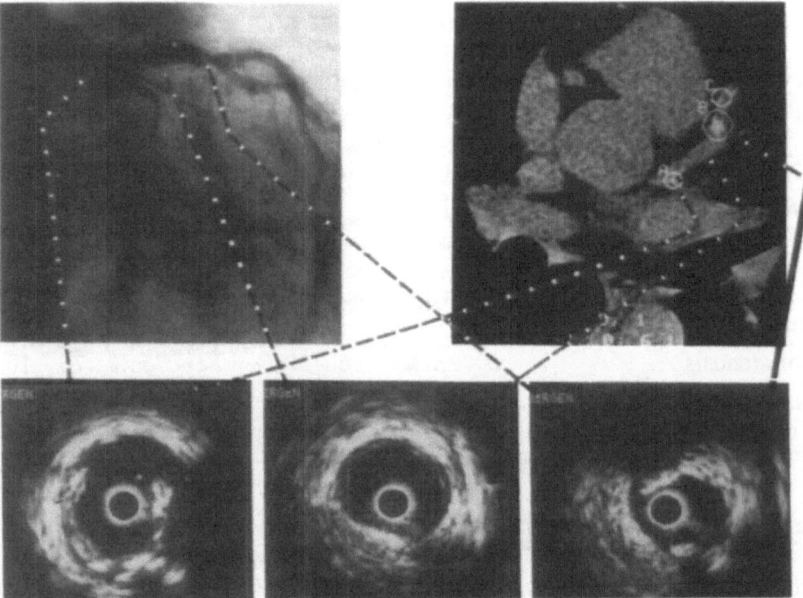

Figure 3. Comparison of left coronary angiogram, electron beam CT (EBCT) scan, and intracoronary ultrasound (ICUS) in a 58-year old patient. The angiogram shows irregular contours and an intermediate stenosis at the level of the first diagonal branch. In the EBCT scan, coronary calcific lesions are seen at the level of the first diagonal branch ('lesion B') and in the left main coronary artery ('lesion A'). The intracoronary ultrasound shows partially calcified plaques at corresponding sites in the left anterior descending and left main coronary arteries.

Association of coronary calcification and coronary risk factors

Whereas coronary risk factors of varied significance known today increase the probability of coronary events, coronary calcification almost invariably signifies coronary atherosclerosis. Thus, even though two different parameters are compared, an association appears obvious. Actually, a significant increase of the EBCT Agatston calcium score was seen with an increasing number of known risk factors [41,49]. In an EBCT study with 865 asymptomtic subjects, high blood pressure, diabetes mellitus, hypercholesterolemia, and a high body mass index were found to be independent predictors of coronary calcification besides age and sex [49]. In another study with inclusion of 650 symptomatic and asymptomatic subjects, only high blood pressure and smoking independently predicted coronary calcification besides age and sex [41]. In an effort to compare both risk factor analysis and EBCT to coronary angiography, 164 selected patients underwent an EBCT examination after risk assessment and coronary angiography [42]. Using multivariate regression analysis, coronary calcification proved to be the single best predictor of (obstructive) CAD. Besides coronary calcification, only fibrinogen and lipoprotein(a) concentrations were of predictive value, because the 'traditional' risk factors, especially hypercholesterolemia, were highly prevalent. The combination of the 'new' risk factors fibrinogen and lipoprotein(a) with the EBCT examination allowed an improved detection of (obstructive) CAD compared to EBCT alone (p < 0,05), so that 86 % of the patients were classified correctly [42].

In 740 asymptomatic participants of the Rochester Family Heart Study (20 - 59 years of age, 378 females) lipoprotein analysis and an EBCT examination were performed. None in the study group had known CAD, high blood pressure, or diabetes mellitus [33]. Of these asymptomatic subjects, 126 (17 %) were considered to be at high risk (current smokers, hypercholesterolemia), and of these high risk subjects, 52 (41 %) showed coronary calcification. Of the 614 subjects (83 %) considered to be at low risk, 89 (14 %) had EBCT calcification. The authors concluded that these individuals not identified by standard screening techniques might represent those asymptomatic persons at increased risk for coronary events who cannot be detected with conventional risk analysis (lipoprotein status, blood pressure, blood glucose, and smoking habits analysis) [33].

Coronary calcification and prognosis

In a prospective study, 1461 asymptomatic high risk subjects were examined with cardiac cinefluoroscopy for coronary calcification and followed for 1 year [11]. Coronary calcification was found in 691 subjects. In this group, 8 persons (1.2 %) had a nonfatal myocardial infarction within the follow-up period, but only 2 persons in the group without coronary calcification found by fluoroscopy (n = 768) (0,3 %). Coronary artery bypass surgery was performed in 10 persons with coronary calcification (1.5 %) and in 3 persons without coronary calcification (0,4 %). In each of the two groups (with/without calcification), 3 persons died from a coronary event (0.4 %, respectively) [11].

A group of 205 asymptomatic subjects was followed for 1 - 2 years after assessment of coronary calcification with EBCT [48]. Coronary events (fatal or nonfatal myocardial infarction, coronary artery bypass surgery) were seen in 6

% of subjects with and in 1 % of persons without coronary calcification. In another study, the data of 848 asymptomatic subjects without increased coronary risk were analyzed about 21 months after an EBCT examination [5]. Subjects with an Agatston calcium score in the upper 30 % developed CAD in 8 %, subjects with calcium scores in the lower percentiles in only 1 %.

Coronary calcification assessed with EBCT can increase by an augmenting volume of preexisting calcified plaques, by the development of new plaques, or by calcification of formerly noncalcified plaques (Figure 4) [15,24]. An increase of the calcium score > 40 in 1 year and > 200 in 5 years was shown to be accompagnied by an increased risk for coronary events [15].

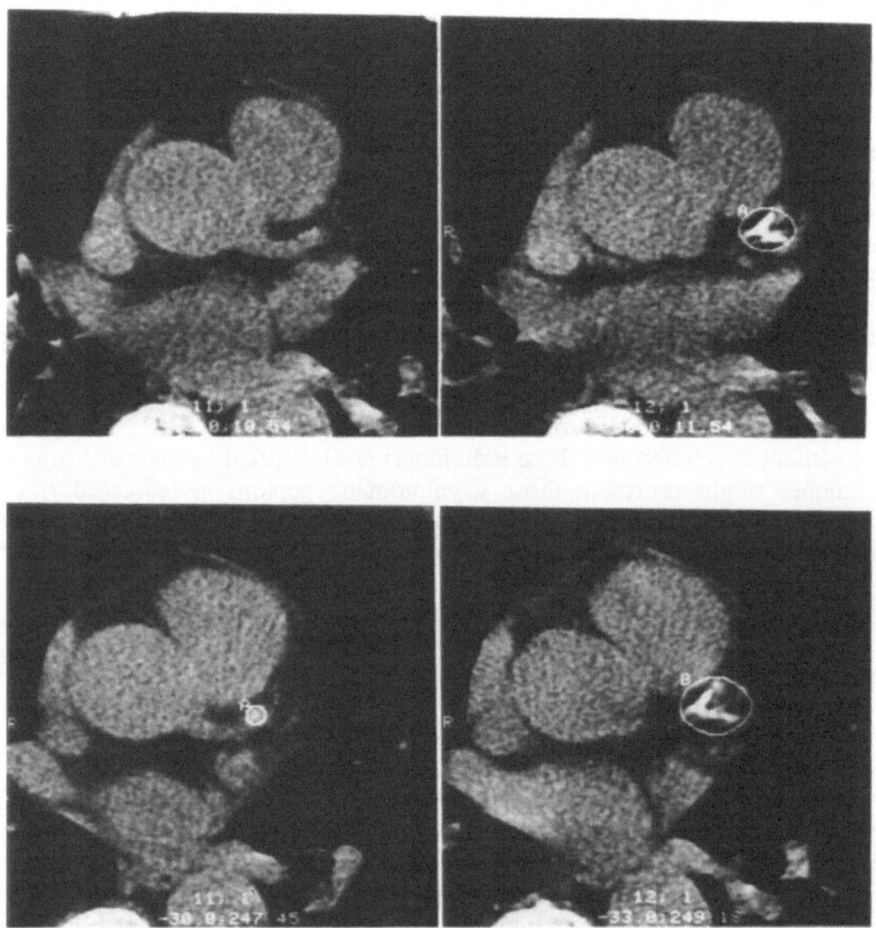

Figure 4. Electron beam CT transversal scans at almost identical levels at the 'trifurcation' of left main, left anterior descending, and left circumflex coronary artery in a 56-year old patient. The time interval between both examinations was 6 months. Due to growth of the calcified lesion, the Agatston calcium-score in the encircled areas has increased from 97 to 126.

Conclusion

EBCT assessment of coronary calcification allows noninvasive, reliable identification of asymptomatic subjects with coronary atherosclerosis. The severeness of coronary stenoses caused by the atherosclerotic process cannot yet be predicted with acceptable precision. Even at present, however, the extent of coronary calcification assessed with EBCT is by far the best noninvasive predictor of obstructive CAD. Additionally, in subjects with nonobstructive plaques, direct signs of the coronary atherosclerotic process are documented. These subjects are not detected by conventional stress tests, although they are known to carry an increased risk for coronary events compared to the general population.

According to preliminary studies, conventional risk analysis and EBCT have an additive value in asymptomatic subjects: subjects with a low risk profile and therefore usually undetected coronary atherosclerosis and increased risk for coronary events can be identified with EBCT. In subjects without coronary calcification, the risk for coronary events is very low. In subjects with an age-related high amount of EBCT coronary calcification, however, morbidity and mortality seem to be significantly increased. This is confirmed by histopathologic investigations and studies using fluoroscopy.

Thus, EBCT seems to represent a valuable new method for the early detection of coronary atherosclerosis and CAD. Since it has only recently been introduced into clinical practice, guidelines for the use of EBCT (who? - when? - what are the consequences?) are not yet available. They are now being developed at several centers. It can be expected that high risk asymptomatic subjects with comparably high coronary calcium scores will be advised intensive risk reduction measures, especially cholesterol lowering, and aspirin. Additionally, stress testing might be recommended in selected cases [22].

References

1. Adams MR, Nakagomi A, Keech A *et al*. Carotid intima-media thickness is only weakly correlated with the extent and severity of coronary artery disease. Circulation 1995;92:2127-34.
2. Agatston AS, Janowitz WR, Hildner FJ, Zusmer NR, Viamonte M Jr, Detrano R. Quantification of coronary artery calcium using ultrafast computed tomography. J Am Coll Cardiol 1990;15:827-32.
3. Agatston AS, Janowitz WR. Coronary calcification: detection by ultrafast computed tomography. In: Stanford W., J.A. Rumberger (eds.): Ultrafast computed tomography in cardiac imaging: Principles and practice. Futura Publishing, Mount Kisco, NY 1992:77-95.
4. American Heart Association: 1993 Heart and Stroke Facts Statistics. American Heart Association, Dallas, 1993.
5. Balogh T, Hoff J, Rich S, Wolfkiel CJ. Development of coronary artery disease in asymptomatic subjects undergoing coronary artery calcification screening by electron beam tomography. Circulation 1995;92(suppl.I):I-650.
6. Baskin KM, Stanford W, Thompson BH, Hoffman E, Tajik J, Heery SD. Comparison of electron beam and helical computed tomography in assessment

of coronary artery calcification. Circulation 1995;92(Suppl.I:I-651.

7. Baumgart D, Schmermund A, Görge G *et al.* Klinischer Stellenwert der Elektronenstrahltomographie - Entdeckung signifikanter Stenosen. Z Kardiol 1995;84(Suppl.1):91.

8. Bielak LF, Kaufmann RB, Moll PP, McCollough CH, Schwartz RS, Sheedy PF. Small lesions in the heart identified at electron beam CT: calcification or noise? Radiology 1994;192:631-6.

9. Breen JF, Sheedy PF, Schwartz RS *et al.* Coronary artery calcification detected with ultrafast CT as an indication of coronary artery disease. Radiology 1992;185:435-9.

10. Detrano RC, Froelicher V. A logical approach to screening for coronary artery disease. Ann Int Med 1987;106:846-52.

11. Detrano RC, Wong ND, Tang W *et al.* Prognostic significance of cardiac cinefluoroscopy for coronary calcific deposits in asymptomatic high risk subjects. J Am Coll Cardiol 1994;24:354-8.

12. Devereux R, Alderman M. Role of preclinical cardiovascular disease in the evolution from risk factor exposure to development of morbid events. Circulation 1993;88:1444-55.

13. Doherty TM, Detrano RC. Coronary arterial calcification as an active process: a new perspective on an old problem. Calcif Tissue Intern 1994;54:224-30.

14. Epstein S, Quyymi A, Bonow R. Sudden cardiac death without warning. Possible mechanisms and implications for screening asymptomatic populations. New Engl J Med 1989;321:320-4.

15. Eusebio J, Chomka EV, Daniels T, Rich S, Brundage BH, Wolfkiel CJ. Five year changes in coronary calcification by ultrafast computed tomography. J Am Coll Cardiol, special issue February 1995:386A.

16. Fallavollita JA, Brody AS, Bunnell IL, Kumar K, Ganty JM. Fast computed detection of coronary calcification in the detection of coronary artery disease. Circulation 1994;89:285-90.

17. Frink RJ, Achor RW, Brown AL Jr, Kincaid OW, Brandenburg RO. Significance of calcification of the coronary arteries. Am J Cardiol 1970;26:241-7.

18. Ge J, Erbel R, Zamorano J *et al.* Coronary remodeling in atherosclerotic disease: An intravascular ultrasonic study in vivo. Coron Art Dis 1993;4:981-6.

19. Glagov S, Weisenberg E, Zarins CK, Stankunavicius R, Kolettis GJ. Compensatory enlargement of human atherosclerotic coronary arteries. New Engl J Med 1987;316:1371-5.

20. Görge G, Baumgart D, Schmermund A *et al.* Erkennung arteriosklerotischer Frühläsionen durch Elektronenstrahltomographie und intravasalen Ultraschall bei Patienten mit normalem Koronarogramm. Z Kardiol 1995;84(Suppl.1):85.

21. Gould RG. Principles of ultrafast computed tomography: Historical aspects, mechanism of action, and scanner characteristics. In: Stanford W., J.A. Rumberger (eds.): Ultrafast computed tomography in cardiac imaging: Principles and practice. Futura Publishing, Mount Kisco, NY 1992:1-15.

22. Guerci AD. Is screening for coronary artery disease with fast computed tomography useful? Cardiol Rev 1995;3):217-24.

23. Harper RW, Kennedy G, de Sanctis RW, Hutter AM. The incidence of angina pectoris before acute myocardial infarction. Am Heart J 1979;97:178-83.

24. Janowitz WR, Agatston AS, Viamonte M. Comparison of serial quantitative evaluation of calcified coronary artery plaque by ultrafast computed tomography

in persons with and without obstructive coronary artery disease. Am J Cardiol 1991;68:1-6.

25. Janowitz WR, Agatston AS, Kaplan G, Viamonte M. Differences in prevalence and extent of coronary artery calcium detected by ultrafast computed tomography in asymptomatic men and women. Am J Cardiol 1993;72:247-54.

26. Kaufmann RB, Sheedy PF, Breen JF *et al.* Detection of heart calcification with electron beam CT: Interobserver and intraobserver reliabilty for scoring quantification. Radiology 1994;190:347-52.

27. Kaufmann RB, Peyser PA, Sheedy PF, Rumberger JA, Schwartz RS. Quantification of coronary artery calcium by electron beam computed tomography for determination of severity of angiographic coronary artery disease in younger patients. J Am Coll Cardiol 1995;25:626-32.

28. Little WC, Constantinescu M, Applegate RJ *et al.* Can coronary angiography predict the site of a subsequent myocardial infarction in patients with mild-to-moderate coronary artery disease? Circulation 1988;78:1157-66.

29. Mautner GC, Mautner SL, Froehlich J *et al.* Coronary artery calcification: assessment with electron beam CT and histomorphometric correlation. Radiology 1994;192:619-23.

30. Mautner SL, Mautner GC, Froehlich J, Feuerstein IM, Proschan MA, Roberts WC. Coronary artery disease: prediction with in vitro electron beam CT. Radiology 1994;192:625-30.

31. Mc Carthy JH, Palmer FJ. Incidence and significance of coronary artery calcification. Br Heart J 1974;36:499-506.

32. Oliver MF. Strategies for preventing and screening for coronary heart disease. Br Heart J 1985;54:1-5.

33. Peyser PA, Kaufmann RB, Maher JE, Bielak LF, Sheedy PF, Schwartz RS. Progress in assessment of CAD markers: the epidemiology of coronary artery calcification. Athersclerosis 1995;X:159-62.

34. Proudfit WL, Bruschke AVG, Sones FMJ. Clinical course of patients with or slightly or moderately abnormal coronary angiograms: 10 year follow-up of 521 patients. Circulation 1980;62:712-7.

35. Rienmüller R, Lipton MJ. Detection of coronary artery calcification by computed tomography. Dynam Cardiovasc Imaging 1987;1:139-45.

36. Rifkin RD, Parisi AF, Folland E. Coronary calcification in the diagnosis of coronary artery disease. Am J Cardiol 1979;44:141-7.

37. Rumberger JA, Schwartz RS, Simons DB, Sheedy PF, Edwards WD, Fitzpatrick LA. Relation of coronary calcium determined by electron-beam computed tomography and lumen-narrowing determined at autopsy. Am J Cardiol 1994;73:1169-73.

38. Rumberger JA, Sheedy PF, Breen JR, Schwartz RS. Coronary calcium, as determined by electron beam computed tomography, and coronary disease on arteriogram: Effect of patient's sex on diagnosis. Circulation 1995;91:1363-7.

39. Rumberger JA, Simons DB, Fitzpatrick LA, Sheedy PF, Schwartz RS. Coronary artery calcium area by electron-beam computed tomography and coronary atherosclerotic plaque area. A histopathologic correlative study. Circulation 1995;92:2157-62.

40. Schmermund A, Baumgart D, Görge G *et al.* Arteriosklerotische Veränderungen bei Patienten mit koronarer Herzkrankheit - Elektronenstrahltomographie und IVUS. Z Kardiol 1995;84(Suppl.1):31.

41. Schmermund A, Lange S, Sehnert C *et al.* Elektronenstrahltomographie bei

koronarer Herzkrankheit. Prävalenz und Verteilung von Koronarkalk und Assoziation mit koronaren Risikofaktoren bei 650 Patienten. Dtsch Med Wschr 1995;120:1229-35.

42. Schmermund A, Lange S, Baumgart D *et al.* Risk factors, coronary calcium, coronary artery disease, and need for intervention. Am J Cardiac Imaging 1995;9(Suppl.1):6.

43. Shepherd J, Cobbe SM, Ford I *et al.* Prevention of coronary artery disease with pravastatin in men with hypercholesterolemia. N Engl J Med 1995;333:1301-7.

44 Simons DB, Schwartz RS, Edwards WD, Sheedy PF, Breen JF, Rumberger JA. Noninvasive definition of anatomic coronary artery disease by ultrafast CT: a quantitative pathologic study. J Am Coll Cardiol 1992;20:1118-26.

45. Stary HC. The sequence of cell and matrix changes in atherosclerotic lesions of coronary arteries in the first forty years of life. Eur Heart J 1990;11(Suppl.E):3-19.

46. The Scandinavian Simvastatin Survival Study Group: Randomised trial of cholesterol lowering in 4444 patients with coronary heart disease: the Scandinavian Simvastatin Survival Study (4S). Lancet 1994;344:1383-9.

47. Wolkoff K. Über die Atherosklerose der Coronararterien des Herzens. Beitr Path Anat Allg Path 1929;82:555-96.

48. Wong ND, Vo A, Abrahamson D, Eisenberg H, Tobis JM. Prediction of coronary events from noninvasive screening by ultrafast CT. Circulation 1993;88(Suppl.I):I-15.

49. Wong ND, Kouwabunpat D, Vo AN *et al.* Coronary calcium and atherosclerosis by ultrafast computed tomography in asymptomatic men and women: Relation to age and risk factors. Am Heart J 1994;127:422-30.

Colour section

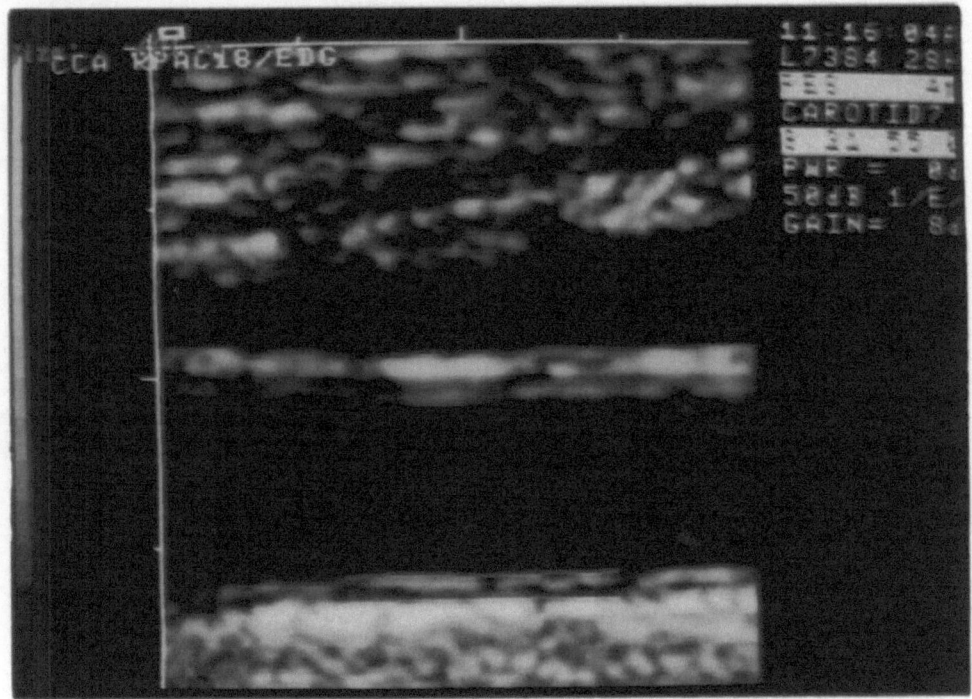

Figure 4. (Chapter 11) RES 2 x 2 cm. B-mode ultrasound image of the common carotid arterial segment. In the far wall, a measurement of approximately 10 mm along the arterial wall has been performed. The MEAN thickness of this specific segment was denoted as 0.681 mm.

Quantitative 3D Reconstruction of ICUS

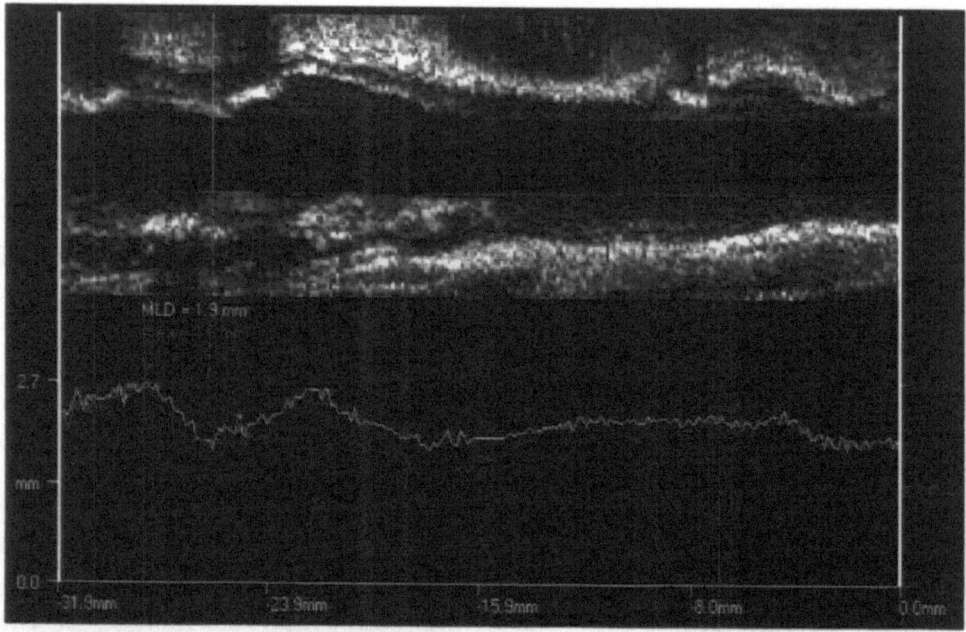

Figure 4. (Chapter 21) Longitudinal view of the proximal left anterior descending coronary artery after slow pass of a 2.15 mm Rotablator burr. The reconstructed image, obtained after acquisition and segmentation of multiple tomographic ICUS images obtained during a motorized pull-back at 0.5 mm/sec, shows the presence of a large calcific plaque with residual calcification in the proximal vessel, an intermediate normal segment and a new mild stenosis at 5 cm from the coronary ostium. Note that the reconstruction process, including the automatic recognition of the blood pool, encoded in red, and display of the diameter (yellow line) and area (green line) measurements, was completed in 90 seconds after the end of the ICUS examination (EchoLong, Indec, Capitula, CA).

3-D Reconstruction after Coronary Stenting

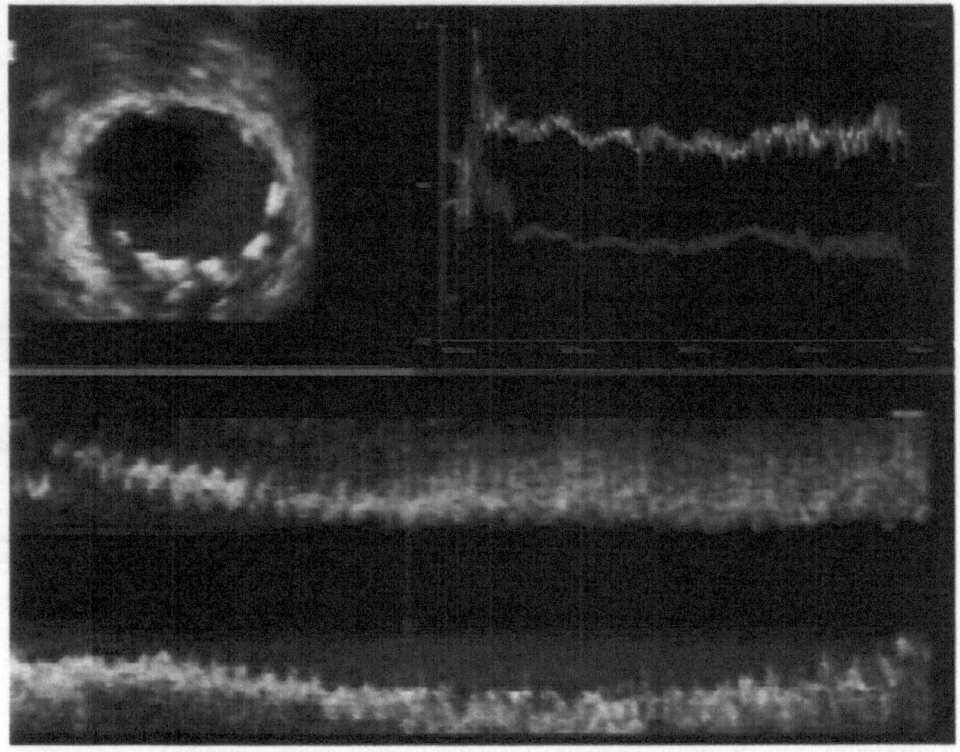

Figure 5. Longitudinal view of the proximal left anterior descending coronary artery after implantation of 3 NIR stenst. Note the perfect matching of the diameter of the proximal reference segment and of the stented segment.

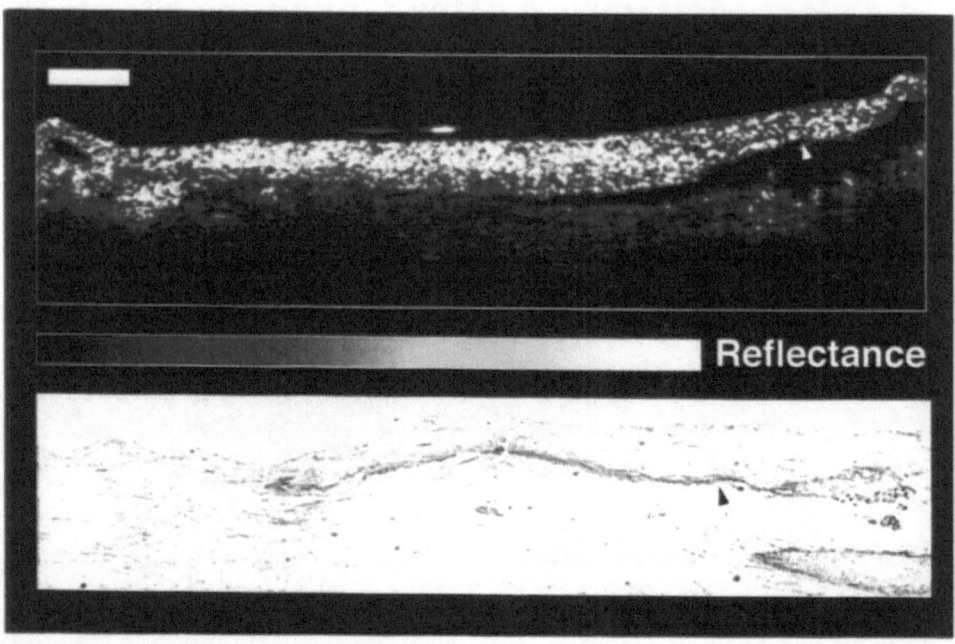

Figure 9. (Chapter 21) Optical coherence tomographic (OCT) image of a human coronary artery and corresponding histology. The reflectance pattern not only shows a striking difference at tissue transitions zones (arrow) but also tissue type is clearly noted by intensity differences. Courtesy of Dr. Neal Weissman (Georgetown University), and Dr. Mark Brezinski (Massachusetts General Hospital).

Plaque Rupture Left Main

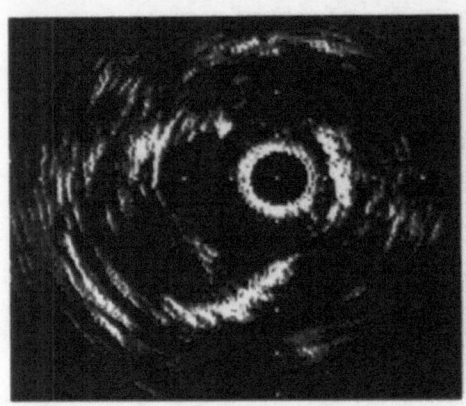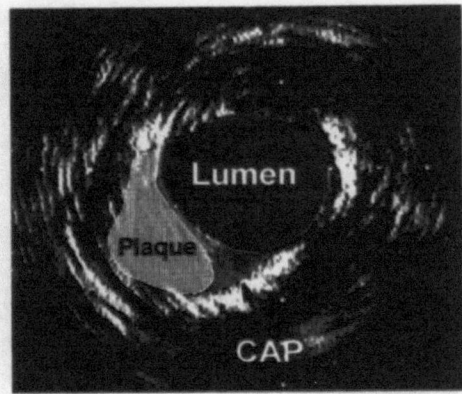

Figure 3. (Chapter 23) Plaque rupture in the left main in a patient with unstable angina. Ruptured lipid cap and remodelling of the left main with large total vessel area.

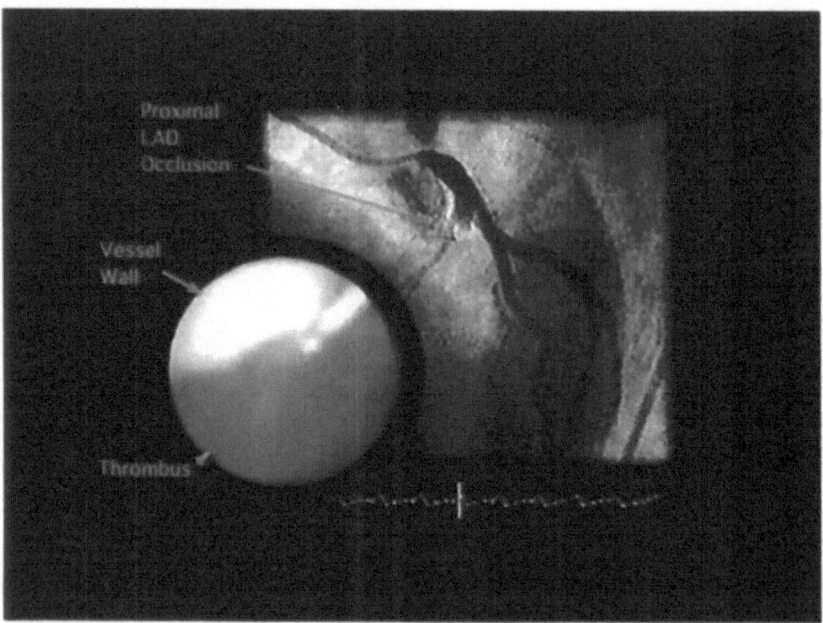

Figure 4. (Chapter 29) Coronary angiogram in Cranial LAO view showing abrupt LAD occlusion caused by trauma. Angioscopy reveals a large, red, occluding thrombus.

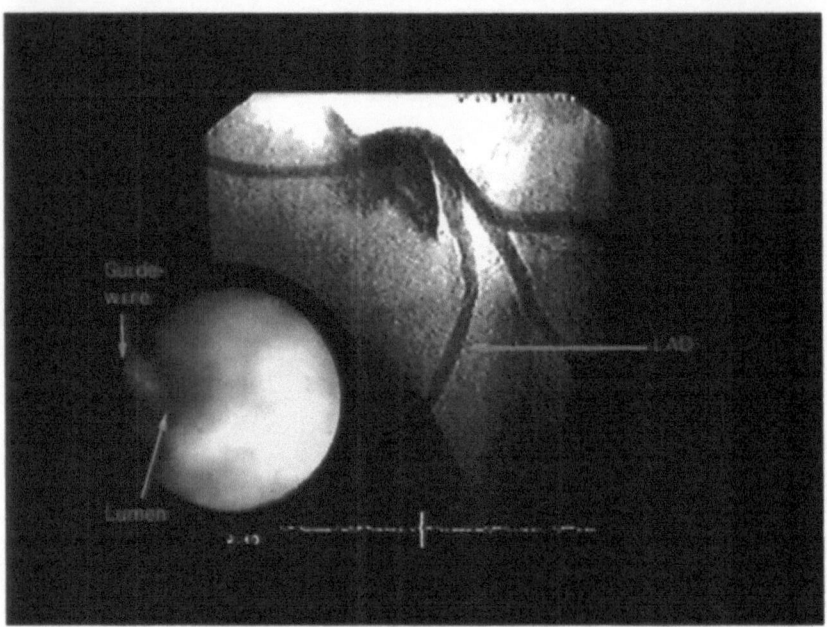

Figure 5. (Chapter 29) The same patient, 10 days following PTCA and intravenous heparin treatment. The patency of the LAD is fully restored. Angioscopy shows brown/yellow discoloration, probably remnants from balloon dilatation, but absence of thrombus.

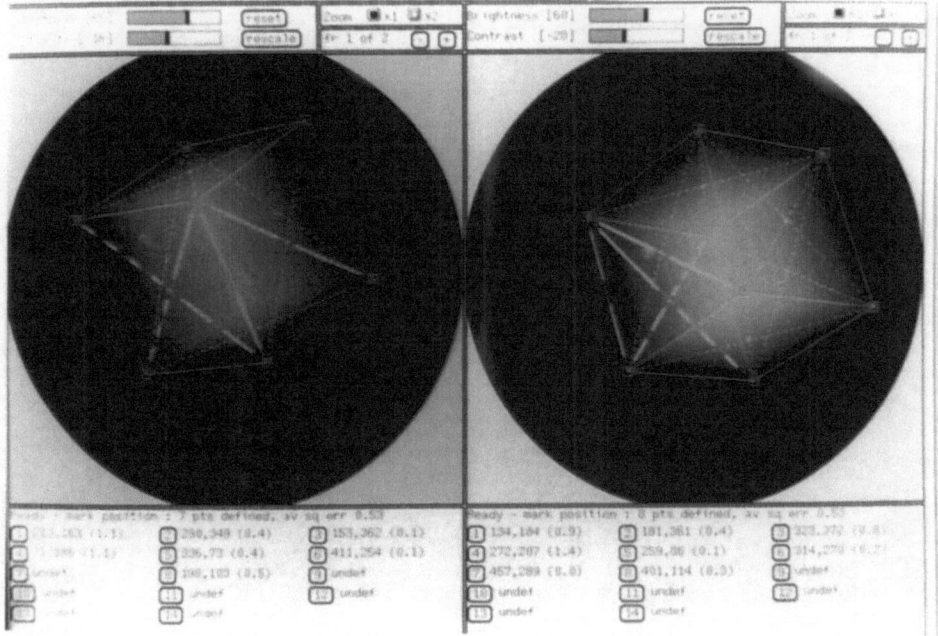

Figure 1. (Chapter 33) A pair of x-ray images of the cube with graphical superimposition of the cube lines showing the generation of the transformation matrices.

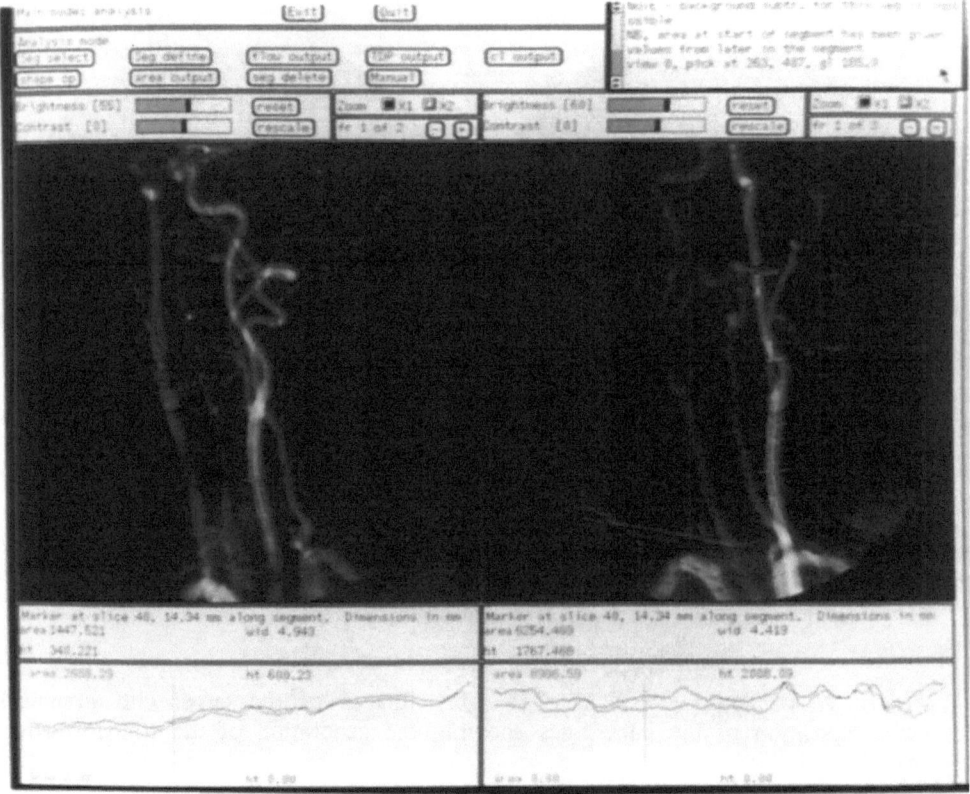

Figure 2. (Chapter 33) A biplanar digital x-ray angiogram of the aortic arch and the major arteries leading towards the head, with the detected edges superimposed on the angiograms (see Table 4, patient MB).

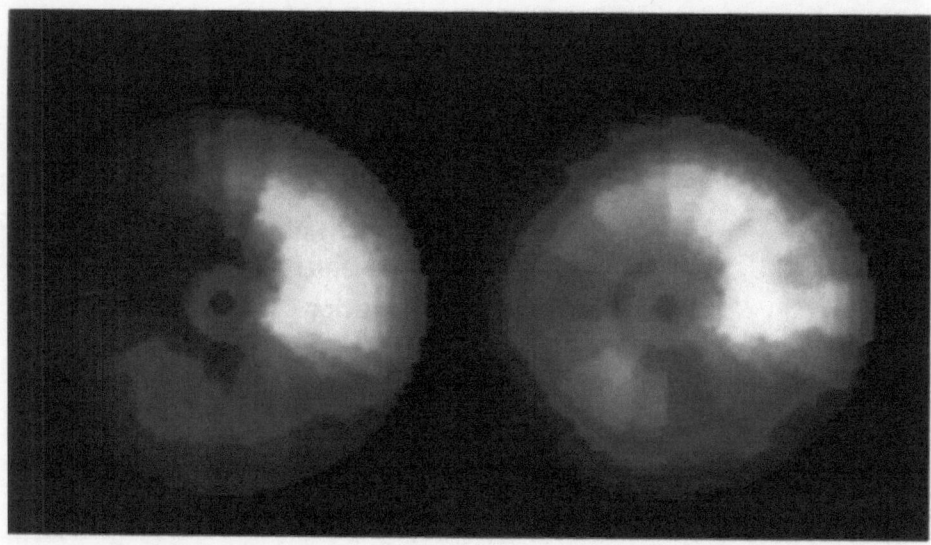

Figure 3. (Chapter 38) Bull's eye plot of ^{99m}Tc-tetrofosmin images obtained during stress before (*left*) and during diltiazem medication (*right*). Before medication the anteroseptal area shows a significant perfusion defect which is almost completely resolved during diltiazem therapy.

Index

96. I. Cikes (ed.): *Echocardiography in Cardiac Interventions.* 1989
ISBN 0-7923-0088-2
97. E. Rapaport (ed.): *Early Interventions in Acute Myocardial Infarction.* 1989
ISBN 0-7923-0175-7
98. M.E. Safar and F. Fouad-Tarazi (eds.): *The Heart in Hypertension.* A Tribute to Robert C. Tarazi (1925-1986). 1989 ISBN 0-7923-0197-8
99. S. Meerbaum and R. Meltzer (eds.): *Myocardial Contrast Two-dimensional Echocardiography.* 1989 ISBN 0-7923-0205-2
100. J. Morganroth and E.N. Moore (eds.): *Risk/Benefit Analysis for the Use and Approval of Thrombolytic, Antiarrhythmic, and Hypolipidemic Agents.* Proceedings of the 9th Annual Symposium on New Drugs and Devices (1988). 1989 ISBN 0-7923-0294-X
101. P.W. Serruys, R. Simon and K.J. Beatt (eds.): *PTCA - An Investigational Tool and a Non-operative Treatment of Acute Ischemia.* 1990 ISBN 0-7923-0346-6
102. I.S. Anand, P.I. Wahi and N.S. Dhalla (eds.): *Pathophysiology and Pharmacology of Heart Disease.* 1989 ISBN 0-7923-0367-9
103. G.S. Abela (ed.): *Lasers in Cardiovascular Medicine and Surgery.* Fundamentals and Technique. 1990 ISBN 0-7923-0440-3
104. H.M. Piper (ed.): *Pathophysiology of Severe Ischemic Myocardial Injury.* 1990
ISBN 0-7923-0459-4
105. S.M. Teague (ed.): *Stress Doppler Echocardiography.* 1990 ISBN 0-7923-0499-3
106. P.R. Saxena, D.I. Wallis, W. Wouters and P. Bevan (eds.): *Cardiovascular Pharmacology of 5-Hydroxytryptamine.* Prospective Therapeutic Applications. 1990
ISBN 0-7923-0502-7
107. A.P. Shepherd and P.A. Öberg (eds.): *Laser-Doppler Blood Flowmetry.* 1990
ISBN 0-7923-0508-6
108. J. Soler-Soler, G. Permanyer-Miralda and J. Sagristà-Sauleda (eds.): *Pericardial Disease.* New Insights and Old Dilemmas. 1990 ISBN 0-7923-0510-8
109. J.P.M. Hamer: *Practical Echocardiography in the Adult.* With Doppler and Color-Doppler Flow Imaging. 1990 ISBN 0-7923-0670-8
110. A. Bayés de Luna, P. Brugada, J. Cosin Aguilar and F. Navarro Lopez (eds.): *Sudden Cardiac Death.* 1991 ISBN 0-7923-0716-X
111. E. Andries and R. Stroobandt (eds.): *Hemodynamics in Daily Practice.* 1991
ISBN 0-7923-0725-9
112. J. Morganroth and E.N. Moore (eds.): *Use and Approval of Antihypertensive Agents and Surrogate Endpoints for the Approval of Drugs affecting Antiarrhythmic Heart Failure and Hypolipidemia.* Proceedings of the 10th Annual Symposium on New Drugs and Devices (1989). 1990 ISBN 0-7923-0756-9
113. S. Iliceto, P. Rizzon and J.R.T.C. Roelandt (eds.): *Ultrasound in Coronary Artery Disease.* Present Role and Future Perspectives. 1990 ISBN 0-7923-0784-4
114. J.V. Chapman and G.R. Sutherland (eds.): *The Noninvasive Evaluation of Hemodynamics in Congenital Heart Disease.* Doppler Ultrasound Applications in the Adult and Pediatric Patient with Congenital Heart Disease. 1990
ISBN 0-7923-0836-0
115. G.T. Meester and F. Pinciroli (eds.): *Databases for Cardiology.* 1991
ISBN 0-7923-0886-7
116. B. Korecky and N.S. Dhalla (eds.): *Subcellular Basis of Contractile Failure.* 1990
ISBN 0-7923-0890-5
117. J.H.C. Reiber and P.W. Serruys (eds.): *Quantitative Coronary Arteriography.* 1991
ISBN 0-7923-0913-8
118. E. van der Wall and A. de Roos (eds.): *Magnetic Resonance Imaging in Coronary Artery Disease.* 1991 ISBN 0-7923-0940-5
119. V. Hombach, M. Kochs and A.J. Camm (eds.): *Interventional Techniques in Cardiovascular Medicine.* 1991 ISBN 0-7923-0956-1
120. R. Vos: *Drugs Looking for Diseases.* Innovative Drug Research and the Development of the Beta Blockers and the Calcium Antagonists. 1991 ISBN 0-7923-0968-5

Developments in Cardiovascular Medicine

121. S. Sideman, R. Beyar and A.G. Kleber (eds.): *Cardiac Electrophysiology, Circulation, and Transport*. Proceedings of the 7th Henry Goldberg Workshop (Berne, Switzerland, 1990). 1991   ISBN 0-7923-1145-0
122. D.M. Bers: *Excitation-Contraction Coupling and Cardiac Contractile Force*. 1991
                                                                 ISBN 0-7923-1186-8
123. A.-M. Salmasi and A.N. Nicolaides (eds.): *Occult Atherosclerotic Disease*. Diagnosis, Assessment and Management. 1991   ISBN 0-7923-1188-4
124. J.A.E. Spaan: *Coronary Blood Flow*. Mechanics, Distribution, and Control. 1991
                                                                 ISBN 0-7923-1210-4
125. R.W. Stout (ed.): *Diabetes and Atherosclerosis*. 1991   ISBN 0-7923-1310-0
126. A.G. Herman (ed.): *Antithrombotics*. Pathophysiological Rationale for Pharmacological Interventions. 1991   ISBN 0-7923-1413-1
127. N.H.J. Pijls: *Maximal Myocardial Perfusion as a Measure of the Functional Significance of Coronary Arteriogram*. From a Pathoanatomic to a Pathophysiologic Interpretation of the Coronary Arteriogram. 1991   ISBN 0-7923-1430-1
128. J.H.C. Reiber and E.E. v.d. Wall (eds.): *Cardiovascular Nuclear Medicine and MRI*. Quantitation and Clinical Applications. 1992   ISBN 0-7923-1467-0
129. E. Andries, P. Brugada and R. Stroobrandt (eds.): *How to Face 'the Faces' of Cardiac Pacing*. 1992   ISBN 0-7923-1528-6
130. M. Nagano, S. Mochizuki and N.S. Dhalla (eds.): *Cardiovascular Disease in Diabetes*. 1992   ISBN 0-7923-1554-5
131. P.W. Serruys, B.H. Strauss and S.B. King III (eds.): *Restenosis after Intervention with New Mechanical Devices*. 1992   ISBN 0-7923-1555-3
132. P.J. Walter (ed.): *Quality of Life after Open Heart Surgery*. 1992
                                                                 ISBN 0-7923-1580-4
133. E.E. van der Wall, H. Sochor, A. Righetti and M.G. Niemeyer (eds.): *What's new in Cardiac Imaging?* SPECT, PET and MRI. 1992   ISBN 0-7923-1615-0
134. P. Hanrath, R. Uebis and W. Krebs (eds.): *Cardiovascular Imaging by Ultrasound*. 1992   ISBN 0-7923-1755-6
135. F.H. Messerli (ed.): *Cardiovascular Disease in the Elderly*. 3rd ed. 1992
                                                                 ISBN 0-7923-1859-5
136. J. Hess and G.R. Sutherland (eds.): *Congenital Heart Disease in Adolescents and Adults*. 1992   ISBN 0-7923-1862-5
137. J.H.C. Reiber and P.W. Serruys (eds.): *Advances in Quantitative Coronary Arteriography*. 1993   ISBN 0-7923-1863-3
138. A.-M. Salmasi and A.S. Iskandrian (eds.): *Cardiac Output and Regional Flow in Health and Disease*. 1993   ISBN 0-7923-1911-7
139. J.H. Kingma, N.M. van Hemel and K.I. Lie (eds.): *Atrial Fibrillation, a Treatable Disease?* 1992   ISBN 0-7923-2008-5
140. B. Ostadel and N.S. Dhalla (eds.): *Heart Function in Health and Disease*. Proceedings of the Cardiovascular Program (Prague, Czechoslovakia, 1991). 1992
                                                                 ISBN 0-7923-2052-2
141. D. Noble and Y.E. Earm (eds.): *Ionic Channels and Effect of Taurine on the Heart*. Proceedings of an International Symposium (Seoul, Korea , 1992). 1993
                                                                 ISBN 0-7923-2199-5
142. H.M. Piper and C.J. Preusse (eds.): *Ischemia-reperfusion in Cardiac Surgery*. 1993
                                                                 ISBN 0-7923-2241-X
143. J. Roelandt, E.J. Gussenhoven and N. Bom (eds.): *Intravascular Ultrasound*. 1993
                                                                 ISBN 0-7923-2301-7
144. M.E. Safar and M.F. O'Rourke (eds.): *The Arterial System in Hypertension*. 1993
                                                                 ISBN 0-7923-2343-2
145. P.W. Serruys, D.P. Foley and P.J. de Feyter (eds.): *Quantitative Coronary Angiography in Clinical Practice*. With a Foreword by Spencer B. King III. 1994
                                                                 ISBN 0-7923-2368-8

Developments in Cardiovascular Medicine

Developments in Cardiovascular Medicine

Previous volumes are still available

KLUWER ACADEMIC PUBLISHERS – DORDRECHT / BOSTON / LONDON